MEDICAL
THERAPEUTICS

MEDICAL
THERAPEUTICS

Second Edition

PAUL G. RAMSEY, MD

Professor and Chairman
Department of Medicine
University of Washington School of Medicine
Seattle, Washington

ERIC B. LARSON, MD, MPH

Associate Dean for Clinical Affairs and Professor of Medicine
University of Washington School of Medicine
Medical Director
University of Washington Medical Center
Seattle, Washington

W.B. SAUNDERS COMPANY
A Division of Harcourt Brace & Company

hiladelphia   London   Toronto   Montreal   Sydney   Tokyo

W.B. SAUNDERS COMPANY
A Division of
Harcourt Brace & Company

The Curtis Center
Independence Square West
Philadelphia, Pennsylvania 19106

Library of Congress Cataloging-in-Publication Data

Medical therapeutics / [edited by] Paul G. Ramsey, Eric B. Larson. — 2nd ed.

   p. cm.

Includes bibliographical references.

ISBN 0–7216–3496–6

1. Internal medicine.   2. Therapeutics.   I. Ramsey, Paul G.
   II. Larson, Eric B.

[DNLM: 1. Therapeutics—handbooks.   WB 39 M488]

RC46.M4754   1993

616–dc20
DNLM/DLC   92-17196

MEDICAL THERAPEUTICS   ISBN   0–7216–3496–6

Printed in the United States of America.

Last digit is the print number: 9   8   7   6   5   4   3   2

CONTRIBUTORS
CONTRIBUTORS
CONTRIBUTORS

RICHARD K. ALBERT, M.D.
Professor of Medicine, University of Washington School of Medicine; Section Head, Pulmonary and Critical Care Medicine, University of Washington Medical Center, Seattle, Washington
Pulmonary Conditions

KENNETH A. ARNDT, M.D.
Professor of Dermatology, Harvard Medical School; Dermatologist-in-Chief, Beth Israel Hospital, Boston, Massachusetts
Dermatologic Diseases

JEFFREY P. BAKER, M.D.
Assistant Professor of Medicine, University of Toronto; Staff Gastroenterologist, St. Michael's Hospital, Toronto, Canada
Nutritional Therapeutics

EDWARD A. BENSON, M.D.
Clinical Assistant Professor, University of Washington School of Medicine; Attending Physician, Virginia Mason Hospital, Seattle, Washington
Endocrinologic Diseases and Related Metabolic Disorders

MARK BERNHARDT, M.D.
Consultant in Dermatology, Broward General Medical Center and Holy Cross Hospital, Fort Lauderdale, Florida
Dermatologic Diseases

ROBERT L. CARITHERS, Jr., M.D.
Professor of Medicine, University of Washington School of Medicine; Director of Hepatology Section, Division of Gastroenterology; Medical

Director, Liver Transplantation Program, University of Washington Medical Center, Seattle, Washington
Liver Diseases

CAROLYN COLLINS, M.D.
Assistant Professor, Division of Medical Oncology, Department of Medicine, University of Washington School of Medicine, Seattle, Washington
Oncologic Therapeutics

WILLIAM L. DALEY, M.D., M.P.H.
Clinical Instructor, Harvard Medical School; Physician, West Roxbury Veterans Administration Medical Center, Boston, Massachusetts
Cardiovascular Disease

ALLAN S. DETSKY, M.D., Ph.D., FRCPC
Professor of Medicine, University of Toronto; Chief, Division of General Internal Medicine, The Toronto Hospital, Toronto, Canada
Nutritional Therapeutics

DAVID C. DUGDALE, M.D.
Assistant Professor of Medicine, University of Washington School of Medicine; Attending Physician; University of Washington Medical Center, Seattle, Washington
General Medical Care; Fluid and Electrolyte Therapy; Hypertension

LESLIE S. T. FANG, M.D., Ph.D.
Assistant Professor of Medicine, Harvard Medical School; Chief, Walter Bauer Firm, Medical Service, Massachusetts General Hospital, Boston, Massachusetts
Renal Diseases

GREGORY C. GARDNER, M.D.
Assistant Professor of Medicine, Division of Rheumatology, and Adjunct Assistant Professor, Department of Orthopaedic Surgery, University of Washington School of Medicine; Attending Physician, University of Washington Medical Center, Seattle, Washington
Rheumatic Disorders

BRUCE C. GILLILAND, M.D.
Professor of Medicine and Professor of Laboratory Medicine, Associate Dean for Clinical Affairs, University of Washington School of Medicine, Seattle, Washington
Rheumatic Disorders

ERIC B. LARSON, M.D., M.P.H.
Associate Dean for Clinical Affairs and Professor of Medicine, University of Washington School of Medicine; Medical Director and Attending Physician, University of Washington Medical Center, Seattle, Washington
General Medical Care

W. CONRAD LILES, M.D., Ph.D.
Senior Fellow in Allergy and Infectious Diseases and Acting Instructor in Medicine, Department of Medicine, University of Washington School of Medicine; Attending Physician, University of Washington Medical Center, Seattle, Washington
Infectious Diseases

ROBERT B. LIVINGSTON, M.D.
Professor of Medicine and Head of Division of Oncology, University of Washington School of Medicine; Staff Attending Physician, University of Washington Medical Center, Seattle, Washington
Oncologic Therapeutics

TERRY J. MENGERT, M.D.
Assistant Professor of Medicine, University of Washington School of Medicine; Attending Physician, Emergency Medicine Service, University of Washington Medical Center, Seattle, Washington
Pulmonary Conditions

JOANNE MORTIMER, M.D.
Associate Professor of Medicine, Washington University School of Medicine; Attending Physician, Barnes Hospital and Jewish Hospital, St. Louis, Missouri
Oncologic Therapeutics

OLIVER W. PRESS, M.D., Ph.D.
Associate Professor of Medicine/Oncology, Adjunct Associate Professor of Biological Structure, University of Washington School of Medicine, Associate Member, Fred Hutchinson Cancer Research Center, Seattle, Washington
Oncologic Therapeutics

THOMAS H. PRICE, M.D.
Associate Professor of Medicine, University of Washington School of Medicine; Director Clinical Services, Puget Sound Blood Center, Seattle, Washington
Hematology and Transfusion Medicine

PAUL G. RAMSEY, M.D.
Professor and Chairman, Department of Medicine, University of Washington School of Medicine; Physician-in-Chief, University of Washington Medical Center, Seattle, Washington
General Medical Care; Infectious Diseases

NORMAN R. ROSENTHAL, M.D.
Clinical Assistant Professor of Medicine, University of Washington School of Medicine; Staff Physician, Endocrinology Section, Virginia Mason Medical Hospital, Seattle, Washington
Endocrinologic Diseases and Related Metabolic Disorders

LAWRENCE R. SOLOMON, M.D.
Associate Clinical Professor of Medicine, Yale University School of Medicine, New Haven; Medical Director, The Connecticut Hospice, Branford, Connecticut
Hematology and Transfusion Medicine

A. HILLARY STEINHART, M.D., F.R.C.P.(C)
Assistant Professor, Department of Medicine, University of Toronto; Staff Gastroenterologist, Mount Sinai Hospital, Toronto, Ontario, Canada
Nutritional Therapeutics

PHILLIP D. SWANSON, M.D., Ph.D.
Professor of Medicine, Head, Division of Neurology, University of Washington School of Medicine; Attending Physician, University of Washington Affiliated Hospitals, Seattle, Washington
Neurologic Diseases

GEORGE E. THIBAULT, M.D.
Associate Professor of Medicine, Harvard Medical School; Chief of Medicine, Brockton/West Roxbury Veterans Affairs Medical Center; Vice-Chairman, Department of Medicine, Brigham and Women's Hospital; Physician, Massachusetts General Hospital, Boston, Massachusetts
Cardiovascular Diseases

MARGARET THORNTON, M.D.
Senior Fellow, Division of Nephrology, Seattle Veterans Affairs Medical Center, Seattle, Washington
Hypertension

THOMAS R. VIGGIANO, M.D.
Assistant Professor of Medicine, Mayo Clinic, Mayo Medical School; Staff Consultant, Mayo Clinic, St. Mary's Hospital, Rochester Methodist Hospital, Rochester, Minnesota
Gastrointestinal Diseases

KENNETH K. WANG, M.D.
Assistant Professor, Mayo Medical School; Consultant, Mayo Clinic and Foundation, Rochester, Minnesota
Gastrointestinal Diseases

PREFACE
PREFACE

PREFACE

Medical Therapeutics is designed to guide both seasoned and apprentice clinicians as they apply available therapies to a broad range of medical disorders. In this second edition of *Medical Therapeutics,* an outline format has been introduced to enable the reader to identify quickly specific recommendations for treatment. Descriptions of disease manifestations and pathophysiology are brief. *Medical Therapeutics* is intended to help the health professional in everyday patient care, whether in the hospital or in the outpatient setting. The information presented in this manual should be used as a practical supplement to a comprehensive textbook of medicine, such as *The Cecil Textbook of Medicine* or *Harrison.*

The first edition of the *Cecil Textbook of Medicine* was published in 1927. In the subsequent six decades, biomedical research has revolutionized the practice of medicine, and scientific advances have led to dramatic improvements in therapeutic skills. Paul Beeson, a former editor of *Cecil,* described this revolution in medical therapeutics in his paper, "Changes in Medical Therapy During the Past Half Century." This paper documents the vastly expanded range of effective therapies available in all areas of medicine. Treatments recommended for 60% of diseases covered in the first edition of *Cecil* were classified as "harmful," "useless," "of questionable value," or merely "symptomatic." In 1927, only 6% of diseases had treatments considered to be "effective," "helpful," or "highly effective." In striking contrast, these ratings for effective therapy could be applied to more than 50% of diseases a half century later. The therapeutic revolution analyzed by Dr. Beeson continues, as documented in subsequent editions of *Cecil* and other texts.

As editors, we have endeavored to emphasize effective treatments and to provide guidelines to administer and monitor treatments. In addition to a new outline format, this second edition of *Medical Therapeutics* contains new information reflecting advances and changes in therapeutics since the first edition. Continued advances will occur, however, and we urge the user of *Medical Therapeutics* to stay current by using information available in journals, in drug handbooks such as the *Physicians' Desk Reference* and the *Medical Letter,* and through participation in continuing medical education programs.

PAUL G. RAMSEY, M.D.
ERIC B. LARSON, M.D.

Reference

Beeson, PB: Changes in Medical Therapy During the Past Half Century, Medicine 59:79–99, 1980

CONTENTS
CONTENTS
CONTENTS

STAT DRUGS (ADULT DOSAGES)

CARDIAC ARRHYTHMIAS

1. **Ventricular fibrillation or pulseless ventricular tachycardia**
   a. Defibrillate 200 joules, 200-300 joules, up to 360 joules.
   b. Start CPR, establish IV access.
   c. Epinephrine 1:10,000, 0.5-1.0 mg IV (repeat every 5 min.)
   d. Intubate if possible.
   e. Difibrillate up to 360 joules.
   f. Lidocaine 1 mg/kg IV.
   g. Defibrillate up to 360 joules.
   h. Lidocaine 0.5 mg/kg IV or bretylium 5 mg/kg IV.
   i. Consider bicarbonate 1 mEq/kg IV.
   j. Alternate defibrillatory shocks (up to 360 joules) with additional antiarrhythmic, lidocaine 0.5 mg/kg IV every 5 min up to max of 3 mg/kg or bretylium 10 mg/kg.

2. **Ventricular tachycardia (pulse and stable)**
   a. Lidocaine: 1 mg/kg IV (repeat 0.5 mg/kg every 5-10 min up to 3 mg/kg).
   b. Procainamide 20 mg/min up to 1000 mg.
   c. Cardiovert 50, 100, 200, 360 joules.

3. **Ventricular tachycardia (pulse and unstable)**
   a. Consider sedation, oxygen, IV access.
   b. Cardiovert 50, 100, 200, 360 joules.
   c. Lidocaine 1 mg/kg IV (repeat 0.5 mg/kg every 5-10 min up to 3 mg/kg).

4. **Asystole**
   a. Start CPR, establish IV access.
   b. Epinephrine 1:10,000 0.5-1.0 mg IV (repeat every 5 min).
   c. Intubate if possible.
   d. Atropine 1.0 mg IV.
   e. Consider bicarbonate 1 mEq/kg IV.
   f. Consider pacing.

5. **Electromechanical dissociation**
   a. Start CPR, establish IV access.
   b. Epinephrine 1:10,000 0.5-1.0 mg IV.
   c. Intubate if possible.
   d. Consider bicarbonate 1 mEq/kg IV.
   e. Consider correctable causes (hypovolemia, cardiac tamponade, tension pneumothorax, hypoxemia, acidosis, pulmonary embolism).

STAT DRUGS (ADULT DOSAGES)—*continued*

6. **Bradycardia**

   a. Atropine 0.5–1.0 mg IV (may repeat every 5 min up to 2.0 mg).

   b. Consider isoproterenol 2–10 mg/min IV.

   c. Pacer.

7. **Paroxysmal supraventricular tachycardia (PSVT) stable**

   a. Vagal maneuvers.

   b. Adenosine 6 mg IV push (repeat with12 mg IV push if no response) or verapamil 5 mg IV (repeat with 5–10 mg IV in 15 min if no response).

   c. Consider cardioversion, beta blockers (esmolol), digoxin, or overdrive pacing.

8. **Paroxysmal supraventricular tachycardia (PSVT) unstable**

   a. Consider sedation.

   b. *Synchronous* cardioversion: 75–100, 200, 360 joules.

9. **Premature ventricular contractions (PVCs)**

   a. Lidocaine 1 mg/kg (repeat 0.5 mg/kg every 5–10 min up to 3 mg/kg).

   b. Procainamide 20 mg/min up to 1000 mg.

   c. Bretylium 5–10 mg/kg over 10 min.

SHOCK

1. **Cardiogenic**

   a. Dobutamine (250 mg in 500 ml D_5W = 500 µg/ml). Start at low dose and increase according to hemodynamic response (2.0–10 µg/kg/min).

   b. Dopamine (200 mg in 250 ml D_5W = 800 µg/ml). Start at low dose and increase according to hemodynamic response (2.0 to 5.0 µg/kg/min initially, may increase to 50 µg/kg/min).

   c. Consider nitroprusside (50 mg in 250 ml D_5W = 200 µg/ml) start at 0.25–2.5 µg/kg/min and titrate according to hemodynamic response, to a maximum dose of 10 µg/kg/min.

2. **Septic**

   a. Support BP with fluid (crystalloid or colloid).

   b. Dopamine as above or:

   c. Norepinephrine: levarterenol bitartrate (levophed) (4 mg in 500 ml D_5W = 8 µg/ml). Start at low dose and increase according to hemodynamic response. (2–32 µg/min).

3. **Anaphylactic**

   a. Epinephrine 0.3–0.5 mg (0.3–0.5 ml of a 1:1000 dilution) given SC or IM or 0.1–0.25 mg (1.0-2.5 ml of a 1:10,000 dilution) given IV if hypotension present.

   b. Support BP with fluids, or vasopressors if necessary.

   c. Consider corticosteroids.

STAT DRUGS (ADULT DOSAGES)—*continued*

STATUS ASTHMATICUS

a. Albuterol or metoproterenol inhaled via nebulizer: repeat p.r.n.

b. Methyl prednisolone 125 mg IV.

c. Epinephrine 0.3–0.5 mg (0.3 cc of 1:1000 dilution) SC or IM or Terbutaline 0.25 mg SC: may repeat once in 15–30 minutes.

d. Aminophylline: 6 mg/kg IV over 20–30 minutes, followed by infusion at 0.5 mg/kg/hr.

PULMONARY EDEMA

a. Furosemide (Lasix) 40–80 mg IV.

b. Morphine sulfate 4–8 mg IV.

c. Nitroglycerin: 5–25 μg/min IV or 1–2 inches of paste.

HYPERKALEMIA

a. Calcium gluconate (10 ml or 1 ampule) IV over 1–2 minutes.
(Use if K + > 8 mEq/L or ECG changes are present).

b. Sodium bicarbonate (50 mEq or 1 ampule) IV over 2–5 minutes.

c. Glucose (250 ml of 20% glucose) IV *and* regular insulin 10 units IV.

d. Sodium polystyrene sulfonate (Kayexalate) 15–30 gm in 50–100 cc water given orally *or* 50 gm of Kayexalate *plus* 50 gm sorbitol in 250 ml of water rectally (retain for 30–45 minutes).

e. Consider hemodialysis.

HYPERTENSIVE ENCEPHALOPATHY

a. Nifedipine: 10–20 mg p.o. or:

b. Furosemide (Lasix) 40–80 mg IV or:

c. Nitroprusside: 50 mg in 250 ml D_5W = 200 μg/ml. Start at 0.25–02.5 μg/kg/min and titrate according to hemodynamic response. Invasive arterial monitoring recommended or:

d. Labetalol: 20 mg IV initially, then 40–80 mg IV every 10 minutes. May also be given as continuous infusion of 2 mg/min IV. Do not exceed a total cumulative dose of 300 mg IV or:

e. Esmolol: 5 gm diluted in 480 ml D_5W. Loading dose of 500 μg/kg/min for 30 seconds (250 μg/kg total) followed by maintenance infusion dose of 25 μg/kg/min for 4 minutes. May increase infusion by increments of 50 μg/kg/min for 4 minutes up to a maximum rate of 300 μg/kg/min; each preceded by a loading dose of 500 μg/kg/min for 1 minute.

STATUS EPILEPTICUS

a. Benzodiazepines for immediate control: Diazepam (valium) 5–10 mg IV or lorazepam (Ativan) 2 mg IV.

b. Phenobarbital or phenytoin for prolonged control: Phenobarbital: 150–400 mg IV (may repeat in 20 minutes with 150-250 mg IV) *or* phenytoin (Dilantin): 1000 mg IV loading dose. (Do not exceed 50 mg/min; monitor BP closely for hypotension and do not mix Dilantin with solution other than sodium chloride.)

MEDICAL
THERAPEUTICS

GENERAL MEDICAL CARE

DAVID C. DUGDALE
PAUL G. RAMSEY
ERIC B. LARSON

1111111111111111111111111111

I. INTRODUCTION

A. Therapeutic plans should be individually tailored for patients, taking into consideration factors such as age, underlying diseases, and psychosocial issues.

B. Evaluation of therapeutic efficacy, compliance, potential drug interactions, adverse effects, and cost should be routine as part of the planning and monitoring of medical care. Unexpected or new adverse effects of a medication should be reported to the Food and Drug Administration.

II. MEDICAL ORDER WRITING

A. Medical orders communicate essential patient information and therapeutic plans. If you use a systematic approach to order-writing, and if you write legibly and avoid ambiguity and confusing abbreviations, you will minimize errors. The mnemonic "ADCA VAN DIMLS" stands for the essential order categories:

A–**ADMITTING ORDER:** noting physician(s) responsible for the patient

D–**DIAGNOSIS**

C–**CONDITION**

A–**ALLERGIES**

V–**VITAL SIGNS:** frequency of monitoring and conditions for which the physician(s) should be notified

A–**ACTIVITY LEVEL**

N–**NURSING:** instructions for general care

D–**DIET**

I–**INTRAVENOUS (IV) ORDERS**

M–**MEDICATION ORDERS**

L–**LABORATORY STUDIES**

S–**SPECIAL ORDERS:** miscellaneous instructions

B. Personal discussion of medical orders with the person who will do them improves patient care. Regular review of orders—especially medications—helps ensure appropriate care.

III. DRUG INTERACTIONS AND ADVERSE EFFECTS

A. Many adverse effects occur when dosages inappropriate for a patient's size or physiologic status are ordered. Others are mediated by interactions between medications. Constant attention to detail is required to maintain therapeutic effect while minimizing adverse effects. The following information may be useful in calculating drug doses:

1. Creatinine clearance = [(140 − age)/serum creat (mg/dL)] × weight (kg)/72 × 0.85 (for women)
(A good estimate if serum creat is less than 5 mg/dL)

2. Ideal body mass:
  a. Women: 45 kg for first 152 cm (60 inches) + 0.9 kg/cm over 152 *or* 2.3 kg/inch over 60
  b. Men: 48 kg for first 152 cm (60 inches) + 1.1 kg/cm over 152 *or* 2.8 kg/inch over 60

3. Body surface area nomogram.

4. Alteration of drug dose in renal dysfunction. See page 216.

B. Morbidity from drug interactions (Table 1–1) may be avoided by using only essential drugs, monitoring compliance and adverse effects, and measuring drug levels and effects when appropriate. Drug interactions include:

1. ADDITIVE EFFECTS (e.g., sedation using both narcotics and benzodiazepines).

2. ABSORPTIVE EFFECTS (enteral route) may be mediated by binding (e.g., cholestyramine and digoxin) or pH (e.g., antacids and tetracycline) effects.

3. CLEARANCE EFFECTS may occur with medications that induce (barbiturates and rifampin) or inhibit (cimetidine, isoniazid) the hepatic microsomal enzyme system, altering the clearance of other medications. Cessation of a microsomal inducer may allow toxic accumulation of another medication (e.g., rifampin and theophylline).

4. PROTEIN-BINDING EFFECTS may occur with medications that are greater than 90% protein bound. Drug effects generally correlate with free drug levels, which may be altered by competition for protein binding. For example, sodium valproate may increase free serum phenytoin levels. The onset of such an interaction may be delayed, depending on the level of the second drug required to produce it.

5. METABOLIC EFFECTS may cause an increased risk of toxicity (e.g., furosemide-induced hypokalemia causing digoxin toxicity). Induction of hypothyroidism by a medication may alter the clearance of many drugs.

McInnes GT, Brodie MJ: Drug interactions that matter: A critical reappraisal. Drugs 36:83–110, 1988.
Szoa PR, Edgren RA: Drug interactions with oral contraceptives: Compilation and analysis of an adverse experience report database. Fertil Steril 49(suppl):31S–38S, 1988.

TABLE 1–1A. SELECTED DRUG INTERACTIONS

AGENT	DRUGS THAT MAY INCREASE EFFECT OR LEVEL OF AGENT	DRUGS THAT MAY DECREASE EFFECT OR LEVEL OF AGENT	DRUGS WITH UNPREDICTABLE EFFECT
Oral contraceptives (combination)	—	Barbiturates, carbamazepine, chloramphenicol, griseofulvin, phenytoin, rifampin; antibiotic-induced diarrhea may decrease absorption; prolonged course of sulfonamides may decrease effect; failure may be heralded by breakthrough bleeding and may be managed by use of a higher estrogen dose	—
Warfarin	Aspirin, cimetidine, disulfiram, methyldopa, metronidazole, quinidine, sulfinpyrazone, sulfonylureas, trimethoprim-sulfamethoxazole, fluconazole, ketoconazole; clofibrate and nonsteroidal anti-inflammatory drugs (NSAIDs) may increase bleeding risk due to different hemostatic defects	Adrenocorticosteroids, antacids, antihistamines, barbiturates, carbamazepine, chlordiazepoxide, cholestyramine, combination oral contraceptives, glutethimide, haloperidol, rifampin	Diuretics, ranitidine, phenytoin, ethanol
Phenytoin	Chlordiazepoxide, cimetidine, diazepam, disulfiram, estrogens, isoniazid, phenothiazines, salicylates, sulfonamides, tolbutamide, warfarin, fluconazole	Calcium-containing antacids, carbamazepine	Barbiturates, valproic acid, ketoconazole
Carbamazepine	Calcium channel blockers, cimetidine, erythromycin, isoniazid, propoxyphene	Phenobarbital, phenytoin	—
Digoxin	Diphenoxylate, propantheline, quinidine, amiodarone, verapamil, diltiazem, spironolactone, triamterene, tetracycline, erythromycin	Antacids, bleomycin, cholestyramine, cyclophosphamide, cytarabine, doxorubicin, kaolin-pectin, neomycin, procarbazine, sulfasalazine, vinblastine, vincristine	—
Quinidine	Acetazolamide, hydrochlorothiazide, cimetidine	Phenobarbital, phenytoin, rifampin	—
Procainamide	Cimetidine	Phenobarbital, phenytoin, rifampin	—
Diisopyramide	—		—
Sulfonylureas	Chloramphenicol, NSAIDs, probenecid, salicylates, sulfonamides, warfarin, fluconazole	Calcium channel blockers, estrogens, isoniazid, phenothiazines, phenytoin	—

Table continued on the following page

5

TABLE 1–1B. DRUGS THAT MAY INDUCE OR INHIBIT THE HEPATIC OXYGENASE SYSTEM

INDUCERS	INHIBITORS
Barbiturates	Allopurinol
Carbamazepine	Amiodarone
Ethanol (chronic)	Cimetidine
Glutethimide	Diltiazem
Griseofulvin	Disulfiram
Phenytoin	Erythromycin
Rifampin	Ethanol (acute)
	Isoniazid
	Ketoconazole
	Metoprolol
	Metronidazole
	Oral contraceptives
	Phenothiazines
	Propranolol
	Quinidine
	Sodium valproate
	Sulfonamides
	Tricyclic antidepressants
	Verapamil

IV. MANAGEMENT OF PAIN

A. Pain, the most common presenting symptom, suggests anatomic or physiologic derangement. Symptomatic treatment should not be offered until diagnostic possibilities have been considered and, if necessary, evaluated. Treatment with narcotics is contraindicated in undiagnosed acute abdominal pain and in head injuries. It may complicate assessment and management. The proper management of pain depends on the underlying disease, chronicity of pain, and psychosocial factors. Non-pharmacologic treatment may be useful.

B. Acetaminophen (Table 1–2) is widely used for mild to moderate pain. Phenacetin is a related compound that is metabolized to acetaminophen but is rarely employed singly as an analgesic agent. The mechanism of action of acetaminophen is not clearly defined, and its anti-inflammatory effect is weak. Acetaminophen is especially useful in the presence of aspirin allergy, warfarin treatment, upper GI sensitivity to anti-inflammatory agents, and bleeding disorders.

Acetaminophen is absorbed rapidly from the GI tract, and 90% is excreted in the urine after conjugation by the liver. Its primary toxic effect, hepatic necrosis, is seen in acute overdosage. Liver damage may occur with chronic acetaminophen therapy in patients with prior liver disease (Ann Intern Med 104:399–404, 1986).

Although acetaminophen can induce synthesis of hepatic microsomal enzymes, this does not occur with standard doses, and significant drug interactions are unusual.

The **salicylates** and **nonsteroidal anti-inflammatory drugs** (NSAIDs;

Table 1–2) are widely used to control pain and inflammation. Although the medications are used interchangeably, not all are approved by the FDA for both indications.

C. **Salicylates** are the most commonly used analgesics. Some formulations include caffeine, sedatives, or antihistamines, but there is no evidence of an enhanced analgesic effect when these agents are added.

The most common route of administration is oral. Rectal (absorption erratic) and parenteral formulations are available.

1. ADVERSE EFFECTS

The most common adverse effect of these agents is gastric intolerance. **Gastritis** and **peptic ulcer disease** may occur. Enteric-coated preparations (e.g., Ecotrin) and combinations with antacids (e.g., Ascriptin) are available but may achieve lower salicylate blood levels.

Aspirin sensitivity (bronchospasm, rhinosinusitis, urticaria, and anaphylaxis) can occur as part of a triad including asthma and nasal polyps. Some degree of aspirin sensitivity may occur in 10–20% of asthmatics. Other NSAIDs usually cause the same reactions. Normal sinus x-rays predict a low risk of sensitivity and less severe reactions if they do occur. Desensitization protocols are available (J Allerg Clin Immunol 74:617–622, 1984).

Other adverse effects are: an **antiplatelet effect** that lasts for the lifetime of the platelet. Nonacetylated salicylates have less antiplatelet effect, similar to NSAIDs. **Tinnitus** at high doses. Aspirin treatment is associated with the development of **Reye's syndrome** in children and teenagers with viral infections such as influenza and varicella (N Engl J Med 313:849–857, 1985).

Significant **drug interactions with salicylates** include increase of prothrombin time in warfarin-treated patients, decrease of the uricosuric effect of probenecid and sulfinpyrazone, and increase in methotrexate plasma levels due to decreased renal clearance.

D. **The NSAIDs** (Table 1–2), while more convenient than salicylates, are more expensive, and their clear superiority over aspirin as analgesic/anti-inflammatory agents has not been established. In general, the shorter-acting agents are preferred as analgesics; longer-acting agents are easier for chronic use as anti-inflammatories. Parenteral forms are available. NSAIDs are metabolized in the liver and excreted in urine. In some cases there is a fecal component of excretion.

Adverse effects include:

Reversible **platelet inhibition.**

Gastric intolerance that may be associated with gastritis and peptic ulcer disease.

Acute renal failure (especially in the elderly and patients with "prerenal" conditions) due to a decrease in glomerular filtration rate caused by alteration in renal prostaglandins. Nephrotoxicity may be less common with sulindac (Arch Intern Med 150:268–270, 1990).

Hyperkalemia due to a hyporeninemic-hypoaldosteronemic state.

Central nervous system effects, including confusion, delirium, and dizziness, are most common in the elderly.

TABLE 1–2. NON-NARCOTIC ANALGESICS

AGENT	USUAL ADULT ORAL DOSE RANGE (mg)	MAXIMAL DAILY DOSE (mg)	COMMENT
Acetaminophen	325–650 q 4 hr po or pr	4000	*See text*
Salicylates			
Aspirin	325–975 q 4 hr	6000	*See text*
Choline magnesium trisalicylate (Trilisate)	500–1000 q 12 hr	3000	Available as a liquid; increases effects of sulfonylureas
Salsalate (Disalcid)	500–1000 q 8 hr 750–1500 q 12 hr	3000	Absorbed from intestines; increases effects of sulfonylureas
Short-acting NSAIDs			
Diclofenac (Voltaren)	25–75 bid–tid	200	15% of patients develop transaminitis (4% elevated above 3 times normal level)
Fenoprofen calcium (Nalfon)	300–600 q 6 hr	3200	May displace protein-bound drugs and increase effect of phenytoin, sulfonamides, and sulfonylureas
Ibuprofen (Motrin, Rufen)	400–600 q 6 hr	3200	Available in nonprescription strength, 200 mg; also approved for primary dysmenorrhea
Indomethacin (Indocin)	25–50 q 8 hr	200	Available as suspension, suppository, and sustained release; high frequency of headache (10%) and CNS side effects; may elevate lithium levels; approved for gout
Ketoprofen (Orudis)	50–75 q 6–8 hr	300	High rate of dyspepsia
Meclofenamate sodium (Meclomen)	50–100 q 6 hr	400	High rate of diarrhea (10–33%); may increase warfarin effect

Drug	Dosage	Comments
Mefanamic acid (Ponstel)	500, then 250 q 6 hr	Also approved for primary dysmenorrhea
Tolmetin sodium (Tolectin)	400 q 6–8 hr	High rate of nausea (11%)
Intermediate-acting NSAIDs		
Diflunisal (Dolobid)	500 q 12 hr	May increase serum level of acetaminophen; do not use with indomethacin
Flurbiprofen (Ansaid)	50–100 bid–tid	May cause CNS stimulation
Naproxen (Naprosyn)	250–500 q 12 hr	Also approved for primary dysmenorrhea, acute gout; may increase effect of protein-bound drugs including warfarin, phenytoin, sulfonamides, and sulfonylureas; may increase lithium and methotrexate levels
Sulindac (Clinoril)	150–200 q 12 hr	Also approved for acute gout; decreases uricosuric effect of probenecid; may increase warfarin effect
Long-acting NSAID		
Piroxicam (Feldene)	10–20 q 24 hr	High rate of gastric upset; may increase lithium level; may increase effect of warfarin
Parenteral NSAID		
Ketorolac (Toradol)	30 or 60 initially, then 15–30 q 6 hr (all IM) 150 1st day; 120 qd afterward	Peak effect 2 hr after dose; in some studies, 30 mg equal to 6–12 mg of morphine sulfate or 50–100 mg of meperidine; no respiratory depression; 10 times as expensive as morphine sulfate

TABLE 1–3. NARCOTIC ANALGESICS

AGENT	PARENTERAL (SC/IM) DOSE EQUAL TO 10 MG MORPHINE (mg)	ORAL DOSE (mg) EQUAL TO LISTED PARENTERAL DOSE	COMMON DOSES (mg) AND ROUTES	COMMENT
Fentanyl (Sublimaze)	0.125	NA	0.05–0.1 q 1–2 hr IM	Primary use is IV and epidurally for anesthesia
Oxymorphone (Numorphan)	1.0–1.5	NA	1.0–1.5 q 4–6 hr IM; 5 q 4–6 hr pr	Major use is perioperative
Hydropmorphone (Dilaudid)	1.5	7.5	2 q 4–6 hr po; 1–2 q 4–6 hr IM; 3 q 6–8 hr pr	High abuse potential
Levorphanol (Levo-Dromoran)	2–3	4	2 q 6–8 hr po	Long acting: T½ up to 12 hr
Butorphanol (Stadol)	2–3	NA	1–4 q 3–4 hr IM	Mixed agonist-antagonist; not cross tolerant with morphine but associated with a withdrawal syndrome; major use is perioperative; not a controlled substance
Methadone (Dolophine)	8–10	20	5–10 q 4–6 hr po	Different T½ for analgesia and prevention of opiate withdrawal
Morphine sulfate (Roxanol)	10	60	5–20 q 4 hr IM; 5–20 q 6 hr pr	Oral bioavailability is poor; long-acting oral form (Roxanol SR) is available: dose is 20–60 po (equal to 10 IM) q 6–12 hr
Oxycodone (Percocet, Percodan, Tylox)	10–15	25	5–10 q 6 hr po	Percodan is a combination with aspirin; Percocet and Tylox are with acetaminophen
Hydrocodone (Vicodin)	NA	30	5–10 q 4–6 hr po	Approximately 6 times as potent as codeine
Pentazocine (Talwin)	30–60	135	30–60 q 3–4 hr IM; 50–100 q 4 hr po	Mixed agonist-antagonist; some oral forms contain naloxone to prevent parenteral abuse
Meperidine (Demerol)	75–100	250	50–125 q 3–4 hr IM; 50–100 q 4 hr po	May be used IV; oral bioavailability is poor; the metabolite normeperidine may accumulate with prolonged use, causing excitation, seizure
Codeine	120	180	15–60 q 4 hr po	Usually combined with aspirin or acetaminophen
Propoxyphene (Darvon)	140–180	270–360	32–100 q 4 hr po	Less abuse potential than codeine at common doses; withdrawal syndrome may occur with daily doses above 500 mg; often combined with aspirin or acetaminophen

Impaired antihypertensive effects of diuretics (due to sodium retention) and beta blockers.

E. Narcotic use for analgesia (Table 1–3) always should be carefully controlled. However, less than 1% of cases of narcotic addiction begin with physician prescriptions. In general, narcotics are underused for acute pain and overused for chronic pain.

Narcotic orders often specify as needed or "prn" use. A more effective technique for inpatients is to give the medication unless the patient refuses it or unless somnolence or respiratory depression occurs. A "trough" in analgesic effect is avoided, and the "pain behavior" that is central to the addictive process is minimized.

Adverse effects of narcotics include:

Respiratory depression is unlikely to occur in a patient still in pain. It can be reversed with IV naloxone injected over 10–15 seconds; bolus dosing should be avoided in patients using narcotics chronically.

Excess narcotic use is a common cause of **postoperative confusion.**

All narcotics may cause direct histamine release and a non-IgE–mediated **anaphylactoid response.** This is most graphically illustrated by appearance of perivenous erythema after IV narcotic injection.

Nausea, more common in ambulatory patients, can usually be managed by choosing an alternative narcotic. Narcotics have a direct central effect that is antagonized by antidopaminergic agents such as prochlorperazine. A vestibular component, if present, may respond to meclizine or dimenhydrinate. Gastric stasis responsive to metoclopramide may occur, especially in patients receiving chronic narcotics.

Narcotics may cause **smooth muscle spasm** leading to abdominal cramps, urinary retention, or worsening of biliary colic. Meperidine and codeine have less pharmacologic effect on biliary tract pressure than does morphine.

Constipation may result due to decreased propulsive contraction.

1. **ADJUNCTIVE AGENTS**

   Addition of 650 mg of aspirin or acetaminophen to 30 mg of codeine causes analgesic effect equal to 60 mg of codeine.

   Hydroxyzine 25–100 mg IM is also used to potentiate narcotic effect but appears to act primarily as a sedative.

2. **ADMINISTRATION**

   The standard initial dose of morphine sulfate in a 70-kg adult is 10 mg IM. Peak analgesia occurs at 1 hour with onset in 30 minutes.

   When immediate effect is required, morphine sulfate may be used IV. Peak analgesia occurs at 20 minutes and peak respiratory depression at 10 minutes. The usual starting dose is 2–8 mg (higher for pain).

   Patient-controlled analgesia may be the best strategy in selected postoperative patients (Arch Intern Med 150:1897–1903, 1990).

3. **CHRONIC PAIN**

   Chronic pain management differs in many ways from that of acute pain management. Psychosocial issues are often paramount; however, they may be concealed by the patient or may be otherwise unapparent clinically. Somatic pathology is often less apparent. Regional (i.e., nerve blocks) and nonpharmacologic approaches may be helpful in the management of selected chronic pain syndromes.

Narcotics usually should be avoided in chronic pain management. The major exception is patients with **terminal malignant disease** in whom narcotic dependence may be expected. Required doses may be very high.

When narcotics are used chronically, longer-acting agents (e.g., methadone, long-acting oral morphine) should be given on a fixed schedule. One method is the "pain cocktail" that may also contain acetaminophen and hydroxyzine. With this technique the patient is unaware of minor dosage adjustments, which is useful in some circumstances.

A variety of medications that are not traditional analgesics are useful in chronic pain management.

Tricyclic antidepressants, most commonly amitriptyline and doxepin, have been used, especially if neuropathic pain is suspected. The typical dose is 25–100 mg qd. Fluphenazine (a neuroleptic) 2 mg qd or bid may also be effective.

Phenytoin and **carbamazepine** (starting doses 100 mg qd and 200 mg bid, respectively) are useful for neuropathic pain, sometimes as the sole agent. They may be effective in dosages that yield serum levels below quoted "therapeutic levels."

Etidronate disodium (5 mg/kg/day) may help the bone pain associated with cancer and Paget's disease.

Beta blockers, notably propranolol and nadolol, are used for headache disorders, either therapeutically or prophylactically, solely or adjunctively.

Dextroamphetamine (5–20 mg bid) may reverse sedation in cancer patients using narcotics chronically.

Belladonna and opium suppositories (30 mg of opium qd or bid) may help the pain associated with rectal or bladder tenesmus (e.g., postprostatectomy and in rectal or bladder cancer).

Perlman SL: Modern techniques of pain management. West J Med 148:54–61, 1988.

V. FEVER

A. Definition and Manifestations. Fever, a body temperature (measured orally) above 38°C, often requires diagnostic testing before symptomatic treatment is begun. Although fever may be a part of the host defense system, some patients benefit from antipyresis.

If fever is not controlled, elderly patients may become confused, children and epileptic patients may have seizures, and the increased metabolic rate may aggravate heart disease. Furthermore, patients with fever are often uncomfortable.

B. Management

   1. ASPIRIN and **ACETAMINOPHEN** are both effective in lowering body temperature in doses of 325 to 650 mg po or pr. Acetaminophen is the drug of choice in children and teenagers when viral illnesses are suspected.

In patients with prolonged or recurrent fever, the drugs may be given every 3–4 hours until the underlying illness resolves (unless temperature must be monitored as a measure of therapeutic efficacy). When antipyretics are used irregularly only for a specified temperature elevation, the patient may needlessly be subjected to the discomforts of recurrent sweating and chilling.

2. **IBUPROFEN, INDOMETHACIN,** and **CORTICOSTEROIDS** are potent antipyretics useful in selected circumstances.

3. **PHYSICAL MEASURES** for treatment of fever (sponge baths and cooling blankets) are usually reserved for treatment of heat stroke.

Styrt B, Sugarman B: Antipyresis and fever. Arch Intern Med 150:1589–1597, 1990.

VI. CONSTIPATION

A. Causes. Constipation is common among inpatients because of inactivity, dietary change, and medication side effects. Commonly implicated medications include narcotics, aluminum- or calcium-containing antacids, tricyclic antidepressants, phenothiazines, calcium channel blockers, and iron salts.

B. Management. Constipation should not be treated without consideration of possible underlying causes such as metabolic and bowel abnormalities. There are few contraindications to transient laxative use in inpatients, but chronic use in outpatients should be discouraged. Classes of laxatives (Table 1–4) include:

Bulking agents, usually the drugs of choice for outpatients, may be less useful for inpatients due to delayed onset of effect. Increased bulk causes increased peristaltic activity and decreased transit time. Bulk laxatives may affect medication absorption.

Emollient laxatives are also safe, except for mineral oil, which may lead to fat-soluble vitamin deficiency and lipid pneumonitis. Emollients are the drugs of choice for hard, dry stools.

Cathartic laxatives induce hyperosmolarity in the intestinal lumen and decrease water absorption. They are contraindicated in patients with abdominal pain of uncertain cause. Injudicious use can induce fluid and electrolyte abnormalities.

Stimulant laxatives promote fluid accumulation in the gut lumen and enhance intestinal motility. All stimulant laxatives are contraindicated in patients with abdominal pain of uncertain cause. They are habit-forming; chronic use may cause neurologic damage with colonic atony, dilation, and hypomotility.

Suppositories and enemas are useful to prepare the bowel for x-rays but should not be used in other circumstances if oral agents are effective.

Bisacodyl, an effective stimulant available as a suppository, acts in 15–30 minutes and is usually better tolerated than enemas.

Enemas increase rectal peristalsis by distention; some preparations (e.g., potassium bitartrate) produce carbon dioxide to enhance this

TABLE 1–4. LAXATIVES

AGENT	USUAL ADULT DOSE AND ROUTE	TIME TO EFFECT	COMMENT
Bulk agents			
Methylcellulose (Citrucel)	4–6 gm tid po	Onset 12–24 hr; full effect, 2–3 days	May reduce absorption of digoxin, salicylates, and nitrofurantoin if given simultaneously
Psyllium (Metamucil, Perdiem Plus)	3–6 gm qd–tid po	Same as above	Same as above, may also reduce absorption of warfarin; some preparations contain sugar
Bran	6 gm qd po	Same as above	Cheap; no drug interactions
Emollient agents			
Dioctyl sodium sulfosuccinate (DSS, Colace)	50–360 mg qd po	1–3 days	Available as capsule, solution, and tablet
Dioctyl potassium sulfosuccinate (Dialose)	100–240 mg qd po	Same as above	Available as capsule
Dioctyl calcium sulfosuccinate (Surfak)	50–240 mg qd po	Same as above	Available as capsule

	Dose	Onset/Duration	Comments
Cathartic agents			
Magnesium hydroxide (Milk of Magnesia)	30–60 mL qd po (82–164 mEq Mg)	3–6 hr; low dose: 6–8 hr	Avoid in renal failure; commonly used at hs in low dose; double-strength formulations available; may decrease tetracycline absorption
Lactulose (Chronulac)	10–20 gm qd po (15–30 mL)	24 hr	Poorly absorbed disaccharide also used in hepatic encephalopathy; often used in elderly patients
Sorbitol	15–30 mL of 70% solution qd po	3–6 hr	Nonabsorbable; less expensive than lactulose but as effective; also given rectally to treat hyperkalemia
Magnesium citrate	100–200 mL qd po (77–154 mEq Mg)	3–6 hr	Avoid in renal failure; induces watery stool
Sodium sulfate (Golytely)	2–4 liters po	1–3 hr	Induces watery stool; commonly used in bowel prep
Stimulant agents			
Senna (Senokot)	5–15 mL qd po	Onset 6 hr; 12–24 hr to full effect	May induce melanosis coli; available as powder or liquid
Cascara sagrada	5 mL qd po	Onset 8 hr	May induce melanosis coli
Bisacodyl (Dulcolax)	5–15 mg qd po; 10 mg qd pr	6–12 hr po 15–30 min pr	Tablets contain tartrazine dye; do not give orally within 1 hour of antacids; suppository may cause mild proctitis
Castor oil	15–60 mL po	1–6 hr	Induces semifluid stool; active in small intestine; cramping common; should be reserved for bowel prep

effect. Other substances used as enemas include glycerin, sorbitol, and tap water. The main criterion for selection is ease of administration.

VII. DIARRHEA

A. **Causes.** Diarrhea is a common symptom of disease, but it also can be a medication side effect. Common offenders include magnesium-containing antacids, antibiotics (with and without *Clostridium difficile* infection), laxatives, quinidine, and colchicine. Diarrhea should not be treated symptomatically before other possible causes are ruled out. Drugs that inhibit motility usually should be withheld if acute mucosal inflammation is suspected.

B. **Management** (Table 1–5). Adequate fluid intake should be ensured (oral or IV) while avoiding excessive osmotic loads. Acute diarrheal illnesses may decrease intestinal lactase activity and lactose restriction for 3 to 5 days is often helpful. Oral glucose-electrolyte solutions are useful in some circumstances, especially in pediatrics.

Bulking agents (Table 1–4) lead to formed stools by absorption of water but may increase electrolyte losses. Bulking agents are more useful in management of chronic diarrhea associated with irritable bowel syndrome, colostomy, and ileostomy.

Kaolin (hydrated aluminum silicate) and pectin (polygalacturonic acid) are combined for their supposed adsorbent and mucosal-protective properties. Stool fluidity decreases, but overall stool weight or frequency does not. Adverse effects, except for drug interactions, are usually minimal.

Bismuth subsalicylate (Pepto-Bismol) decreases intestinal fluid secretion by affecting the intestinal prostaglandins. It works in traveller's diarrhea (usually due to enterotoxogenic *Escherichia coli;* Gastroenterology 73:715–718, 1977). It is contraindicated in patients with a history of aspirin hypersensitivity or when Reye's syndrome is possible. Significant salicylate absorption may occur. In one study use of 8 ounces of Pepto-Bismol over 3.5 hours caused absorption of salicylate equivalent to 2600 mg of aspirin (J Pediatr 99:654–656, 1981).

Preparations that contain **natural antimuscarinics** (e.g., atropine, scopolamine) or **synthetic anticholinergics** inhibit intestinal motility and cramping. However, they involve anticholinergic risks (acute glaucoma, urinary retention, CNS side effects). At dosages low enough to avoid adverse effects, these agents are not effective in severe diarrhea and should not be used if acute mucosal inflammation is suspected.

All **narcotics** exert an antidiarrheal effect by decreasing intestinal motility and reducing secretory activity mediated by opioid receptors. At standard doses, the antidiarrheal narcotics do not cause analgesia, but doses above recommended levels can cause euphoria and physical dependence. This risk is highest with camphorated tincture of opium, less with diphenoxylate, and even less with loperamide.

Diphenoxylate and loperamide are equally effective for acute diarrhea. However, loperamide is more effective in chronic diarrhea due to inflammatory bowel disease. These agents should be avoided if acute mucosal inflammation is suspected (JAMA 226:1525–1528, 1973).

TABLE 1–5. ANTIDIARRHEALS

AGENT	USUAL ADULT DOSE	DRUG INTERACTIONS	COMMENT
Bulk or adsorbent agents			
Psyllium (Metamucil, Perdiem Plus)	3 gm qd–tid	*See Table 1–4*	Must be given with water
Methylcellulose (Citrucel)	4–6 gr bid–tid	*See Table 1–4*	Must be given with water
Kaolin-pectin (Kaopectate)	60–120 mL after each bowel movement	May reduce absorption of digoxin and tetracyclines	Kaopectate tablets contain a different adsorbent
Prostaglandin synthesis inhibitor			
Bismuth subsalicylate (Pepto-Bismol)	524 mg (2 pills or 30 mL) every 30 min; maximum 8 doses qd	Increased risk of bleeding in those taking warfarin	Changes stool color to black
Antimuscarinic agents			
Kaolin, pectin, hyoscyamine, atropine, scopolamine (Donnagel)	30 mL, then 15 mL every 3 hr, up to 60 mL qd	Decreased absorption of digoxin and chloroquine	Anticholinergic side effects; available with paregoric
Opioid agents			
Tincture of opium (Paregoric)	5–10 mL up to qid	Increased depression with CNS depressants	5 mL equivalent to 2 mg morphine
Diphenoxylate, 2.5 mg and atropine 0.025 mg (Lomotil)	2 tablets up to qid	Increased depression with CNS depressants	Contraindicated in invasive infectious diarrhea and acute ulcerative colitis
Loperamide (Imodium)	4 mg, then 2 mg after each stool; maximum 16 mg qd	Increased depression with CNS depressants	Same as above; more potent than diphenoxylate; available without prescription
Bile acid binder			
Cholestyramine (Questran)	4 gm tid–qid	Decreased absorption of many drugs, e.g., chlorothiazide, digoxin, thyroxine, warfarin, and phenobarbital	Must be given with water; give other drugs 1 hr before or 4 hr after dose

In acute ulcerative colitis, opiates may increase the risk of toxic megacolon.

Cholestyramine, a bile acid binder, should be considered for diarrhea due to excessive intraluminal bile acids (e.g., ileal resection) and in patients with pseudomembranous colitis.

DiJohn D, Levene MM: Treatment of diarrhea. Infect Dis Clin North Am 2:719–745, 1988.

Barrett KE, Dharmsathapom K: Pharmacological aspects of therapy in inflammatory bowel disease. J Clin Gastroenterol 10:57–63, 1988.

Brownlee HJ (ed): Management of acute nonspecific diarrhea. Am J Med 88(suppl 6A):1S–37S, 1990.

VIII. NAUSEA AND VOMITING

A. **Causes.** Nausea is the most common adverse drug effect. Nausea and vomiting are mediated by a medullary center that receives afferents from the GI tract, the cortical centers, the vestibular system, and the dopaminergic chemoreceptor trigger zone (CTZ), a medullary center.

After possible diagnoses have been considered, symptomatic treatment should be used to reduce patient discomfort, to avoid electrolyte disturbances, to reduce risk of aspiration of gastric contents, and to avoid gastroesophageal injury.

B. **Management. Airway protection** is important in the management of nausea and vomiting; a stuporous patient may require an endotracheal tube. A nasogastric tube and positioning the patient with the head elevated by 15 to 30 degrees may help.

C. **Antiemetics** (Table 1–6). **Emetrol** is a mixture of dextrose, levulose, and phosphoric acid that may be effective in mild nausea or motion sickness. It is the only antiemetic judged safe during pregnancy.

Antacids may help when there is a peptic component, as in reflux esophagitis.

Some **antihistamines** with H_1 specificity are effective for nausea associated with motion sickness or vestibular disorders. They are less effective than the neuroleptics in nausea due to other causes. The antihistamines depress labyrinthine excitability and vestibulocerebellar pathways. They may cause sedation and such anticholinergic symptoms as dry mouth and urinary retention.

Meclizine and dimenhydrinate are used primarily for nausea of motion sickness or vestibular dysfunction. The latter is more effective for motion sickness, and prophylactic use is superior. Parenteral preparations of hydroxyzine and diphenhydramine are available. The IV route (diphenhydramine only) is preferred in patients receiving cancer chemotherapy. Drug interactions, aside from additive sedative effects, are unusual for this class of medications.

Scopolamine, a natural antimuscarinic, is the most potent agent available for motion sickness but is not useful for nausea of other causes. It is best used prophylactically and is available in transdermal form. This delivers 0.5 mg qd for up to 72 hours.

Metoclopramide has central antidopaminergic and peripheral cholinergic activities. It stimulates gastric emptying and decreases gastroesoph-

TABLE 1-6. ANTIEMETICS

AGENT	CLASS	USUAL ADULT DOSE AND ROUTE	ANTI-CHOLINERGIC EFFECT	POTENTIAL FOR DYSTONIA	COMMENT
Dextrose, levulose, phosphoric acid (Emetrol)		15–30 mL po q 15 min	0	0	Available without prescription; safe in pregnancy
Dimenhydrinate (Dramamine)	Histamine$_1$ (H$_1$) blocker	50–100 mg po, IM, or IV q 4 hr	1–2+	0	Available without prescription
Diphenhydramine (Benadryl)	H$_1$ blocker	25–100 mg po, IM q 6 hr; 25–75 mg IV q 4 hr	3+	0	Most sedating of the H$_1$ blockers; available as elixir
Hydroxyzine (Vistaril, Atarax)	H$_1$ blocker	25–100 mg po, IM q 6 hr	2+	0	Mild anxiolytic; not for IV use; available as elixir
Meclizine (Antivert)	H$_1$ blocker	12.5–37.5 mg po tid	1–2+	0	Single daily dose useful as motion sickness prophylaxis
Scopolamine (Transderm-Scop)	Antimuscarinic	See text	4+	0	Sedation is common; used transdermally
Trimethobenzamide (Tigan)	Chemoreceptor trigger zone (CTZ) effect	250 mg po tid-qid; 200 mg pr, IM tid-qid	1+	1+	Suppository contains benzocaine; pregnancy category B
Metoclopramide (Reglan)	CTZ effect	10–20 mg po qid; 1–2 mg/kg IV q 2 hr; see text	0	2–4+	Risk of dystonia is dose dependent: 0.2% for low dose, 25% for very high dose
Droperidol (Inapsine)	CTZ effect	1.25–2.50 mg IV or IM q 4 hr	1+	2+	High rate of sedation; onset in 3–10 min
Chlorpromazine (Thorazine)	Phenothiazine	10–25 mg po q 4–6 hr; 25–50 mg IM q 3–4 hr; 25–100 mg pr q 8 hr	3+	2–3+	Also useful for hiccups; more sedating and higher frequency of hypotension than with prochlorperazine
Prochlorperazine (Compazine)	Phenothiazine	5–10 mg po, IM, or IV q 6 hr; 25 mg pr q 12 hr	2+	3+	Available as elixir
Promethazine (Phenergan)	Phenothiazine	12.5–25.0 mg po, pr, or IM q 4–6 hr	3+	2+	More sedating than prochlorperazine; also useful for motion sickness and as an antihistamine; available as elixir
Dexamethasone (Decadron)	Steroid	10–20 mg IV q 12 hr 8 mg po q 6 hr	0	0	Used as 2–3 day course of adjunctive treatment for nausea of chemotherapy
Methylprednisolone (Solumedrol)	Steroid	250–500 mg IV q 6 hr	0	0	Used similarly to dexamethasone
Dronabinol (Marinol)	Cannabinoid	5–10 mg/m^2 po q 4–6 hr	0	0	Schedule II

ageal reflux. The usual starting dose is 10 mg qid. For chemotherapy-induced nausea, the dosage may be up to 2 mg/kg every 2 hours for 2 doses, then 1 mg/kg every 3 hours for 3 doses. Doses should be halved if the creatinine clearance is less than 40 cc/min.

Sedation is a common side effect (10% for 10 mg qid; 70% for 1–2 mg/kg). Other common adverse effects include dystonic reactions and pseudoparkinsonism. Metoclopramide potentiates the risk of dystonic reactions to phenothiazines and may precipitate a hypertensive crisis in patients taking MAO inhibitors. It may decrease absorption of drugs absorbed from the stomach (e.g., digoxin).

Neuroleptic drugs act at the CTZ, where they have antidopaminergic effects. All neuroleptics except thioridazine have some antiemetic effect, but usually at doses substantially below their neuroleptic dosage. These drugs are less useful in nausea due to local action on the GI tract or vestibular dysfunction. They have sedative, alpha-adrenergic blocking, and anticholinergic actions.

Acute dystonic reactions, which may occur with any of these agents, can be treated with diphenhydramine 25–50 mg or benztropine mesylate 1–2 mg IM or IV followed by a course of oral therapy. The neuroleptics are metabolized in the liver; their effect may be diminished by microsomal inducers.

Tetrahydrocannabinol is available for oral use at selected centers in the United States for cancer patients refractory to other agents. It is as effective as prochlorperazine or metoclopramide. The main adverse effects of tetrahydrocannabinol are depersonalization, dysphoria, and somnolence.

Prophylactic combination treatment of nausea should be considered in patients receiving chemotherapy. High doses of metoclopramide, droperidol, prochlorperazine, and promethazine are effective prophylactically. IV diphenhydramine is also used commonly, though not as a single agent. It prevents dystonic reactions. Brief courses of dexamethasone or methylprednisolone may be useful adjuncts. Low doses of lorazepam may be helpful also in decreasing discomfort of nausea associated with chemotherapy.

Recently developed **serotonin antagonists** may prove to be as effective as metoclopramide with fewer side effects.

Morrow GR: Chemotherapy-related nausea and vomiting: Etiology and management. CA 39(2):89–104, 1989.
Merrifield KR, Chaffee BJ: Recent advances in the management of nausea and vomiting caused by antineoplastic agents. Clin Pharm 8:187–199, 1989.

IX. NEUROLEPTICS

A. **Drugs used to treat psychosis** (Table 1–7) belong to the phenothiazine, thioxanthine, or butyrophenone classes. Collectively, they are called neuroleptic agents; all are equally effective antipsychotics at equipotent doses. All have greater or lesser antidopaminergic, anticholinergic, and alpha-adrenergic blocking properties. The agent should be chosen on the basis of possible side effects. In general, the less potent

TABLE 1-7. NEUROLEPTICS

AGENT	USUAL* ADULT TOTAL DAILY ORAL DOSE (mg) AND SCHEDULE	MAXIMAL* ORAL DAILY DOSE (mg)	SINGLE* IM DOSE (mg)	SEDATION	RELATIVE MAGNITUDE OF EXTRA-PYRAMIDAL EFFECT	RELATIVE MAGNITUDE OF HYPO-TENSIVE EFFECT	COMMENT
Chlorpromazine (Thorazine)	100–800 bid–tid	2000	25–100	3+	2+	3+	Increases level of tricyclic antidepressants; increases renal clearance of lithium; decreases effect of warfarin; absorption decreased by antacids
Fluphenazine (Prolixin)	1–20 tid–qid	30	1.25–2.50	1+	3+	1+	Increases effect of propranolol; same effect on lithium and warfarin as chlorpromazine; available as decanoate or enanthate for long-acting therapy
Mesoridazine (Serentil)	50–300 tid	400	25	3+	1+	2+	Absorption decreased by antacids
Perphenazine (Trilafon)	4–32 bid	64	5–10	2+	2+	1+	Absorption decreased by antacids
Thioridazine (Mellaril)	100–600 tid–qid	800	NA	3+	1+	2+	Absorption decreased by antacids
Trifluoperazine (Stelazine)	4–20 bid	60	1–2	1+	3+	1+	Same effects on propranolol, lithium, and warfarin as fluphenazine
Thiothixene (Navane)	4–30 qd–bid	60	2–4	2+	2+	2+	Absorption decreased by antacids
Haloperidol (Haldol)	0.5–15.0 bid–tid	100	2–5	1+	3+	1+	Available as decanoate for long-acting therapy
Loxapine (Loxitane)	40–100 bid–qid	250	12.5–50.0	1+	2+	1+	Increases serum level of tricyclic antidepressants

*Lower doses are recommended for frail elderly persons. Doses listed are "antipsychotic doses" usually used in conjunction with a psychiatrist.

neuroleptics are more sedating, cause more postural symptoms, have more anticholinergic effects, and have fewer associated movement disorders (with the exception of tardive dyskinesia).

B. Treatment of acute major psychosis consists of frequent doses of parenteral drugs. Haloperidol, 5 mg IM, or chlorpromazine, 50–100 mg IM, may be used hourly until control is achieved, followed by additional doses every 4–8 hours for the first 24–72 hours.

In most cases, lower doses or a parenteral benzodiazepine should be used initially in frail elderly persons. Patients must be monitored for development of hypotension or acute dystonia.

Patients with **confusion** or **delirium** should not be treated symptomatically with neuroleptics until underlying conditions such as medication toxicity, electrolyte imbalance, infection, hypoxia, hepatic insufficiency, and cardiovascular disease have been ruled out or treated primarily. General supportive measures are also important in management of psychosis, delirium, and confusion.

Disturbance of the patient should be minimized and the room lights should be dimmed at night. Attendants may be required and are preferred to restraints. Restraints are used for the safety of patients and staff.

Family members may help reassure the patient. They need to know that the patient's bizarre behavior is not willful and that it will in most cases resolve without sequelae.

After complicating medical illnesses have been ruled out, symptomatic treatment with low doses (0.5–2 mg hs) of haloperidol may be helpful. In agitated critically ill patients, higher doses or a parenteral benzodiazepine may be necessary. All neuroleptics have the potential to cause several extrapyramidal syndromes. **Acute dystonia** is more common in young patients. It may be treated with diphenhydramine 25–50 mg IM or benztropine mesylate 1–2 mg IM; subsequent oral therapy may be required for days to several weeks. A syndrome identical to **Parkinson's disease** may occur, especially in the elderly. Usually the offending drug must be discontinued. **Tardive dyskinesia** is a late complication of neuroleptics for which there is no effective treatment.

Neuroleptic malignant syndrome is a potentially fatal emergency characterized by fever, stupor, catatonia, hemodynamic instability, and myoglobinemia (Quart J Med 56:421–429, 1985). Recognition with immediate discontinuation of the neuroleptic and prompt treatment are essential.

Dubin WR: Rapid tranquilization: Antipsychotics or benzodiazepines? Clin Psychiatry 49(suppl):5–12, 1988.
Kane JM: The current status of neuroleptic treatment. J Clin Psychiatry 50:322–328, 1989.

X. SEDATIVES AND HYPNOTICS

A. Possible underlying disorders, ranging from metabolic diseases to sleep apnea, should be considered before undertaking symptomatic treatment of **insomnia** (Table 1–8).

Short-term treatment of insomnia is safe if side effects of hypnotic drugs are carefully monitored. Chronic use of hypnotics for insomnia is not recommended because of difficulties with habituation, side effects, and questionable efficacy. Objective improvement in daytime functioning due to hypnotic use has never been demonstrated.

Many nonprescription sleeping aids contain an **antihistamine** such as diphenhydramine, hydroxyzine, or pyrilamine. These agents are minimally effective, with tolerance developing rapidly; however, they have no addiction potential. Anticholinergic side effects may occur.

B. **Benzodiazepines** are usually the drugs of choice for insomnia and anxiety. They have a favorable therapeutic index with minimal effects on respiration at commonly used dosages.

Addiction and withdrawal syndromes may occur. Dangerous withdrawal syndromes are rare with daily doses of less than 20 mg diazepam. Moderate symptoms such as dysphoria, irritability, and insomnia may occur in up to one third of patients.

The shorter-acting agents are more likely to produce withdrawal symptoms as well as rebound insomnia after only short-term use. The **benzodiazepines should be avoided during pregnancy** because of the risk of fetal abnormalities.

The selection of one benzodiazepine agent over another is based on pharmacokinetic differences. All are well absorbed orally, but only lorazepam is consistently and rapidly absorbed when given IM.

All are metabolized by the liver. Lorazepam and oxazepam are cleared solely by glucuronidation, which is less affected by age and co-morbidity, and are preferred for patients with underlying liver disease. Some have long-lived active metabolites that are responsible for part of their effect. Lorazepam, oxazepam, and temazepam have no active metabolites; alprazolam and triazolam have only short-lived ones.

Diazepam has the most rapid onset of action of all benzodiazepines, reaching peak concentration within 30–60 minutes of an oral dose. It is generally not used as a hypnotic because of long-lived active metabolites.

Agents marketed as hypnotics include triazolam and temazepam, which act within 1–2 hours. Flurazepam reaches peak effect in 1–3 hours and has long-lived active metabolites. It is widely used for insomnia and is more effective after the first night. Its effect persists for 1–2 days after discontinuation.

C. **Barbiturates.** The only major indications for barbiturates are as adjuncts to anesthesia and as anticonvulsants. When these drugs are used as hypnotics, tolerance begins to develop within a few days; the effect on total sleep time is halved after 2 weeks. Their therapeutic index is low.

D. **Chloral hydrate** is a hypnotic that, in commonly used doses (500–1000 mg), shortens time to sleep but does not change total time asleep. It is useful for sleep induction before electroencephalographic recording due to its relatively slight effect on EEG patterns. Its therapeutic index is between that of the benzodiazepines and the barbiturates.

E. **Glutethimide** is a sedative that has significant anticholinergic action as well as long-lived active metabolites. **Meprobamate** is also used as a hypnotic. These uses of both drugs should be abandoned owing to their potential for dependence and abstinence syndromes and their lack of advantages over the benzodiazepines.

TABLE 1–8. SEDATIVES AND HYPNOTICS

AGENT	HALF-LIFE OF EFFECT INCLUDING ACTIVE METABOLITES (hr)	ADULT DOSE, mg* (ORAL UNLESS STATED) FOR HYPNOTIC USE	COMMENT
Antihistamines			
Diphenhydramine (Benadryl)	4–6	25–50	Highest rate of anticholinergic effects; most sedating of the antihistamines
Hydroxyzine (Vistaril, Atarax)	6–24	25–50	Used as an anxiolytic at higher dose, up to 100 mg
Pyrilamine (Rynatan)	4–6	25–50	Relatively little anticholinergic effect
Barbiturates			
Pentobarbital (Nembutal)	15–48	100 po or 120–200 pr	Barbiturates should not be used as hypnotics for more than 2 consecutive weeks; all have been linked to fetal abnormalities, though they are safer in pregnancy than benzodiazepines; drug interactions common due to induction of hepatic microsomal system (e.g., warfarin, corticosteroids, phenytoin, estrogens)
Secobarbital (Seconal)	15–40	100 po or 200 pr	
Amobarbital (Amytal)	8–42	65–200	
Benzodiazepines			All benzodiazepines are contraindicated in the 1st trimester of pregnancy; chlordiazepoxide, lorazepam, and oxazepam are commonly used in treatment of alcohol withdrawal syndrome
Short-acting			
Oxazepam (Serax)	5–10	15–30	Not used as an anxiolytic
Triazolam (Halcion)	1.5–3.0	0.125–0.25	
Intermediate-acting			
Alprazolam (Xanax)	11–19	1–2	Not commonly used as a hypnotic; used for panic disorder (2–4 mg per day)
Lorazepam (Ativan)	10–20	2–4	Only benzodiazepine that is useful IM: use 1 mg q 1–2 hr for acute agitation (fewer side effects than haloperidol)
Temazepam (Restoril)	10–17	15–30	Not used as an anxiolytic; half-life in elderly women greater than in elderly men

Drug			Comments
Long-acting			
Chlordiazepoxide (Librium)	30–60	25–100	Long-acting form, Tranxene-SD, available for use as anxiolytic
Chlorazepate (Tranxene)	50–80	15–30	
Clonazepam (Klonopin)	18–50	1–2	FDA approved as adjunctive anticonvulsant
Diazepam (Valium)	30–60	5–10	Also used as a muscle relaxant and for treatment of alcohol withdrawal; used IV for seizures and as premedication for procedures; maximal rate of administration is 5 mg/min due to risk of collapse; available in long-acting form, Valrelease
Flurazepam (Dalmane)	50–100	15–30	Not used as an anxiolytic; 15 mg as effective as 30 mg for most patients
Prazepam (Centrax)	50–100	20–40	Primarily used as an anxiolytic
Miscellaneous Drugs			*See text for further comments*
Chloral hydrate (Noctec)	4–10	500–1000	Many patients may require up to 2000 mg; may affect pro time in warfarin-treated patients
Glutethimide (Doriden)	5–22	250–500	Decreases effect of warfarin
Meprobamate (Miltown)	6–17	800	Approved by the FDA only for anxiety
Paraldehyde (Paral)	—	4–8 mL	Rapid onset of action; used in alcohol withdrawal, 5–10 mL q 2–4 hr
Pure Anxiolytic			
Buspirone (Buspar)	—	5–20 mg tid	May be a selective anxiolytic; minimal sedative activity; may displace digoxin from plasma proteins

*Lower doses recommended for frail elderly persons.

F. Paraldehyde is a liquid medication that is rapidly absorbed, metabolized by the liver, and partly excreted by exhalation. Its most common use is as a sedative during alcohol withdrawal; however, it is not better than the benzodiazepines. Paraldehyde may induce dependence. If stored in partially filled bottles, it may degrade to acetic acid.

G. Anxiety may be a symptom of depression, psychosis, substance abuse, or panic disorder. Any of the agents discussed above may be used to treat anxiety symptomatically, but only hydroxyzine, buspirone, and the benzodiazepines are widely employed.

Hydroxyzine has the advantage of lack of dependence or abstinence syndromes, though high doses (50–100 mg qid) may be required to treat anxiety.

The **benzodiazepines** are effective as anxiolytics and are commonly used at one third to one half of the hypnotic dose administered bid–qid. The agents with active long-lived metabolites have the advantage of less frequent dosing once effect has been established. Benefit for 4 months of continuous use has been documented. The effectiveness of longer-term use has not been proved, and dependence can occur.

A new class of drugs, represented by **buspirone,** is available to treat anxiety with minimal sedation and possibility for dependence. The anxiolytic effect may have a latency of onset of 1–2 weeks. Its role in the treatment of anxiety disorders is not yet clearly defined.

Hauri PJ, Esther MS: Insomnia. Mayo Clin Proc 65:869–882, 1990.
Prinz PN, Vitiello MV, Raskind MA, Thorpy MJ: Geriatrics: Sleep disorders and aging. N Engl J Med 323:521–526, 1990.
Roy-Byrne PP, Hommer D: Benzodiazepine withdrawal: Overview and implications for treatment of anxiety. Am J Med 84:1041–1052, 1988.
Cole JO: The drug treatment of anxiety and depression. Med Clin North Am 72(4):815–830, 1988.

XI. AFFECTIVE DISORDERS

A. Depression, with a prevalence of 3–9%, may be a manifestation of a major affective disorder or a bipolar illness. Metabolic disorders or drugs may cause depression. Commonly implicated drugs include alcohol, sedatives, cimetidine, alphamethyldopa, reserpine, beta blockers, and corticosteroids.

B. Assessment of the risk of **suicide** is a critical part of managing depression. Features that suggest a high risk include detailed thought to a suicide plan, coexistence of alcoholism, social isolation, male gender, and advanced age.

A high risk of suicide usually mandates hospital admission.

C. Antidepressant Medications. Antidepressants (Table 1–9) are effective in all types of depression. A medication is usually selected to address the most bothersome symptom(s) with a minimum of side effects. Which drug will be the most effective is not predictable.

All antidepressants have a latency of antidepressant effect of up to 4 weeks. Because the average duration of an untreated depressive event is 9 months, antidepressants are usually given for 8–12 months and then tapered.

There are several important side effects of antidepressants. Anticholinergic effects, sedation, a fine tremor, and postural hypotension are the most common. **Cardiotoxicity** includes heart block, bundle branch block, and brady- or tachyarrhythmias. Atrial arrhythmias and premature ventricular contractions are not contraindications to therapy, but concomitant therapy with type I antiarrhythmics should be given cautiously due to similar actions. Tricyclic antidepressants (TCAs) are contraindicated in acute MI.

Significant additive effects may occur with other CNS sedatives. Cimetidine increases the pharmacologic effects of most TCAs. The TCAs are well absorbed orally and have half-lives long enough to allow once-daily administration if side effects permit.

There is a roughly linear correlation between therapeutic effect and serum levels for most agents. Routine drug level monitoring is not necessary, however, except for nortriptyline, which may have a narrow therapeutic "window." Lower dosages of all TCAs (Table 1–9) are recommended in frail elderly persons.

Monoamine oxidase (MAO) inhibitors are rarely used as first-line antidepressant agents and appear to be more effective in atypical depression, panic disorder, and depression with psychomotor retardation. Due to inhibition of MAO in the GI tract, foods rich in tyramine or tryptophan are contraindicated. Implicated foods include cheese, wine, beer, yogurt, chicken liver, chocolate, bananas, avocados, and sour cream (Arch Intern Med 151:873–884, 1991).

Many medications, such as amphetamines, caffeine, sympathomimetics, alphamethyldopa, and L-dopa, should not be given simultaneously with the MAO inhibitors. Consumption of the above foods, beverages, and medications may cause severe hypertension. Orthostatic hypotension, tremor, and insomnia may occur with all of the MAO inhibitors.

Lithium, usually in the form of lithium carbonate, is the mainstay of chronic treatment for mania. Acute treatment may also require sedatives or neuroleptics. Lithium carbonate is well absorbed orally and is usually administered 2 or 3 times per day. Lithium has a half-life of 20–24 hours in patients with normal renal function. Sodium depletion may decrease lithium clearance.

The average daily dose of lithium carbonate is 900–1500 mg, and an increment of 300 mg corresponds to a change in serum level of 0.2 mEq/L. *Monitoring of serum levels is essential,* due to a narrow therapeutic range. A level of 0.8–1.2 mEq/L (10 hours after the previous dose) is considered optimal.

With therapeutic lithium concentrations, thyroxine synthesis may be impaired, although most patients remain euthyroid. Nephrogenic diabetes insipidus, leukocytosis, ECG abnormalities, and neurologic symptoms may also result from lithium use.

Potter WZ, Rudorfer MV, Manji H: The pharmacologic treatment of depression. N Engl J Med 325:633–642, 1991.

TABLE 1–9. DRUGS USED IN THE AFFECTIVE DISORDERS

AGENT	ADULT ORAL DAILY DOSE RANGE (mg),* ACUTE (MAINTENANCE DOSE IS ½–⅔ OF THIS)	RELATIVE MAGNITUDE OF SEDATION	RELATIVE MAGNITUDE OF ANTI-CHOLINERGIC EFFECT	RELATIVE MAGNITUDE OF DELAY OF CARDIAC CONDUCTION	RELATIVE MAGNITUDE OF POSTURAL HYPOTENSION	COMMENT
Tricyclic Antidepressants (TCAs)						
Amitriptyline (Elavil, Endep)	75–300; starting IM dose is 20 mg qid	3	2	3	3	Most common agent for chronic pain
Desipramine (Norpramin, Pertofrane)	75–300	1	1	3	1	Metabolite of imipramine
Doxepin (Sinequan, Adapin)	75–300	3	3	1	3	Potent antihistamine: H_1 and H_2
Imipramine (Tofranil)	50–300	2	2	3	2	May decrease antihypertensive effect of clonidine; also used in panic disorder
Nortriptyline (Pamelor, Aventyl)	75–150	1	1	2	1–2	Metabolite of amitriptyline; apparent narrow therapeutic "window"
Protriptyline (Vivactil)	15–60	0	2	2	1	May decrease effect of warfarin and clonidine
Trimipramine (Surmontil)	50–300	2–3	2	3	1–2	May decrease effect of clonidine

	Dosage					Comments
Tetracyclic						
Amoxapine (Asendin)	200–600	2	1	1	1	Metabolite has neuroleptic side effect
Maprotiline (Ludiomil)	75–300	2	1	1	1	May lower seizure threshold
Heterocyclic						
Trazodone (Desyrel)	50–600	2–3	1	0	2	Should be given in divided doses; risk of priapism; may increase serum levels of digoxin and phenytoin; may decrease effect of clonidine
Fluoxetine (Prozac)	20–80	0	0	0	0	May cause insomnia or akathisia; may increase serum levels of warfarin, TCAs, and digoxin; should not be given with MAO inhibitors
Monoamine Oxidase (MAO) Inhibitors						
Phenelzine (Nardil)	10–30	0	1	0	3	Also used in panic disorder
Tranylcypromine (Parnate)	20–30	0	1	0	3	May be more stimulating

*Lower doses recommended for frail elderly persons.

XII. PRESSURE SORES

A. The pressure sore ("decubitus ulcer") has a prevalence among hospital inpatients of 3–11% (Ann Intern Med 105:337–342, 1986). Patients with hypoalbuminemia, fecal incontinence, and fractures are at greatest risk of developing pressure sores. Pathophysiologic factors (Ann Intern Med 94:661–666, 1981) include external pressure sufficient to close the cutaneous capillaries exerted for more than 2 hours, shear forces on the skin producing damage to dermal structures, and external friction causing damage to the stratum corneum. The presence of moisture accelerates epidermal breakdown by interfering with natural reparative processes.

B. Preventive measures should be used for all patients at risk of pressure sores. Frequent turning of a patient (every 1–2 hours) normally permits adequate blood supply, though underlying microvascular disease may further impair capillary function.

Although cushioning systems may help, none have consistently lowered pressures below capillary closing pressure. Air-fluidized bed and mattress systems are effective but not practical for general use.

Cutaneous shear forces may be decreased by use of sheepskin and clothing that is free of particulate matter. Proper positioning—whether lying or sitting—also helps minimize shear forces. Skin care to maintain appropriate levels of moisture may require intervention to dry the skin as well as judicious use of emollients to minimize fragility. Heat lamps may help but carry the risk of burns.

Early pressure lesions may be confused with cellulitis. If such lesions progress to ulceration and tissue necrosis, surgical debridement is usually necessary.

C. Management of established pressure sores is similar to the management of ulcerative lesions in general, with debridement of necrotic tissue done by mechanical means (instruments, Water Pik, whirlpool) or by topical means ("wet to dry" dressing with gauze soaked in normal saline or hydrogen peroxide, or biochemical agents such as collagenase, fibrinolysin-deoxyribonuclease, or papain). Studies of alternatives to wet to dry dressings have been poorly controlled, and no convincing advantages have been demonstrated.

Once the wound is free of necrotic debris, it should be kept moist with minimal trauma. Topical antibiotics (e.g., silver sulfadiazine) or vapor-permeable occlusive dressings should be used.

Patients should receive nutritional support if needed, and measures should be taken to avoid new pressure sores.

Allman RM: Pressure ulcers among the elderly. N Engl J Med 320:850–853, 1989.
Adams-Mondoux LC (ed): Pressure ulcers. Nurs Clin North Am 22:357–492, 1987.

XIII. URINARY INCONTINENCE

A. Urinary incontinence occurs in 20% of hospitalized elderly patients and

50% of nursing home residents. Many events, including hospitalization, may cause transient urinary incontinence.

New medications may promote urinary retention and overflow incontinence (anticholinergics, analgesics, sedatives) or increased flow (diuretics). Alpha-adrenergic agonists and antagonists, theophylline, and calcium channel blockers may also contribute to the development of incontinence.

B. **Evaluation of the Incontinent Patient.** A history, physical examination, and record of the timing of micturition and incontinence may suggest drug reactions or functional incontinence.

Urinalysis may provide evidence of a tumor, stone, or infection, leading to specific evaluation and treatment. **Measurement** of the postvoid residual urine volume ("in and out" catheterization) is important to evaluate for bladder outlet obstruction. Up to 50 mL may be normal in elderly men.

C. Patients with incontinence due to acute medical illness have a good prognosis for recovery of urinary function when their medical problem resolves. Judicious use of **absorptive undergarments** may be helpful, though care must be taken to avoid skin breakdown.

For men, **condom catheters** may help but may cause skin breakdown and contribute to bladder infection and can aggravate confusion. Use of **indwelling bladder catheters** is generally not an appropriate long-term solution, although they may be needed in some cases. Intermittent bladder catheterization is preferred.

D. **Detrusor instability** is the most common cause of chronic incontinence in the elderly. It results from insufficient inhibition of the detrusor muscle by the CNS (e.g., cerebrovascular disease, Alzheimer's disease, normal pressure hydrocephalus) or hyperexcitability of the afferent pathways (e.g., bladder or pelvic infection, tumor, fecal impaction, uterine prolapse, and prostatic hypertrophy).

The pattern of micturition is erratic but usually with voided volumes over 150 mL. There is usually a period of warning sensation before micturition. Bladder training, in which the patient voids voluntarily every 1–2 hours, may keep the bladder volume within the detrusor capacity.

Drug therapy of detrusor instability:

Anticholinergic agents include propantheline bromide (Pro-Banthine) 15–120 mg qd administered bid–qid; imipramine (Tofranil) 25–150 mg qd administered bid–qid; oxybutinin (Ditropan) 5–20 mg qd administered bid–qid.

Detrusor-sphincter dyssynergia may also be present. **Alpha-adrenergic blockers** may help relax the smooth muscle internal sphincter: prazosin (Minipress) 2–20 mg qd administered bid–tid; phenoxybenzamine (Dibenzyline) 10–60 mg qd given bid–tid.

E. Overflow incontinence usually involves frequent small amounts of urinary leakage from a distended bladder.

It may result from bladder outlet obstruction or detrusor weakness, usually from a drug effect or a neurologic lesion such as radiculopathy or neuropathy. After an episode of acute overdistention (600–800 mL or more), the bladder may be hypotonic but may recover its tone after 7–14 days of catheter decompression.

Mechanical obstruction should be treated surgically or with catheter drainage. Maneuvers such as Valsalva or suprapubic compression may also help.

Drug therapy of overflow incontinence: alpha-adrenergic blockers may allow internal sphincter relaxation (see above); detrusor tone may be augmented by bethanechol (Urecholine, Duvoid) 10–50 mg administered tid–qid.

F. Sphincter insufficiency most commonly appears as stress incontinence. It is common in parous postmenopausal women and may occur in men with surgically damaged internal sphincters. Initial management of women is with pelvic floor exercises and, in postmenopausal patients, topical estrogens. Alpha-adrenergic drugs such as phenylpropanolamine 50–100 mg qd given bid–qid, and surgical correction are other potential treatments.

Resnick NM: Management of urinary incontinence in the elderly. N Engl J Med 313:800–805, 1985.

National Institutes of Health Consensus Conference. Urinary incontinence in adults. JAMA 261:2685–2690, 1989.

XIV. DRUG OVERDOSES

A. Incidence. At least 12,000 poisoning deaths occur in the United States each year. Toxic sequelae to drugs may be intentional, accidental, or iatrogenic, and should be considered in any patient with altered mental status, seizures, or cardiac arrhythmias. A thorough history is required to direct therapy. The local Poison Control Center may provide invaluable advice in patient diagnosis and management.

B. Immediate Assessment and Treatment

1. **THE SAFETY OF TREATMENT STAFF SHOULD BE ENSURED**
Patients suffering toxic effects from environmental chemicals such as tear gas and insecticides may pose a hazard to staff (usually due to contaminated clothes). Until decontamination can be completed, staff should wear gowns, gloves, and airway protection (if needed).

2. **THE FIRST STEP IN PATIENT MANAGEMENT IS TO ENSURE ADEQUATE AIRWAY, BREATHING, AND CIRCULATION**
Usually, a large-bore IV catheter should be placed, while blood samples are obtained for analysis. Cardiac rhythm should be monitored continuously.

3. **LABORATORY STUDIES** that should be routine include:

   a. Serum electrolytes, glucose, BUN, and creatinine. Serum drug levels are important in many circumstances, and some blood should be retained for future use. Toxicology screens may help if no history is available.

   b. Arterial blood gases should be determined, including the carboxy-hemoglobin level if applicable.

   c. A 12-lead ECG should be done.

4. **IMMEDIATE TREATMENT IN THE PATIENT WITH AN ALTERED LEVEL OF CONSCIOUSNESS** should include thiamine 100 mg IV, glucose 25 gm IV, and naloxone 0.8–2.0 mg IV (2–5 ampules); use a higher dose if opiate overdose is strongly suspected. The dosage for children is 0.01 mg/kg.

5. **SEIZURES** should be treated by protecting the airway and administering diazepam (5–10 mg IV) or lorazepam (2–4 mg IV or IM). Phenytoin, 15–18 mg/kg, may be given IV at 50 mg/min if these benzodiazepines are not effective.

6. **CARDIAC ARRHYTHMIAS**
   Supraventricular tachycardia occurs in many overdoses, especially if anticholinergic drugs are involved. **Physostigmine,** 0.5–1.0 mg given over 2 minutes and repeated every 15 minutes up to a total of 6 mg, is a specific antagonist. **Atropine,** 0.5 mg for each 1 mg of physostigmine, may be required to treat adverse effects.

   Physostigmine is contraindicated in patients with heart block, widening of the QRS complex, or CHF. It is relatively contraindicated in patients with peptic ulcer disease, asthma, pancreatitis, and GI or GU obstruction, though its adverse effects in these settings usually can be managed with additional therapy.

   Phenytoin is an alternative when physostigmine cannot be used.

   Ventricular ectopy or tachycardia should be treated with IV lidocaine (50–100 mg loading dose followed by 1–4 mg/min). Phenytoin may also be effective. Avoid giving procainamide and quinidine.

7. Measures to decrease absorption of any ingested toxin should be initiated (see below).

8. Other additional treatment should be given based on the initial clinical impression, supplemented by laboratory tests. Co-morbid conditions such as bronchospasm and infections should be treated.

9. A patient with drug toxicity should be considered suicidal until proved otherwise. No patient should be discharged from the emergency department without a psychiatric assessment. When there is doubt, hospital admission is appropriate.

C. Measures to Stop Absorption

1. In patients with topical absorption, contaminated clothes and equipment should be removed and the skin cleaned.

2. In patients who have ingested a toxin, *vomiting should be induced* (except as noted). In an awake patient, give syrup of ipecac (15 mL for children, 30 mL for adults) and water (15 mL/kg for children, 1000 mL for adults). Repeat this in 20 minutes; if no emesis occurs, perform **gastric lavage.** Gastric lavage (36 French tube through mouth or nose) may be done in an awake patient (head down, left lateral decubitus position). Lavage with at least 5 L of warmed water. Use 300 mL aliquots in adults, 10 mL/kg aliquots in children.

There are important **contraindications** to emesis or lavage. Patients with impaired mental status or gag reflex should be lavaged only after endotracheal intubation with a cuffed endotracheal tube. Emesis should not be induced with ipecac.

Patients who have ingested antiemetics should be lavaged without attempting to induce emesis. Patients who have ingested a caustic substance (acid, alkali) should not be lavaged (Table 1–10). Ingestion of long-chain **hydrocarbons** such as gasoline, mineral oil, turpentine, and kerosene is also a contraindication to lavage due to the risk of aspiration pneumonitis. However, patients who have ingested aromatic or halogenated hydrocarbons (benzene, toluene), camphor, phenol, and insecticides should be lavaged.

3. After the stomach is cleared of pill fragments, **activated charcoal** should be given (50–100 gm) unless acetaminophen toxicity is suspected (charcoal binds N-acetylcysteine, the antidote for acetaminophen toxicity). Repeated doses (every 4–6 hours) may be useful in drugs with enterohepatic circulation (e.g., tricyclic antidepressants).

Passage of remaining toxins should be stimulated by **cathartic agents.** Examples include **magnesium citrate:** 150–250 mL in adults, 1 to 2 mL/kg in children; avoid in renal dysfunction. **Sodium sulfate** (Golytely): 150–250 mL in adults, 1–2 mL/kg in children; avoid in congestive heart failure. **Sorbitol** (70%): 100 mL in adults, 1–2 mL/kg in children.

D. Measures to **enhance drug excretion** should also be used for some situations. **Forced diuresis** (3–6 mL of urine/kg/hour) may be helpful. This is done by volume loading followed by furosemide or mannitol, with careful observation of fluid and electrolyte status (especially serum potassium).

Neutral diuresis may aid excretion of isoniazid and bromides.

Acid diuresis (urine pH less than 5.5), induced with ascorbic acid (500–2000 mg po or IV) or ammonium chloride (20 mg/kg po or IV every 6 hours), will help excretion of phencyclidine ("PCP"), strychnine, amphetamines, quinine, and quinidine. It should be avoided in patients who may have myoglobinuria (e.g., drug-induced, prolonged coma with crush injury).

Alkaline diuresis (urine pH greater than 7.5) induced with 1 to 2 mg/kg of sodium bicarbonate IV, increases the excretion of salicylates and phenobarbital (not other barbiturates).

TABLE 1–10. SPECIFIC TOXIN ANTIDOTES

AGENT	ANTIDOTE(S) AND COMMENTS
Acetaminophen	N-acetylcysteine (Mucomyst) usually given based on serum level at 4 hrs after ingestion; best given within 10 hrs of ingestion; severe toxicity likely for doses above 140 mg/kg (child) or 10 gm (adult); some drugs may enhance toxicity
Alcohol	*See specific agent*
Antidepressants	*See Tricyclic antidepressants*
Arsenic	Dimercaprol (BAL), D-penicillamine
Carbon monoxide	Oxygen (at least 100%; hyperbaric depending on carboxyhemoglobin level)
Caustic agents	Avoid vomiting; consider esophagoscopy and corticosteroids
Cyanide	Oxygen, Lilly Cyanide Kit (contains amyl nitrite, sodium nitrite, and sodium thiosulfate)
Digoxin	Digoxin specific antibody fragments
Ethylene glycol	Ethanol (IV) while awaiting and during hemodialysis: 1 mL/kg of 100% ethanol diluted with 5% dextrose in water to make a 10% ethanol solution; maintenance dose is 0.16 mL of 100% ethanol/kg/hr (increase to 0.4 during dialysis) also given as a 10% solution; pyridoxine 50 mg IM every 6 hrs
Insecticides	*See Organophosphates*
Iron	Oral bicarbonate to convert to less absorbable ferrous carbonate; desferrioxamine chelation
Isoniazid	Pyridoxine, dose equal to amount of isoniazid ingested
Lead	Dimercaprol (BAL), EDTA
Mercury	Dimercaprol (BAL)
Methanol	Same as ethylene glycol, except no pyridoxine
Methemoglobinemia	Methylene blue; exchange transfusion; may result from toxins (aniline dyes, benzene) or medications (sulfonamides, phenytoin, dapsone, nitrates)
Opiates	Naloxone; may require many ampules followed by infusion
Organophosphates	Atropine (to control result of cholinergic excess); pralidoxime (to rejuvenate cholinesterase)
Theophylline	Propranolol (if underlying disease permits)
Tricyclic antidepressants	Sodium bicarbonate to increase arterial pH to 7.50 to 7.55 (may affect tissue binding of drug)

Charcoal hemoperfusion is indicated in toxicity due to paraquat (a common insecticide). Patients with overdoses of digitoxin, ethchlorvinyl, phenobarbital, theophylline, and tricyclic antidepressants may also benefit, depending on clinical status.

Hemodialysis. Poisoning by these agents is usually an indication for hemodialysis: ethylene glycol, methanol, heavy metals in soluble compounds or after chelation, *Amanita phalloides* mushrooms.

Many other chemicals are dialyzable, and patients with toxicity from the following agents may benefit from hemodialysis: alcohols, amphetamines, antibiotics, bromides, chloral hydrate, isoniazid, lithium, meprobamate, paraldehyde, phenobarbital, potassium, quinidine, quinine, salicylates, strychnine, theophylline.

E. Specific Antidotes (Table 1–10). Some toxins have specific antidotes which affect the metabolism of toxins to produce less toxic substances (e.g., ethanol for methanol); protect specific organs from damage (e.g., *N*-acetylcysteine for acetaminophen); or enhance excretion (e.g., chelating agents for heavy metals).

In most cases of drug toxicity, however, removal of exposure and supportive therapy are the mainstays of treatment.

XV. MEDICATIONS AND PREGNANCY

Approximately 3% of neonates have recognized congenital malformations, but only 10% of these conditions are linked to specific agents. The time of greatest risk of major morphologic abnormalities is between 18 and 60 days' gestation. Only a few medications have been shown to be teratogenic in humans; likewise, only a small number are known to be safe. Many are known animal teratogens in doses exceeding common clinical use; the majority carry an unknown risk (Table 1–11).

A. The Food and Drug Administration has established 5 **categories of risk** of medication use:

1. Controlled studies in humans failed to demonstrate risk to the fetus.

2. No evidence of risk in humans: either animal findings show risk but human findings do not, or, if no adequate human studies have been done, animal findings are negative.

3. Human studies have not been done; animal studies may be positive or not done.

4. Available data show risk to the fetus, but potential benefits may outweigh the potential risks.

5. Contraindicated in pregnancy.

This classification is helpful at the extreme ranges of risk. Unfortunately, most drugs fall in categories 2 and 3.

Some medications given after the first trimester may cause fetal harm without leading to major malformations. When administered after the

TABLE 1–11. MEDICATION USE DURING PREGNANCY

CLASS OF DRUG	GENERALLY CONSIDERED SAFE[1]	PROBABLY SAFE BUT WITH FEWER DATA AVAILABLE[2]	SOME RISK DOCUMENTED OR SUSPECTED[3]	CONTRAINDICATED[4]
Analgesics	Acetaminophen Codeine[5] Morphine[5] Meperidine[5]	Oxycodone[5] Methadone[5]	Salicylates[6] Indomethacin[6] Naproxen[6] Ibuprofen[6] Sulindac[6]	—
Antiasthmatics	—	Theophylline Oxtriphylline Metaproterenol Terbutaline	Isoetharine[7] Cromolyn sodium	—
Antibiotics	Ampicillin Erythromycin[8] Isoniazid Penicillin	Amphotericin B Cephalosporins Dicloxacillin Ethambutol Methicillin Metronidazole Nafcillin Nitrofurantoin[9] Oxacillin Rifampin Sulfonamides[10] Ticarcillin	Chloroquine Gentamicin[11] Tobramycin[11]	Doxycycline Streptomycin[11] Tetracycline Trimethoprim[12]
Anticoagulants	—	Dipyridamole	Warfarin Heparin[13]	—
Anticonvulsants	—	—	Clonazepam Phenobarbital Phenytoin	Valproic acid
Antidepressants	—	—	Amitriptyline Amoxapine Desipramine[14] Doxepin[14] Imipramine Nortriptyline	—

Table continued on the following page

37

TABLE 1–11. MEDICATION USE DURING PREGNANCY *Continued*

CLASS OF DRUG	GENERALLY CONSIDERED SAFE[1]	PROBABLY SAFE BUT WITH FEWER DATA AVAILABLE[2]	SOME RISK DOCUMENTED OR SUSPECTED[3]	CONTRAINDICATED[4]
Antiemetics	Emetrol	Trimethobenzamide	Prochlorperazine Promethazine	—
Antihistamines	—	Chlorpheniramine Dimenhydrinate Meclizine	Brompheniramine Diphenhydramine Hydroxyzine	—
Antihypertensives	Hydralazine[20] Methyldopa	Atenolol[15] Metoprolol[15] Nadolol[15] Propranolol[15] Clonidine[15] Furosemide[16] Prazosin	Captopril Chlorothiazide[16] Enalapril Spironolactone[16] Triamterene[16] Phenoxybenzamine	Nitroprusside
Cardiac drugs	—	Atropine Digoxin Disopyramide Lidocaine Quinidine Nifedipine	Nitroglycerin Procainamide Verapamil	—
Decongestants	—	Phenylpropanolamine	Pseudoephedrine	—
Hormones	Levothyroxine	Propylthiouracil	Cortisone Dexamethasone Prednisone[17] Methimazole	Estrogens, including diethylstilbestrol
Psychotropics	—	—	Chlorpromazine and other phenothiazines Haloperidol	Lithium
Sedatives	—	Oxazepam Secobarbital	Chlordiazepoxide Diazepam Flurazepam Meprobamate	Alprazolam Triazolam

Miscellaneous

Kaolin-pectin
Milk of Magnesia
Psyllium

Cimetidine
Ranitidine
Dioctyl sodium
  sulfosuccinate
Guaifenesin
Tetanus toxoid
Vaccines:
  Influenza
  Hepatitis B
  Polio
  Purified protein derivative
    for skin

Sulfasalazine[6]

Antineoplastic agents
Bromocriptine
13-cis-retinoic acid
Disulfiram
Live virus vaccines:
  Measles
  Mumps
  Rubella[18]
Oral hypoglycemics[19]

1. No drug can be considered unequivocally safe during pregnancy.
2. Many drugs in this group are new but no consistent adverse effects have been reported.
3. Degree of risk is quite variable in this class; these drugs may be useful if potential benefit outweighs potential risk.
4. Use should be avoided in all but exceptional circumstances.
5. Avoid narcotics near delivery owing to risk of neonatal depression.
6. Not teratogenic, but avoid use during last trimester.
7. Teratogenicity has been shown only in animals; no human studies are available.
8. Avoid erythromycin estolate owing to risk of neonatal hepatic toxicity.
9. Avoid use at term owing to risk of hemolysis in neonates deficient in glucose-6-phosphate dehydrogenase.
10. Avoid sulfonamides near term owing to risk of neonatal hyperbilirubinemia; not 1st-line therapy for urinary tract infections in pregnant patients.
11. Not clearly teratogenic but there is risk of fetal ototoxicity.
12. Should not be used owing to its activity as a folate antagonist.
13. Not teratogenic, but increased rate of fetal loss occurs (see text); however, this is anticonvulsant of choice during pregnancy.
14. Risk of teratogenicity has not been clearly shown for these agents.
15. Neonatal toxicity may occur when used at term.
16. Use of diuretics is usually inappropriate during pregnancy.
17. Little risk has been documented with low doses of prednisone, though it may have the same adverse metabolic effects as cortisone. All corticosteroids may cause fetal growth retardation.
18. Congenital rubella syndrome has never been demonstrated after infection with vaccine virus but is theoretically possible.
19. Use of oral hypoglycemic agents is inappropriate during pregnancy; insulin should be used.
20. Safety during the 1st trimester is not as widely accepted as its safety during the 3rd trimester.

fourth month of pregnancy, tetracycline may cause staining of the teeth. Whereas the deciduous teeth are most frequently involved, the permanent teeth may be affected if tetracycline is used close to term.

Heparin, the anticoagulant of choice during pregnancy, is not associated with congenital defects; however, it carries a 20–30% risk of fetal loss.

Narcotics and barbiturates used late in pregnancy may cause dependence and withdrawal syndromes in the neonate.

B. Since few medications are 100% safe during pregnancy, the best strategy is to use a minimum number for as short a time as possible. Combination products, both prescription and nonprescription, should be avoided. Use of the reference books listed below or consultation with an individual with special interest in teratology may help when choosing medications.

Shepard TH: Catalog of Teratogenic Agents, 6th ed. Baltimore, Johns Hopkins University Press, 1989.

Briggs GG, Freeman RK, Yaffe SJ: Drugs in Pregnancy and Lactation, 2nd ed. Baltimore, Williams & Wilkins, 1986.

Hill LM, Kleinberg F: Effects of drugs and chemicals on the fetus and newborn. Mayo Clin Proc 59:707–716, 757–765, 1984.

Newton ER (ed): Medical problems in pregnancy. Med Clin North Am 73(3):517–752, 1989.

Ginsberg JS, et al: Use of anticoagulants during pregnancy. Chest 95(suppl 2):156S–160S, 1989.

Mortola JF: The use of psychotropic agents in pregnancy and lactation. Psychiatr Clin North Am 3:69–87, 1989.

XVI. PERIOPERATIVE MEDICAL CARE

A. The goals of **preoperative medical evaluations** are to provide an objective prediction of surgical risk, to identify patients whose planned elective surgery should be delayed, and to identify and modify risk factors to minimize perioperative complications. The preoperative evaluation is not a definitive medical workup: many "loose ends" may be uncovered, but only a small fraction will require delay of surgery.

Effective communication between the consultant and the surgeon is essential. An organized and directed consultation note enhances communication and contains the following elements:

1. "Thank you for this consult."

2. "Problem"–a statement of the issue(s) that the consultant is addressing.

3. "Assessment and recommendations"–the consultant's assessment and a list of recommendations, preferably less than 5. They should be as explicit and specific as possible, including drugs, dosage, and contingency recommendations. Failure to state what is obvious to the consultant is a frequent cause of miscommunication.

4. A brief "discussion"–pertinent history, physical findings, laboratory results, and the rationale for the given recommendations.

It is important to remember that recommendations for medications and tests are more likely to be carried out than those for physician or nurse actions. Furthermore, recommendations delivered verbally are more likely to be followed than those communicated by a note in the patient's chart.

B. Cardiovascular Disease. A widely used **scoring system** is available to classify the cardiac risk of noncardiac surgery (Ann Intern Med 98:116–125, 1983). The consultant must judge the presence of factors including:

1. Presence of a third heart sound or jugular venous distention.
2. Myocardial infarction (MI) in the previous 6 months.
3. More than 5 premature ventricular contractions per minute documented at any time.
4. Rhythm other than sinus or presence of premature atrial contractions on the last preoperative ECG.
5. Evidence of significant valvular aortic stenosis.

The first 2 features are the most significant. Age greater than 70 years, emergency or major surgery, and poor medical condition further increase the cardiac risk. A modification of this system considers the degree of angina (J Gen Intern Med 1:211–219, 1986).

1. REDUCTION OF CARDIAC COMPLICATIONS

A plateau in the risk of perioperative myocardial reinfarction occurs if surgery is performed more than 6 months after the initial MI. The risk declines steadily through this period. A patient with a normal post-MI treadmill test and normal left ventricular function has a low risk of perioperative reinfarction even 6 weeks after the initial MI and may be cleared for semielective surgery such as resections for cancer cure. General anesthesia (versus spinal) and stable essential hypertension (with diastolic blood pressure less than 110 mm Hg) do not increase the risk of perioperative MI.

Spinal anesthesia is less likely to exacerbate CHF than is general anesthesia but may be relatively contraindicated in those with hypertrophic cardiomyopathy (JAMA 254:2419–2421, 1985).

Stable angina is not independently associated with an increased risk of perioperative MI. Routine use of cardiac diagnostic testing is not generally helpful, although some groups of surgical patients may benefit, such as those with claudication (Ann Intern Med 10:859–866, 1989). Patients who are more than 30 days post successful coronary artery angioplasty or bypass grafting have a low perioperative cardiac morbidity.

Patients receiving **chronic antiarrhythmic therapy** should receive it up to and including the morning of surgery, with resumption as soon as possible after operation. Prophylactic lidocaine during surgery is reserved for patients with a history of symptomatic ventricular arrhythmias.

The perioperative development of acute **complete heart block** is unusual. Patients with isolated bundle branch or bifascicular block do not require temporary pacing. For asymptomatic patients with complete heart block or bifascicular block with second degree AV block, or with new perioperative bifascicular block, temporary pacing should be instituted. Other indications for temporary perioperative pacing are the same as for permanent pacemakers.

Hemodynamic monitoring is indicated in patients with CHF, aortic stenosis, or recent MI, as well as in patients in whom substantial fluid shifts may be expected. Since postoperative fluid mobilization may require 48 hours, monitoring is usually continued for that period.

Perioperative hypertension may be caused by fluid overload, hypoxia, medication withdrawal, and inadequate sedation and analgesia. Mobilization of tissue fluid may lead to hypertension 24 to 48 hours postoperatively. Hypertension must persist for at least 3 hours before it becomes a risk for cardiac complications.

If the above factors are not present, hypertension may be managed with nitroprusside (IV) or hydralazine (5 mg IV or IM, repeated every 15 minutes as needed).

Patients receiving **antihypertensive medication(s)** chronically should take them up to the morning of surgery and resume them as soon as possible. The only exception is diuretics, which in some cases should be discontinued 2–3 days preoperatively (to allow volume expansion).

In patients with **renovascular hypertension,** surgery is safe as long as normokalemia is maintained. Surgery in patients with undiagnosed **pheochromocytoma,** however, is associated with up to 50% mortality. Effective management strategies rely on meticulous blood pressure control (Clev Clin J Med 57:613–617, 1990).

2. MEDICATION MANAGEMENT

   a. **Beta blockers.** Patients who take propranolol or other beta blockers are at risk of a withdrawal syndrome, which begins 24 hours after the last dose, including hypertension and tachycardia. Propranolol should be continued until the morning of surgery and resumed either orally or via nasogastric tube as soon as possible. Alternative approaches include IV propranolol or the use of preoperative nadolol given at one fourth the usual daily dose of propranolol (Ann Intern Med 98:116–125, 1983).

   b. **Digoxin.** When used in the management of CHF, the indications for perioperative use are the same as for chronic use. Digoxin may be helpful prophylactically in patients at high risk of perioperative supraventricular tachycardia (SVT) such as elderly patients undergoing thoracic surgery and patients with valvular heart disease or a history of SVT.

   c. **Anticoagulants.** For patients with prosthetic heart valves (especially in the presence of mechanical valves), abnormal mitral valves, or atrial fibrillation, warfarin should be discontinued within 24–48 hours preoperatively and vitamin K should be given. Heparin should be given simultaneously and discontinued 8–12 hours preoperatively. (Heparin is stopped later when there is a high risk of embolism and then reversed acutely with protamine). Heparin should be resumed 12 hours postoperatively and warfarin 2–3 days postoperatively. When the prothrombin time is therapeutic, heparin can be discontinued.

   For patients with most other indications for warfarin, a less aggressive approach is reasonable. It may be discontinued 3–4 days preoperatively (so that the preoperative prothrombin time is within 2 seconds of control) and resumed 3–4 days postoperatively.

C. **Pulmonary Disease.** The primary perioperative pulmonary complications are pneumonia and atelectasis. Risk factors for pulmonary complications include specific surgical procedures (e.g., thoracic and upper abdominal operations); chronic obstructive pulmonary disease (COPD) with dyspnea or productive cough; age over 60 years; surgery longer than 3 hours; smoking; obesity; forced expiratory volume (FEV) in 1 second less than 2 liters; and baseline P_{CO_2} greater than 45 mm Hg.

The use of intensive bronchodilators, adequate hydration, incentive spirometry (with preoperative teaching), and early mobilization and avoidance of sedatives minimizes risk in the patient with **COPD.** Chest physiotherapy may be helpful for patient with localized pulmonary infiltrates but is of minimal benefit in others.

For patients with **productive cough,** procedures should be scheduled later in the day to allow clearance of morning sputum. Patients with chronically infected sputum benefit from preoperative antibiotic treatment.

For **cigarette abstinence** to be beneficial, it must begin at least 2 and preferably 4 weeks preoperatively.

D. **Deep Venous Thrombosis and Pulmonary Embolism.** Within the broad scope of general and gynecologic surgery, **heparin,** 5000 units subcutaneously every 12 hours starting 2 hours before surgery, reduces the risk of **deep venous thrombosis (DVT),** clinically significant pulmonary embolism (PE), and fatal PE (NIH Consensus Development Conference, Vol 6, No. 2). The risk of bleeding and wound hematoma is increased, but the risk of serious hemorrhagic complications is minimal.

Intermittent pneumatic compressive devices are as effective as subcutaneous heparin and have no adverse effects.

If no contraindications are present, patients with any of the following risk factors should receive subcutaneous heparin (5000 units every 12 hours): age over 40 years, obesity, presence of malignancy or prior thromboembolic disease, oral contraceptive use, and long surgical procedure.

The proper duration of treatment is unclear, but prophylaxis should continue at least until the patient is ambulatory. Estrogen-containing **oral contraceptives** should be discontinued 3 weeks before elective surgery. Postmenopausal estrogen replacement therapy need not be discontinued.

Knee and hip **arthroplasty** and open **prostatectomy** have a high rate of DVT, and low-dose subcutaneous heparin is less effective than in general surgery. Dextran, warfarin (JAMA 249:374–378, 1983), and adjusted-dose subcutaneous heparin (N Engl J Med 309:954–958, 1983) decrease morbidity but not mortality. The risk of bleeding is clearly increased, and laboratory monitoring is required.

E. **Management of Specific Problems**

   1. NAUSEA

   GI hypomobility may be expected with certain surgical procedures. Unexpected ileus may result from metabolic disturbances or from use of new medications. The phenothiazines or other dopaminergic antagonists are the drugs of choice.

2. **PAIN**

Control of postoperative pain requires careful attention to avoid possible toxic effects: most commonly **excess sedation** (with accompanying risk of pulmonary complication) and confusion. In thoracic and abdominal surgery, adequate pain control may diminish the risk of pulmonary complications due to decrease in splinting. Patient-controlled analgesia should be considered. Use of regional anesthetic techniques (nerve blocks) or epidural narcotics may be indicated.

3. **SEDATION**

Sedatives must be used cautiously in the perioperative period to avoid neurologic and pulmonary complications.

Anxiety or agitation may develop postoperatively as a result of metabolic disturbance or withdrawal from previously unreported drug use, such as alcohol or narcotics. Both warrant specific treatment. Use of a sedative without analgesia increases the risk of confusion or agitation.

4. **FEVER**

Fever in the first 2 to 3 postoperative days is a common sign that may signify infection; it may also result from tissue injury or atelectasis. In the absence of localized physical findings or evidence of toxicity (e.g., hypotension), an extensive laboratory evaluation is not needed. If the patient has had a bladder catheter, a urinalysis should be performed.

5. **MEDICATION**

The doses of many medications should be adjusted or the drugs should be discontinued entirely during the perioperative period. Beta blockers, antihypertensives, digoxin, antiarrhythmics, estrogens, and anticoagulants are discussed above. Other examples include:

  a. **Insulin:** Give half of the patient's usual morning dose of intermediate-acting insulin on the morning of surgery and sliding scale regular insulin, with a dextrose-containing IV solution.

  b. **Oral hypoglycemic agents:** Discontinue 2 to 5 days preoperatively and use insulin as needed.

  c. **Corticosteroids:** Determine need for supplemental doses by cosyntropin stimulation test; when in doubt, give double the chronic dose or hydrocortisone 100 mg IV every 8 hours for 48–72 hours perioperatively. The need for perioperative steroid coverage extends past the date of discontinuation in patients tapered from long-term therapy.

  d. **Antianginal drugs:** Continue through surgery using topical, parenteral, or sublingual routes as needed.

  e. **Aspirin:** Discontinue 10 days preoperatively.

  f. **NSAIDs:** Discontinue 1–3 days preoperatively, depending on pharmacokinetics.

g. Anticonvulsants: Continue perioperatively.

h. Psychiatric medications: Taper and discontinue antidepressants, antipsychotics, anxiolytics, and especially lithium, 5–7 days preoperatively.

Kammerer WS, Gross RJ (eds): Medical Consultation: The Internist on Surgical, Obstetric, and Psychiatric Services, 2nd ed. Baltimore, Williams & Wilkins, 1990.

Bolt RJ (ed): Medical Evaluation of the Surgical Patient. Mt. Kisco, NY, Futura Publishing Company, 1987.

Merli GJ, Weitz HH (eds): Preoperative consultation. Med Clin North Am 71(3):353–590, 1987.

Kroenke K: Preoperative evaluation: The assessment and management of surgical risk. J Gen Intern Med 2:257–269, 1987.

FLUID AND ELECTROLYTE THERAPY

DAVID C. DUGDALE

I. NORMAL FLUID AND ELECTROLYTE PHYSIOLOGY

In healthy persons, the renal, pulmonary, and endocrine systems maintain the body water and electrolytes within the physiologic range. When regulatory mechanisms fail, the physician must supplement or alter natural fluid and electrolyte inputs.

A. **Total Body Water (TBW).** TBW accounts for approximately 50% of body weight in females and 60% in males. Approximately ⅔ of TBW is intracellular.

The **extracellular fluid** comprises intravascular fluid (¼ of extracellular fluid, or 1/12 of TBW) and extravascular fluid composed primarily of interstitial fluid, with small amounts in the bone and dense connective tissues.

Fluids administered IV distribute between the intravascular and extravascular spaces in fractions determined by the fluids' protein and sodium content.

B. **Normal Fluid and Electrolyte Balance** (Table 2–1)
Since the maximal concentrating ability of the renal tubule is 1200 milliosmoles (mOsm)/L, excretion of the daily average production of 600 mOsm requires a minimum urine output of 500 mL. "**Insensible losses**" (skin, respiratory tract) increase by 100–300 mL/day for each degree C of fever. When oral intake is decreased, maintenance fluid and electrolytes must be provided. If feasible, the enteral route is preferred because of its lower rate of complications.

If parenteral supplements are required, IV **dextrose** solutions are used. Administration of 100–200 gm/day (3.4 Kcal/gm) avoids ketosis and lessens body protein catabolism.

Although the renal conservation of **sodium** (Na) is very effective, maintenance Na is usually given, 80–120 mEq/day. Obligatory renal and fecal **potassium** (K) losses must be replaced (60–100 mEq/day).

Total **maintenance** fluid and electrolyte needs are typically met with 2–3 L of 5% dextrose containing either 0.2 or 0.45% sodium chloride (NaCl) and 20–30 mEq of KCl/L. For maintenance longer than 5 days, adding calcium, magnesium, phosphate, and vitamins should be considered (Tables 2–2 and 2–3).

TABLE 2–1. FLUID FLUXES IN A HEALTHY MALE (mL/DAY)

INTAKE	QUANTITY	OUTPUT	QUANTITY
Ingested fluid	1400	Urine	1500
Fluid in food	850	Skin	500
Water of oxidation	350	Respiratory tract	400
		Stool	200

TABLE 2–2. INFORMATION FOR CALCULATION OF FLUID AND ELECTROLYTE REPLACEMENT

COMMON CONVERSIONS

1 mEq Na = 23 mg Na = 58.5 mg NaCl
1 gm Na = 2.54 gm NaCl = 43 mEq Na
1 gm NaCl = 0.39 gm Na = 17 mEq Na

1 mEq K = 39 mg K = 74.5 mg KCl
1 gm K = 1.91 gm KCl = 26 mEq K
1 gm KCl = 0.52 gm K = 13 mEq K

1 mEq Ca = 20 mg Ca
1 gm Ca = 50 mEq Ca

1 mEq Mg = 0.12 gm $MgSO_4$ $7H_2O$
1 gm Mg = 10.2 gm $MgSO_4$ $7H_2O$ = 82 mEq Mg

10 mMol P_i = 0.31 gm P_i
1 gm P_i = 32 mMol P_i

COMMON AMPULES

7.5% $NaHCO_3$	50 mL	44.6 mEq Na
50% Dextrose	50 mL	25 gm dextrose
10% $CaCl_2$ $2H_2O$	10 mL	13.6 mEq Ca
10% Ca gluconate	10 mL	4.6 mEq Ca
50% $MgSO_4$ $7H_2O$	2 mL	8.1 mEq Mg
46% K phosphate	10 mL	30 mMol (930 mg); P_i 44 mEq K
42% Na phosphate	10 mL	30 mMol (930 mg); P_i 40 mEq Na

TABLE 2–3. ELECTROLYTE CONTENT OF INTRAVENOUS FLUIDS (in mEq/L)

INTRAVENOUS FLUID	mOsm/L	Na	K	Ca	Cl	HCO_3 EQUIVALENT
0.45% NaCl (half-normal saline)	154	77	–	–	77	—
0.9% NaCl (normal saline)	308	154	–	–	154	—
3% NaCl	1026	513	–	–	513	—
Lactated Ringer's	272	130	4	30	109	28
5% Dextrose in water	252	50 gm/L of dextrose, no electrolytes				
5% Dextrose with quarter-normal saline	320	34	–	–	34	—
5% Dextrose with half-normal saline	406	77	–	–	77	—

II. DISTURBANCES OF BODY FLUID VOLUME

The management of body fluid volume disturbances is based on 3 principles:

1. Diagnosis and treatment of disorders that create or maintain imbalances;
2. Correction of abnormalities of volume status while providing maintenance therapy;
3. Correction of remaining electrolyte disturbances (unless threatening to life at presentation).

A vast number of disease processes lead to fluid and electrolyte abnormalities. Knowledge of body fluid content (Table 2–4) allows estimation of derangements, but clinical and laboratory measurements are needed for precise assessment.

The **urgency** of volume deficit correction is determined by clinical criteria. Moderate intravascular volume depletion may produce **thirst** as its only symptom. Tachycardia, decreased skin turgor and axillary sweat, decreased urine output, and modest azotemia with the blood urea nitrogen (BUN) elevated disproportionately to the serum creatinine may be seen. Usually deficits should be corrected over 24–48 hours.

More severe volume depletion is associated with **postural hypotension** and **oliguria.**

Initial treatment is the rapid (up to 1000 mL/hour) administration of 0.9% NaCl (normal saline), until postural hypotension has resolved. Only 25% of administered normal saline remains in the intravascular space. Hypertonic saline should not be used just for volume expansion.

Once the severe deficit is corrected, slower replacement continues (e.g., 45% NaCl, 75–150 mL/hour) and electrolyte disturbances can be treated.

Volume loss sufficient to cause **resting hypotension** usually results from **hemorrhage,** which may require infusion of blood or plasma protein products. Use of plasma itself for volume expansion has no advantage over albumin or plasma protein fractions (e.g., Plasmanate) and carries a higher risk of hepatitis.

Clinical criteria may correlate imperfectly with volume status—especially in the face of renal, cardiac, or infectious diseases. Use of central venous

TABLE 2–4. ELECTROLYTE CONTENT OF SELECTED BODY FLUIDS

FLUID	ELECTROLYTE CONCENTRATIONS (mEq/L)				
	Na	**K**	**Cl**	**Hco_3**	**H**
Sweat	30–60	5	40–80	—	—
Gastric	40–80	5–20	80–120	—	10–80
Bile	130–160	5	80–120	40–50	—
Pancreatic	120–150	5	60–80	70–90	—
Ileostomy	60–120	10	60–130	30–50	—
Stool					
Normal	5	50	5	—	—
Diarrhea	50–100	20	20–60	30–50	—

(in absence of cardiopulmonary disease) or pulmonary artery pressure monitoring may help guide therapy.

III. DISTURBANCES OF SERUM SODIUM (Na) CONCENTRATION

Abnormalities of the serum Na concentration result from free water imbalance. In some cases, treatment of an associated volume deficit is an important first step. Symptoms of hypo- or hypernatremia may be mild or may be overshadowed by volume-related symptoms.

A rapidly developed abnormality of serum Na causes more symptoms than a slowly developed one. Hyponatremia with serum Na above 125 mEq/L rarely causes symptoms. The symptoms of hypernatremia correlate better with the degree of hyperosmolality than the serum Na ($Osm_{calculated}$ = 2 × Na + glucose/18 + BUN/2.8; glucose and BUN in mg/dL). Hypo- and hypernatremia produce neurologic symptoms ranging from lethargy and coma to irritability, muscular twitching, and seizures.

A. Hyponatremia. So-called **pseudohyponatremia** may occur with severe hyperlipidemia (lipemic serum) or hyperglobulinemia. The Na concentration per liter of plasma water is normal, and the apparent hyponatremia does not affect the clinical status.

The presence of a large amount of osmotically active solute (glucose is most common) causes true hyponatremia. For each increase by 100 mg/dL of the serum glucose above normal, the serum Na decreases by 1.6 mEq/L (e.g., a serum glucose of 600 mg/dL causes an Na reduction of 8 mEq/L).

Important **causes** of hyponatremia include:

1. Fluid loss with hypotonic replacement;
2. Diuresis induced by drugs or osmotic loads;
3. Edematous states;
4. Endocrine diseases (hypothyroidism, deficiency of gluco- or mineralocorticoids);
5. Syndrome of inappropriate secretion of antidiuretic hormone (SIADH);
6. Extreme polydipsia (usually greater than 15 L/day).

Treatment of hyponatremia depends on its degree and whether symptoms are present. **Hypovolemia** should be corrected if the underlying diseases allow. If **symptoms are minimal** or hyponatremia is moderate (serum Na greater than 120 mEq/L) or chronic, water intake restriction to 1000 mL/day is appropriate initial treatment. The ADH antagonist demeclocycline, 900 to 1200 mg/day, may help in patients with SIADH.

If **symptoms are severe,** the amount of sodium required to raise the serum concentration to 125 mEq/L should be administered over 6 hours as 0.9% or 3% NaCl. The rate should not exceed 2.5 mEq/L/hour or 20 mEq/L/day; extreme cases may require more than 6 hours.

$$Na\ deficit = (125 - Na_{measured}) \times TBW$$

3% NaCl may be given IV with furosemide (20–80 mg IV) to prevent volume overload. Rapid correction to Na above 125 mEq/L is usually unnecessary and is also dangerous since it may cause a central demyelination syndrome.

B. Hypernatremia. This may result from:

1. Hypotonic fluid loss (sweat);
2. Osmotic diuresis (glucose);
3. Adrenal hyperfunction;
4. Diabetes insipidus.

The **goal of treatment** is to provide half of the water deficit in 12 to 24 hours, then the remainder in another 24 hours. During the first 2 days of treatment, the Na should be reduced by no more than ½ mEq/L/hour

$$\text{Free water deficit} = \left[\frac{(\text{serum Na})}{140} - 1 \right] \times \text{TBW}$$

Since volume deficit is usually present, **initial treatment** is with normal saline until the patient becomes euvolemic. Overly rapid correction of the serum Na (or osmolality) may produce cerebral edema and death.

If hyperosmolality is present without hyperglycemia or hypernatremia, toxins such as ethanol or organic acids should be suspected as the cause of the "osmolal gap."

Berl T: Treating hyponatremia: What is all the controversy about? Ann Intern Med 113:417–419, 1990.

Sterns RH: Severe symptomatic hyponatremia: Treatment and outcome. A study of 64 cases. Ann Intern Med 107:656–664, 1987.

Schelling JR, Howard RL, Winters D, Linas SL: Increased osmolal gap in alcoholic ketoacidosis and lactic acidosis. Ann Intern Med 113:580–582, 1990.

IV. DISTURBANCES OF SERUM POTASSIUM CONCENTRATION

A. Hypokalemia. Hypokalemia is usually asymptomatic. In patients with **chronic hypokalemia,** the level of serum K that requires treatment is controversial. In the absence of premature ventricular contractions, ischemic heart disease, and digoxin therapy, one might withhold replacement unless the serum K is less than 3.2 mEq/L. If due to medications (e.g., diuretics taken for hypertension), a potassium-containing salt substitute (50–70 mEq K/teaspoon), change in diet, or change of medication should be considered.

The **symptoms** of hypokalemia are primarily neuromuscular, ranging from weakness to cramps to paralysis. Ventricular arrhythmias, a renal-concentrating defect, ileus, rhabdomyolysis, and aggravation of hepatic encephalopathy may also result from hypokalemia.

Causes of hypokalemia include:

1. Gastrointestinal loss (vomiting, diarrhea);
2. Renal loss (metabolic alkalosis; use of diuretics, gentamicin, carbenicillin, or amphotericin B; excess mineralocorticoid effect; renal tubular acidosis; Mg depletion);

3. Extracellular to intracellular shifts (acute alkalosis, insulin therapy).

The serum K may remain normal even with a total body deficit of 100–200 mEq, as seen typically with acidemia. If the serum K is 2.0–4.0 mEq/L and renal function is normal, each 100–200 mEq of K administered will increase serum K by 1.0 mEq/L.

K can be replaced orally (Table 2–5) or IV. Liquid K supplements have a disagreeable taste and may cause gastric irritation. Slow-release supplements are better tolerated but may cause GI ulcers or may be only partially utilized.

IV administration of more than 10 mEq of K/hr causes **phlebitis.** Central IV lines allow rates up to 20–30 mEq/hr. Such high rates of administration are usually reserved for emergent treatment of arrhythmias. ECG monitoring is mandatory.

B. **Hyperkalemia.** Artifactual elevations (**pseudohyperkalemia**) may occur with thrombocytosis (usually platelet count above 1,000,000/cu mm) or leukocytosis (more than 100,000/cu mm). The plasma K remains normal. Sample hemolysis, usually due to use of small needles or laboratory delay, also elevates K determinations.

Hyperkalemia can lead to **muscle weakness and cardiac arrhythmias.** Common **causes** include:

1. Excessive intake (usually iatrogenic);
2. Poor **renal excretion** (renal failure, obstructive uropathy, adrenal

TABLE 2–5. ORAL POTASSIUM SUPPLEMENTS

FORM	STRENGTH (%)	DOSE	COMMENT
Liquid			
Potassium chloride	5, 7.5, 10, 15, 20	15 mL of 10% liquid contains 20 mEq K	Some brands contain sugar, saccharin, alcohol, flavorings, or tartrazine
Potassium gluconate	10	Same	Some brands contain alcohol or saccharin
Powder			
Potassium chloride	15, 20, 25 mEq K per package		Some brands contain alcohol or saccharin
Tablets			
Potassium chloride	1, 3.3, 4, 6.7, 8, 10, 20 mEq K per tablet		Some brands contain sugar, saccharin, or tartrazine; some are effervescent mixtures of salts; some are chewable; wax matrix formulations have lower risk of GI complications

insufficiency, and many drugs: K-sparing diuretics, NSAIDs, angiotensin-converting enzyme [ACE] inhibitors);

3. Redistribution phenomena (acidemia, rhabdomyolysis, succinyl-choline, digoxin toxicity).

Treatment: The urgency of treatment is dictated by the presence of ECG changes (peaked T waves, prolonged P-R interval, absent P waves, widened QRS complex, ventricular arrhythmias). If ECG changes more severe than peaked T waves are present, cardiac monitoring and frequent serial K measurements are indicated.

IV **Ca gluconate,** 10–20 mL of a 10% solution, injected over 1–5 minutes blunts the effect of hyperkalemia on neuromuscular membranes within 5 minutes. The effect lasts about 30 minutes. It should be used cautiously if the patient has been receiving digoxin.

The administration of **sodium bicarbonate ($NaHCO_3$)** or **insulin** causes movement of extracellular K into the intracellular space. The redistribution effects last several hours. Insulin may be exogenous (5–10 units of regular insulin subcutaneously) or endogenous (stimulated by giving 25 to 50 gm dextrose over 1 hour). Individual ampules of $NaHCO_3$ (44.6 mEq) or 50% dextrose (25 gm) may be used cautiously or 500 mL of 10% dextrose in water with 10 units of regular insulin and 1 to 3 ampules of $NaHCO_3$ (depending on acid-base balance) may be given over 30–60 minutes.

K is removed from the body by the **cation exchange resin Na polystyrene sulfonate** (Kayexelate). 1 gram of resin removes 1 mEq of K in exchange for 1.5 mEq of Na. The oral dose is 15–30 gm with 50–100 mL of 20% sorbitol, up to 4 times per day. 50 gm of resin with 200 mL of 20% sorbitol may also be given as a retention enema.

Hemodialysis may be useful in the patient with renal failure and volume excess.

Ponce SP, Jennings AE, Madins NE, et al: Drug-induced hyperkalemia. Medicine 64:357, 1985.
Alvo M, Warnock DG: Hyperkalemia. West J Med 141:666, 1984.

V. DISTURBANCES OF SERUM CALCIUM CONCENTRATION

Calcium (Ca) is a divalent cation that exists in serum as a free ion and bound to plasma proteins. Alkalemia increases the fraction that is protein bound, lowering the ionized calcium concentration. The ionized Ca is physiologically active and symptoms correlate with its level. Serum Ca is controlled by a complex regulatory system involving the parathyroid gland, kidneys, and vitamin D metabolism.

Most laboratories measure total serum calcium; hypoalbuminemia causes a low total serum Ca without affecting the ionized Ca or causing symptoms. For each 1 gm/dL decrease in serum albumin concentration, the total Ca concentration falls by 0.8 mg/dL.

A. **Hypocalcemia.** The primary **sign** of acute hypocalcemia is **tetany.** It may be elicited by inflating a sphygmomanometer around the arm to cause carpal spasm (Trousseau's sign). Muscle spasm, lethargy, seizures, and Chvostek's sign (elicited by percussion over the facial nerve) may be present.

Major **causes** of hypocalcemia include:

1. Hypoparathyroidism (usually after thyroid or parathyroid surgery);
2. Hypomagnesemia (usually at levels below 0.8 mEq/L);
3. Pancreatitis;
4. Tumor lysis syndrome;
5. Rhabdomyolysis;
6. Vitamin D deficiency;
7. Chronic renal failure.

Treatment of acute hypocalcemia: 10–20 mL of 10% Ca gluconate followed by continuous infusion of 25–50 mg/hr is useful. Underlying disorders must also be treated.

If serum phosphate (P_i) is very high, IV Ca must be used carefully: when the Ca-P_i product (with both in mg/dL units) exceeds 65, there is a risk of metastatic calcification.

If magnesium (Mg) deficiency is present, it must be treated also while monitoring K balance.

Longer-term treatment involves oral Ca supplements (Table 2–6). They are usually well tolerated, though constipation may occur. Non-carbonated Ca salts are better absorbed than Ca carbonate if hypo-chlorhydria is present, but a carbonate is usually less expensive. Measurement of urinary Ca excretion may be indicated in some circumstances.

B. Hypercalcemia. The **symptoms** of hypercalcemia, including fatigue, confusion, nausea, vomiting, constipation, and polyuria (due to a reversible renal tubular defect), usually begin at serum levels between 11 and 12 mg/dL. A shortened Q-T interval, premature ventricular contractions, and an idioventricular rhythm may also occur. Hypercalcemia above 15 mg/dL or severe symptoms require emergency treatment.

Primary hyperparathyroidism or malignancy causes 90% of cases of hypercalcemia. Other causes include:

1. Granulomatous diseases;
2. Hyperthyroidism;
3. Immobilization;
4. Milk-alkali syndrome;
5. Drug effects (lithium, thiazides, vitamin D).

Treatment: Most hypercalcemic patients are volume depleted. Management of the underlying disease is crucial for the long-term treatment of hypercalcemia.

Normal saline to correct volume depletion followed by more normal saline with furosemide-induced diuresis is frequently all the therapy needed. Calciuresis begins promptly, and the serum Ca may fall by 4 mg/dL in 24 hours.

Glucocorticoids (daily dosage equivalent to 60 mg of prednisone) are especially useful in patients with granulomatous diseases, hematologic malignancies, breast cancer, and vitamin D excess. Maximal effect is reached in 24–48 hours.

Oral phosphate should be used if the serum P_i is less than 3 to 4 mg/dL. The initial dose is 250 mg of elemental P_i 3 or 4 times daily. Oral P_i therapy is frequently limited by diarrhea. IV P_i, while extremely effec-

TABLE 2–6. ORAL CALCIUM SUPPLEMENTS

SALT	% ELEMENTAL Ca BY WEIGHT	DOSE AVAILABLE IN mg (TOTAL)	COMMENT
Ca gluconate	9	500, 650, 975, 1000	
Ca lactate	13	325, 650	
Ca citrate	21	950	
Ca carbonate	40	625, 650, 750, 1250, 1500	Chewable and liquid forms available

tive, is risky and should be considered only in extreme emergencies.

Calcitonin (usually as salmon calcitonin) is effective in certain conditions with rapid bone turnover, most notably immobilization, vitamin D excess, and thyrotoxicosis. It is less effective in hypercalcemia due to malignancy or hyperparathyroidism. The initial dose, 4 units/kg subcutaneously or IM, may be repeated every 6–12 hours. It is not useful for long-term therapy of hypercalcemia. Giving a test dose (to exclude allergy) should be considered.

Plicamycin (mithramycin) inhibits osteoclast activity and works in most patients. It is given as an infusion over 4–6 hours at a dose of 25 µg/kg and may be repeated every 2–4 days. It can produce serious toxicity, including thrombocytopenia and renal and hepatic damage.

Strewler GJ, Nissenson RA: Nonparathyroid hypercalcemia. Adv Intern Med 32:235, 1986.
Levine MM, Kleeman CR: Hypercalcemia: Pathophysiology and treatment. Hosp Pract 22:73, 1987.
Mundy GR, Wilkinson R, Heath D: Comparative study of available medical therapy for the hypercalcemia of malignancy. Am J Med 74:421, 1983.

VI. DISTURBANCES OF SERUM PHOSPHORUS CONCENTRATION

Phosphorus is present in the serum in several anionic forms. The content is expressed as mg of elemental inorganic phosphorus (P_i) per dL. In the normal state, P_i concentration decreases by 1.0 to 1.5 mg/dL after meals. Alkalemia also decreases the P_i level.

A. Hypophosphatemia. Mild to moderate hypophosphatemia (1–2.5 mg/dL) is common in hospitalized patients and usually has no clinical consequences. Adequate nutrition and treatment of the underlying illness is usually sufficient therapy. If needed, oral replacement is 250 mg of P_i 2–3 times daily. Diarrhea is the main side effect (Table 2–7).

Patients with P_i concentrations below 1 mg/dL may have severe **symptoms,** including anorexia, bone pain, muscle weakness (including respiratory muscles), CHF, hemolysis, and rhabdomyolysis.

Causes include:

1. Feeding of malnourished patients (e.g., chronic alcoholics);
2. Treatment of diabetic ketoacidosis;
3. Respiratory alkalosis;

TABLE 2–7. ORAL PHOSPHATE SUPPLEMENTS

PREPARATION	FORM	P$_i$ DOSE (mg) PER UNIT	CATIONS PER UNIT
K-Phos Neutral	Tablet	250	1.1 mEq K 13.0 mEq Na
Neutra-Phos	Capsule	250	7.1 mEq K 7.1 mEq Na
Neutra-Phos-K	Capsule	250	14.2 mEq K
Phospho-Soda	Liquid (6.7 mL)	1000	40.0 mEq Na

4. GI malabsorption (may be due to aluminum-containing antacids);
5. Renal wasting (Fanconi syndrome).

Severe hypophosphatemia may be treated IV. 2–6 mg/kg of P$_i$ should be given over 6 hours and repeated until the serum P$_i$ reaches 2 mg/dL. Extra caution is needed for patients with renal failure or hypercalcemia (increased risk of metastatic calcification). Hypocalcemia may result from therapy.

The initial IV fluid management of hospitalized *chronic alcoholics* should include 6–8 gm of P$_i$, as the Na or K salt. Otherwise, resumption of a normal diet is usually sufficient.

B. **Hyperphosphatemia.** Elevated levels of serum P$_i$ occur in chronic renal failure, hypoparathyroidism, vitamin D excess, tumor lysis syndrome, and rhabdomyolysis. Usually there are no symptoms unless hypocalcemia or metastatic calcification develops.

Dietary restriction of phosphate (and protein) and use of phosphate binders (aluminum hydroxide or carbonate suspensions, 15–30 mL tid initially) with meals are helpful.

Knochel JP: The clinical status of hypophosphatemia. N Engl J Med 313:447, 1985.

VII. DISTURBANCES OF SERUM MAGNESIUM CONCENTRATION

Like Ca, magnesium (Mg) is a divalent cation with many actions in the neuromuscular system. Through its effect on parathyroid hormone release and action, Mg is important in Ca regulation. The normal serum concentration is 1.6–2.4 mEq/L (2–3 mg/dL).

A. **Hypomagnesemia.** Hypomagnesemia can produce irritability, confusion, weakness, fasciculations, nystagmus, and seizures. Serious symptoms are rare until the concentration is less than 0.8 mEq/L. Symptoms may be aggravated by coincident hypocalcemia.

Common **causes** include:

1. Poor nutrition (e.g., chronic alcoholism);
2. Intestinal malabsorption;
3. Renal wasting (diuretics, *cis*-platinum, gentamicin, amphotericin B, primary hyperaldosteronism, diabetic ketoacidosis);
4. Acute pancreatitis;
5. Postop hypoparathyroidism.

Urgent **treatment** uses IV Mg sulfate, 1–2 gm (as a 50% solution) diluted to 5% concentration in D_5W and infused over 10–15 minutes. In patients suspected of having Mg deficiency, 1–2 mL of 50% Mg sulfate may be given IM as needed or added to maintenance IV fluids.

Oral Mg supplements may be given in the form of Mg oxide (600-mg pill contains 30 mEq of Mg, taken 1–2 times daily) or milk of magnesia (10 mL contains 30 mEq of Mg, taken 1–2 times daily). Diarrhea is the limiting side effect.

B. Hypermagnesemia. Symptoms and signs of hypermagnesemia:

1. Serum level of 3–5 mEq/L: hypotension and nausea;
2. Serum level of 5–7 mEq/L: hyporeflexia and somnolence;
3. Serum level above 12 mEq/L: coma;
4. Prolongation of the Q-T interval and QRS duration, T-wave peaking, atrioventricular block, and cardiac arrest may also occur at high levels.

Hypermagnesemia results from excess administration or ingestion of a laxative or antacid that contains Mg by a patient with renal insufficiency (serum creatinine above 3–4 mg/dL).

IV Ca gluconate 10–20 mL of a 10% solution given over 5 minutes temporarily reverses the effects of Mg toxicity. In patients with advanced renal failure, dialysis is the only other modality available. In patients with residual renal function, forced diuresis may help.

Cronin RE, Knochel JP: Magnesium deficiency. Adv Intern Med 28:509, 1983.
Whang R: Magnesium deficiency: Pathogenesis, prevalence, and clinical implications. Am J Med 82(suppl 3A):24–29, 1987.
Elin RJ: Magnesium metabolism in health and disease. Dis Mon 34:166, 1988.

VIII. ACID-BASE DISTURBANCES

Acid is continuously produced by normal metabolism. The blood pH is regulated by buffer systems and the excretory ability of the lungs and kidneys.

Buffer systems (bicarbonate, phosphate, proteins) rapidly absorb newly produced acid.

Carbon dioxide, produced from carbonic acid, is excreted by the lungs.

The kidney excretes **hydrogen ions** into the urine, thereby regenerating bicarbonate. Hydrogen ions in the urine are buffered by ammonia and phosphate species.

A pathologic process that causes alveolar hypo- or hyperventilation results in a primary increase or decrease in the partial pressure of carbon dioxide (PCO_2) and leads to **respiratory acidosis or alkalosis,** respectively.

A process that causes a primary increase or decrease in the serum bicarbonate (HCO_3) concentration results in a **metabolic alkalosis or acidosis,** respectively.

When the blood pH goes above or below normal, alkalemia or acidemia is present.

The kidney compensates for respiratory disturbances and the lungs

TABLE 2–8. SIMPLE ACID-BASE DISTURBANCES

DISTURBANCE	PRIMARY CHANGE	pH	COMPENSATORY CHANGE
Metabolic acidosis	Decreased bicarbonate	Decreased	Decreased P_{CO_2}
Metabolic alkalosis	Increased bicarbonate	Increased	Increased P_{CO_2}
Respiratory acidosis	Increased P_{CO_2}	Decreased	Increased bicarbonate
Respiratory alkalosis	Decreased P_{CO_2}	Increased	Decreased bicarbonate

for metabolic disturbances. The compensation is not complete. Thus, the primary disturbance can be identified from evaluating the arterial pH and P_{CO_2} and the serum H_{CO_3} (the "measured" CO_2 of the serum electrolytes).

When arterial blood gases are determined, only 2 of the quantities are measured directly; the 3rd is calculated on the basis of the Henderson-Hasselbalch equation:

$$pH = 6.1 + \log \frac{H_{CO_3}}{0.03 \times P_{CO_2}}$$

Most acid-base disturbances have only one primary pathophysiologic process. Compensation by the lung (change in minute ventilation) occurs rapidly; renal compensation requires several hours to days. Inadequate or inappropriate compensation produces a mixed acid-base disturbance. Predictive rules are available to make this distinction (Tables 2–8 and 2–9).

TABLE 2–9. EXPECTED COMPENSATORY CHANGES IN ACID-BASE DISTURBANCES

Normal arterial blood pH: 7.35–7.45
Normal arterial P_{CO_2}: 35–45 mm Hg
Normal total CO_2: 24–30 mEq/L

EXPECTED COMPENSATORY CHANGE
ΔH_{CO_3} = change in measured bicarbonate (mEq/L)
ΔP_{CO_2} = change in arterial P_{CO_2} (mm Hg)

DISORDER	EXPECTED CHANGE
Metabolic acidosis	$\Delta P_{CO_2} = (1.0–1.5) \times \Delta H_{CO_3}$
Metabolic alkalosis	$\Delta P_{CO_2} = (0.25–1.00) \times \Delta H_{CO_3}$
Respiratory acidosis	
Acute	$\Delta H_{CO_3} = 0.1 \times \Delta P_{CO_2} \pm 3$
Chronic	$\Delta H_{CO_3} = 0.4 \times \Delta P_{CO_2} \pm 4$
Respiratory alkalosis	
Acute	$\Delta H_{CO_3} = (0.1–0.3) \times \Delta P_{CO_2}$*
Chronic	$\Delta H_{CO_3} = (0.2–0.5) \times \Delta P_{CO_2}$†

*Change to below 18 mEq/L is unusual.
†Change to below 14 mEq/L is unusual.

A. **Metabolic Acidosis.** Generation of excess acid or loss of alkali results in metabolic acidosis. Calculation of the **anion gap** [AG = Na − (Cl + CO_2)] allows a simplified **diagnostic approach.** The traditional normal AG range is 8–16 mEq/L, but variations in laboratory techniques may lower the reference range by up to 5 mEq/L.

Causes of metabolic acidosis with **increased AG** include:

1. Renal failure
2. Ketoacidosis (diabetic or alcoholic)
3. Lactic acidosis
4. Drug intoxication (methanol, paraldehyde, salicylate, ethylene glycol).

Causes of metabolic acidosis with a **normal AG** include:

1. Gastrointestinal loss of alkali (diarrhea, ureteroileostomy)
2. Renal tubular acidosis
3. Acetazolamide
4. Cholestyramine
5. Obstructive uropathy
6. Administration of HCl or NH_4Cl
7. Sulfur ingestion
8. Hyperparathyroidism.

In acute metabolic acidosis, correction of the underlying cause is crucial. If arterial pH falls below 7.15, or hemodynamic collapse occurs, $NaHCO_3$ may be given on the basis of an estimate of the **bicarbonate deficit:**

$$HCO_3 \text{ deficit} = \text{weight} \times 0.4 \times (\text{"target" } HCO_3 - \text{actual } HCO_3)$$

To avoid **overshoot alkalemia,** the "target" HCO_3 is usually 15–18 mEq/L. One half of the deficit is given over 3–4 hours, using D_5W with 1–3 ampules of $NaHCO_3$ added.

The endpoint of treatment is determined by clinical and laboratory data because the volume of distribution of HCO_3 is variable, and acid production may be ongoing. Bicarbonate replacement is not important in toxin ingestion (e.g., salicylates, methanol) and is rarely needed for diabetic ketoacidosis. Rapid correction may lead to hypokalemia or hypocalcemia, with their attendant morbidity.

Respiratory muscle fatigue may require mechanical ventilation to maintain appropriate respiratory compensation.

Treating chronic metabolic acidosis often requires administration of bicarbonate or citrate.

B. **Respiratory Acidosis.** Respiratory acidosis is caused by **alveolar hypoventilation.** It may result from neuromuscular disease, sedative drugs, mechanical airway obstruction, or severe intrinsic lung disease. The treatment is restoration of ventilation. If acidemia is life-threatening and ventilatory support must be delayed, small amounts of IV $NaHCO_3$ may be given.

C. Metabolic Alkalosis. Metabolic alkalosis can occur with **volume depletion,** when the urinary chloride concentration is usually less than 10 mEq/L. **Causes** include:

1. Vomiting
2. Nasogastric suction and fluid loss
3. Excessive diuresis.

Metabolic alkalosis may also be associated with **mineralocorticoid excess,** usually with urinary chloride levels above 20 mEq/L. Examples include:

1. Cushing's syndrome
2. Primary hyperaldosteronism
3. Bartter's syndrome.

Treatment of the first group is aimed at the underlying disorder. Volume restoration with NaCl allows bicarbonate excretion. Potassium deficits are often present and should be treated, since they help promote and maintain metabolic alkalosis. If prolonged nasogastric suction is expected, cimetidine or other histamine$_2$ blockers may lessen the alkalosis.

Treatment of the mineralocorticoid excess is aimed at the underlying disorder. KCl is given. Excess alkali consumption should be avoided. Sodium should be replaced with NaCl.

If alkalemia is causing cardiac arrhythmias (usually pH greater than 7.6), 0.15 molar HCl in sterile water may be given IV through a central venous catheter.

The bicarbonate excess may be calculated as described above for metabolic acidosis. Half of the acid may be given over 4 hours or until signs of alkalemia abate.

Acetazolamide, 250–500 mg tid, which increases renal alkali excretion, is also useful.

D. Respiratory Alkalosis. Hyperventilation leads to an increased blood pH. Causes include:

1. Sepsis
2. Salicylate toxicity
3. Hepatic disease
4. Pregnancy
5. Excessive mechanical ventilation
6. Anxiety
7. Pain
8. Hypoxia
9. Intrinsic pulmonary disease
10. CNS disease (e.g., encephalitis).

Treatment is aimed at the underlying cause. If complications appear, the respiratory drive may be blunted with a sedative such as IV lorazepam (1–2 mg), midazolam (2–5 mg), or morphine sulfate (5–10 mg).

E. Mixed Acid-Base Disturbances. Diagnosis of mixed disorders is based on the clinical setting and results of laboratory studies. Once diagnosed, the disturbances are treated as described previously in this chapter, with priority determined by clinical criteria.

Emmett M, Narins RG: Clinical use of the anion gap. Medicine 56:38–54, 1977.

Narins RG, Emmett M: Simple and mixed acid-base disorders: A practical approach. Medicine 59:161–187, 1980.

Gabow PA: Disorders associated with an altered anion gap. Kidney Int 27:472–483, 1985.

Winter SD, Pearson JR, Gabow PA, et al: The fall of the serum anion gap. Arch Intern Med 150:311–313, 1990.

INFECTIOUS DISEASES

W. CONRAD LILES
PAUL G. RAMSEY

3333333333333333333

The clinical management of infectious disease has become increasingly complex with new pathogens, new patterns of antimicrobial resistance, and larger numbers of immunocompromised patients. Antimicrobial therapy selection is based on many factors, including established efficacy in the clinical situation at hand, host factors, drug toxicity, pharmacokinetics, and the relative cost of a given antimicrobial agent compared with other agents.

I. SELECTION AND USE OF ANTIMICROBIAL AGENTS: GENERAL CONSIDERATIONS

Empiric antimicrobial therapy directed against the spectrum of probable infecting organisms must often be given before definitive microbiologic identification and antimicrobial susceptibility information are available. In certain instances broad-spectrum antimicrobial therapy is warranted. If the clinical situation is acute, empiric therapy via the IV route is usually begun immediately after specimens are collected. In less serious, stable clinical circumstances, therapeutic decisions may be delayed until the results of microbiologic culture are in, and initial therapy may be oral or parenteral.

A. Host Factors. Several factors about the patient should be considered in selecting antibiotics.

  1. AGE
  In young children and the elderly, **gastric pH is decreased,** allowing increased absorption of agents such as penicillins and other orally administered beta-lactams. Absorption of weak acids such as ketoconazole may be decreased. Young age and inadequate glucuronyl transferase production can lead to "**gray syndrome**" in neonates and young children treated with chloramphenicol. When given to pregnant women or newborns, **sulfonamides** displace bilirubin and may result in **kernicterus. Tetracycline** given to children younger than age 8 years may cause **tooth discoloration.**

  2. RENAL FUNCTION
  Toxic levels of penicillins, aminoglycosides, tetracyclines, and quinolones may develop as renal function declines, leading possibly to **nephrotoxicity** and **ototoxicity,** particularly with **aminoglycosides. Neurotoxic reactions** may result with increased levels of **penicillins and cephalosporins.**

  3. HEPATIC DYSFUNCTION
  Hepatic dysfunction may lead to **impaired metabolism** of macrolides, rifamycins, imidazoles, chloramphenicol, and linconoid drugs. The risk of aminoglycoside-induced nephrotoxicity is increased in patients with underlying cirrhosis or hepatic failure.

4. METABOLIC ABNORMALITIES

Slow acetylation of isoniazid is genetically determined and is associated with **polyneuritis**. **Glucose-6-phosphate dehydrogenase (G-6-PD) deficiency** may predispose patients to hemolysis when antibiotics such as sulfonamides, nitrofurantoin, furazolidone, chloramphenicol, and pyrimethamine are used. The action of sulfonylurea hypoglycemics may be potentiated by sulfonamides and chloramphenicol.

5. SITE OF INFECTION

The site of infection determines the route and dose of antibiotic to be given. To treat meningitis effectively, the agent must be lipid soluble to cross the **blood-brain barrier.** The vegetations of bacterial endocarditis and devitalized bone or tissue are other areas where penetration may be poor. Local conditions such as pH or the presence of a foreign body also alter the choice of antimicrobial therapy (e.g., aminoglycosides are ineffective at pH < 7.0).

6. HISTORY OF PREVIOUS ADVERSE EFFECTS

A history of adverse effects from a particular class of antibiotics must be considered before prescribing a similar antibiotic.

7. PREGNANCY

Pregnant patients should be identified before antibiotics are prescribed. Virtually all antibiotics cross the placenta and are excreted in breast milk to some extent. Most penicillins (except ticarcillin), cephalosporins, and erythromycins can be used safely in pregnant women.

B. **Drug Interactions and Dosing Recommendations.** Major adverse effects and drug interactions are summarized in Table 3–1, and dosing recommendations for antimicrobial agents are found in Table 3–2.

C. **Identification of the Infecting Organism.** The **Gram stain** is one of the simplest, quickest, and least expensive methods of identifying bacteria and fungi. In normally sterile body fluids (pleural, pericardial, peritoneal, cerebrospinal, and synovial fluids, urine, and the buffy coat component of blood), the morphologic characteristics of microorganisms provide specific information to guide therapy. For body substances that contain "normal" flora as well as potential pathogens (sputum, stool, and vaginal secretions), findings from Gram stains are more difficult to interpret. Gram stains may reveal polymorphonuclear leukocytes in an infected fluid even when the etiologic agent is not apparent. Immunologic methods for antigen detection can be useful as a rapid diagnostic tool (e.g., fluorescent antibody stains for *Legionella* and selected viruses, such as herpes simplex virus and cytomegalovirus).

D. **Antimicrobial Susceptibility.** Antimicrobial agents listed as "preferred agents" (blue shading) or "alternative agents" (gray shading) in Table 3–3 should be used when the suspected pathogen has been isolated from culture and the organism has been shown to be sensitive. Since some preferred agents may not be active against all strains of a suspected pathogen, more broad-spectrum coverage provided by other antimicrobial agents (gray shading) may be considered before culture results are obtained in appropriate acute clinical situations. For example, since all strains of *Hemophilus influenzae* are not sensitive to ampicillin, another agent should be used initially in the setting of suspected *H. influenzae* meningitis (e.g., ceftriaxone or chloramphenicol) until the antimicrobial sensitivity pattern is known. If the isolate is sensitive to ampicillin, then the antibiotic coverage can be narrowed to the appropriate "preferred agent." A number of methods are available to determine antimicrobial susceptibility.

1. **DISC DIFFUSION**

   The disc diffusion method involves placing antibiotic-permeated paper discs on a solid medium that has been inoculated with a pure culture of the patient's organism. The method is simple and inexpensive and has been standardized for most organisms. Within 24 hours, most bacteria can be rated as susceptible, intermediate, or resistant, on the basis of the size of the zone of inhibition around each antibiotic disc. This technique cannot be applied to fastidious or slow-growing organisms and has not been standardized for anaerobes.

2. **AGAR OR BROTH DILUTION**

   Agar or broth dilution techniques provide quantitative susceptibility information about an organism. These serial dilution methods are used to determine the lowest concentration of antibiotic that will inhibit visible bacterial growth after an 18- to 24-hour period. This level is called the **minimal inhibitory concentration (MIC).** An organism is considered sensitive to an antibiotic when the MIC of the antibiotic to that organism is no more than one fourth of the obtainable peak serum concentration. The **minimal bactericidal concentration (MBC)** may be found by subculturing the dilution tubes that do not show growth into antibiotic-free media. The subculture from the lowest antibiotic concentration that suppresses overnight growth is designated as that organism's MBC.

E. **Combination Antimicrobial Therapy.** Most infections can be treated with a single antimicrobial agent. The simultaneous use of two or more antimicrobial agents has effects on the host and the flora. Combination therapy is appropriate only in specific situations. In vitro, an antimicrobial combination can have one of three different effects on a microorganism: (1) **additive,** in which the activity of the drugs in combination is equal to the sum of their separate activities; (2) **synergistic,** in which the activity of the drug combination is greater than the sum of their separate activities; and (3) **antagonistic,** in which the combined activity of the agents is less than the sum of their independent effects. Although these effects can be demonstrated by several methods in the laboratory, clinical trials documenting the in vivo effects of the in vitro findings are limited.

There are several commonly cited reasons for using combination antimicrobial therapy:

1. **PREVENTION OF EMERGENCE OF RESISTANT ORGANISMS**

   If the spontaneous mutation of microorganisms were the most common method of acquiring resistance, then combination therapy would decrease this occurrence. However, tuberculosis and, perhaps, infec-

Text continued on page 75

TABLE 3–1. ADVERSE EFFECTS AND DRUG INTERACTIONS

ANTIMICROBIAL	MAJOR ADVERSE EFFECTS	DRUG INTERACTIONS
Acyclovir	Possible bone marrow suppression	Probenecid: ↑ acyclovir toxicity
Amantadine	Central nervous system effects (e.g., disorientation)	Anticholinergics: hallucinations, confusion
Aminoglycosides	Ototoxicity, maculopapular rash, neuromuscular blockade ↑ Nephrotoxicity with amphotericin B, cephalosporins, loop diuretics	Inactivated by high levels of carbenicillin, ticarcillin ↑ Effects of neuromuscular blocking agents
Amphotericin B	Acute tubular necrosis ↑ Nephrotoxicity with aminoglycosides Hypokalemia Hypomagnesemia Phlebitis, eosinophilia	↑ Digitalis toxicity ↑ Effects of neuromuscular blocking agents
Aztreonam	Bleeding disorders	↓ Effect of aminoglycosides
Carbenicillin and ticarcillin	Hypokalemia	
Cephalosporins	Anaphylaxis, serum sickness, leukopenia, pseudomembranous colitis, maculopapular rash, erythema multiforme ↑ Bleeding, hypoprothrombinemia ↑ Nephrotoxicity with aminoglycosides, loop diuretics Interstitial nephritis	Disulfiram-like reaction with alcohol and cefamandole, moxalactam, cefoperazone, cefotetan
Chloramphenicol	Pseudomembranous colitis Aplastic anemia, hemolysis in glucose-6-phosphate dehydrogenase (G-6-PD) deficiency	Acetaminophen: ↑ chloramphenicol level Barbiturates: ↑ effects → chloramphenicol effect Warfarin: ↑ anticoagulant effect Phenytoin: ↑ toxicity ↓ chloramphenicol effect Sulfonylureas: ↑ effect
Clindamycin	Pseudomembranous colitis	↑ Effects of neuromuscular blocking agents
Erythromycin	Diarrhea, cholestatic jaundice	Carbamazepine, digoxin, theophylline: ↑ levels
Imipenem with cilastatin	Thrombocytopenia, encephalopathy, seizures, phlebitis, nausea, diarrhea	

Drug	Adverse Effects	Drug Interactions
Isoniazid (INH)	Anemia, peripheral neuropathy, drug-induced lupus Chronic hepatitis, cytotoxic effects ↑ INH hepatotoxicity with rifampin	Aluminum: ↓ INH absorbed Carbamazepine: ↑ toxicity of both Disulfiram: psychosis ataxia
Ketoconazole	Possible inhibition of adrenal corticosteroid synthesis with prolonged use	Antacids, cimetidine: ↓ ketoconazole levels Cyclosporine: ↑ cyclosporine levels Alcohol: disulfiram-like reaction
Metronidazole	Peripheral neuropathy	Anticoagulants: ↑ anticoagulant effect Disulfiram: organic brain syndrome Barbiturates: ↓ metronidazole effect
Penicillins	Maculopapular rash, photosensitivity, erythema multiforme, anaphylaxis, serum sickness, anemia, leukopenia, diarrhea, pulmonary infiltrates, drug-induced lupus, encephalopathy (with high doses) Interstitial nephritis (especially with methicillin), glomerulonephritis Hepatitis with oxacillin Pseudomembranous colitis Seizures with high-dose therapy	↓ Effect of aminoglycoside in renal failure Oral contraceptives: ↓ effect with ampicillin
Pentamidine	Nephrotoxicity, hepatotoxicity Hypoglycemia, hypotension, phlebitis, bone marrow depression	
Quinolones	Dizziness, headache, nausea, leukopenia, eosinophilia, rash	↑ Effect of theophylline with ciprofloxacin, enoxacin ↓↓ Effect of anticoagulants, barbiturates, beta blockers, oral contraceptives, corticosteroids, digoxin, quinidine, sulfonylureas
Rifampin	Anemia Orange coloration of body secretions	↑ INH hepatotoxicity ↑↑ Effect of warfarin, phenytoin, sulfonylureas, theophylline
Sulfonamides	Anaphylaxis, serum sickness, aplastic anemia, pulmonary infiltrates, maculopapular rash, photosensitivity. drug-induced lupus Glomerulonephritis	↑ Effect of warfarin, digoxin, lithium
Tetracyclines	Photosensitivity, discoloration of developing teeth, nausea, epigastric distress Prerenal azotemia	Antacids, iron: ↓ tetracycline absorption Barbiturates, phenytoin: ↓ doxycycline levels
Trimethoprim	Rash, bone marrow depression	
Vancomycin	Ototoxicity	Aminoglycosides: ↑ nephrotoxicity

TABLE 3–2. DOSING RECOMMENDATIONS FOR ANTIMICROBIAL AGENTS

	STANDARD DOSAGE (NORMAL RENAL FUNCTION)	DOSAGE INTERVAL FOR CREATININE CLEARANCE (ML/MIN)			SUPPLEMENT AFTER DIALYSIS*
		80–50	50–10	<10	
Aztreonam	0.5–2.0 gm IV q 6–12 hr	8–12 hr	12–24 hr	24–36 hr	Yes (H)
Aminoglycosides†‡					
Amikacin	5.0–7.5 mg/kg IV q 8–12 hr	12 hr	24–36 hr	36–72 hr	Yes (H,P)
Gentamicin	1.0–2.0 mg/kg IV q 8 hr	8–12 hr	12–24 hr	24–72 hr	Yes (H,P)
Tobramycin	1.0–2.0 mg/kg IV q 8 hr	8–12 hr	12–24 hr	24–72 hr	Yes (H,P)
Amphotericin B	Initial test dose, 1 mg IV, then 0.5–1.0 mg/kg IV q 24 hr	24 hr	24 hr	24–48 hr	No
Cephalosporins					
First generation:					
Cefadroxil	0.5–1.0 gm po q 12–24 hr	12–24 hr	24 hr	36–48 hr	Yes (H)
Cephradine	0.5 gm po q 6 hr	6 hr	8 hr	12–24 hr	Yes (H,P)
Cephalexin	0.25–0.50 gm po q 6 hr	6 hr	8–12 hr	24–48 hr	Yes (H)
Cephalothin	1–2 gm IV q 4–6 hr	6 hr	8 hr	12 hr	Yes (H,P)
Cephapirin	1 gm IV q 4–6 hr	6 hr	8 hr	12 hr	Yes (H)
Cefazolin	1–2 gm IV q 6–8 hr	8 hr	12 hr	24–48 hr	Yes (H)
Second generation:					
Cefaclor	0.25–0.50 gm po q 8 hr	8 hr	8 hr	8 hr	Yes (H)
Cefonicid	1–2 gm IV q 24 hr	24 hr	24 hr	3–5 days	No (H,P)
Cefotetan	1–2 gm IV q 12 hr	12 hr	24 hr	48 hr	Yes (H)
Cefoxitin	1–2 gm IV q 4–6 hr	8 hr	12 hr	24–48 hr	Yes (H), No (P)
Cefuroxime	0.75–1.50 gm IV q 8 hr	8–12 hr	24–48 hr	24 hr	Yes (H,P)
Third generation:					
Cefoperazone	1–2 gm IV q 8–12 hr	8–12 hr	8–12 hr	8–12 hr	Yes (H)
Cefotaxime	1–2 gm IV q 4–6 hr	4–6 hr	6–12 hr	12–24 hr	Yes (H)
Ceftazidime	1–2 gm IV q 6–8 hr	8–12 hr	12–24 hr	24–48 hr	Yes (H,P)
Ceftizoxime	1–2 gm IV q 6–8 hr	8 hr	12 hr	12–24 hr	Yes (H,P)
Ceftriaxone	1–2 gm IV q 12–24 hr	12–24 hr	24 hr	24 hr	No

Chloramphenicol†	1 gm IV q 6 hr	6 hr	6 hr	6 hr	Yes (H), No (P)
Clindamycin	0.15–0.45 gm po q 6 hr 0.15–0.90 gm IV q 6 hr	6 hr	6 hr	6 hr	No (H,P)
Erythromycin	0.25–0.50 gm po q 6 hr 0.25–1.0 gm IV q 6 hr	6 hr	6 hr	6 hr	No (H,P)
Imipenem	0.5–1.0 gm IV q 6–8 hr	6–8 hr	6–12 hr	12–24 hr	Yes (H)
Metronidazole	0.25–0.50 gm po q 8 hr 0.50–0.75 gm IV q 8 hr	8 hr	8–12 hr	12–24 hr	Yes (H), No (P)
Penicillins					
Penicillin G	1–3 MU IV q 4–6 hr	6–8 hr	8–12 hr	12–24 hr	Yes (H), No (P)
Penicillin V	0.25–0.50 gm po q 6 hr	6–8 hr	8–12 hr	12–24 hr	Yes (H), No (P)
Penicillinase-Resistant Penicillins					
Dicloxacillin	0.5 gm po q 6 hr	6 hr	6 hr	6 hr	No (H)
Nafcillin§	0.5–2.0 gm IV q 4–6 hr	4–6 hr	4–6 hr	4–6 hr	No (H)
Methicillin	1–2 gm IV q 4–6 hr	6 hr	8 hr	12 hr	No (H,P)
Broad-Spectrum Penicillins					
Amoxicillin	0.25–0.50 gm po q 8 hr	8 hr	12 hr	12–24 hr	Yes (H), No (P)
Amoxicillin/clavulanate	One tablet (250 or 500 mg amoxicillin/ 125 mg clavulanate) po tid	8 hr	12 hr	12–24 hr	N/A
Ampicillin	0.5–1.0 gm po q 6 hr 1–2 gm IV q 4–6 hr	6 hr	8 hr	12 hr	Yes (H), No (P)
Ampicillin/sulbactam	1–2 gm/0.5–1.0 gm IV q 6 hr	6–8 hr	12 hr	24 hr	Yes (H), No (P)
Carbenicillin	4–5 gm IV q 4–6 hr	6–8 hr	12–24 hr	24–48 hr	Yes (H,P)
Ticarcillin	2–3 gm IV q 4–6 hr	8–12 hr	12–24 hr	24–48 hr	Yes (H,P)
Ticarcillin/clavulanate	One (3 gm ticarcillin/0.1 gm clavulanate) vial q 4–6 hr	8–12 hr	12–24 hr	24–48 hr	N/A
Azlocillin	2–3 gm IV q 4–6 hr	4–6 hr	6–8 hr	12 hr	Yes (H)
Mezlocillin	2–4 gm IV q 4–8 hr	4–6 hr	6–8 hr	8–12 hr	Yes (H)
Piperacillin	3–4 gm IV q 4–6 hr	4–6 hr	6–8 hr	12 hr	Yes (H)

Table continued on the following page

69

TABLE 3–2. DOSING RECOMMENDATIONS FOR ANTIMICROBIAL AGENTS Continued

	STANDARD DOSAGE (NORMAL RENAL FUNCTION)	DOSAGE INTERVAL FOR CREATININE CLEARANCE (ML/MIN)			SUPPLEMENT AFTER DIALYSIS*
		80–50	50–10	<10	
Trimethoprim-Sulfamethoxazole	160/800 mg po q 12 hr; 10–20 mg/kg/day IV based on trimethoprim component divided into q 6-hr or q 12-hr schedule	12 hr	18 hr	24–48 hr	Yes (H); No (P)
Tetracyclines	0.25–0.50 gm po q 6 hr		— Contraindicated —		
	0.50 to 1.0 gm IV q 12 hr				
Doxycycline	0.1 gm po or IV q 12 hr	12–24 hr	12–24 hr	12–24 hr	No (H,P)
Vancomycin†	0.5–1.0 gm IV q 12–24 hr	1–2 days	2–4 days	4–7 days	No (H,P)
Quinolones					
Ciprofloxacin	0.25–0.75 gm po q 12 hr	12 hr	12–24 hr	24 hr	Yes (H,P)
Norfloxacin	0.4 gm po q 12 hr	12 hr	12–24 hr	24 hr	N/A

*H = hemodialysis; P = peritoneal dialysis; N/A = not applicable.

†Levels should be followed.

‡For more specific dosing information see Hull JH, Sarubbi FA: Gentamicin serum concentrations: Pharmocokinetic predictions. Ann Intern Med 85:183–189, 1976. Patients with moderate-to-severe renal insufficiency should receive a loading dose of 1.0–2.0 mg/kg of all aminoglycosides (except amikacin, which is 5.0–7.5 gm/kg).

§Dose should be reduced in combined renal and hepatic failure.

For further information, see Bennett WM, Aronoff GR, Morrison G, et al.: Drug prescribing in renal failure: Dosing guidelines for adults. Am J Kidney Dis 3:155, 1983; and Van Scoy RE, Wilson WR: Antimicrobial agents in adult patients with renal insufficiency: Initial dosage and general recommendations. Mayo Clin Proc 62:1142, 1987.

TABLE 3-3. ANTIMICROBIAL AGENTS OF CHOICE AGAINST SELECTED ORGANISMS

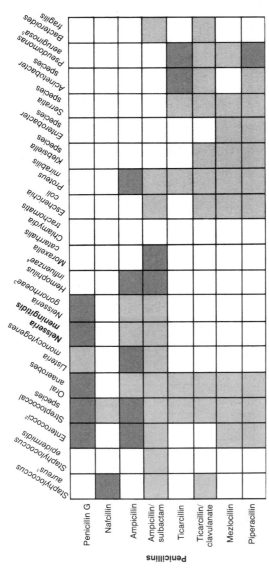

Penicillins: Penicillin G, Nafcillin, Ampicillin, Ampicillin/sulbactam, Ticarcillin, Ticarcillin/clavulanate, Mezlocillin, Piperacillin

Organisms (columns): Staphylococcus aureus[1], Staphylococcus epidermidis, Enterococci[2], Streptococcal species, Oral anaerobes, Listeria monocytogenes, Neisseria meningitidis, Neisseria gonorrhoeae[3], Hemophilus influenzae[4], Moraxella catarrhalis, Chlamydia trachomatis, Escherichia coli, Proteus mirabilis, Klebsiella species, Enterobacter species, Serratia species, Acinetobacter species, Pseudomonas aeruginosa[5], Bacteroides fragilis

KEY: Appropriate antibiotics for treatment of clinical infections caused by various bacteria are depicted. Blue-shaded squares denote "preferred agent(s)" for therapy; "alternate agents" are designated by the gray-shaded squares. These choices of antimicrobial therapy are based in part on antibiotic sensitivity data from the University of Washington Medical Center. Since these data represent solely the experience from a single hospital, information in this table may not be accurate for other hospitals. It is important to be aware of local antimicrobial sensitivity patterns when choosing antibiotic therapy. [1]"Methicillin-resistant" strains of Staphylococcus aureus (MRSA) are found in some hospitals and will be resistant to multiple beta-lactams. In general, infections due to MRSA should be treated with vancomycin. [2]Use penicillin (or ampicillin or vancomycin) with an aminoglycoside for systemic infections. [3]In regions where penicillinase producers are prevalent, use a cephalosporin (e.g. ceftriaxone) or ciprofloxacin. [4]For penicillinase producers, use a second- or third-generation cephalosporin (e.g. cefuroxime or ceftriaxone), ampicillin/sulbactam, or TMP/SMX. [5]Combination therapy is optimal: an aminoglycoside plus an extended-spectrum penicillin or a third-generation cephalosporin. TMP/SMX, Trimethoprim-sulfamethoxazole.

Table continued on the following page

TABLE 3-3. ANTIMICROBIAL AGENTS OF CHOICE AGAINST SELECTED ORGANISMS *Continued*

Cephalosporins	Staphylococcus aureus[1]	Staphylococcus epidermidis	Enterococci[2]	Streptococcal species	Oral anaerobes	Listeria monocytogenes	Neisseria meningitidis	Neisseria gonorrhoeae[3]	Hemophilus influenzae[4]	Moraxella catarrhalis	Chlamydia trachomatis	Escherichia coli	Proteus mirabilis	Klebsiella species	Enterobacter species	Serratia species	Acinetobacter species	Pseudomonas aeruginosa[5]	Bacteroides fragilis
Cefazolin	▓			▓	▓		▓					▓	▓	▓					
Cefoxitin	▓			▓	▓		▓					▓	▓	▓					▓
Cefotetan	▓			▓	▓		▓	▓				▓	▓	▓		▓			▓
Cefuroxime	▓			▓	▓		▓	▓	▓	▓		▓	▓	▓					
Cefotaxime				▓	▓		▓	▓	▓			▓	▓	▓	▓	▓			
Cefoperazone				▓	▓				▓				▓	▓	▓			▓	
Ceftriaxone				▓	▓		▓	▓	▓			▓	▓	▓	▓	▓			
Ceftazidime				▓	▓							▓	▓	▓	▓	▓	▓	▓	

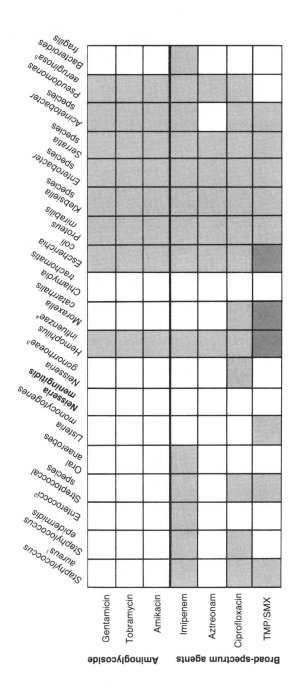

Table continued on the following page

TABLE 3–3. ANTIMICROBIAL AGENTS OF CHOICE AGAINST SELECTED ORGANISMS *Continued*

Miscellaneous agents	Staphylococcus aureus[1]	Staphylococcus epidermidis	Enterococci[2]	Streptococcal species	Oral anaerobes	Listeria monocytogenes	**Neisseria meningitidis**	Neisseria gonorrhoeae[3]	Hemophilus influenzae[4]	Moraxella catarrhalis	Chlamydia trachomatis	Escherichia coli	Proteus mirabilis	Klebsiella species	Enterobacter species	Serratia species	Acinetobacter species	Pseudomonas aeruginosa[5]	Bacteroides fragilis
Erythromycin																			
Clindamycin																			
Tetracycline																			
Vancomycin																			
Metronidazole																			
Chloramphenicol																			

74

tions due to *Pseudomonas aeruginosa* are the only diseases for which this rationale should routinely lead to the use of multiple agents.

2. **TREATMENT OF POLYMICROBIAL INFECTIONS**
Intra-abdominal, pelvic, and genital tract infections, as well as abscesses in other locations, are caused by aerobic and anaerobic flora. These infections may require combination therapy to cover the broad variety of organisms involved.

3. **THERAPY FOR INFECTIONS OF UNKNOWN ETIOLOGY IN SEVERELY ILL OR IMMUNOCOMPROMISED PATIENTS**
Broad-spectrum initial coverage may be necessary until the causative pathogen or pathogens become apparent. A commonly employed regimen is a third-generation cephalosporin or extended-spectrum penicillin combined with an aminoglycoside.

4. **DECREASED TOXICITY**
Theoretically, it may be possible to lower the dose of a potentially toxic agent when used in combination with another effective antimicrobial.

5. **SYNERGISM**
Although many synergistic antimicrobial combinations have been demonstrated in the laboratory, combination therapy has been proved more effective than a single agent in only a few clinical situations. The most widely accepted combination is penicillin plus an aminoglycoside for enterococcal endocarditis. A combination of an antipseudomonal penicillin with an aminoglycoside against *Pseudomonas aeruginosa* is also widely accepted. Fixed drug combinations, such as trimethoprim with sulfamethoxazole, work by inhibiting 2 steps in the folic acid cycle. Beta-lactam agents in combination with beta-lactamase inhibitors, such as amoxicillin or ticarcillin plus clavulanate (Augmentin and Timentin, respectively), act synergistically.

F. **Assessment of Antimicrobial Therapy.** Effective antimicrobial therapy should result in clinical improvement of the patient, as evidenced by normalization of temperature and white blood cell count, accompanied by subjective improvement and disappearance of the pathogen from the infection site. The duration of antibiotic therapy should be determined on the basis of clinical response. Not enough well-controlled studies are available to make decisions concerning length of therapy in most situations. In general, most acute bacterial infections for which antibiotics penetrate well to the site of infection should be treated for at least 3 to 5 days *after* clinical signs of infection have resolved. Some chronic infections such as osteomyelitis and infections involving sites that are penetrated poorly by antibiotics such as vegetations in bacterial endocarditis may require much longer antibiotic courses after symptoms and signs of infection have resolved.

The **serum bactericidal titer** has been used to monitor therapy in bacterial endocarditis. Serial dilutions of the patient's serum are incubated with a standardized inoculum of the infecting organism. The highest dilution that inhibits growth is determined. A serum bactericidal titer of 1:8 or greater correlates with successful outcome in most serious infections. In bacterial endocarditis, a titer greater than 1:64 is desirable. The lack of standardization and consistency of this test has made its use controversial.

Measurements of antimicrobial serum concentrations are useful to avoid toxicity from elevated levels of agents such as the aminoglycosides and vancomycin, especially in patients with impaired renal function. Measurement can also be used to ensure adequate peak levels of these agents.

If a patient does not improve clinically, there are several factors to consider. These include the following:

1. Inadequate drug delivery resulting from poor compliance or poor absorption of the agent;

2. Inadequate dosage or prolonged antibiotic-free intervals between doses;

3. Poor antibiotic penetration to the site of infection, as, for example, in endocarditis;

4. Presence of abscess or abscesses that require drainage;

5. Presence of a foreign body;

6. Emergence of a resistant pathogen or superinfection with a new pathogen;

7. A new infection site, such as pneumonia, urinary tract infections, or phlebitis in the hospitalized patient;

8. Drug fever;

9. Altered host defenses.

II. PROPHYLACTIC USE OF ANTIMICROBIAL AGENTS

A. Antimicrobial Prophylaxis for Surgery. Preop prophylactic antibiotics are used in some situations (Table 3–4). The antibiotic chosen should have a narrow spectrum of coverage directed against the most likely infecting pathogen or pathogens. Its cost, safety, and efficacy must be considered and the prophylaxis tailored to each situation. Prophylactic antibiotics must reach high tissue levels during the operation. For this reason, a dose should usually be given "on call" to the operating room and repeated only if the surgery is delayed or prolonged. A maximum of 3 doses should be given for most operations, except for "contaminated cases" (e.g., a perforated viscus), when a longer course is indicated. It is also common practice to give more than 3 doses when prosthetic joints and heart valves are to be implanted, though additional benefit has not been established clearly in these situations. Administration beyond 72 hours increases the risk of bacterial resistance and drug toxicity without decreasing the risk of infection.

Appropriate prophylactic antimicrobial use must be coupled with proper surgical technique and judgment. Factors that contribute to the development of wound infection in "clean" surgical procedures include prolonged hospitalization before the procedure, extended operative time, excessive use of wound drains, and razor shaving of the operative field the night before surgery. A preoperative shower with an antiseptic soap has been shown to decrease the incidence of wound infection.

TABLE 3-4. ANTIMICROBIAL PROPHYLAXIS FOR SURGERY

TYPE OF SURGERY	LIKELY PATHOGENS	DOSAGE BEFORE SURGERY*
Cardiovascular	*Staphylococcus epidermidis,* *S. aureus, Corynebacterium* sp.	Cefazolin or vancomycin,† 1 gm IV
Orthopedic (including prosthetic joint placement)	*S. aureus, S. epidermidis*	Cefazolin or vancomycin,† 1 gm IV
Head and neck	*S. aureus,* streptococci, oral anaerobes	Cefazolin, 1 gm IV
High-risk gastroduodenal or biliary tract	Enteric gram-negative bacilli, gram-positive cocci, group D streptococci, *Clostridium*	Cefazolin, 1 gm IV
Colorectal	Enteric gram-negative bacilli, anaerobes	Oral: neomycin, plus erythromycin base, 1 gm of each at 1 PM, 2 PM, and 11 PM the day before surgery‡ Parenteral: cefoxitin, 1 gm IV
Appendectomy	Enteric gram-negative bacilli, anaerobes	Cefotetan, 1 gm IV
Vaginal or abdominal hysterectomy; high-risk cesarean section	Enteric gram-negative bacilli, anaerobes, group B and D streptococci	Cefazolin, 1 gm IV
Abortion	As above, but test for *Chlamydia*	Tetracycline, 500 mg po qid, or doxycycline, 100 mg po bid; continue for 7 days if *Chlamydia* culture positive
Ruptured viscus	Enteric gram-negative bacilli, anaerobes, group D streptococci	Clindamycin, 600 mg IV q 6 hr, plus gentamicin or tobramycin, 1.5 mg/kg IV or IM, with or without ampicillin, 1.5 gm IV q 6 hr; *or* cefotetan alone or with gentamicin or tobramycin; *or* imipenem, 500 mg IV q 6 hr.
Traumatic wounds§	*S. aureus,* group A streptococcus, *Clostridium, Pasteurella*	Ampicillin-sulbactam, 1.5–3.0 gm IV q 4–6 hr, with or without gentamicin or tobramycin; *or* cefazolin, 1 gm q 6–8 hr IM or IV; *or* ticarcillin/clavulanate, 3.1 gm IV q 4–6 hr.

*Parenteral prophylactic antimicrobials for "clean" and "clean-contaminated" surgery can be given as a single dose just before the operation. For prolonged operations, additional intraoperative dosages should be given q 4–8 hr for the duration of the procedure. For "dirty" surgery, therapy should usually be continued for 5 to 10 days.

†For hospitals in which methicillin-resistant *S. aureus* and *S. epidermidis* frequently cause wound infection, or for patients with penicillin or cephalosporin allergy.

‡After appropriate diet and catharsis (see Nichols RL: Postoperative infections and antimicrobial prophylaxis. *In* Mandell GL, Douglas RG, Bennett JE, et al. (eds): Principles and Practice of Infectious Diseases. 2nd ed. New York, Wiley, 1985, p 1641.)

§For bite wounds, in which likely pathogens may also include oral anaerobes, *Eikenella corrodens* (humans), and *Pasteurella multocida* (dogs and cats), some consultants recommend use of amoxicillin-clavulanic acid (Augmentin) or ampicillin-sulbactam (Unasyn).

Adapted from recommendations presented in Med Lett Drugs Ther 29: 91–94, 1987. Modifications based on local usage.

Hirschman JV, Inui TS: Antimicrobial prophylaxis: A critique of recent trials. Rev Infect Dis 2:1–23, 1980.
Hull JH, Sarubbi FA: Gentamicin serum concentrations: Pharmacokinetic predictions. Ann Intern Med 85:183, 1976.
Medical Letter: The choice of antimicrobial drugs. Med Lett Drugs Ther 28:33–40, 1986.
Sarubbi FA, Hull JH: Amikacin serum concentrations: Predication of levels and dosage guidelines. Ann Intern Med 89:612–618, 1978.
Symposium on antimicrobial agents. Mayo Clin Proc 62:789–1031, 1987.

B. Antimicrobial Prophylaxis for Prevention of Endocarditis. The American Heart Association issued new recommendations for the prevention of bacterial endocarditis in dental and medical procedures in 1990. Endocarditis prophylaxis is recommended for patients with:

1. Prosthetic cardiac valves, including bioprosthetic and homograft valves;
2. Most congenital cardiac anomalies;
3. Hypertrophic cardiomyopathy;
4. Mitral valve prolapse with associated audible murmur of valvular regurgitation;
5. A history of previous bacterial endocarditis, even in the absence of heart disease;
6. A history of rheumatic and other acquired valvular dysfunction, even following corrective valvular surgery.

Prophylaxis is not recommended for patients with:

1. Isolated secundum atrial septal defect;
2. Mitral valve prolapse without valvular regurgitation;
3. Physiologic, functional, or innocent heart murmurs;
4. Cardiac pacemakers and implantable defibrillators;
5. A history of previous coronary artery bypass graft surgery;
6. A history of previous rheumatic fever or Kawasaki's disease without valvular dysfunction;
7. A history of surgical repair without residua beyond 6 months of secundum atrial septal defect, ventricular septal defect, or patent ductus arteriosus.

Patients with increased risk of bacterial endocarditis should receive antibiotic prophylaxis when undergoing the following procedures:

1. Dental procedures likely to result in gingival bleeding (including professional dental cleaning);
2. Tonsillectomy;
3. Adenoidectomy;
4. Rigid bronchoscopy;
5. Surgical procedures involving manipulation of the respiratory mucosa;
6. Cholecystectomy and biliary tract surgery;
7. Cystoscopy;
8. Urethral surgery;
9. Prostatic surgery;
10. Incision and drainage of infected tissue;

11. Vaginal hysterectomy;

12. Urethral catheterization, urinary tract surgery, and vaginal delivery when infection is present.

The recommended **prophylactic regimen** for **dental, oral, or upper respiratory tract procedures is amoxicillin, 3.0 gm po 1 hour before the procedure, followed by 1.5 gm po 6 hours after the initial dose.** In penicillin-allergic patients, either erythromycin (1.0 gm po 2 hours before the procedure, followed by 500 mg po 6 hours after the initial dose) or clindamycin (300 mg po 1 hour before the procedure, followed by 150 mg 6 hours after the initial dose) may be employed.

For genitourinary or gastrointestinal procedures, the recommended regimen for prophylaxis against endocarditis is: **ampicillin, 2.0 gm IV or IM, plus gentamicin, 1.5 mg/kg (not to exceed 80 mg) 30 minutes before the procedure, followed by amoxicillin, 1.5 gm po 6 hours after the initial dose (or the parenteral regimen may be repeated once 8 hours after the initial dose).** In penicillin-allergic patients, the recommended regimen is: vancomycin 1.0 gm IV, plus gentamicin 1.5 mg/kg (not to exceed 80 mg) 1 hour before the procedure. Repeat administration of vancomycin and gentamicin can be considered 8 hours after the initial doses. An alternate regimen for low-risk patients is: amoxicillin 3.0 gm po 1 hour before the procedure, followed by 1.5 gm po 6 hours later.

Dajani AS et al: Prevention of bacterial endocarditis: Recommendations by the American Heart Association. JAMA 264:2919–2922, 1990.

III. OTITIS AND SINUSITIS

A. Otitis Externa. Otitis externa, infection of the external auditory canal, can be divided into 4 categories, as follows:

1. Acute localized otitis externa usually occurs as a pustule or furuncle caused by *Staphylococcus aureus.* Erysipelas due to group A streptococcus may also be present in the canal. **Treatment** for both conditions is **local heat and systemic antibiotics** (dicloxacillin or erythromycin). Incision and drainage may be needed for some patients.

2. Acute diffuse otitis externa (swimmer's ear) occurs in warm, humid environments. **Treatment** consists of local **irrigation with hypertonic saline (3%) and cleansing with mixtures of alcohol (70 to 95%) and acetic acid.** Burow's solution (50%) may reduce inflammation. Topical treatment with solutions containing antibiotics (neomycin and polymixin) and a steroid is effective also (e.g., Cortisporin Otic). Systemic antibiotics are not necessary unless "invasive otitis" is suspected.

3. Chronic otitis externa is secondary to irritating drainage from chronic suppurative otitis media, and **treatment is that of a middle ear infection.**

4. Invasive otitis externa (also called malignant otitis externa) occurs most frequently in the elderly diabetic patient and results from the spread of infection into the adjacent soft tissues, cartilage, and bone.

Treatment includes surgical debridement of the canal, along with topical application of antipseudomonal antibiotics and steroids. Systemic therapy directed against *Pseudomonas aeruginosa* (an aminoglycoside and a beta-lactam antibiotic, such as carbenicillin or ticarcillin) for 4 to 6 weeks is also necessary. Hemorrhagic external otitis caused by *P. aeruginosa* has also been described in association with hot tub use and also may require IV antibiotic administration.

B. **Otitis Media.** **Acute** otitis media characterized or accompanied by symptoms of an upper respiratory tract infection, ear pain, drainage, and decreased hearing is commonly due to *Streptococcus pneumoniae* and nontypable *Hemophilus influenzae*. Less frequent pathogens include group A streptococcus, *Staphylococcus aureus,* and *Moraxella catarrhalis.* Gram-negative bacilli may have a role in chronic suppurative otitis and in infections in immunosuppressed patients. Therapy is usually initiated without knowledge of the pathogen and should be directed toward covering *Streptococcus pneumoniae* and *H. influenzae.* **Ampicillin, 250 mg po qid, or amoxicillin, 250 mg po tid,** is the initial agent of choice for adults. **Amoxicillin-clavulanate, 250 mg po tid,** is an option when the prevalence of ampicillin-resistant *H. influenzae* is appreciable or when *M. catarrhalis* is suspected. In the **penicillin-allergic patient, trimethoprim-sulfamethoxazole, 1 double-strength tablet 160 mg/800 mg po bid or an oral cephalosporin (i.e., cefaclor 250 mg qid)** can be administered. Decongestants and antihistamines are of no proven benefit. The presence of bullous myringitis suggests possible infection by *Mycoplasma pneumoniae.* **Erythromycin, 250 mg qid, is the treatment of choice.**

Chronic otitis media following recurrent episodes of acute infection and prolonged duration of middle ear effusion has been managed by chemoprophylaxis and immunoprophylaxis. Chemoprophylaxis with once-a-day antimicrobial therapy has been successful in children. Immunoprophylaxis with pneumococcal vaccine may reduce the incidence of acute otitis media due to serotypes of *Streptococcus pneumoniae* included in the vaccine. Persistent middle ear effusion is most successfully treated by insertion of tympanostomy tubes.

Mastoid infection may accompany otitis media, and tympanocentesis cultures are useful to guide antibiotic selection. Initial therapy should include antimicrobial coverage for *Streptococcus pneumoniae* and *H. influenzae,* with additional coverage for *Staphylococcus aureus* and gram-negative enteric bacilli if the clinical course has been prolonged.

Doroghazi RM, Nadol JB, Hyslop NE: Invasive external otitis: Report of 21 cases and review of the literature. Am J Med 71:603–614, 1981.
Nelson JD: Changing trends in the microbiology and management of acute otitis media and sinusitis. Pediatr Infect Dis 5:749–753, 1986.

C. **Maxillary Sinusitis.** Over 90% of acute (<3 weeks in duration) sinusitis involves the maxillary sinuses. Treatment is usually empiric and is directed toward *Streptococcus pneumoniae,* nonencapsulated *H. influenzae,* and *M. catarrhalis.* **Amoxicillin-clavulanate (Augmentin) 250– 500 mg po tid, or trimethoprim-sulfamethoxazole 160 mg/800 mg, 1 tablet twice a day for a 10-day course, is recommended.** Oxymetazoline hydrochloride nasal spray 3 times a day (not to be used for more than 3 days) may reduce mucosal swelling. Follow-up with repeat transillumination and sinus radiographs or computerized tomography is indicated for patients who do not respond to therapy. Consultation with an ENT specialist should be considered for patients with chronic symptoms, especially if sinus x-rays show persistent air-fluid levels or complete opacification of the airspace.

D. **Nosocomial Sinusitis.** Nosocomially acquired sinusitis, a common problem in ICU patients with indwelling nasal or oral tubes, is usually caused by antibiotic-resistant gram-negative rods. Effective treatment depends on the results of cultures from material obtained by direct sinus puncture. Initial treatment should cover *Pseudomonas aeruginosa* until culture results are available and indwelling tubes are removed, if possible.

E. **Chronic Sinusitis.** Cultures of material obtained by direct maxillary sinus puncture in patients with sinusitis of longer than 3 months' duration usually show a predominance of anaerobic flora or *Staphylococcus aureus*. Antimicrobial therapy directed at oral anaerobic flora and *Staphylococcus aureus* may be helpful in these individuals, but no well-controlled studies are available to guide antibiotic use. Surgical procedures to create better drainage should be considered if symptoms do not respond to antimicrobial therapy. Patients with chronic sinusitis and severe asthma may respond well to surgical drainage, often with considerable improvement in their response to treatment for bronchospasm.

F. **Complications of Sinusitis.** Untreated **frontal sinusitis** can lead to cranial osteomyelitis, frontal subperiosteal abscess, epidural abscess, subdural abscess, and brain abscess. Initial antimicrobial therapy for mild frontal sinusitis is the same as that for maxillary sinusitis. Close observation is necessary, however, as these patients may require hospitalization for IV therapy or surgical intervention.

Orbital cellulitis is a complication of **ethmoid sinusitis.** The causative bacteria that have been described include *Staphylococcus aureus, H. influenzae, Streptococcus pneumoniae,* and *Streptococcus pyogenes.* Early treatment with IV antibiotics is essential, and these patients should be followed carefully by an otolaryngologist.

Sphenoid sinusitis is rare but is associated with severe complications because of the proximity of the sphenoid sinus to several important structures. **Cavernous sinus thrombosis,** pituitary insufficiency, bitemporal hemianopsia, subdural abscess, internal carotid infection, and meningitis can result from extension of infection.

Septic cavernous sinus thrombosis is most frequently caused by *S. aureus*. **Initial antimicrobial therapy should include IV administration of a semisynthetic penicillin or vancomycin in the penicillin-allergic patient. Broad-spectrum coverage** directed against aerobic gram-negative rods is also indicated, pending culture results. Heparin therapy is controversial.

Mucormycosis and *aspergillosis,* caused by opportunistic organisms, are types of **fungal sinusitis** seen in diabetic and immunosuppressed patients. **Surgical treatment is usually necessary, along with administration of systemic amphotericin B.** Unless these fungal infections are diagnosed very early in the clinical course, osteomyelitis is usually present in affected patients. Aggressive early surgical therapy may improve the prognosis of fungal sinusitis.

Hamory BH, Sande MA, Sydnor A, et al: Etiology and antimicrobial therapy of acute maxillary sinusitis. J Infect Dis 139:197–202, 1979.
Daley CL, Sande M: The runny nose: Infections of the paranasal sinuses. Infect Dis Clin North Am 2:131–147, 1988.

IV. PHARYNGEAL INFECTIONS

A. Pharyngitis. The goal in the diagnosis and treatment of acute pharyngitis is to separate pharyngitis due to group A streptococcal disease and other serious throat infections from those that are benign and self-limited. Most pharyngitis is caused by a virus. A throat culture should be done in adults who have a history of rheumatic fever, contact with a person known to have streptococcal pharyngitis, or clinical signs suggesting possible streptococcal infection such as fever, pharyngeal exudate, and cervical adenopathy.

1. **GROUP A STREPTOCOCCAL PHARYNGITIS**
   Treatment may be initiated on the basis of either a positive throat culture or high clinical suspicion and then discontinued if the culture is negative. **Penicillin V 250 mg po qid for 10 days or benzathine penicillin G, 1.2 MU in a single IM dose is recommended.** The latter treatment, while painful, eliminates the problem of the patient's compliance. **The penicillin-allergic patient can be given erythromycin, 250 mg po qid for 10 days.** Initiation of treatment within 1 week of the onset of streptococcal pharyngitis should prevent rheumatic fever. A repeat throat culture after clinically successful treatment is not necessary. Oral therapy suffices for most patients with pharyngitis. Hospitalization and parenteral therapy are required if adequate hydration cannot be maintained or there is danger of airway compromise. Severe odynophagia suggests possible complications (e.g., epiglottitis or peritonsillar abscess). Pharyngitis due to other beta-hemolytic streptococci is rare and does not require antimicrobial therapy.

2. **GONOCOCCAL PHARYNGITIS**
   Treatment is described on p. 95.

3. **VIRAL PHARYNGITIS**
   Viral pharyngitis caused by type A influenza may benefit from early use of amantadine, 100 mg po bid or 200 mg po qd. Herpetic oropharyngeal infection in the immunosuppressed patient can be treated with acyclovir 250 mg/m^2 every 8 hours IV for 7 days.

4. **LUDWIG'S ANGINA (ANAEROBIC PHARYNGITIS)**
   This type of pharyngitis can be treated with an oral penicillin or cephalosporin initially. It may, however, spread to the soft tissues of the neck and require surgical drainage and IV antibiotics.

B. Epiglottitis. When epiglottitis is suspected on the basis of clinical findings or lateral neck radiographic abnormalities, **initial IV antibiotic therapy should be directed against** *Hemophilus influenzae*. However, *Streptococc-*

cus pneumoniae, other streptococci, *Staphylococcus aureus,* and *H. parainfluenzae* also have been implicated in cases of epiglottitis in normal hosts, and *Pseudomonas aeruginosa* may cause epiglottitis in the immunosuppressed patient. Hospitalization for IV antimicrobial therapy and close observation is indicated for adults with epiglottitis.

C. **Peritonsillar Abscess.** *Streptococcus pyogenes* is the organism most frequently associated with peritonsillar abscess, but other pathogens, including *Staphylococcus aureus,* have been noted. Drainage, along with appropriate antimicrobial therapy, is often needed for successful treatment.

Ramsey PG, Weymuller EA: Complications of bacterial infection of the ears, paranasal sinuses, and oropharynx in adults. Emerg Med Clin North Am 3:143–159, 1985.

V. TRACHEOBRONCHITIS

A. **Acute Bronchitis.** Most cases of acute bronchitis are associated with viruses (rhinovirus, coronavirus, influenza A and B viruses, adenovirus, measles virus) or are due to *Mycoplasma pneumoniae.* Treatment is symptomatic with cough suppressants, rest, and hydration. Antibiotics are not recommended unless infection with *M. pneumoniae* or *Bordetella pertussis* is suspected. During influenza A epidemics, treatment with amantadine may be considered if the illness is of less than 48 hours' duration.

B. **Chronic Bronchitis: Acute Infectious Exacerbations.** Respiratory viruses frequently cause exacerbations of chronic bronchitis. Since patients with chronic bronchitis are often colonized with *Streptococcus pneumoniae,* unencapsulated *Hemophilus influenzae,* and *Moraxella catarrhalis,* a sputum Gram stain will usually reveal these organisms during periods of acute exacerbation. After a sputum culture has been obtained, antimicrobial therapy may be directed against *H. influenzae* and *S. pneumoniae.* **Amoxicillin 250 mg po tid, tetracycline 500 mg po qid, or trimethoprim-sulfamethoxazole, 1 double-strength tablet (160 mg/800 mg) po bid, may be chosen.** If *Moraxella catarrhalis,* which often produces penicillinase, is suspected by Gram stain, **amoxicillin-clavulanate 250 mg po tid** should be employed. Prophylactic and chronic antibiotic therapy is controversial and should be considered only in selected patients with frequent exacerbations. Influenza and pneumococcal vaccines should be given to these patients.

C. **Bacterial Tracheitis.** Bacterial tracheitis is uncommon in adults, with the exception of patients who have had tracheal injury due to viral infection or intubation. Community-acquired organisms include *Staphylococcus aureus,* group A beta-hemolytic streptococci, and *Hemophilus influenzae* type B. Hospital-acquired infection is more likely to be caused by gram-negative pathogens. In the ICU, it is important to differentiate colonization from infection. Fever, stridor, dyspnea, or grossly purulent sputum suggests infection. Empiric therapy should be directed toward the organisms seen on the Gram stain, when infection is suspected.

VI. PNEUMONIA

Initial antimicrobial therapy for pneumonia is often based on limited information and may be empiric. A sputum Gram stain and subsequent culture provide the most valuable information to guide therapy. The method of sputum collection (expectorated, nasotracheal, transtracheal needle aspiration, bronchoscopic, or open lung biopsy) should be tailored to the condition of the individual patient. A satisfactory sputum sample contains fewer than 10 epithelial cells and more than 25 white blood cells per low-power field with a predominating organism. When an expectorated sputum specimen is inadequate and does not enable the clinician to detect an etiologic agent, a more invasive method for obtaining sputum may be considered before beginning therapy. Alternatively, in selected patients, other information, such as age group, predisposing conditions, and where the pneumonia was acquired, can be used to guide initial antibiotic selection.

A. Community-Acquired Pneumonia: Factors to Consider in Antibiotic Selection

1. **YOUNG ADULTS**
   Mycoplasma pneumoniae, respiratory viruses, *Chlamydia pneumoniae*, and pneumococcus are the major etiologic agents. *Legionella* may cause approximately 1% of cases in this population. Empiric therapy with erythromycin is often employed if sputum is not available and the patient is not severely ill.

2. **OLDER ADULTS**
   Bacterial pathogens are more common than in younger adults (*Streptococcus pneumoniae*, *Legionella pneumophila*, *Hemophilus influenzae*, and *Staphylococcus aureus*). Vigorous attempts to identify the etiologic agent are indicated.

3. **NURSING HOME RESIDENTS AND THE ELDERLY**
   Pneumonia is more likely to be due to gram-negative organisms, including *Klebsiella pneumoniae*, *H. influenzae,* and *Enterobacter-aerogenes*. Pneumococcal and staphylococcal pneumonias are also prevalent.

4. **ALCOHOLISM**
   As the causative agent of pneumonia associated with alcoholism, *S. pneumoniae* is most common, followed by anaerobes, *H. influenzae*, *K. pneumoniae,* and *Mycobacterium tuberculosis*.

5. **ASPIRATION PNEUMONIA**
   When consciousness is altered or normal airway protective reflexes are impaired, the resulting pneumonia reflects the flora of the oropharynx. *Bacteroides melaninogenicus, Fusobacterium* spp., and anaerobic gram-positive cocci are the most common anaerobes isolated. *Streptococcus* spp. are the most common aerobes isolated in community-acquired aspiration pneumonia, while gram-negative bacilli and *S. aureus* are the most common aerobic isolates in the hospital setting.

6. **Chronic Obstructive Pulmonary Disease**

   H. influenzae, S. pneumoniae, and *Moraxella catarrhalis* predominate as the causes of pneumonia associated with chronic obstructive pulmonary disease.

7. **Cystic Fibrosis**

   In pneumonia associated with cystic fibrosis, *S. aureus* and *H. influenzae* prevail in younger patients, followed later by *Pseudomonas aeruginosa.*

8. **Postinfluenza Bacterial Pneumonias**

   S. pneumoniae, S. aureus, or *H. influenzae* may cause this type of pneumonia.

B. **Hospital-Acquired Pneumonia: Factors to Consider in Antibiotic Selection.** The oropharynx is often colonized with gram-negative organisms. Anaerobes are also in high concentration and may be aspirated. Colonization with these organisms must be distinguished from infection and therapy directed accordingly. *Mechanical ventilation* markedly increases the risk of pulmonary superinfection and nosocomial pneumonia. The presence of radiographic infiltrates, fever, and purulent sputum strongly suggests pneumonia, but infection may be difficult to distinguish from bacterial colonization in the severely ill patient. Misguided, prolonged broad-spectrum antibiotic therapy may result in colonization and subsequent infection with multiply resistant organisms. Most nosocomial pneumonias occurring in the setting of mechanical ventilation are caused by enteric and nonenteric aerobic gram-negative rods.

C. **Principles of Therapy.** For most patients with pneumonia, hospitalization is indicated for IV antibiotics and hydration, monitoring of respiratory status, and good pulmonary toilet. Oxygen should be given, if indicated by respiratory status. Young people with mycoplasmal, mild pneumococcal, or viral pneumonia may be followed closely as outpatients and treated with oral antibiotics.

   After appropriate cultures are obtained, initial antibiotic coverage should be directed at the most likely pathogen or pathogens indicated by the sputum Gram stain, considering the mode of acquisition and host factors. Initial coverage should be broader in the seriously ill patient, pending results of diagnostic studies.

D. **Therapy by Organism for Pneumonia**

   1. **Gram-Positive Organisms**

      a. *Streptococcus pneumoniae.* In the young, healthy adult, erythromycin or penicillin V, given orally, may be adequate. If extrapulmonary sites are involved or the patient is seriously ill, **aqueous penicillin G, 1 to 2 MU IV every 4 hours,** should be given. **Procaine penicillin G, 300,000 to 600,000 U every 12 hours IM,** can be used if the patient is not hospitalized. Therapy should be continued for at least 2 to 3 days after the temperature returns to normal. Elderly individuals and patients with extrapulmonary sites should receive at least 7 days of parenteral therapy.

    b. *Staphylococcus aureus.* A beta-lactamase stable penicillin (e.g., nafcillin) should be used initially until the organism's susceptibilities are known. Treatment is usually continued for 3–4 weeks.

2. GRAM-NEGATIVE ORGANISMS
Most gram-negative pneumonias are hospital-acquired and result from aspiration of oropharyngeal contents. Two antimicrobial agents should be used initially when the pathogen is unknown. Treatment is usually continued for 2–3 weeks, guided by the response of the patient.

    a. *Klebsiella pneumoniae.* **Mild disease may be treated with a single agent (e.g., a first-generation cephalosporin, such as cefazolin 1 gm IV every 8 hours or cephalothin 2 gm IV every 6 hours).** An **aminoglycoside** should be added for synergy in more seriously ill patients, especially for the first few days of therapy. Depending on susceptibility data, a single second-generation or third-generation cephalosporin (e.g., ceftriaxone) may be used.

    b. *Pseudomonas aeruginosa.* **Combination therapy with an antipseudomonal penicillin (e.g., ticarcillin) or cephalosporin (e.g., ceftazidime) plus an aminoglycoside (e.g., gentamicin) is indicated.** A third-generation cephalosporin alone is not adequate, and the role of other single agents (e.g., imipenem) remains unproved.

    c. *Hemophilus influenzae.* **Known beta-lactamase–negative strains should be treated with ampicillin, 1–2 gm IV every 4–6 hours for 10 days.** Patients with a penicillin allergy may receive **cefuroxime.** If cephalosporins cannot be given, chloramphenicol is an alternative. Ampicillin-resistant organisms can be treated with cefuroxime, a third-generation cephalosporin, ampicillin/sulbactam, or chloramphenicol.

3. ASPIRATION PNEUMONIA WITH MIXED ORGANISMS

    a. Community-Acquired Infection. Penicillin G, 1–2 MU IV every 4 hours, is usually adequate. The patient with a penicillin allergy may receive a first-generation cephalosporin or clindamycin.

    b. Hospital-Acquired Infection. Broad-spectrum antibiotics (e.g., cephalosporin and aminoglycoside combinations) are usually begun to cover gram-negative organisms until culture results are known. Newer antibiotics, such as ticarcillin-clavulanate and imipenem-cilastatin, also provide excellent coverage.

4. OTHER INFECTIONS

    a. *Mycoplasma pneumoniae.* Infection with this organism may be treated with erythromycin or tetracycline, 250–500 mg po every 6 hours for 2 weeks.

    b. Legionnaires' Disease (*L. pneumophila* **and** *L. micdadei***).** Erythromycin, 0.5–1.0 gm IV or po every 6 hours for 3 weeks, should be given to patients with this disease.

    c. Q Fever and Psittacosis. Either tetracycline 500 mg po qid, doxycycline 100 mg po bid, or chloramphenicol 50 to 100 mg/kg/day po or IV (divided into q 6-h doses) given for 2 weeks is effective against these diseases.

   d. Viral Pneumonia. Influenza is the most common cause of viral pneumonia in adults. Amantadine may speed improvement (Table 3–5).
   e. *Pneumocystis carinii.* Infection with this organism is discussed under "Acquired Immunodeficiency Syndrome (AIDS)" (Table 3–6, p. 90).
   f. *Pseudomonas pseudomallei.* This agent is endemic to Southeast Asia and the South Pacific. Therapy should be based on susceptibility data. Tetracycline 500 mg qid or trimethoprim-sulfamethoxazole, 1 double-strength tablet (160 mg/800 mg) po bid, is often effective. Ceftazidime (1.5 gm IV q 8 h) should be administered to the severely ill patient.
   g. *Yersinia pestis* (Plague) and *Francisella tularensis* (Tularemia). An aminoglycoside (streptomycin or gentamicin) is the agent of choice. Tetracycline may also be effective, but relapses or treatment failures have been observed with short courses (e.g., those less than 2 weeks).

Donowitz GR, Mandell GL: Empiric therapy for pneumonia. Rev Infect Dis 5:S40–S50, 1983.

E. Lung Abscess. Lung abscesses appear radiographically as one or more large cavities with air-fluid levels or as multiple small cavities, as seen in necrotizing pneumonia. Most abscesses form after aspiration of oropharyngeal organisms. Necrotizing pneumonias are usually caused by anaerobes, *Klebsiella,* other gram-negative bacteria, or *Staphylococcus aureus.* Septic emboli to the lung may also result in abscess formation. Transtracheal aspiration, empyema fluid, blood cultures, or percutaneous transthoracic aspiration is often needed to obtain useful specimens for culture. Therapeutic options include:

   1. BRONCHOSCOPY may be required therapeutically, as well as diagnostically, if the patient is not expectorating sputum and improving. Postural drainage is also helpful. Patients not responding to these methods and to antibiotics may need surgical drainage.

   2. HIGH-DOSE PENICILLIN (6 to 12 MU/day) can be successful in the mildly ill patient. Because of the increased incidence of penicillin-resistant anaerobes, **metronidazole** should be added in serious anaerobic infections, pending susceptibility data. **Clindamycin** is a good choice in the penicillin-allergic patient. Imipenem, ticarcillin-clavulanate, ampicillin-sulbactam, and chloramphenicol are also active against most anaerobes.

   3. A penicillinase-resistant penicillin is preferred for known staphylococcal abscesses. Vancomycin or a cephalosporin may be appropriate in the patient allergic to penicillin. For group A streptococcal infection, penicillin G is the agent of choice. Two agents (an aminoglycoside and a cephalosporin) should be used for infection due to *K. pneumoniae* or other facultative or aerobic gram-negative bacilli in the seriously ill patient.

Bartlett JG, Gorbach SL, Tally FP et al: Bacteriology and treatment of primary lung abscess. Am Rev Respir Dis 109:510, 1974.

Text continued on page 92

TABLE 3–5. ANTIVIRAL CHEMOTHERAPY

VIRUS	DISEASE OR GOAL OF TREATMENT	TREATMENT
Nonimmunocompromised Host		
Herpes simplex virus (HSV)	Primary genital HSV	Topical: 5% acyclovir (ACV) ointment 5/day for 7 days
		Oral: ACV, 200 mg 5/day for 10 days*
		IV: ACV, 5 mg/kg q 8 hr for 5 days
	Recurrent	Oral: ACV, 200 mg 5/day for 5 days
	Suppression	Oral: ACV, 200 mg bid–tid for 4–6 mo
	Encephalitis	IV: ACV 10–15 mg/kg q 8 hr for 10 days
	Keratoconjunctivitis	Topical: 1% trifluorothymidine ophthalmic solution, 1 drop q 2 hr while awake (9 drops/day maximum) After re-epithelialization, 1 drop 5/day for 7 days
		Oral: ACV, 800 mg 5/day for 10 days
		IV: ACV, 5 mg/kg q 8 hr (rarely indicated)
Varicella zoster virus (VZV)	Prophylaxis against varicella	IM: varicella zoster immune globulin, 625 U (5 vials)
Immunocompromised Host		
HSV	Prophylaxis	Oral: ACV, 400 mg 5/day
		IV: ACV, 250 mg/m^2 q 8 hr
	Treatment	Oral: ACV, 400 mg 5/day for 10 days (or until 3 days after healing)
		IV: ACV, 250 mg/m^2 q 8 hr for 7 days
	Suppression	Oral: ACV, 200 mg 2–3/day; increase if reactivation occurs

Virus	Indication	Regimen
VZV	Zoster or varicella	IV: ACV, 500 mg/m^2 q 8 hr for 7 days
	Prophylaxis	IM: varicella zoster immune globulin, 625 U (5 vials)
Influenza A	Prophylaxis	Oral: amantadine, 200 mg/day for 5–7 wk† or only for 10–14 days after influenza vaccination
	Treatment	Oral: amantadine, 200 mg/day for 3–5 days† (start within 24–48 hr of disease onset)
Influenza A and B, respiratory syncytial virus	Treatment	Aerosol: ribavirin (diluted to 20 mg/ml) given 12 hr/day for 3 days
Human immunodeficiency virus (HIV)	Suppression	Oral: azidothymidine (AZT), 100 mg po 5/day
Cytomegalovirus (CMV) retinitis, pneumonia, hepatitis, GI tract	Treatment	IV: ganciclovir, 5 mg/kg q 12 hr for 14 days
	Relapse	IV: ganciclovir, 6 mg/kg qd

*Adjustments for renal impairment:
1. Acyclovir: for the following creatinine clearance ranges, give 1.73 mg/m^2 at these adjusted intervals:
   >50 ml/min, dose q 8 hr
   24–50 ml/min, dose q 12 hr
   10–25 ml/min, dose q 24 hr
   <10 ml/min, halve dose q 24 hr
2. Amantadine: daily amantadine dose (in mg) = 200 × (patient's creatinine clearance in ml/min ÷ 120).

In elderly, use 1.4 mg/kg/day, if normal renal function.

†For additional information, see the following references: Dorsky DI, Crumpacker CS: Drugs five years later: Acyclovir. Ann Intern Med 107:859–874, 1987. Hermans PE, Cockerill FR: Antiviral chemotherapy. Infect Dis Clin North Am 1: vol 1, no 2, 1987. Gold D, Corey L: Acyclovir prophylaxis for herpes simplex virus infection. Antimicrob Agents Chemother 31:361–367, 1987. Knight V, Gilbert BE (eds): Antiviral agents. Mayo Clin Proc 62:1108–1115, 1987.

TABLE 3–6. TREATMENT OF OPPORTUNISTIC INFECTIONS IN PATIENTS WITH AIDS

INFECTION	TREATMENT	DURATION	COMMENTS
Pneumocystis carinii pneumonitis	TMP-SMZ (TMP 20 mg/kg/day; SMZ 100 mg/kg/day) po or IV in 4 divided doses TMP, 20 mg/kg/day po, in 4 divided doses and dapsone, 100 mg/day po Pentamidine isethionate, 4 mg/kg/day IV	14–21 days	Side effects: rash, fever, neutropenia, thrombocytopenia, hepatitis Side effects: hemolysis in G-6-PD deficiency, methemoglobinemia Side effects: neutropenia, hypoglycemia, renal/hepatic toxicity, orthostatic hypotension Maintenance therapy: TMP-SMZ, 1 double-strength tablet po bid 3 × /week or aerosolized pentamidine, 300 mg/month
Cryptococcal meningitis	Amphotericin B, 0.5–1.0 mg/kg/day IV with or without Fluconazole	To 1.5 grams over 6 wk	Maintenance therapy: Fluconazole, 100–200 mg po qd Avoid 5-FC in patients with bone marrow suppression
Toxoplasmosis	Sulfadiazine sodium, 6–8 gm/day po (after 6 wk reduce to 2 gm), *and* Pyrimethamine, 100–200 mg loading dose and then 75–100 mg/day po (after 6 wks, reduce to 25–50 mg), *with* Leucovorin, 10–50 mg/day po	Indefinite	Biopsy if no clinical response; if neutropenia develops: pyrimethamine (50 mg/day) alone or with clindamycin (450–600 mg qid)

Condition	Therapy	Duration	
Mycobacterium avium-intracellulare infection	No standard effective therapy	—	Investigational drugs: ansamycin, clofazimine, ciprofloxacin, with other antituberculous agents
Mycobacterium tuberculosis infection	See "Tuberculosis," p 92	—	
Cryptosporidiosis	No effective therapy	—	Supportive plus antidiarrheal agents
Oral candidiasis	Clotrimazole troche, 10 mg 5/day Nystatin, gargle and swallow 100,000 U qid If refractory to above, then ketoconazole, 200 mg po qd, or fluconazole, 100–200 mg po qd	Until resolved	Suppression: clotrimazole 1–2 troches/day, ketoconazole, 200 mg/day, or fluconazole, 100–200 mg po qd
Esophageal candidiasis	Ketoconazole, 400 mg/day po Fluconazole, 200–400 mg/day po	Until resolved	Maintenance: ketoconazole, 200 mg/day or clotrimazole troche 5/day
Cytomegalovirus infection (disseminated, pulmonary, GI tract, retina)	Ganciclovir 5 mg/kg IV bid	Unknown	Maintenance dose 6 mg/kg/day Side effects: leukopenia
Herpes simplex infection (mild) (severe)	Acyclovir 200–400 mg 5/day po Acyclovir 10 mg/kg IV q 8 hrs, or 800 mg 5/day po	7–10 days 7–10 days	Maintenance: acyclovir, 200 mg bid or tid
Herpes zoster infection	Acyclovir 10–15 mg/kg IV q 8 hrs, or 800 mg 5/day po	Minimum of 5 days, until crusted	—

For further information, see Sande MA, Volberding PA (eds): The Medical Management of AIDS. 3rd ed. Philadelphia. W. B. Saunders Company, 1992.

F. Tuberculosis. Pulmonary disease is the most common clinical manifestation of *Mycobacterium tuberculosis* infection. The diagnosis is suggested by chest x-ray and is confirmed by isolation of the organism from sputum. Newer culture techniques have shortened the time needed to demonstrate the organism. Acid-fast bacilli (AFB) can often be visualized on stained sputum smears. Fluorochrome smears have improved the sensitivity and specificity of sputum examination. Skin test reactivity identifies those who have been exposed to the organism but who have subclinical disease. However, there are a number of reasons that patients have false-negative skin test reactions, including overwhelming tuberculosis.

1. **THERAPY**

Antimicrobial therapy for *active* tuberculosis should always include at least 2 agents to which the organism is known to be susceptible. More than one active agent appears to be necessary to prevent the emergence of resistant strains. Therapy for active tuberculosis must always be prolonged, because of the slow growth of the organism.

   a. 9-Month Therapy. The standard therapy for patients with pulmonary tuberculosis and for many patients with extrapulmonary tuberculosis is **isoniazid (INH) (300 mg) plus rifampin (600 mg) and pyridoxine (50 mg)** taken po qd on an empty stomach. **One additional agent** (either ethambutol 15 mg/kg or streptomycin 1 gm) is given daily during the first 6–8 weeks while awaiting sensitivity data. For the remainder of the 9 months, INH and rifampin can be given either daily or twice weekly (increase the dose of INH to 900 mg when given twice weekly).

   b. 6-Month Therapy. Short-course chemotherapy for pulmonary tuberculosis was developed to optimize patient compliance and thereby increase the likelihood of therapeutic success. One currently accepted 6-month regimen for uncomplicated tuberculosis consists of an **initial 2 months of daily rifampin (600 mg), INH (300 mg), pyrazinamide (30 mg/kg), and pyridoxine (50 mg) followed by 4 months of daily rifampin, isoniazid, and pyridoxine.** While awaiting sensitivity data, ethambutol (15 mg/kg/day) should be added to the treatment regimen for patients with a history of previous INH therapy or emigration within the past 30 years from a country with a high rate of drug-resistant tuberculosis.

   c. Special Treatment Circumstances. The following guidelines are useful in specific situations:

   (1). When INH cannot be used because of suspected or documented resistance or other reasons, rifampin and ethambutol may be used for 18 months.

   (2). When rifampin cannot be used, INH and ethambutol can be used for 18 months, with streptomycin for the first 6–8 weeks.

   (3). When neither INH nor rifampin is an option, at least 3 drugs to which the organism is sensitive should be used for at least 18 months.

(4). *In patients with renal disease,* neither ethambutol nor streptomycin is recommended. Pyrazinamide or ethionamide
should be considered.

(5). *In end-stage renal disease,* INH and rifampin can be used in
the usual doses and given after dialysis. Pyridoxine supplementation is necessary.

(6). *Pregnancy.* 9-month therapy can be used. INH, rifampin,
and ethambutol should be given during the first 6–8 weeks.
Streptomycin and pyrazinamide should be avoided.

(7). *HIV Infection or AIDS.* 9-month therapy is recommended:
INH (300 mg qd) and rifampin (600 mg qd), with either
pyrazinamide (30 mg/kg qd) or ethambutol (15 mg/kg qd) for
the initial 2 months.

2. FOLLOW-UP

Uncomplicated pulmonary tuberculosis can be managed in the outpatient setting. Contacts of the patient have usually been exposed
before diagnosis. A patient's sputum is usually not infectious after 2
weeks of effective therapy. Sputum smears and cultures should be
performed monthly until 3 consecutive specimens are negative. Cultures are then obtained at 2- to 3-month intervals and at 6 months
after therapy is completed. Chest x-rays are often done monthly until
sputum cultures yield negative findings and then at 2- to 3-month
intervals. Follow-up radiographs are obtained at the completion of
therapy and if reactivation is suspected. *The local public health
department should be involved in the follow-up of patients and in
contact tracing.* Contacts with evidence of active disease should be
identified and treated.

3. ISONIAZID THERAPY FOR SUBCLINICAL INFECTION

INH may be given for subclinical infection when a positive skin test
indicates the presence of viable bacilli with potential for reactivation.
Preventive chemotherapy involves INH 300 mg with pyridoxine 50
mg po qd for 6–12 months. High-dose INH (15 mg/kg), given twice
weekly, may also be considered for some patients. Patients should
be made aware of the signs of hepatitis, and liver function tests
should be performed if symptoms develop. Because of the risks of
INH-related hepatitis, preventive chemotherapy in those 21–35 years
of age is controversial. Hepatotoxicity is rare in patients under 20
years of age. For patients over the age of 35, chemotherapy without
signs of active disease may not be indicated. INH is contraindicated
in patients with a history of INH-related hepatitis.

Dutt AK, Moers D, Stead WW: Short-course chemotherapy for extrapulmonary tuberculosis.
Ann Intern Med 104:7–12, 1986.

Van Scoy RE, Wilkowske CJ: Antituberculous agents. Mayo Clin Proc 62:1129–1136, 1987.

Combs DL, O'Brien RJ, Geiter LJ: USPHS tuberculosis short-course chemotherapy trial 21:
Effectiveness, toxicity, and acceptability. Ann Intern Med 112:397–406, 1990.

Cohn DL, Catlin BJ, Peterson KL, et al: A 62-dose, 6-month therapy for pulmonary and
extrapulmonary tuberculosis. Ann Intern Med 112:407–415, 1990.

VII. CELLULITIS AND ANIMAL BITES

A. Cellulitis. Cellulitis is most frequently caused by group A streptococci and *Staphylococcus aureus*. Cultures of the "leading edge" rarely yield the causative agent but may be useful to identify rare pathogens (e.g., gram-negative rods) in some patients. Skin biopsies more frequently yield the causative organism but are rarely used except in complicated cases. Blood cultures seldom reveal the pathogen.

Initial antimicrobial therapy should be based on clinical presentation and a patient's underlying risk factors. Therapy can be adjusted based on the clinical response or according to blood and skin culture results, if positive. Antibiotics are usually given for 7–10 days. When there is clinical improvement, the course can be completed with oral agents. Patients with **cellulitis of the lower extremity can usually be treated effectively with a semisynthetic penicillin** such as nafcillin or with a **cephalosporin.** *Hemophilus influenzae* should be suspected in children or in adults with facial cellulitis. Aerobic gram-negative organisms may occasionally cause cellulitis in patients with diabetes or in immunosuppressed individuals. More broad-spectrum therapy is indicated for these patients, especially if they are severely ill.

Hook EW, Hooton TM, Horton CA, et al: Microbiologic evaluation of cutaneous cellulitis in adults. Arch Intern Med 146:295–297, 1986.

B. Animal Bites. Therapy for animal bites primarily consists of local care and tetanus prophylaxis (Table 3–7). Prophylactic antibiotics should be considered as adjunctive therapy. Local care consists of adequate wound irrigation and debridement. The risk of bacterial infection increases with delay in local care. Infections resulting from animal bites are often caused by *Pasteurella multocida,* whereas human bites are often complicated by *Staphylococcus aureus* infections. Aerobic and anaerobic cultures should be obtained from wound exudate. Gram stain may reveal the infecting organism. Penicillin is the antibiotic of choice for *Pasteurella multocida.*

VIII. SEXUALLY TRANSMITTED DISEASES

A. Gonorrhea. The increasing incidence of penicillin-resistant strains has made alternatives to penicillin important in the treatment of gonorrhea. Penicillin can still be used in areas where resistance is not a problem. Gram stains and cultures should be obtained from all sites that may be potentially infected because of the patient's sexual practices. Rectal cultures should be standard procedures for all women because of the potential for inoculation of this area from infected cervicovaginal secretions. Pharyngeal Gram stains are unreliable. For treatment recommendations listed below, tetracycline 500 mg po qid may be substituted for doxycycline.

1. UNCOMPLICATED ANOGENITAL GONORRHEA IN WOMEN AND HETEROSEXUAL MEN

   Ampicillin 3.5 gm po plus probenecid 1.0 gm po, followed by doxycycline 100 mg po bid given for 7 days, may be used in regions where penicillinase-producing strains of gonococcus are not a problem. Otherwise, either cefixime 400 mg po or ceftriaxone 125–250 mg IM, followed by doxycycline, 100 mg po bid for 7 days, is recommended. In patients with a history of anaphylaxis to beta-lactam antibiotics, give spectinomycin 2.0 grams IM or ciprofloxacin 500 mg po followed by doxycycline as above.

2. **UNCOMPLICATED ANOGENITAL GONORRHEA IN HOMOSEXUAL AND BISEXUAL MEN**
Cefixime 400 mg po, ceftriaxone 125–250 mg IM, or ciprofloxacin 500 mg po may be given, but ampicillin and probenecid should be avoided.

3. **PHARYNGEAL GONOCOCCAL INFECTION**
Cefixime 400 mg po, ceftriaxone 125–250 mg IM, or ciprofloxacin, 500 mg po may be used; *or* ampicillin 3.5 gm po, plus probenecid 1.0 gm po, followed by doxycycline 100 mg po bid given for 7 days.

4. **UNRELIABLE PATIENTS**
Ceftriaxone 125–250 mg IM can be selected for therapy, but ampicillin and probenecid should be avoided; ceftriaxone may be followed by doxycycline 100 mg po bid for 7 days, depending on perceived likelihood of compliance.

5. **PERSISTENT GONOCOCCAL INFECTION AFTER PREVIOUS TREATMENT; OR KNOWN CASES OF PENICILLIN RESISTANCE**
Ceftriaxone 250 mg IM may be used. As an alternative, spectinomycin 2 gm IM may be administered but is not effective for pharyngeal infection.

6. **PENICILLIN-ALLERGIC PATIENTS**
   a. **History of Late Onset, Atypical, or Undocumented Penicillin Allergy.** Cefixime 400 mg po, or ceftriaxone 125–250 mg IM, plus doxycycline 100 mg po bid for 7 days, can be used; the patient should be observed for 30 minutes after being given cephalosporin. Alternatively, ciprofloxacin 500 mg po followed by doxycycline may be employed.
   b. **History of Anaphylaxis or Immediate Urticaria.** Spectinomycin 2 gm IM or ciprofloxacin 500 mg po, plus doxycycline (100 mg bid) for 7 days, may be selected.

7. **MANAGEMENT OF CONTACTS**
All partners at risk should be examined, cultured, and treated; although there is no time period that will encompass all circumstances, in most cases the following should be considered *minimal* criteria.
   a. **Symptomatic Patients.** All partners within *2 weeks* before *onset* of symptoms should be examined.
   b. **Asymptomatic Patients.** All partners within *4 weeks* before *diagnosis* should be examined.

B. **Syphilis.** Penicillin remains the drug of choice for syphilis, and there are no resistant strains. *Treponema pallidum* cannot be cultured. Diagnosis is made by darkfield examination of any lesions and by serology.

TABLE 3–7. IMMUNIZATIONS

DISEASE	VACCINE TYPE	SCHEDULE
Routine Immunizations		
Measles	LV*	Routine childhood
Mumps	LV*	Routine childhood
Rubella	LV*	Routine childhood; if not, before pregnancy
Poliomyelitis (oral poliovaccine, or OPV)	LV*	Routine childhood
Poliomyelitis (inactivated polio vaccine, or IPV)	KV	Nonimmunized adults
Pertussis	KB	Routine childhood
Diphtheria	BT	Routine childhood, booster every 10 yr
Tetanus	BT	Routine childhood, booster every 10 yr, and if tetanus-prone wound occurs, *with* tetanus immune globulin
Hemophilus influenzae type b	BP	Routine childhood
Travel Immunizations		
Yellow fever	LV*	Single shot every 10 yr
Rabies, Human diploid cell vaccine (HCDV)	KV	Pre-exposure: 3 doses; booster every 2 yr
		Postexposure: 5 doses with rabies immune globulin
Japanese encephalitis	KV	Limited availability: 3 shots, booster every 4 yr
Cholera	KB	2 shots, booster every 6 mo (single dose fulfills most travel requirements)
Typhoid	KB	2 shots (Note: oral vaccine now available)
Plague	KB	3 shots, booster every 6–12 mo
Meningococcus infection	BP	Single shot, no boosters (rarely needed)
Hepatitis A and B	IG	Single shot, booster every 3–6 mo (Hepatitis B KV vaccine provides better hepatitis B protection; see below)

Special Immunizations

Influenza A and B	KV	Single shot annually, for elderly, those with chronic diseases, and those with high exposure risk
Hepatitis B	KV	3 shots (at 0, 1, and 6 mo); need for boosters unknown; indicated for those at risk of exposure; postexposure in unimmunized person, give with HBIG
Pneumococcus infection	BP	Single shot, booster not needed for at least 5 yr; indicated for elderly and chronically ill
Hepatitis B immune globulin (HBIG)	IG	Give within 24–48 hr of exposure to blood containing high titer of HB_sAg or within 14 days of sexual contact; give with hepatitis B vaccine (additional HBIG needed 1 mo later if given without vaccine)
Immune globulin	IG	Give within 14 days of exposure to hepatitis A
Rabies immune globulin (RIG)	IG	Give postexposure in those unimmunized with rabies vaccine
Tetanus immune globulin	IG	Give postexposure with tetanus toxoid
Varicella zoster immune globulin	IG	Give postexposure in immunocompromised patients

LV = live virus; KV = killed virus; KB = killed bacteria; BT = bacterial toxoid; BP = bacterial polysaccharide; IG = immune globulin.
*Live virus vaccines are generally contraindicated in pregnancy and immunocompromised patients.

For all stages of syphilis, penicillin is the treatment of choice; if tetracycline is given, it is extremely important to counsel the patient firmly about adherence to the regimen, since deletion of only a few doses or slight shortening of therapy significantly increases the failure rate.

1. **EARLY SYPHILIS (PRIMARY, SECONDARY, AND EARLY LATENT SYPHILIS UP TO 1 YEAR IN DURATION)**
   Benzathine penicillin G 2.4 MU IM in a single dose should be given; *or* tetracycline 500 mg qid for 15 days (if there is well-documented allergy to penicillin) may be used. In addition, patients should be counseled about the possibility of a Jarisch-Herxheimer reaction.

2. **LATE SYPHILIS (MORE THAN 1 YEAR IN DURATION), EXCLUDING NEUROSYPHILIS**
   Benzathine penicillin G 2.4 MU IM weekly for 3 doses (total, 7.2 MU) is the treatment of choice. Tetracycline 500 mg qid for 30 days (if there is well-documented allergy to penicillin) is an alternative.

3. **NEUROSYPHILIS IN PATIENTS INFECTED 1 YEAR OR MORE, BOTH SYMPTOMATIC AND ASYMPTOMATIC**

   a. **Treatment of Choice.** Hospitalization is required for administration of penicillin G, 2 to 3 MU IV every 4 hours for 10 days, followed by benzathine penicillin G, 2.4 MU IM weekly for 3 doses.

   b. **Outpatient Alternative.** The following is effective: procaine penicillin G 2.4 MU IM once daily, plus probenecid 500 mg qid, both for 10 days, followed by benzathine penicillin G 2.4 MU IM weekly for 3 doses.

   c. **Patients with History of Penicillin Allergy.** The patient should be referred for penicillin skin testing; if skin testing confirms an allergy, penicillin desensitization should be considered; a 10-day course of ceftriaxone may be an effective alternative, but data are incomplete; the efficacy of erythromycin and tetracycline is not established for neurosyphilis.

4. **FOLLOW-UP**

   a. **Syphilis in Pregnancy.** The follow-up of pregnant patients with syphilis is individualized, but most patients should be seen on the following schedules.

   b. **Early Syphilis (Primary, Secondary, and Early Latent).** A clinical examination should be performed 1 week after treatment; the serology (quantitative Venereal Disease Research Laboratory [VDRL]) should be repeated 1, 3, 6, and 12 months after treatment.

   c. **Neurosyphilis.** The serology should be repeated as for late syphilis, and follow-up lumbar punctures should be given at 3- to 4-month intervals until results are normal (includes patients having early syphilis with abnormal cerebrospinal fluid).

5. **MANAGEMENT OF CONTACTS**

Contacts of patients with early syphilis should receive routine history, examination, and syphilis serology, including rapid plasma reagin (RPR); treatment should be administered for all contacts within the preceding 3 months. In **contacts of patients with late syphilis,** serologic studies should be performed (including fluorescent treponemal antibody absorption [FTA-ABS] even if the VDRL is negative) in all chronic (e.g., marital) contacts and in the children of infected women.

C. **Nongonococcal and Postgonococcal Urethritis.** The major causes of nongonococcal urethritis (NGU) and postgonococcal urethritis (PGU) are *Chlamydia trachomatis* and, less often, *Ureaplasma urealyticum*. A Gram stain should be performed, along with culture for *Neisseria gonorrhoeae* and *C. trachomatis*.

1. **INITIAL OR ISOLATED EPISODE (NO EPISODE WITHIN THE PREVIOUS 6 WEEKS)**

Doxycycline 100 mg bid (or tetracycline, 500 mg qid) may be given for 7 days; *or* erythromycin stearate or base 500 mg qid (or enteric-coated erythromycin base 666 mg tid), can be used for 7 days when a tetracycline is contraindicated or not tolerated.

Trimethoprim-sulfamethoxazole (Bactrim, Septra), one double-strength tablet bid for 7 days, can be administered if neither tetracycline nor erythromycin is tolerated.

Sexual abstention should be advised until symptoms have resolved and treatment of both patient and partner is complete.

2. **IMMEDIATE TREATMENT FAILURE (PERSISTENT URETHRITIS WHILE ON THERAPY OR RECRUDESCENCE IMMEDIATELY AFTER TREATMENT COMPLETION)**

Urethritis must be confirmed by examination and laboratory studies. A urethral wet mount and culture for *Trichomonas* should be obtained; if the wet mount is negative, the patient should be re-treated with erythromycin, as above (or with tetracycline, as above, if erythromycin was used initially), pending the results of the *Trichomonas* culture.

3. **RECURRENCE OF URETHRITIS WITHIN 6 WEEKS FOLLOWING APPARENT RESOLUTION**

It should be confirmed that the treatment regimen was followed and that sexual contact limitations were followed (or that the partner was examined and treated). The patient should be treated with erythromycin 500 mg qid for 2–4 weeks or with doxycycline 100 mg bid for 2–4 weeks (if the original treatment was erythromycin).

4. **MANAGEMENT OF CONTACTS**

For regular partners and source contacts, these persons should be examined and treated with doxycycline, tetracycline, or erythromycin. In contacts of men with recurrent NGU, the need and value of treatment are unknown.

D. Mucopurulent Cervicitis. The leading cause of nongonococcal muco-purulent cervicitis (MPC) is *Chlamydia trachomatis*. However, other considerations include herpetic cervicitis, trichomoniasis, candidiasis, vaginitis due to foreign bodies or chemical irritation, and IUDs, all of which may be associated with polymorphonuclear neutrophils (PMNs) in endocervical smears and occasionally with other signs suggestive of MPC. The diagnosis of MPC should be made with caution when any of these conditions is present.

1. **TREATMENT OF NONGONOCOCCAL MUCOPURULENT CERVICITIS**
Doxycycline 100 mg bid may be administered for 7 days; or erythromycin base or stearate 500 mg qid (or enteric-coated erythromycin base 666 mg tid) may be given for 7 days; in the case of severe gastrointestinal intolerance, erythromycin should be given with food, the dose should be halved, and therapy should be extended to 14 days.
    Persistent or recurrent MPC should be **re-treated** if therapeutic compliance appears to have been suboptimal. If the patient has a new or untreated partner, or if the initial antibiotic was erythromycin, a switch to tetracycline or doxycycline is in order.

2. **MANAGEMENT OF CONTACTS**
When NGU or gonorrhea is present, the condition should be treated accordingly. In those with no urethritis, regular and source contacts should be treated as for NGU; treatment of other contacts should be deferred, pending culture results.

E. Pelvic Inflammatory Disease. *Neisseria gonorrhoeae* and *Chlamydia trachomatis* are the most common causes of pelvic inflammatory disease (PID). A cervical Gram stain, plus cultures for *N. gonorrhoeae* and *C. trachomatis* should be performed. Culturing the cervix for other bacteria is not necessary. When PID is suspected, IUDs should be removed, if present. Hospitalization is recommended when patients are unable or unwilling to follow outpatient regimens, as well as when pregnancy, pelvic abscess, or an unclear diagnosis is a consideration.

1. **INPATIENTS**
Doxycycline 100 mg IV bid and cefoxitin 2 gm IV qid should be given for at least 48 hours after the patient's fever subsides. Doxycycline 100 mg po bid should be continued to complete a 10–14 day course. An alternative treatment is clindamycin 600 mg IV qid plus gentamicin or tobramycin IV for at least 48 hours after the patient improves. Then, clindamycin 450 mg po qid should be continued to complete a 10- to 14-day total course.

2. **OUTPATIENTS**
Ceftriaxone 250 mg IM, followed by doxycycline 100 mg bid or tetracycline 500 mg qid may be given for 10 days. Alternative loading regimens that may be substituted for ceftriaxone include cefoxitin 2 gm IM plus probenecid 1 gm po or spectinomycin, as for uncomplicated gonorrhea.

3. **Management of Contacts**

Examination and urethral smear and culture for *Neisseria gonorrhoeae* and *Chlamydia trachomatis* are imperative for all contacts within the preceding 4 weeks, regardless of symptoms. When gonorrhea or NGU is present, the condition should be treated accordingly. Persons in whom no urethritis is present should be treated as for NGU.

F. **Bacterial Vaginosis.** Bacterial vaginosis (BV) is associated with an overgrowth of *Gardnerella vaginalis* and anaerobic bacteria, with a decrease in the normal *Lactobacillus* flora. Saline wet mount or Gram stain of the vaginal secretions does not indicate BV, since it is frequently isolated in low numbers from normal women. Asymptomatic patients are usually not treated, unless the discharge is especially profuse.

1. **Treatment of Symptomatic Patients**

Metronidazole 500 mg bid should be administered for 7 days. Alcohol consumption should be avoided for 12 hours before and 24 hours after completion of therapy. This drug is contraindicated in pregnancy. As an alternative, amoxicillin-clavulanate 500 mg tid or clindamycin 300 mg po tid may be given for 7 days (effective in 50% of patients). These drugs may be used if the patient is pregnant or cannot tolerate metronidazole.

2. **Resistant or Recurrent BV**

The optimal treatment for recurrent BV is unknown; options include re-treatment with metronidazole or amoxicillin and simultaneous re-treatment of the patient and her regular sexual partner. If an IUD is present, its removal should be considered.

G. **Trichomonal Vaginitis.** *Trichomonas vaginalis* can be identified by microscopic examination of a saline wet mount of vaginal secretions. Culture should also be performed. The **treatment for trichomonal vaginitis is metronidazole, 2 gm po in a single dose.** Alcohol consumption should be avoided for 12 hours before and 24 hours after completion of therapy. In addition, sexual abstention is recommended until symptoms have improved and the partner or partners have been treated.

1. **Treatment Failure (Persistence or Recurrence Despite Sexual Abstention or After Intercourse Only with a Treated Partner)**

Metronidazole 500 mg bid may be administered for 7 days in cases of continued persistence or if there are 2 or more recurrences when reinfection is unlikely.

2. **Pregnant Women**

Clotrimazole vaginal tablets or 1% cream, 1 tablet or 1 applicatorful daily, can be used for 7 days; metronidazole is contraindicated in the first trimester and is of uncertain safety in the second and third trimesters.

3. **Management of Contacts**

Treatment should not be dispensed or prescribed for unexamined partners, nor should it be given to patients for distribution to partners.

In regular partners or source contacts a routine genitourinary examination should be performed; the contact should be treated with metronidazole, 2 gm in a single dose.

H. Candida Vulvovaginitis. Candidiasis is usually due to *Candida albicans*. Diagnosis is by microscopic examination of a wet mount or Gram stain of vaginal secretions. Culture is not routinely advised. Clotrimazole vaginal tablets or 1% cream, 1 dose daily, may be given for 7 days. Miconazole nitrate 2% vaginal cream, 1 application daily at bedtime, can be used for 7 days. Alternatively, in nonpregnant patients, fluconazole 200 mg po may be employed.

I. Acute Epididymitis. Acute epididymitis is often due to *Neisseria gonorrhoeae* or *Chlamydia trachomatis*. A Gram stain, as well as cultures of urethral swabs for these organisms, should be performed. Treatment recommendations are:

1. **CHLAMYDIAL EPIDIDYMITIS (PROVEN OR SUSPECTED)**
Doxycycline 100 mg bid (or tetracycline 500 mg qid) can be administered for 10 days.

2. **GONOCOCCAL EPIDIDYMITIS**
An effective treatment is ceftriaxone 250 mg IM (single dose), plus doxycycline or tetracycline, as described above, for 10 days.

3. **NONCHLAMYDIAL, NONGONOCOCCAL EPIDIDYMITIS**
Begin therapy with 250 mg of ceftriaxone IM (single dose), followed by doxycycline 100 mg bid, while awaiting urinalysis and culture results; a case of documented bacterial epididymitis should be referred for urologic consultation.

Handsfield HH (ed): Sexually transmitted diseases. Infect Dis Clin North Am Vol 1, No 1, 1987.
Handsfield HH, Schwebke JR: Sexually Transmitted Disease Clinic Clinical Practice Guidelines. Seattle, Seattle-King County Department of Public Health, 1991.
Holmes KK, Mardh P-A, Sparling PF, et al: Sexually Transmitted Diseases. New York, McGraw-Hill, 1984.

IX. URINARY TRACT INFECTIONS

The most commonly isolated pathogens infecting the urinary tract are from the Enterobacteriaceae family. Most uncomplicated urinary tract infections (UTI) are caused by *Escherichia coli*. Other frequently isolated bacteria are *Klebsiella, Enterobacter, Serratia, Proteus,* and *Providencia*. Coagulase-negative staphylococci, particularly *Staphylococcus saprophyticus*, are becoming more widely recognized as urinary tract pathogens, especially in young women. Infections with *Pseudomonas* spp., enterococci, and *Staphylococcus aureus* are associated with use of urinary tract instrumentation. *Chlamydia trachomatis* is linked with acute urethral syndrome (AUS) in women.

A Gram stain and culture of the urine are key in directing antimicrobial therapy. Colony counts of greater than 100,000/mL constitute "significant bacteriuria." Lower colony counts (10^2 to 10^4/mL) may be considered significant if obtained as a midstream urine specimen from a symptomatic female with pyuria. Sterile pyuria in a symptomatic woman suggests AUS. A yield of 3 or more types of bacteria in a culture probably is due to contamination. Blood cultures are essential for the patient with suspected pyelonephritis.

A. Acute Uncomplicated Urinary Tract Infection: Therapy. Traditional therapy for women with an acute, uncomplicated UTI has been a 7–10 day course of antibiotics. Single-dose and 3-day therapies may be as effective as 10-day therapy. Most UTIs in healthy, young, nonpregnant women without genitourinary tract abnormalities are due to *Escherichia coli* or *Staphylococcus saprophyticus*.

1. **REGIMEN OF CHOICE**
   The therapy of choice is trimethoprim-sulfamethoxazole, one double-strength tablet po bid for 3 days. If the patient is allergic to sulfonamides, amoxicillin 500 mg tid may be given for 3 days. If the patient is allergic to sulfonamides and penicillin, doxycycline 100 mg bid can be administered for 3 days. For more resistant organisms, the following can be considered: amoxicillin-clavulanate (250/125 mg po tid), oral cephalosporins (cephalexin 250–500 mg po qid), or a quinolone.

2. **FOLLOW-UP**
   A urinalysis of a midstream specimen and culture should be performed 3–7 days after completion of treatment. Women who have been given 3 days of trimethoprim-sulfamethoxazole should return if symptoms persist or recur. Men with UTI should be referred for urologic evaluation.

B. Acute Urethral Syndrome (AUS). Acute urethral syndrome, characterized by sterile pyuria, is often due to *Chlamydia trachomatis* (*Neisseria gonorrhoeae* and other causes of vaginitis must also be considered). Treatment is a 7-day course of doxycycline 100 mg po bid or tetracycline 500 mg po qid. An empiric trial may also be useful in patients with sterile cultures and no pyuria. Although tuberculosis should be considered in an older individual with sterile pyuria, *Mycobacterium tuberculosis* genitourinary infection is rare in young women.

C. Urinary Tract Infection in Males. A UTI in a male is considered complicated. Gonorrhea and NGU must be ruled out. In addition, a urine Gram stain and culture must be performed. Many infections have a prostatic focus, and a localization test should be considered. While awaiting culture results, **empiric treatment** may be begun with **trimethoprim-sulfamethoxazole (1 double-strength tablet po bid for 12–14 days).** Urologic evaluation is recommended.

D. Pyelonephritis. Pyelonephritis (fever, chills, flank pain, and white blood cell casts in the urine) may be treated on an outpatient or inpatient basis, depending on factors involving the patient.

1. **OUTPATIENTS**
   Recommended therapy includes either trimethoprim-sulfamethoxazole (1 double-strength tablet po bid) or ciprofloxacin (500 mg po bid) for 14–21 days to ensure eradication of infection.

2. INPATIENTS

Ampicillin (1 gm IV q 4–6 hours) with IV aminoglycoside therapy should be initiated pending culture results. Vancomycin may be substituted for ampicillin in the case of penicillin allergy. Patients may be discharged soon after clinical improvement but should receive oral antibiotics on an outpatient basis to complete a 14–21 day course.

3. FOLLOW-UP

The urine culture should be repeated 1–2 weeks after completion of therapy. Ultrasound examination of the kidneys and urologic evaluation should be considered in those patients not responding to appropriate antimicrobial therapy.

Asymptomatic bacteriuria often clears spontaneously in healthy nonpregnant females and does not require treatment. It should, however, be treated in pregnant women. Therapy for asymptomatic bacteriuria in the elderly is controversial.

Patients with bacteriuria and indwelling catheters should not be treated unless they are symptomatic. Symptomatic UTIs should be treated with antibiotics for short periods of time to sterilize the urine, but long courses should not be used to avoid selecting resistant organisms. Chronic antibiotic suppression is not effective in patients with chronic indwelling catheters.

E. **Acute Bacterial Prostatitis.** In acute bacterial prostatitis (fever and perineal discomfort), the urinalysis and culture generally yield positive findings. **Trimethoprim-sulfamethoxazole, 1 double-strength tablet bid for at least 14 days, is recommended.**

F. **Chronic Bacterial Prostatitis.** Chronic bacterial prostatitis may cause recurrent UTIs in men. Localization studies and urologic evaluation are recommended. **Prolonged treatment (6–12 weeks) with trimethoprim-sulfamethoxazole (1 double-strength tablet po bid) or ciprofloxacin (500 mg po bid)** may be effective.

Andriole VT (ed): Urinary tract infections. Infect Dis Clin North Am Vol 1, No 4, 1987.
Andriole VT: Urinary tract infections: Recent developments. J Infect Dis 156:865–869, 1987.
Gleckman RA: Treatment duration for urinary tract infections in adults. Antimicrob Agents Chemother 31:1–5, 1987.
Latham RH, Wong ES, Larson A, et al: Laboratory diagnosis of urinary tract infection in ambulatory women. JAMA 254:3333–3337, 1987.
Lipsky BA, Ireton RC, Fihn SD, et al: Diagnosis of bacteriuria in men: Specimen collection and culture interpretation. J Infect Dis 155:847–854, 1987.
Johnson JR, Stamm WE: Urinary tract infections in women: Diagnosis and treatment. Ann Intern Med 111:906–917, 1989.

X. INFECTIOUS DIARRHEA

Infectious diarrhea is diagnosed largely on the basis of stool cultures. Special techniques may be necessary to isolate likely pathogens based on clinical history. Gram stains of stool are generally not useful to identify specific organisms, with the exception of patients with *Campylobacter* gastroenteritis and *Staphylococcus aureus* enterocolitis. Gram stains, however, may reveal PMNs that would raise the possibility of an infectious cause requiring specific treatment.

Therapy is supportive in most cases of infectious diarrhea. The majority of patients can be rehydrated orally. Antispasmodics may actually be harmful in some cases, and in general, drugs such as diphenoxylate hydrochloride with atropine (Lomotil) should be avoided.

Treatment of diarrhea due to the following diseases is mainly supportive and does not require antimicrobials: viral gastroenteritis; infection with *Clostridium perfringens, S. aureus, E. coli 0157:H7, Bacillus cereus, Vibrio parahaemolyticus,* and *Aeromonas hydrophila;* and Ciguatera, scombroid, and shellfish poisoning. Table 3–8 provides recommendations for treating specific infections.

XI. BONE AND JOINT INFECTIONS

A. Infectious Bursitis. Infectious bursitis usually involves the prepatellar or olecranon bursa and is characterized by pain and swelling. A Gram stain of the bursa aspirate often provides an etiologic diagnosis even when the culture is negative. *Staphylococcus aureus* is the most common agent. Streptococci are the next most common bacteria involved, especially group A beta-hemolytic strains. Other organisms, such as atypical mycobacteria, are uncommon.

In most cases, the initial therapy should be parenteral with a semisynthetic penicillinase-resistant penicillin (nafcillin 1.0 to 1.5 gm IV every 4–6 hours). In patients with mild disease, oral therapy (dicloxacillin 250 to 500 mg po qid) may be used. The duration of treatment should be 14–21 days. Adequate drainage is required in all patients.

B. Intervertebral Disc Space Infections. Most intervertebral disc space infections in adults occur postoperatively. The operative site is often healed, with no signs of infection at presentation. Blood cultures should be done, and material for culture should be obtained from the disc space by needle aspiration. Cultures from the wound rarely reflect the true pathogen. *Staphylococcus aureus* is the most common pathogen, followed by *Staphylococcus epidermidis* and enteric gram-negative organisms.

Therapy is guided by the Gram stain and by culture of the material obtained by needle aspiration. If gram-positive cocci are involved, nafcillin should be given empirically. For infection with gram-negative bacteria a cephalosporin or a penicillinase-resistant penicillin plus an aminoglycoside should be used. If cultures are negative, therapy should be directed against *S. aureus.* If no improvement is noted after 2–3 weeks of appropriate antimicrobial therapy, aspiration should be reattempted. Surgery to obtain tissue for culture and to provide adequate drainage should be considered. The duration of therapy should be at least 4–6 weeks.

C. Infectious Arthritis. The most important step in the diagnosis of infectious arthritis is examination of fluid obtained by direct joint aspiration. A Gram stain and aerobic and anaerobic cultures should be obtained; in addition, a total leukocyte count and differential, a glucose level determination, and examination for crystals should be done. In patients with chronic arthritis and in immunosuppressed patients, mycobacterial and fungal cultures may be useful. Synovial tissue biopsy may be required for diagnosis of chronic arthritis (e.g., tuberculous arthritis).

TABLE 3–8. TREATMENT OF INFECTIOUS DIARRHEA

ORGANISM	THERAPY
Salmonella	
S. *choleraesuis*	Uncomplicated gastroenteritis: supportive only
S. *enteritidis*	Antibiotics prolong the carrier state
	Septicemia: treat as for enteric fever
S. *typhi*	Enteric fever: chloramphenicol, 500 mg IV or po q 4 hr for 21 days
	Alternates: ampicillin, 1–2 grams IV q 6 hr, or trimethoprim-sulfamethoxazole (TMP-SMZ), one double-strength tablet po q 12 hr, ciprofloxacin, 500 mg po q 12 hr
	Carriers (excreting >6 mo) with cholelithiasis: cholecystectomy, failing alternative antibiotics for 30 days
	Avoid antidiarrheal agents
Shigella	
S. *sonnei*	Bacillary dysentery: ampicillin (do not use
S. *flexneri*	amoxicillin), 500 mg IV or po q 6 h for 5–7 days, or TMP-SMZ, one double-strength tablet po q 12 hr for 5 days (for ampicillin-resistant strains), or ciprofloxacin, 500 mg po q 12 hr
	Avoid antidiarrheal agents
Yersinia sp.	
Y. *enterocolitica*	Enterocolitis and mesenteric adenitis: supportive care only
	Septicemia: tetracycline, 500 mg po q 6 h, or doxycycline, 100 mg po q 6 hr, TMP-SMZ, one double-strength tablet po q 12 hr
Y. *pseudotuberculosis*	Septicemia: ampicillin, 1–2 grams IV q 6 hr
Enteropathogenic	
Escherichia coli	Traveler's diarrhea: ciprofloxacin, 500 mg po bid, or TMP-SMZ, one double-strength tablet po bid, for 5 days, reduces duration
Campylobacter	Protracted symptoms: ciprofloxacin, 500 mg po bid, or erythromycin, 500 mg po qid for 3–4 wk
Clostridium difficile	Antibiotic-associated diarrhea: vancomycin, 125–500 mg po qid for 7 days, or metronidazole, 500 mg po tid for 10 days; oral cholestyramine may be used as adjunctive symptomatic therapy

For further information, see Gorbach SL (ed): Infectious diarrhea. Infect Dis Clin North Am, vol 2, no 3, 1988.

1. **ETIOLOGIC AGENTS**

   Of **bacterial agents,** gonococcal infection is the most common cause of monoarticular arthritis in those 15 to 40 years old. In adults with nongonococcal arthritis, *Staphylococcus aureus* is implicated in the majority of cases. *Streptococcus* spp. are the next most common causative agents. Gram-negative bacilli cause infectious arthritis in patients who are immunosuppressed or chronically debilitated and in those who are IV drug users. Anaerobic infections rarely occur. Of the **nonbacterial agents,** viral hepatitis and rubella are often complicated by arthritis. Parvovirus B19 has recently been recognized as a cause of acute arthritis. *Mycobacterium kansasii* and *M. tuberculosis* are uncommon causes of infectious arthritis. *Sporothrix schenckii* is the most common fungus that produces infectious arthritis. Arthritis is a feature of Lyme disease due to *Borrelia burgdorferi* (see under Lyme disease section, below).

2. **THERAPY**

   Appropriate therapy includes both adequate drainage of the joint (aspiration or open) and antimicrobial administration. Repeated aspiration is important both for removal of purulent material and to assess the effectiveness of antimicrobial therapy by repeat Gram stain, culture, and leukocyte count. Initial therapy should be parenteral. Oral antibiotics may be used later in the course, if adequate serum levels can be obtained. The duration of therapy should be at least 2–3 weeks and should be longer in gram-negative infections and those that do not respond promptly. Intra-articular installation of antibiotics is of dubious clinical value.

   a. *Staphylococcus aureus.* For arthritis produced by this organism, nafcillin 9–12 gm/day may be given in divided doses every 4 hours.

   b. **Streptococci.** Penicillin G 10 MU/day may be administered in divided doses every 4 hours. In penicillin-allergic patients, vancomycin or clindamycin may be substituted.

   c. **Gonococcal Arthritis.** In areas where there are no penicillin-resistant strains of *Neisseria gonorrhoeae,* the following may be given: penicillin G, 10 MU/day for 3 days, followed by amoxicillin 500 mg po tid for a total of 7 days of antibiotic therapy. When penicillin-resistant *N. gonorrhoeae* is a possibility, ceftriaxone is the drug of choice. In the patient allergic to penicillin, spectinomycin is an alternative.

   d. **Gram-Negative Bacilli.** Gentamicin (4.5 to 5.0 mg/kg/day in divided doses every 8 hours) and ticarcillin (15 to 18 gm/day in divided doses every 4 hours) may be administered.

   e. **Initial Treatment if Gram Stain Is Negative.** If no organisms are seen on the initial Gram stain in a young, healthy adult, therapy with penicillin should be started. In a patient with risk factors for *S. aureus* and gram-negative infections, nafcillin and gentamicin should be given, pending culture results.

   f. **Lyme Arthritis.** Arthritis develops late in the disease and is treated with high-dose IV penicillin or IV ceftriaxone (see below).

g. Fungal Arthritis. Arthritis caused by fungi is treated with amphotericin B, with the addition of 5-flucytosine if the organism is sensitive.

h. Prosthetic Joint Infections. These infections are best eradicated by removal of the prosthesis, together with debridement and antibiotic therapy. If detected very early, some infections may be cured with prolonged parenteral therapy (6 weeks), followed by oral antibiotics (3 months). Therapy must be individualized.

Goldenberg DL, Reed JI: Bacterial arthritis. N Engl J Med 312:764–771, 1985.

D. Lyme Disease. Lyme disease, a multisystem inflammatory disorder caused by the spirochete *Borrelia burgdorferi,* is transmitted via the bite of Ixodes ticks. Three clinical stages of illness are described. Stage 1 disease (localized disease) consists of constitutional flulike symptoms and a characteristic expanding skin lesion (erythema chronicum migrans). This lesion develops at the site of the tick bite and may be associated with regional lymphadenopathy. Stage 2 disease (disseminated) is characterized by additional skin lesions, migratory joint and muscle pains, regional or generalized lymphadenopathy, hepatitis, cardiac abnormalities (conduction system abnormalities, myocarditis, and pericarditis), and neurologic manifestations (meningitis, cranial neuropathies, and peripheral radiculopathy) that occur from weeks to months after the tick bite. Stage 3 disease (persistent), which may develop weeks to years after exposure to the spirochete, is associated with arthritis, and, less commonly, chronic neurologic symptoms or skin disease (acrodermatitis chronicum atrophicus).

Oral antibiotic therapy generally shortens stage 1 disease and prevents development of later stages in most patients. **Doxycycline (100 mg po bid) or tetracycline (250 mg po qid) for 10–30 days is recommended for most patients with stage 1 disease,** although treatment failures have been reported. **Amoxicillin (500 mg po qid) or erythromycin (250 mg po qid) for 10–30 days** can be used also. A Jarisch-Herxheimer reaction may occur in some patients. **Mild stage 2 disease** (e.g., facial palsy alone or a cardiac abnormality limited to first-degree atrioventricular block) should be treated with a course of oral antibiotics. For **advanced stage 2 or stage 3 disease,** therapy with ceftriaxone (1–2 gm IV qd) or penicillin G (3 MU IV q 4 hours) for 14–21 days is recommended and appears to be effective for many patients. Chronic arthritis seen in stage 3 disease may respond to prolonged oral doxycycline (100 mg po bid for 30 days).

Steere AC: Lyme disease. N Engl J Med 321:586, 1989.

E. Acute Osteomyelitis. Osteomyelitis is classified by its presumed pathogenesis as hematogenous, contiguous, or associated with peripheral vascular disease, each with its unique microbiology. In all cases of osteomyelitis, vigorous attempts should be made to determine the etiologic agent. Blood cultures are particularly important in hematogenous osteomyelitis. Needle aspiration of soft tissue or bone, joint fluid analysis, and open biopsy may be necessary to identify the organism.

1. **HEMATOGENOUS OSTEOMYELITIS**
Staphylococcus aureus is the most common pathogen. Gram-negative bacilli occur frequently in patients with sickle cell disease (*Salmonella*), in heroin addicts (*Pseudomonas*), and in patients with debilitating diseases. Anaerobic osteomyelitis is rare but can occur after anaerobic bacteremia.
Treatment consists of parenteral bactericidal agents in high doses. Therapy is usually continued for at least 4 weeks. Oral therapy may be attempted if the causative agent has been isolated and bactericidal levels can be attained with an appropriate oral antibiotic. Initial therapy, pending culture results, should be directed against *S. aureus* with a penicillinase-resistant semisynthetic penicillin. If gram-negative organisms are suspected on the basis of the clinical situation (e.g., in an IV drug user), an aminoglycoside should be added. Most cases of hematogenous osteomyelitis will be cured without surgery, unless there is poor clinical response or the hip joint is involved. Immobilization should be dictated by local symptoms.

2. **CONTIGUOUS FOCI OSTEOMYELITIS**
Osteomyelitis due to a nearby focus of infection develops indolently in older adults, often postoperatively, or with the presence of adjacent soft tissue infections. Blood cultures do not frequently yield positive results in this form of osteomyelitis but are indicated. Draining wounds often yield mixed cultures, and open biopsy or needle aspiration is necessary to determine the pathogen. *S. aureus* is still the most common agent isolated, but cultures are frequently mixed. *Staphylococcus epidermidis* is considered a pathogen, especially when prosthetic devices are present. Mixed infections often involve gram-negative bacteria. *Pseudomonas aeruginosa* is associated with puncture wounds of the feet and *Pasteurella multocida* with animal bites.
Therapy should be parenteral and directed toward the suspected pathogen. The duration of therapy should be at least 4 weeks. Surgical debridement of adjacent wounds is an important component of proper management.

3. **OSTEOMYELITIS ASSOCIATED WITH PERIPHERAL VASCULAR DISEASE**
This type of osteomyelitis most commonly occurs in the small bones of older diabetic patients, who are predisposed to tissue ischemia and trauma. Blood cultures are usually not helpful. Bone cultures obtained by needle aspiration or open biopsy are necessary to define the pathogens. Most infections are mixed, often staphylococci and streptococci, or a combination of staphylococci, streptococci, and organisms of the Enterobacteriaceae family. Anaerobes may also be present.
Antimicrobial therapy should be directed toward the etiologic agent for 4–6 weeks. Often surgical intervention is necessary, especially that involving limited amputations in diabetics.

F. **Chronic Osteomyelitis.** Persistent pain may be the only symptom of chronic osteomyelitis, and sinus tract or wound drainage may be the only clinical sign. Blood culture and wound sinus cultures are generally not helpful. Needle aspiration or open biopsy should be performed before antimicrobial therapy is started. Surgery is also often necessary for debridement. Staphylococcal and gram-negative infections are common. The optimal length of therapy has not been well defined. Parenteral agents may be given for 4–6 weeks, followed by oral agents for 6 months or longer.

G. Vertebral Osteomyelitis. This disease is a form of hematogenous osteomyelitis that is usually associated with UTI or pelvic infection in older adults or IV drug use in younger adults. Blood cultures are frequently not positive but should be done. It is essential to obtain material for culture by needle aspiration or open biopsy. *Staphylococcus aureus* is the most common pathogen. After a UTI, gram-negative organisms may be involved. *Pseudomonas aeruginosa* is a common infecting organism in IV drug users. Parenteral antibiotics effective against the identified pathogen are recommended for 4–6 weeks.

H. Tuberculous Osteomyelitis. Bone is a common extrapulmonary site of tuberculosis. A chest x-ray, a tuberculin skin test, and needle or open biopsy are part of the workup. The organism implicated is usually *Mycobacterium tuberculosis*, although rare cases of "atypical" mycobacteria have been reported. The recommended treatment is isoniazid and rifampin plus possibly other antimycobacterial agents for a prolonged period of 1–2 years.

I. Fungal Osteomyelitis. Fungal osteomyelitis caused by *Candida, Aspergillus,* or *Rhizopus* spp. is most frequently seen in the immunosuppressed host as part of a disseminated infection. Amphotericin B is indicated, but surgical intervention is often necessary for successful therapy.

Waldvogel FA, Vasey H: Osteomyelitis: The past decade. N Engl J Med 303:360–370, 1980.

XII. INFECTIVE ENDOCARDITIS

The majority of patients with infective endocarditis (IE) have a history of underlying heart disease, of either rheumatic or congenital origin. Some have no detectable valvular abnormalities but experience bacteremia, which leads to infection of the normal valve. The clinical presentation of endocarditis may be nonspecific (fever, fatigue, and arthralgia) or more suggestive of the diagnosis (fever, new heart murmur, and peripheral stigmata). The disease is described as "acute" or "subacute" based on the onset of symptoms. The key to laboratory diagnosis is the blood culture. Bacteremia is usually low grade and continuous. The urgency with which blood cultures must be obtained before instituting antimicrobial therapy depends on the presentation of the patient.

A. **Etiologic Agents.** The majority of IE cases are caused by streptococci or staphylococci. Of the streptococci, viridans streptococci predominate, followed by nonenterococcal group D streptococci and the enterococci. Previously damaged valves are infected with more virulent organisms, such as *Staphylococcus aureus,* pneumococci, gonococci, and group A beta-hemolytic streptococci. Infections caused by enterococci and *Hemophilus* spp. are variable in presentation. Coagulase-positive staphylococci are the most common staphylococci isolated from patients with IE who had previously normal valves. Coagulase-negative staphylococci frequently cause prosthetic valve IE. Less common causes are gram-negative bacilli, anaerobic bacteria, and fungi.

B. **Therapy.** All patients should be hospitalized for high-dose IV antibiotics and observed carefully for arrhythmias and hemodynamic deterioration. Antimicrobial therapy is based on isolation of the etiologic agent and determination of antimicrobial susceptibility. Initial treatment of the patient presenting with acute IE should be directed toward *S. aureus* with **nafcillin (2 gm every 4 hours) plus gentamicin (1 mg/kg every 8 hours). Vancomycin (1 gm every 12 hours)** may be substituted for nafcillin in the penicillin-allergic patient. Presumed IE with negative blood cultures is usually treated with penicillin or ampicillin plus an aminoglycoside for 4 weeks. When an organism is isolated, the MIC and MBC of the appropriate antibiotics should be ascertained. Knowing serum bactericidal levels may be helpful when somewhat resistant organisms are involved or if a course of therapy will be completed with oral antibiotics. In vitro killing should be achieved with peak serum dilutions of at least 1:8 and preferably 1:16 or more.

C. **Specific Therapy Based on Isolated Organism**

1. VIRIDANS STREPTOCOCCI

   Viridans streptococci sensitive to penicillin are most successfully killed with a combination of **aqueous penicillin G 2 to 4 MU IV every 4 hours or procaine penicillin 1.2 MU IM every 6** hours, combined with **gentamicin** 1 mg/kg body weight IV every 8 hours for the initial 1–2 weeks, followed by **penicillin** alone for a total antibiotic treatment duration of 4 weeks. Patients particularly susceptible to aminoglycoside toxicity may be treated with IV penicillin alone for 4 weeks. The second 2 weeks of penicillin therapy alone may be given orally if the patient is reliable and serum bactericidal levels are adequate on the usual dose of penicillin V, 1 gm po q 6 hours, with 0.5 gm of probenecid with each dose. Resistant viridans streptococci should be treated like enterococci. In the patient with a history of severe penicillin allergy or positive skin testing, cephalothin, 8 to 12 gm per day in divided doses every 4 hours, may be given. Vancomycin 1 gm every 12 hours is another alternative. Therapy should be continued for 4 weeks.

2. GROUP D STREPTOCOCCI

   These are classified as nonenterococcal or enterococcal. Infection with nonenterococcal *Streptococcus bovis* can be treated like that with susceptible viridans streptococci if the MICs are similar. For patients with enterococcal endocarditis, an aminoglycoside should be added for the full course of therapy. **Penicillin 3 MU IV every 4 hours, along with gentamicin 1 mg/kg IV every 8 hours** (or **streptomycin 0.5 gm every 12 hours IM**), is suggested for at least 4–6 weeks. In the patient with a history of penicillin allergy, skin testing and desensitization, if necessary, should be performed. Vancomycin, 1 gm every 12 hours, plus an aminoglycoside for 4–6 weeks is an alternative treatment. Recently, enterococci isolated from patients in Michigan, Massachusetts, and other locations have shown "high-level" resistance to all aminoglycosides. At present, endocarditis with these highly resistant enterococcal isolates cannot be treated effectively with antibiotics.

3. STAPHYLOCOCCI

   Nafcillin 2 gm IV every 4 hours or a **cephalosporin** (cephalothin 2 gm IV every 4 hours) should be started initially. If the isolate is subsequently found to be penicillin sensitive, penicillin G, 3 MU IV every 4 hours, may be substituted. The addition of gentamicin, 1 mg/kg every 8 hours, for the first 3–7 days may clear the bacteremia more rapidly. Therapy should continue for 6 weeks. If the patient is allergic to penicillin or the staphylococci are resistant to methicillin, vancomycin, 1 gm IV every 12 hours, is recommended. "Tolerant" staphylococci may be more difficult to treat. Concomitant gentamicin therapy or the addition of rifampin may be indicated.

4. ENTERIC GRAM-NEGATIVE RODS

   Infection with *Escherichia coli* or *Proteus mirabilis* can be treated with a combination of either ampicillin (2 gm IV every 4 hours) or penicillin (3 MU IV every 4 hours) with gentamicin (1.7 mg/kg IV every 8 hours). *Klebsiella* spp. require a combination of a cephalosporin and an aminoglycoside. Infection with *Serratia marcescens* is often refractory to medical therapy alone, and valve replacement may be required. *Pseudomonas* endocarditis is treated with gentamicin or tobramycin (1.7 mg/kg every 8 hours) plus ticarcillin (18 grams per day). Left-sided *Pseudomonas* endocarditis usually requires a combined medical-surgical approach. Medical therapy should be continued for 6 weeks.

5. OTHER AEROBIC BACTERIA

   Endocarditis attributable to *Hemophilus* spp. (non–beta-lactamase producers) may be treated successfully with 2–3 gm of ampicillin IV every 6 hours for 4 weeks. Infection with *H. parainfluenzae* can be managed with 200–300 mg/kg/day of ampicillin plus 4.5 to 5.0 mg/kg/day of gentamicin, in divided doses every 8 hours for 6 to 8 weeks. Pneumococcal, gonococcal, and meningococcal endocarditis should be treated with penicillin G, 3 MU IV every 4 hours for 4 weeks.

6. ANAEROBIC BACTERIA

   Penicillin G 3 MU IV every 4 hours is usually the drug of choice, except for patients with infection caused by *Bacteroides fragilis*. Metronidazole is the drug of choice in these patients.

7. **FUNGAL ENDOCARDITIS**

A combined medical-surgical approach is warranted. Amphotericin B, 0.5 mg/kg/day plus 5-flucytosine, 150 mg/kg/day po, is recommended pending results of sensitivity tests.

D. **Prosthetic Valve Endocarditis.** Prosthetic valve endocarditis (PVE) is often divided into early PVE (within 2 months of valve replacement) and late PVE (more than 2 months postoperatively). *Staphylococcus epidermidis* is the most common cause of early PVE. Late PVE is usually produced by viridans streptococci. There may be a delayed appearance of microorganisms acquired in the perioperative period, such as *S. epidermidis, Candida* spp., diphtheroids, or gram-negative bacilli.

Antimicrobial therapy for PVE follows the same guidelines as that for native valve endocarditis. However, **initial therapy while cultures are pending should be directed toward** *S. epidermidis,* **with vancomycin plus gentamicin.** Surgery should be considered on an individual basis.

E. **Endocarditis in Intravenous Drug Users.** *S. aureus* is the most frequently isolated organism in IV drug users with endocarditis. Other organisms include streptococci, including enterococci; gram-negative bacilli, including *Pseudomonas;* and fungi, usually *Candida.* There is some regional variation. Treatment is the same as for native valve endocarditis. **Empiric coverage, pending culture results, should be directed against** *S. aureus* **and aerobic gram-negative rods (e.g., nafcillin 2 gm IV every 4 hours and gentamicin 1.7 gm/kg IV every 8 hours).** Recent evidence indicates that uncomplicated right-sided *S. aureus* endocarditis may be effectively treated with a 2-week course of nafcillin (1.5 gm IV every 4 hours) and tobramycin (1 mg/kg IV every 8 hours). Vancomycin may be substituted for nafcillin for patients allergic to penicillin.

Chambers, HF, Miller RT, Newman MD: Right-sided *Staphylococcus aureus* endocarditis in intravenous drug abusers: 2-week combination therapy. Ann Intern Med 109:619–624, 1988.
Coleman DL, Horwitz RI, Andriole VT: Association between serum inhibitory and bactericidal concentration and therapeutic outcome in bacterial endocarditis. Am J Med 73:260–267, 1982.
Kaye D: Prophylaxis for infective endocarditis: An update. Ann Intern Med 104:419–423, 1986.
Sande MA, Scheld WM: Combination antibiotic therapy of bacterial endocarditis. Ann Intern Med 92:390–395, 1980.
Wilson WR, Guilani ER, Danielson GK: Symposium on infective endocarditis. Mayo Clin Proc 57:145–148, 1982.

XIII. PERITONITIS

A. **Spontaneous Bacterial Peritonitis.** The majority of cases of spontaneous bacterial peritonitis occur in patients with alcoholic cirrhosis and ascites. The most commonly isolated organisms are *Escherichia coli*, pneumococci, other streptococci, and *Pseudomonas, Enterobacter, Klebsiella,* and *Clostridium* spp. Nephrotic patients are most commonly infected with pneumococci. Gram stain and culture of the peritoneal fluid are essential. Culture yield is enhanced by bedside inoculation of peritoneal fluid into blood culture bottles. Blood cultures often are positive for the same organism. Empiric therapy should be directed at the organism suggested by the Gram stain, if positive. **Empiric therapy**

with ampicillin plus an aminoglycoside has been traditionally recommended. However, concerns regarding aminoglycoside-associated nephrotoxicity have led to alternative empiric regimens such as ampicillin plus aztreonam, a third-generation cephalosporin such as cefotaxime or ceftriaxone, or ampicillin-sulbactam.

B. Secondary Peritonitis. Secondary peritonitis is usually polymicrobial and caused by organisms from the GI tract. The facultative organisms commonly isolated are *Bacteroides fragilis, Bacteroides melaninogenicus, Peptococcus, Peptostreptococcus, Fusobacterium, Eubacterium lentum,* and *Clostridium.* Peritoneal fluid Gram stain and culture, as well as blood cultures, are important in isolating the pathogen. After the appropriate specimens for culture are obtained, antimicrobial therapy should be started. There are several alternatives:

    1. **Clindamycin** (600 mg IV every 6 to 8 hours) or **metronidazole** (a loading dose of 15 mg/kg, then 7.5 mg/kg IV every 6 hours) with **ampicillin** (1.5 to 2.0 gm IV every 4 hours) or **penicillin** (2 MU IV every 4 hours) and an **aminoglycoside** (tobramycin or gentamicin 1.7 mg/kg IV every 8 hours);

    2. **Ampicillin-sulbactam** (1.5 gm IV every 4–6 hours) with or without an aminoglycoside;

    3. **Cefotetan** (2 gm IV every 12 hours) and an aminoglycoside;

    4. **Chloramphenicol** (50–100 mg/kg IV/day divided into doses every 6 hours) and an **aminoglycoside;**

    5. **Imipenem-cilastatin,** 0.5 to 1.0 gm IV every 6 hours.

Weinstein MP, Iannini PB, Stratton CW, et al: Spontaneous bacterial peritonitis: A review of 28 cases with emphasis on improved survival and factors influencing prognosis. Am J Med 64:592–598, 1978.

C. Peritonitis During Continuous Ambulatory Peritoneal Dialysis (CAPD). The most frequently isolated organism is *S. epidermidis,* followed by *S. aureus, Streptococcus* spp., and then gram-negative enteric pathogens. Intraperitoneal administration of cephalothin may be given. Vancomycin should be given both intraperitoneally and IV. Antimicrobials should be given for 10 days to 3 weeks. Fungal peritonitis due to *Candida* spp. may also be encountered.

XIV. CNS INFECTIONS

A. Meningitis. When a patient presents with symptoms suggestive of meningitis (fever, headache, altered mental states, and stiff neck), the first consideration should be therapy, not specific diagnosis. Antimicrobial therapy based on the most likely pathogen should be initiated within 30 minutes of presentation. In the absence of papilledema and other signs of increased intracranial pressure, a lumbar puncture should be obtained rapidly. The results of cerebrospinal fluid studies can be used, along with additional clinical information, to alter the initial therapy, if necessary.

1. LIKELY ORGANISMS BASED ON CHARACTERISTICS OF THE PATIENT

a. Age. *Streptococcus pneumoniae* is the most common cause of bacterial meningitis in adults over the age of 40 years, and *Neisseria meningitidis* is the most common causative agent in individuals aged 18 to 40. *Hemophilus influenzae,* enteric gram-negative bacilli, streptococci, staphylococci, and *Listeria monocytogenes* are much less frequently seen in normal hosts but must be considered more likely in specific situations.

b. Shunt-Associated Meningitis. Up to 30% of all ventricular shunts become infected. The most common organisms found are *Staphylococcus epidermidis, Staphylococcus aureus,* streptococci, diphtheroids, *Bacillus* spp., gram-negative enteric organisms, *Propionibacterium acnes,* and mixed groups. Antimicrobial therapy should be given systemically and intraventricularly in most cases. *Staphylococcus aureus* shunt infection can usually be treated with cephalothin IV and intraventricularly (0.3 mg/mL of estimated cerebrospinal fluid volume) once or twice a day. *S. epidermidis* infections will usually require vancomycin therapy. Gram-negative bacilli-associated shunt infections should be treated with a systemic third-generation cephalosporin, or systemic plus intraventricular aminoglycoside with systemic ticarcillin or piperacillin. Decisions about shunt removal depend on the patient's response to therapy and serial culture results.

c. The Postoperative Neurosurgical Patient. Nosocomially acquired pathogens include gram-negative enteric bacilli, *Pseudomonas* spp., *S. aureus, S. epidermidis,* and streptococci.

d. Head Trauma. Patients are predisposed to acute or recurrent meningitis. *S. pneumoniae,* other streptococci, or gram-negative bacilli are found most frequently.

e. Recurrent Meningitis. *S. pneumoniae* is the most common causative organism. Also found are *Hemophilus* spp., streptococci, *Neisseria* spp., staphylococci, and, especially after prophylactic antibiotic therapy, gram-negative rods.

f. The Immunosuppressed Host. Potential pathogens include *Listeria monocytogenes, Pseudomonas aeruginosa, S. aureus, S. pneumoniae,* gram-negative enteric bacilli, streptococci, anaerobes, *Acinetobacter* spp., *Cryptococcus neoformans,* and coagulase-negative staphylococci. Patients who are neutropenic (e.g., following chemotherapy) may develop central nervous system infections with any of these pathogens. *Listeria, S. pneumoniae,* and *Cryptococcus* are most commonly found in patients with malignancies who have *normal* neutrophil counts in peripheral blood (e.g., patients with Hodgkin's disease).

2. THERAPY FOR BACTERIAL MENINGITIS

When the cerebrospinal fluid Gram stain and/or bacterial culture yields positive findings, therapy specific to the infecting organism should be instituted.

a. **Pneumococcal and Meningococcal Meningitis.** There should be prompt initiation of a 10- to 14-day course of penicillin (18 to 24 MU/day IV in divided doses every 2–4 hours) or ampicillin (12 gm/day IV in divided doses every 2–4 hours). Chloramphenicol (75–100 mg/kg/day IV in divided doses) or ceftriaxone 1–2 gm IV every 12 hours) can be used in the penicillin-allergic patient. Most first- and second-generation cephalosphorins do *not* cross the blood-brain barrier. In cases of meningococcal meningitis, respiratory isolation of the patient is suggested for the first 24 hours of treatment, and prophylaxis of close contacts with rifampin (adult dose: 600 mg bid for 2 days) should be given.

b. *Hemophilus influenzae* **Meningitis.** Ampicillin, 2–4 gm IV every 4 hours, plus chloramphenicol, 75 to 100 mg/kg/day IV every 6 hours, or ceftriaxone, 1.0 to 2.0 gm IV every 12 hours, should be initiated for all patients until it has been determined whether the individual isolate produces beta-lactamase. Ampicillin may be continued alone for beta-lactamase–negative strains, for a minimum course of 10 days. Chloramphenicol, ceftriaxone, and cefotaxime are effective for patients with a beta-lactamase–positive isolate. Failure to improve on appropriate therapy may indicate the presence of subdural effusions (especially in children) or a parameningeal focus of infection (e.g., sinusitis).

c. **Gram-Negative Bacillary Meningitis.** The most likely organisms causing meningitis in adults are *Klebsiella, Escherichia coli,* and *Pseudomonas.* Initial therapy of community-acquired gram-negative meningitis should be a third-generation cephalosporin in high doses (e.g., cefotaxime 50 mg/kg IV every 6 hours). An aminoglycoside should be added (IV and intrathecally) in the severely ill patient or if *Pseudomonas* infection is suspected (0.03 mg of tobramycin or gentamicin or 0.10 mg of amikacin/mL of estimated cerebrospinal fluid volume every 24 hours). The volume of cerebrospinal fluid in adults is estimated at 1 ml per pound of body weight. In hospital-acquired meningitis not involving neurosurgery, a third-generation cephalosporin should be administered. If the meningitis was acquired in the hospital following neurosurgery, nafcillin should be added to a third-generation cephalosporin and aminoglycoside. In the penicillin-allergic patient, vancomycin may be substituted for nafcillin. Therapy should be continued for at least 10 days after the last sterile cerebrospinal fluid culture.

d. *Listeria monocytogenes* **Meningitis.** Ampicillin, 2 gm IV every 4 hours (or penicillin, 18 to 24 MU/day IV in divided doses every 4 hours), should be given for at least 3 weeks. In the patient allergic to penicillin, chloramphenicol, 75 to 100 mg/kg/day in divided doses every 6 hours (or trimethoprim-sulfamethoxazole) may be effective, but there has been little clinical experience with agents other than ampicillin or penicillin.

e. *Staphylococcus aureus* **Meningitis.** Nafcillin, 2 to 3 grams IV every 4 hours, may be given, or vancomycin, 1 gram every 12 hours, can be used in the penicillin-allergic patient. Vancomycin may also be administered intrathecally at a dose of 20 mg/day. Penicillin may be used for penicillin-susceptible organisms. A careful search for associated abscesses (e.g., parameningeal) should be considered.

   f. *Staphylococcus epidermidis* **Meningitis.** Infection with this organism is usually associated with the presence of an infected ventricular shunt. Vancomycin, 1 gm IV every 12 hours, is the drug of choice. Rifampin may be added and may improve the possibility of curing this infection without removal of the shunt.

3. **THERAPY FOR NONBACTERIAL MENINGITIS**

   a. **Tuberculous Meningitis.** The clinical presentation of this type of meningitis often includes cranial nerve palsies and is similar to the presentation of cryptococcal meningitis. Treatment is with isoniazid, 600 mg/day (with pyridoxine), and rifampin, 600 mg/day, often with a third agent, pyrazinamide, for the initial 2 months of therapy. The dosage of isoniazid may be reduced after one month of therapy. The optimal total duration of therapy has not been well defined, and the use of corticosteroids, especially for basilar meningitis, remains controversial.

   b. **Fungal Infections**
      (1). Cryptococcal Meningitis. Amphotericin B (0.3 mg/kg/day) plus 5-flucytosine (150 mg/kg/day) for 6 weeks is the combination of choice. The level of 5-flucytosine should not exceed 100 μg/mL when measured 1–2 hours after oral administration (see Table 3–6 for treatment in patients with AIDS).
      (2). Coccidioidal Meningitis. Amphotericin B 0.5 to 0.6 mg/kg/day should be administered IV and intrathecally.
      (3). Candidal Meningitis. Amphotericin B with 5-flucytosine is the recommended therapy.

   c. **Amebic Meningitis.** Though recovery from this type of meningitis is uncommon, systemic and intraventricular administration of high-dose amphotericin B is recommended.

Schlech WF, Ward JI, Band JD, et al: Bacterial meningitis in the United States, 1978 through 1981. JAMA 253:1749–1754, 1985.

B. **Brain Abscess.** Prompt recognition of brain abscess should lead to early administration of parenteral antibiotics and neurosurgical evaluation. Few patients present with the classic triad of fever, headache, and focal neurologic defect, and a high index of suspicion should prompt CT scans of the head in patients with any suggestive symptoms or signs. Physical examination and laboratory findings are often nonspecific. Lumbar puncture is contraindicated when brain abscess is suspected. CT of the head, with contrast enhancement, is the most sensitive diagnostic test. If a CT scan is not immediately available to confirm the diagnosis, appropriate antibiotics should be started without delay.

1. **BACTERIOLOGY**
   When material is available from a brain abscess, Gram stain and aerobic, anaerobic, mycobacterial, and fungal cultures should be performed. The most common aerobes isolated are streptococci, followed by organisms of the Enterobacteriaceae family and *Pseudomonas* spp., *Staphylococcus aureus, Hemophilus* spp., and coagu-

lase-negative staphylococci. Anaerobes are usually found in mixed infections, with *Bacteroides* and *Peptostreptococcus* being the most common. Much less common are *Propionibacterium acnes* and others such as *Veillonella* and *Actinomyces* spp. Some abscesses may appear sterile if the handling of material for anaerobic cultures is not adequate. Fungal and parasitic infections are appearing more frequently in the immunosuppressed patient.

2. THERAPY

Studies of antibiotic penetration and activity in brain abscesses are incomplete. Therapy should be parenteral and high dose. Penicillin (20 MU/day) and chloramphenicol (1 gm every 6 hours) have been commonly used. However, metronidazole has advantages over chloramphenicol in that it is bactericidal against *Bacteroides fragilis*, attains high concentrations in brain abscess pus, and is not degraded in pus. If gram-negative bacilli are suspected, especially when the patient has a prior history of otic infection, a third-generation cephalosporin should be added.

If staphylococci are suspected, nafcillin (2 gm IV every 4 hours) should be substituted for penicillin. Vancomycin may be used if a methicillin-resistant strain is isolated.

The duration of parenteral therapy should be at least 4–6 weeks, often followed by a prolonged course of oral therapy (2–6 months). Sequential CT scans may be helpful in determining the duration of therapy.

The role of **surgical therapy** must be individualized, and neurosurgical consultation should be obtained early. Recent experience has suggested that some patients may be treated without extensive neurosurgery.

Boom WH, Tuazon CU: Successful treatment of multiple brain abscesses with antibiotics alone. Rev Infect Dis 7:189–199, 1985.
Kaplan K: Brain abscess. Symposium on infections of the central nervous system. Med Clin North Am 69:345–360, 1985.

XV. THE IMMUNOCOMPROMISED HOST

Fever, particularly in the leukopenic patient, should be presumed due to infection, and therapy should be started immediately after appropriate cultures are obtained. When searching for infection in the neutropenic patient, it is important to remember that local signs of purulence and inflammation may be subtle. If no obvious primary site can be found, bacteremia must be assumed.

The most common causes of bacteremia are *Escherichia coli, Klebsiella* spp., *Pseudomonas aeruginosa,* and *Staphylococcus aureus. Staphylococcus epidermidis* infections are becoming more common, especially in patients with Hickman (or other indwelling) catheters. There is no ideal empiric antibiotic combination. A third-generation cephalosporin with an aminoglycoside or another beta-lactam provides effective initial empiric therapy for most neutropenic patients. Vancomycin may be added to this regimen, especially if a patient has a Hickman catheter. If blood cultures are positive, therapy is usually continued for 14 days, with extension until the neutropenia resolves. If blood cultures are negative, antibiotics may be stopped when the granulocyte count is greater than 500/cu mm. If a patient remains febrile after 5–7 days of antimicrobial therapy, superinfection, particularly with fungi, must be considered. Amphotericin B therapy is often recommended at dosages of 0.5 mg/kg/day, along with antibiotics, until the granulocytopenia resolves.

Treatment recommendations for viral infections are shown in Table 3–5, and recommendations for fungal infections are given in Table 3–9.

Hathron JW, Rubin M, Pizzo PA: Empirical antibiotic therapy in the febrile neutropenic cancer patient: Clinical efficacy and impact of monotherapy. Antimicrob Agents Chemother 31:971–977, 1987.

Hughes WT: Guidelines for the use of antimicrobial agents in neutropenic patients with unexplained fever. J Infect Dis 161:381–396, 1990.

Masur HM, Shelhamer J, Parrillo JE: The management of pneumonias in immunocompromised patients. JAMA 253:1769–1773, 1985.

Schimpff SC: Overview of empiric antibiotic therapy for the febrile neutropenic patient. Rev Infect Dis 7(suppl 4):734–740, 1985.

XVI. ACQUIRED IMMUNODEFICIENCY SYNDROME (AIDS)

All HIV-infected individuals should receive a **pneumococcal vaccine (one time only)** and **yearly influenza vaccination** unless specifically contraindicated. **Hepatitis B vaccine** should be administered to all HIV-infected individuals who are HBsAb-negative and at risk for acquiring infection. All patients should be screened with a VDRL or RPR and treated appropriately for syphilis (see p. 98) if screening values are elevated. Skin testing with PPD and anergy controls should be performed on all HIV-infected individuals. Patients with PPD reactions ≥ 5 mm and normal chest x-rays should receive isoniazid prophylaxis, 300 mg po qd for 6–12 months.

Although there is no known cure for human immunodeficiency virus (HIV) infection, the antiviral agent **zidovudine (AZT)** has been shown to slow the progression of HIV-related disease, reduce the number of opportunistic infections, and prolong the lives of patients with established AIDS. Currently, **therapy with AZT, 100 mg po 5 times/day, is indicated for HIV-infected patients with CD4 lymphocyte counts less than 500/cu mm.** The initiation of AZT therapy in individuals with CD4 counts greater than 500/cu mm and following significant exposure to HIV is controversial as of this writing. Side effects and toxicity to AZT include nausea, elevation of liver function tests, myopathy, and bone marrow suppression with anemia, leukopenia, and thrombocytopenia. In patients unable to take AZT, therapy with ddI, a related dideoxynucleoside with antiretroviral activity, should be considered. The toxicity of ddI includes pancreatitis and peripheral neuropathies.

Antiretroviral chemotherapy, supportive care, and the treatment of opportunistic infections are the main therapeutic approaches to HIV infection and AIDS. The management of AIDS-related opportunistic infections is complicated by the lack of expected response to treatment, the need for prolonged courses of therapy, simultaneous opportunistic infections, and a high incidence of toxic drug reactions.

TABLE 3–9. ANTIFUNGAL THERAPY

FUNGUS	INFECTION	THERAPY
Candida	Oropharyngeal	Nystatin (100,000 U/ml), gargle and swallow 4–6 ml qid
		Clotrimazole troches, 10 mg 5/day
		Ketoconazole, 200–400 mg po qd
		Fluconazole, 100–200 mg po qd
	Gastrointestinal	Nystatin (100,000 U/ml), 30–60 ml q 2–4 hr alternating with nystatin troches
		Ketoconazole, 200 mg po qd-bid
		Fluconazole, 200 mg po qd
		If no improvement: low-dose amphotericin, 10–20 mg qd
	Disseminated	Fluconazole, 200–400 mg po/IV qd
		Amphotericin B, 0.4–1.0 mg/kg/day IV over 4–6 hr to cumulative dose of 2–3 gm
		If blood cultures remain positive, add 5–flucytosine (5-FC), 12.5–37.5 mg/kg po q 6 hr
	Transient candidemia	Remove all intravascular catheters
		Ophthalmologic and dermatologic examination
		Repeat blood cultures
	Endocarditis	Surgical intervention plus aggressive therapy for disseminated candidiasis
	Candiduria (lower tract)	Change indwelling catheter; most clear spontaneously
		Fluconazole: 200 mg po/IV qd for 5–7 days
		Continuous bladder irrigation with amphotericin B, 50 mg/L qd for 5 days, or 5-FC, 200 mg po qd
	Candiduria (upper tract)	Fluconazole, 200 mg po/IV qd
		Amphotericin, 1.0–1.5 gm (total dose), plus 5-FC (see under disseminated)
	Central nervous system (CNS)	See under "Disseminated"
	Pulmonary	See under "Disseminated"
	Peritonitis	See under "Disseminated"
	Chronic mucocutaneous	Fluconazole, 100–200 mg po qd
	Suppurative thrombophlebitis	Vein excision; treat for disseminated candidiasis

Organism	Condition	Treatment
Torulopsis glabrata	Fungemia	Remove IV catheters and repeat blood cultures Consider fluconazole or amphotericin B therapy
	Renal infection	Alkalinize urine Fluconazole, 100–200 mg po/IV qd Instill mycostatin or amphotericin Consider systemic amphotericin B and 5-FC
Histoplasma capsulatum	Systemic	Usually benign and self-limited Severe infection: amphotericin B (2–4 wk)
	Progressive dissemination	Amphotericin B, total of 2 grams IV over 10 wk
	Chronic	If cavities are large (>3 mm) or persistent, use amphotericin B Surgery is controversial
Cryptococcus neoformans	Pulmonary only	No therapy if no extrapulmonary sites and falling serum titer
	Disseminated (skin, bone, CNS)	Amphotericin B, 2 gm total, plus 5-FC; acquired immunodeficiency syndrome (AIDS) patients require indefinite maintenance therapy with fluconazole Cerebrospinal fluid (CSF) india ink stain, cryptococcal antigen titer, and culture every week until negative Antigen titer q 3–4 wk; CSF exam q 3 mo for 1 yr after therapy is completed Intrathecal administration of amphotericin B may be necessary
Coccidioides immitis	Pulmonary	No therapy for acute, self-limited disease If persistent, chronic progressive, miliary, or cavitary, particularly in the immunocompromised patient, consider amphotericin B or ketoconazole
	Disseminated	Amphotericin B for at least 1 mo; follow complement-fixing antibodies
	CNS	Systemic plus intrathecal amphotericin B

Table continued on the following page

TABLE 3-9. ANTIFUNGAL THERAPY Continued

FUNGUS	INFECTION	THERAPY
Aspergillus spp.	Sputum colonization	None
	Allergic bronchopulmonary aspergillosis	None for mild disease; may use disodium cromoglycate or beclomethasone diproprionate
		Prednisone, 0.5 gm/kg po every other day
	Aspergillomas	If massive hemoptysis, consider surgery
	Invasive aspergillosis (pulmonary, extrapulmonary)	Amphotericin B, optimal duration unknown
		Consider thoracotomy and resection
Blastomyces dermatitidis	Pneumonitis	Antifungal therapy is controversial
	Chronic (pulmonary, skin, genitourinary, bone, mucosa)	Amphotericin B, 1.5 to 2.0 gm (total dose)
		Surgical excision of local lesions
Mucorales	Rhinocerebral and cutaneous	Amphotericin B, 0.75 to 1.00 mg/kg/day, 3–6 gm total dose over 2–3 mo
		Surgical debridement
	Pulmonary and gastrointestinal	Amphotericin B (as above)
	Disseminated	Aggressive use of amphotericin B (as for rhinocerebral)
Sporothrix schenckii	Cutaneous-lymphatic	Fluconazole, 200 mg po qd
		Potassium iodide solution, 3–4 mg po q 8 hr (begin with 1 ml and gradually increase)
		Continue for 1 mo after signs resolve
		For deep infection: amphotericin B or fluconazole
	Pulmonary	Amphotericin B
	Disseminated	Amphotericin B, 1.5–2.5 gm (total dose)
		Surgical drainage of osteomyelitic and synovial lesions
Bacterial Infections Often Confused with Fungi:		
Actinomyces israelii (anaerobe)	Cervicofacial, thoracic, and abdominal	Penicillin G, 10–20 million U/day IV for 4–6 wk, followed by oral penicillin for 6–12 mo
		Surgical drainage of abscesses and excision of sinus tracts
Nocardia asteroides	Pulmonary systemic	Sulfadiazine, 8–12 gm/day po for 6–12 mo

Treatment recommendations for the most common **opportunistic infections** in patients with AIDS are shown in Table 3–6, pp. 90–91. *Pneumocystis carinii* pneumonia (PCP) continues to be a major cause of morbidity and mortality in the AIDS patient population. *Corticosteroid treatment* is now recommended in addition to antimicrobial therapy in the treatment of moderate-to-severe PCP (paO$_2$ ≤ 70 mm Hg). The current accepted regimen is prednisone, 40 mg po bid for 5 days, followed by 40 mg po qd for 5 days, followed by 20 mg po qd for 11 days. An equivalent dose of a parenteral corticosteroid (i.e., methylprednisolone) can be used for intravenous therapy. Corticosteroids should be started within 24–72 hours of initiating antimicrobial chemotherapy against *P. carinii*. Prophylactic therapy against *P. carinii* is now recommended indefinitely for all patients following an episode of PCP and for those HIV-infected individuals with CD4 levels less than 200/cu mm or less than 20% of the total lymphocyte count. Currently accepted regimens include:

1. Trimethoprim-sulfamethoxazole, 1 double-strength tablet po bid 3–7 days/week;
2. Dapsone, 100 mg po 2 times per week (with or without trimethoprim); and
3. Pentamidine, 300 mg via nebulizer every 4 weeks. Recurrence of *P. carinii* in the lung apices and at extrapulmonary sites has emerged as a problem with the aerosolized pentamidine regimen.

Bozette SA, et al: A controlled trial of early adjunctive treatment with corticosteroids for *Pneumocystis carinii* in the acquired immunodeficiency syndrome. N Engl J Med 323:1451–1456, 1990.

Fischl MA, et al: The safety and efficacy of zidovudine (AZT) in the treatment of subjects with mildly symptomatic human immunodeficiency virus type I (HIV) infection. Ann Intern Med 112:727–737, 1990.

Gagnon S, et al: Corticosteroids as adjunctive therapy for severe *Pneumocystis carinii* pneumonia in the acquired immunodeficiency syndrome—a double-blind, placebo-controlled trial. N Engl J Med 323:1444–1450, 1990.

Glatt AE, Chirgwin K, Landesman SH: Treatment of infections associated with human immunodeficiency virus. N Engl J Med 318:1439–1448, 1987.

Sande MA, Volberding PA (eds): The Medical Management of AIDS. Philadelphia, WB Saunders Co, 1990.

Volberding PA, et al: Zidovudine in asymptomatic HIV infection. N Engl J Med 322:941–949, 1990.

XVII. TRAVEL AND MALARIA

For the majority of travelers, only routine immunizations are recommended (Table 3–7, pp. 96–97). Information on which immunizations are needed and whether a country requires an International Certificate of Vaccination can be obtained from many sources. *Health Information for International Travel* (published by the CDC yearly) and the "Blue Sheet" (published biweekly by the CDC) are most useful.

A. Malaria. Since the risk of acquiring malaria in different areas changes frequently, it is important to obtain recent information from the sources listed above, as well as from the *Morbidity and Mortality Weekly Report,* local health departments, and the CDC. In addition to chemoprophylaxis, it is important to reduce exposure to mosquitoes by the use of protective screening, clothing, and mosquito repellent (e.g., N,N-diethylmetatoluamide [DEET]).

1. CHEMOPROPHYLAXIS recommendations are:

   a. **For *Plasmodium ovale, P. vivax, P. malariae,* and Chloroquine-Sensitive Strains of *P. falciparum.*** Chloroquine phosphate, 300 mg po of base, is recommended once a week on the same day, beginning 1 week prior to travel, continuing every week during travel, and for 4 weeks following departure from the malarious area.

   b. **For a Presumed Attack of Chloroquine-Resistant *P. falciparum* Malaria.** In addition to the above course of therapy, the traveler should take Fansidar tablets (3 tablets: 75 mg of pyrimethamine and 1500 mg of sulfadoxine po) or mefloquine 1250 mg po, as a single dose. Medical attention should be sought immediately. (Note: The combination of chloroquine and Fansidar sometimes causes potentially fatal cutaneous reactions, such as the Stevens-Johnson syndrome; Fansidar should not be taken late in pregnancy or by sulfa-allergic patients.)

   c. **For Long-Term Travel in Areas with High Risk of Chloroquine-Resistant *P. falciparum.*** Mefloquine, 250 mg po once weekly, starting 1 week before entering the endemic area, continuing every week during travel, and for 4 weeks after leaving the endemic region. Alternatively, chloroquine prophylaxis may be combined with doxycycline, 100 mg po qd starting 1–2 days before departure, continuing during travel in an endemic region, and continuing for 4–6 weeks following return from an endemic region.

2. THERAPY

Most patients with acute malaria can be treated with oral medications. The initial treatment is the same for all forms of malaria, unless the patient has acquired chloroquine-resistant *P. falciparum* malaria. Even chloroquine-resistant malaria will have some response to chloroquine but will recur. If the patient is seriously ill, treatment should be directed as though the malaria were chloroquine resistant. Oral therapy for chloroquine-sensitive malaria is chloroquine phosphate, 600 mg (active base), followed by 300 mg (base) 6, 24, and 48 hours later. For *P. vivax* and *P. ovale* malaria, chloroquine therapy should be followed by primaquine 15 mg (base) po qd for 14 days starting around the fourth day. For parenteral therapy of a severe attack, quinidine gluconate should be used, 10 mg/kg (maximum, 600 mg) IV loading dose over 1 hour, followed by continuous administration of 0.02 mg/kg/min IV (maximum, 10 mg/kg every 8 hours) until oral chloroquine therapy is possible. Administration of intravenous quinidine requires hospitalization in an ICU with continuous hemodynamic and cardiac monitoring; widening of the QRS interval or significant lengthening of the QT segment requires discontinuation of drug infusion. Recommended oral therapy for *P. falciparum* (chloroquine-resistant) malaria is quinine sulfate, 540 mg (active base) tid for 3–7 days plus one of the following:

1. Fansidar, 3 tablets (pyrimethamine 75 mg and sulfadoxine 1500 mg) once; or
2. Tetracycline, 250–500 mg qid for 7 days; or
3. Doxycycline, 100 mg bid for 7 days; or
4. Clindamycin, 900 mg tid for 3 days.

Alternatively, mefloquine 1250 mg alone may be given once. (Note: mefloquine must not be given with quinine.) For the severely ill patient, IV quinidine gluconate may be given as above, and oral therapy with quinine plus a second drug (as above) begun as soon as possible. For additional information on side effects, contraindications, and alternate agents, *The Travel and Tropical Medicine Manual* (see reference list at end of section) may be consulted. The Malarial Branch, Centers for Disease Control, in Atlanta, Georgia, may be contacted for information regarding the therapy of malaria: for recorded information on prophylaxis, (404) 332–4555; for questions about management of acute attacks or on prophylaxis, (404) 488–4046 [emergency, (404) 639–2888].

B. **Traveler's Diarrhea.** The majority of cases of traveler's diarrhea are caused by bacteria such as enteropathogenic *Escherichia coli, Shigella, Salmonella,* and *Campylobacter.* Most of these pathogens can be avoided by the use of only chlorinated, boiled, or carbonated water (and ice). Raw vegetables and fruits may be contaminated when washed in water.

1. CHEMOPROPHYLAXIS
Bismuth subsalicylate (Pepto-Bismol), 60 ml po qid, may prevent symptomatic infection. Prophylactic antibiotics for most travelers have more associated risks than benefits. Trimethoprim-sulfamethoxazole 1 double-strength tablet po qd bid, or doxycycline 100 mg po qd bid, or ciprofloxacin 500 mg po qd bid may be considered for short-term (less than 2 weeks) prophylaxis in special cases. However, it is recommended that antibiotics be taken only when symptoms occur.

2. THERAPY
When diarrhea does occur, bismuth subsalicylate (Pepto-Bismol, 30 ml every 30 min for 8 doses) or an antimotility agent (diphenoxylate hydrochloride with atropine [Lomotil] or loperamide hydrochloride [Imodium]) may be taken for no longer than 2 days. For **bloody diarrhea with fever, ciprofloxacin, 500 mg po bid for 5 days, trimethoprim-sulfamethoxazole, 1 double-strength tablet po bid for 5 days, or trimethoprim, 200 mg po bid for 5 days,** is suggested.

Other helminthic, protozoal, and arthropod-borne diseases are discussed elsewhere (Med Lett Drugs Ther 30:15–22, 1988). Table 3–10 provides a summary of treatment recommendations for some common parasitic infections.

TABLE 3–10. TREATMENT RECOMMENDATIONS FOR SELECTED PARASITIC INFECTIONS

ORGANISM	THERAPY
Entamoeba histolytica (Amebiasis)	
Asymptomatic disease	Iodoquinol,* 650 mg po tid for 20 days
Intestinal disease	
Mild to moderate	Metronidazole, 750 mg po tid for 5–10 days, plus iodoquinol, as above, or tetracycline, 500 mg po tid for 5 days
Severe	Above regimen plus emetine, 1 mg/kg/day IM (maximum of 60 mg/day) for up to 5 days
Extraintestinal disease	Metronidazole plus iodoquinol, as above, or chloroquine phosphate, 1 gm po qd for 2 days, then 500 mg po qd for 4 wk plus emetine, as above, for 10 days
Ascaris lumbricoides (round worm)	Mebendazole, 100 mg po bid for 3 days, or pyrantel pamoate, 11 mg/kg once (maximum of 1.0 gm)
Enterobius vermicularis (pinworm)	Pyrantel pamoate, 11 mg/kg po once (maximum of 1.0 gram), or mebendazole, 100 mg po once†
Giardia lamblia Giardiasis	Metronidazole,‡ 2 gm po qd for 3 days or 750 mg tid for 5 days, or quinacrine HCl, 100 mg po tid for 5 days
Strongyloides	Thiabendazole, 25 mg/kg po bid (maximum of 3 gm/day for 2–3 days)
Tapeworms	
Diphyllobothrium latum (fish)	Niclosamide, 2 gm chewed thoroughly as a single dose
Taenia saginata (beef)	As above
Taenia solium (pork)	As above; praziquantel for neurocysticercosis
Trichuris (whipworm)	Mebendazole, 100 mg po bid for 3 days

*Maximal dose of 2 gm/day. Increased dose or duration may result in optic neuritis. Available from Glenwood Laboratories, Inc., 83 North Summit St., Tenafly, NJ 07670.
†Repeat either agent in 2 wk if in heavily contaminated area.
‡Not currently licensed for giardiasis.

Medical Letter: Mefloquine for malaria. Med Lett Drugs Ther 31:13, 1990. Centers for Disease
    Control: Recommendations for the prevention of malaria among travelers. MMWR 39:1, 1990.
Jong EC (ed): The Travel and Tropical Medicine Manual. Philadelphia, WB Saunders Co, 1987.
Medical Letter: Advice for travelers. Med Lett Drugs Ther 29:53–56, 1987.
Medical Letter: Drugs for parasitic infections. Med Lett Drugs Ther 30:15–22, 1988.

XVIII. FEVER OF UNKNOWN ORIGIN

Infections account for 30–40% of fevers of unknown origin (FUO). In
one series, the infectious etiologies found were as follows: mycobacterial
infection, intra-abdominal abscess, UTI, cytomegalovirus infection, sinusitis,
osteomyelitis, catheter infections, candidiasis, amebic hepatitis, and wound
infection. After a thorough investigation of the FUO, including cultures of
blood and other potentially infected sources, drug fever resulting from use
of antimicrobial agents should be considered. Likely agents that cause fever
include isoniazid, nitrofurantoin, novobiocin, penicillin, streptomycin, sulfonamides, and vaccines.

If no apparent etiology for FUO is found, **symptomatic therapy** may be
tried, first with the use of antipyretics such as acetylsalicylic acid or
acetaminophen. If effective, these agents can be continued for a prolonged
period. Prostaglandin synthetase inhibitors, such as indomethacin or ibuprofen, are alternatives. Prednisone may also be tried, if no evidence of
infectious or neoplastic processes has been found.

There are a few diseases that warrant a therapeutic trial of antimicrobial
agents in the absence of a firm diagnosis. If tuberculosis or granulomatous
hepatitis is suspected, a short course (2–3 weeks) of antimycobacterial
chemotherapy can be tried. Penicillin and an aminoglycoside may be used
if clinical findings suggest culture-negative endocarditis.

Jacoby GA, Swartz MN: Fever of undetermined origin. N Engl J Med 289:1407–1410, 1973.
Larson EB, Featherstone JH, Petersdorf RG: Fever of undetermined origin: Diagnosis and
    follow-up of 105 cases, 1979–1980. Medicine 61:269–292, 1982.
Petersdorf RG, Beeson PB: Fever of unexplained origin: Report on 100 cases. Medicine 4:1–30,
    1961.

4 4 4 4 4 4 4 4 4 4 4 4 4 4 4 4

CARDIOVASCULAR DISEASES

GEORGE THIBAULT
WILLIAM DALEY

4444444444444444

I. ANGINA

Angina is a symptom of **transient myocardial ischemia** resulting from an imbalance between myocardial oxygen (O_2) demand and myocardial O_2 supply. Observations made during coronary angioplasty indicate that angina is usually a late symptom in the sequence of events that occur when myocardial blood flow is reduced from occlusion of a coronary blood vessel. Initial findings include impaired relaxation of the ventricle and left ventricular systolic dysfunction, followed by elevation of the filling pressures. Later, ECG changes indicating ischemia are seen. (ST depression occurs with subendocardial ischemia, and transmural ischemia is associated with ST elevation.)

In many cases, angina is due to several factors. Clinically, myocardial O_2 demand correlates with the product of heart rate and systolic blood pressure (double product). This calculation is a useful index to measure myocardial O_2 demand, particularly during exercise. Diminished flow is more difficult to document. Radioisotopes such as thallium and rubidium have improved our ability to document decreased flow in clinically significant coronary artery disease. But we still have no clinically applicable tool to measure acute changes in myocardial blood flow.

Patients with fixed coronary artery obstruction may have superimposed vasoconstriction or platelet fibrin deposition that can further decrease flow. At peak exercise, luminal diameter must be reduced by 50% before flow is reduced and ischemia develops. At rest, a decrease in luminal diameter of 90% is usually needed for ischemia.

The differential diagnosis of angina is extensive, including anxiety hyperventilation, mitral valve prolapse (Barlow's syndrome), Tietz's syndrome, pericarditis, aortic dissection, pulmonary infarction, aortic stenosis, and hypertrophic cardiomyopathy. In aortic stenosis and hypertrophic cardiomyopathy the coronary arteries may be normal, but demand is heightened due to increased muscle mass and elevated left ventricular systolic pressure. Furthermore, the flow to subendocardial regions may be lessened owing to elevated end-diastolic pressure.

A. Treatment. Treatment of angina pectoris should be individualized according to symptoms. The goal of therapy is to modify favorably the balance of myocardial O_2 supply and demand. Beta blockers, calcium channel antagonists, and nitrates are all useful in preventing episodes of angina and in increasing exercise capacity. Comparative effects are shown in Table 4–4.

1. **BETA-BLOCKING AGENTS** (Table 4–1)

Beta blockers reduce heart rate both at rest and during exercise. They also lower blood pressure and reduce myocardial contractility. The net result is a reduction in myocardial oxygen demand. Beta-blocking agents may be "nonselective" (affinity for both beta$_1$ and

TABLE 4–1. PROPERTIES OF VARIOUS β-ADRENERGIC RECEPTOR ANTAGONIST AGENTS

GENERIC (AND TRADE) NAMES	PLASMA HALF-LIFE	LIPID SOLUBILITY	METABOLIZED BY	USUAL ORAL DOSE FOR ANGINA	IV DOSAGE
Noncardioselective					
Propranolol* (Inderal)	1–6	+ + +	Liver	20–80 q 6–8 hr; 1–10 mg* start 10–20 mg	1–10 mg* (0.1 mg/kg)
(Inderal-LA)	8–11	+ + +	Liver	80–320 mg 1 × day	—
Oxprenolol* (Trasicor)	2	+ +	Liver	As propranolol	1–12 mg
Timolol* (Blocadren)	4–5	+	Liver, kidney	5–20 q 12 hr bid; 15–45 mg 3–4 × day	0.4–1 mg
Nadolol* (Corgard)	16–24	0	Kidney	40–240 mg 1 × day; mean 100 mg	—
Sotalol (Sotacor)	15–17	0	Kidney	240–480 mg 1 × day	10–20 mg
Penbutolol* (Levatol)	27	+ + +	Liver	Not studied	—
Cardioselective					
Acebutolol* (Sectral)	8–12	0	Liver, kidney	200–400 mg PO q 8 hr; 900 mg optimal	12.5–50 mg
Atenolol* (Tenormin)	6–9	0	Kidney	50–100 mg 1 × day	5–10 mg*

Betaxolol* (Kerlone)	15	++	Liver, kidney	10–20 mg 1 × day†	—
Metoprolol* (Lopressor) (Betaloc)	3	+	Liver	50–100 mg/PO q 8–12 hr	5–15 mg*
Vasodilatory Beta Blockers, nonselective					
Cartelol* (Cartrol)	5–6	0/+	Kidney	Dose not available for angina	—
Labetalol* (Trandate) (Normodyne)	3–4	+++	Liver	100–200 mg; PO q 8–12 hr 3× day, max 2400 mg/day	1–2 mg/kg* for severe HT
Pindolol* (Visken)	4	+	Liver, kidney	5–15 mg/PO tid	—
Vasodilatory Beta Blockers, selective					
Celiprolol† (Selecor)	6–8	0/+	Chiefly kidney	400 mg 1 × day	—

*Approved by FDA.
†Pending approval by FDA.
Modified from Opie L.H.: Drugs for the Heart, 3rd ed. Philadelphia, W. B. Saunders Co., 1991.

131

beta$_2$ receptors) or "selective" for cardiac (beta$_1$ receptors) only. Beta$_1$ receptors are located in the myocardium, with small amounts of beta$_2$ in the atrium. Beta$_2$ receptors are primarily located in pulmonary tissue (particularly the bronchioles), peripheral arterial vessels, and such specialized sites as pancreatic islet cells. This is important because patients with asthma, chronic obstructive pulmonary disease, diabetes, or intermittent claudication may benefit from a low dose of beta$_1$ selective agents administered with caution. Though beta-selectivity does not appear to be important for antianginal efficacy, it is important for the profile of side effects. Another property of some beta blockers is intrinsic sympathomimetic activity. This property limits the efficacy for treating patients with angina because, at higher doses, heart rate is not decreased and may even be increased. The major effect of beta blockers with sympathomimetic activity is lowering of blood pressure. Pindolol is an example of a blocker with sympathomimetic activity. Labetolol is a drug that has both beta- and alpha-blocking actions. This drug can be used to treat patients with angina as well as those with significant hypertension.

Another potentially important feature of the beta-blocking agents is their lipid solubility. Those that are lipid soluble readily cross the blood-brain barrier and are more likely to cause CNS side effects (depression and nightmares). Patients should also be cautioned not to suddenly discontinue beta-blocker therapy. This has the potential to increase anginal symptoms and may lead to myocardial infarction.

2. **Calcium Channel Blocking Agents** (Table 4–2)
Calcium channel antagonists are standard agents in treating hypertension and angina pectoris. They selectively inhibit the influx of calcium into the calcium-L channel in both smooth muscle and myocardial cells. All have a peripheral arteriolar and coronary dilating effect and a negative inotropic effect.

Verapamil and diltiazem slow the heart rate mildly. A further effect of these agents is their ability to prevent coronary vasoconstriction. In general, verapamil or diltiazem is preferred over the dihydropyridines (e.g., nifedipine) for monotherapy since agents in the latter group may cause a reflex tachycardia.

When adding a calcium channel blocking agent to ongoing beta-blocker therapy, a dihydropyridine is preferred because the potential for reflex tachycardia is prevented by the beta blocker and the problem of unmasking an underlying conduction disorder is avoided. Symptomatic sinus slowing or AV block can occur with the combination of verapamil or diltiazem and a beta blocker. Clinically, this appears to be more common with verapamil. Either agent should be used with caution in patients taking beta blockers but may be safely used in selected patients without sinus node or AV node disease.

The differences between the calcium antagonists result from their structure. Verapamil is a papaverine derivative, nifedipine is a dihydropyridine derivative, and diltiazem a benzothiazine (Table 4–2).

TABLE 4–2. PROTOTYPICAL CALCIUM ANTAGONISTS: INDICATIONS AND DOSAGE

AGENT	INDICATIONS	DOSAGE
Verapamil (Isoptin, Calan)	PSVT with narrow QRS complexes	IV bolus 5–10 mg repeated after 10 min
	Atrial flutter/fibrillation	5–10 mg IV bolus repeated after 10 min; or 80–120 mg 3× day increasing to 80–120 mg 4× day; beware of digitalis toxicity
	Prophylaxis of PSVT	80–120 mg PO; tid
Sustained release	Hypertension	80–120 mg PO tid; or 240–360 mg PO, QD
	Hypertrophic cardiomyopathy*	240–480 mg PO tid
Diltiazem (Cardizem) (Herbesser) (Tildiem) (Tilazem)	Angina Prinzmetal's angina Non–Q-wave infarction*	30–120 mg PO 3–4× day 60 mg PO qid
IV Diltiazem	Atrial flutter/fibrillation*	IV 20–25 mg bolus then 5–15 mg/min infusion
Nifedipine (Procardia) (Adalat) (Procardia SL)	Angina of effort Prinzmetal's angina Severe hypertension	30–80 mg PO 3–4× day Procardia SL 30–150 mg day 10–20 mg PO 3–4× day 10 mg SL (sublingually) or bite and swallow

*Not FDA-approved.
Modified from Opie L.H.: Drugs for the Heart, 3rd ed. Philadelphia, W. B. Saunders Co., 1991.

3. NITRATES (Table 4–3)

Nitrates have several mechanisms of action. They produce arteriolar and venous dilating effects. The arteriolar effect may, however, cause a reflex tachycardia. The venodilating effect of the drug is very potent and plays a major role in alleviating pain by decreasing O_2 demand when used in an acute anginal episode. Coronary vasodilation is induced through the production of nitric oxide (NO), which is presently thought to be an endothelium-derived relaxing factor (EDRF). Nitrates may also play a major role in platelet disaggregation.

A major drawback to the use of nitrates is the development of **tolerance.** There are numerous studies showing that tolerance develops in a few days with continuous exposure. This explains why nitrate patches do not provide a sustained antianginal effect after a 24-hour period. One method of overcoming tolerance is to use the drug intermittently. Because of these problems, nitrates are not recom-

TABLE 4-3. NITRATES

DRUG	ROUTE	FORMULATION	DOSAGE	DURATION OF ACTION*	SIDE EFFECTS
Nitroglycerin	Sublingual	Nitrostat Tabs	0.3–0.6 mg prn	30 min	All nitrates have the potential to cause side effects related to vasodilating properties—e.g., headaches, flushing, reflex tachycardia, postural hypotension, dizziness
	Buccal	Nitrogard (sustained-release tablets, capsules)	1–2 mg tid	4–5 hr	
	Oral		2.5–6.5 mg tid	4–8 hr	
	Transdermal	Ointment (2%)	1.5–2.0 in q 4–6 h	3–4 hr	
		Nitrodisc	8–16 cm^2	Up to 24 hr	Tolerance
		Nitro-Dur	5–30 cm^2/day		
		Transderm-Nitro	2.5–15 mg/day		
		Deponit	16–32 cm^2/day	Up to 24 hr	Tolerance
	Nasal mucosa;	Spray;	0.4/dose	5–10 min	
	intravenous	solution	10–200 μg/min		
Isosorbide dinitrate		Sublingual	5–15 mg	Onset 5–10 min, effect up to 60 min	
		Oral	5–80 mg 2–3× daily	2–8 hr	
		Spray	1.25 mg on tongue	2–3 min	
		Chewable	5 mg qd	2 min–2½ hr	
		Oral; sustained release	40 mg 1–2× daily	2–6 hr	
		Intravenous	1.25–5 mg/hr		
		Ointment	100 mg/24 hr	Not effective during continuous therapy; tolerance	
Pentaerythritol tetranitrate	Oral	Tablets	10–60 mg q 6 hr	4–6 hr	Same
Erythrityl tetranitrate	Sublingual	Tablets	5–15 mg q 6 hr	3–6 hr	Same
	Oral	Tablets	10–30 mg q 6 hr	4–6 hr	

*Period of time that a dose has antianginal effect.

mended as primary or monotherapy for patients with angina. Examples of the use of nitrates would be the application of paste for 4–8 hours in a 24-hour period, the use of a patch overnight, and the use of isosorbide dinitrate (Isordil) tablets on an 8-hour rather than a 6-hour schedule.

Nitrates can be effectively combined with beta blockers. The combination of nitrates with calcium channel antagonists should be used cautiously since postural hypotension may occur.

B. Therapy in Specific Syndromes

1. CHRONIC STABLE ANGINA

a. **Clinical Classification.** A careful history to evaluate the chest pain is the key to diagnosis. The discomfort is classically described as central chest tightness, pressure, or a squeezing sensation. The sensation may radiate to the arm, neck, or jaw. Provoking factors include exertion, cold exposure, and emotional stress. Prompt relief with sublingual nitroglycerin or rest is an additional hallmark of angina. When all these features are present, the pain is "typical," or definite angina. If any one of the features is not present, the pain is probably angina. If more than one feature is absent, the pain is "atypical." A stable pattern of pain in terms of frequency, severity, duration, and provocation is a feature of chronic stable angina. The **classification of pain** as atypical, probable, or definite angina indicates whether significant coronary artery disease may be present. In men, the presence of angiographically demonstrable coronary artery disease for atypical, probable, and definite angina is 22, 60, and 88%, respectively. In women, the incidence is 5, 35, and 58%.

The **Canadian Cardiovascular Society Classification** is useful in describing the severity of angina to guide therapy (Table 4–5). Formal assessment of exercise capacity helps define the severity of incapacity; it also identifies factors sometimes associated with a poor prognosis. Such factors include short exercise duration, marked ST depression at low work loads, and a hypotensive or poor (failure of systolic pressure to exceed 130 mm Hg) blood pressure response during exercise. Although some studies have suggested that the results of scintigraphy or rest/exercise gated blood pool studies enhance risk stratification, these procedures are not recommended for most patients. In selected patients, the results of thallium scintigraphy or single-photon emission computed tomography (SPECT) can be helpful to establish a diagnosis of coronary artery disease or to quantitate the extent of ischemia, particularly in patients in whom the exercise ECG may be uninterpretable owing to baseline abnormalities.

b. **Treatment.** Medical therapy includes **attention to risk factors** as well as specific antianginal therapy. Either a **beta blocker** or a **calcium channel antagonist** for **monotherapy** is recommended initially. Use of a long-acting medication that needs once-daily administration may improve compliance, but this decision must be

TABLE 4–4. COMPARATIVE EFFECTS OF ANTIANGINAL AGENTS

AGENT	ARTERIAL DILATOR	VENODILATOR	PREVENTS CORONARY VASOCON-STRICTION	HEART RATE	SYSTOLIC BLOOD PRESSURE	AV CONDUCTION	TACHY-PHYLAXIS
Beta Blockers							
Nonselective	0	0	–	– –	– –	–	No
Selective	0	0	–	– –	– –	–	No
Intrinsic sympathomimetic activity	0	0	–	–/0	– –	0	No
Calcium Channel Blockers							
Nifedipine	+ + +	0	+ + +	+ +	– –	0	No
Nicarpidine	+ + +	0	+ + +	+ +	– –	0	No
Verapamil	+ +	0	+ + +	–/0	– –	–	No
Diltiazem	+	0	+ + +	– –	–/0	0/–	No
Nitrates	+ +	+ +	+ + +	+	– –	0	Yes (long-acting nitrates)

AV = atrioventricular; + = increase effect; – = decrease/negative effect; 0 = no effect.

136

TABLE 4–5. GRADING OF ANGINA OF EFFORT BY THE CANADIAN CARDIOVASCULAR SOCIETY

I. Ordinary physical activity does not cause angina. Angina occurs with unusually strenuous or prolonged exertion at work or recreation.
II. Slight limitation of ordinary activity. Angina may occur with walking or climbing stairs rapidly, walking uphill, walking or stair climbing after meals, in cold, in wind, under emotional stress, or only during the few hours after awakening. Walking more than 2 blocks on the level and climbing more than 1 flight of ordinary stairs at a normal pace and in normal conditions may cause angina.
III. Marked limitation of ordinary physical activity. Walking 1 to 2 blocks on the level and climbing 1 flight of stairs in normal conditions and at normal pace may cause angina.
IV. Inability to carry on any physical activity without discomfort. Anginal syndrome may be present at rest.

balanced against the possible increased costs and/or side effects of long-acting preparations. If symptoms are not adequately controlled, a combination of the 2 or 3 classes of antianginal agents is recommended. An exception is the patient with a significant vasospastic element. Pain that occurs only at rest, with emotion, or with cold exposure suggests **coronary vasospasm.** Documentation of transient ST elevation during pain is strong support for this diagnosis. A calcium channel blocker may be useful when this proposed physiologic mechanism is suspected.

A **disadvantage** of beta blockers is that they sometimes cause fatigue, impotence, and depression and/or nightmares in the elderly. Therefore, in young patients with active lifestyles, or in the elderly when side effects occur, a calcium channel blocker may be preferable.

In addition to antianginal pharmacologic therapy, care should be taken to identify and treat other factors that may alter the supply/demand balance, such as anemia, hypoxemia, CHF, thyroid dysfunction, and use of sympathomimetic drugs.

   c. **Indications for Mechanical Therapy (Angioplasty or Coronary Bypass).** In chronic stable angina, there are 3 major indications for intervention with mechanical therapy:

   (1). Symptoms. Patients with symptoms not adequately controlled with medical therapy are candidates for intervention with mechanical therapy.

   (2). Functional Impairment. Patients with very abnormal exercise test results may require mechanical therapy, depending on their coronary anatomy and response to medical therapy.

   (3). Anatomy. Patients with left main coronary artery stenosis or patients with 3-vessel disease and impaired left ventricular function may benefit from mechanical therapy for improved survival.

2. UNSTABLE ANGINA (CRESCENDO ANGINA)

a. **Clinical Findings.** The term *unstable angina* is used to describe a variety of clinical syndromes, including cases of patients with chronic angina whose pattern of angina changes in frequency, severity, provoking factors, or responsiveness to nitroglycerin. In some patients the pain comes on at rest or at night. The pain can be so prolonged that it may be indistinguishable from that of an acute MI. The mechanism responsible for development of unstable angina usually involves a change in myocardial O_2 supply as a result of increased coronary vasomotor tone and/or thrombus development at the site of plaque fissure or hemorrhage.

Since the symptoms of unstable angina may be similar to those of acute MI, these patients should be admitted to a monitored unit, and serial ECGs and cardiac enzyme determinations should be performed. ECGs recorded during episodes of pain will often show ischemic changes. The presence of transient ST elevation should raise the possibility of a vasospastic element.

b. **Treatment.** Patients presenting with unstable angina often are receiving therapy that will affect therapeutic choices. Dosage of antianginal medications should be adjusted to achieve optimal heart rate and blood pressure control. Vasoconstriction and the local endothelial damage secondary to plaque and thrombus formation are important precipitating factors in unstable angina. Therefore, an approach that counteracts both is advocated.

In patients whose pain is not initially controlled with bed rest and optimization of oral medications, a nitroglycerin infusion and heparinization (to keep partial thromboplastin time 1.5–2 times the control value) are advised. Nitroglycerin is administered IV with an initial dose of 10 μg/minute, which is titrated up every 5–10 minutes to control pain or until the systolic blood pressure is less than 110 mm Hg. Hypotension should be managed by reducing the infusion rate, elevating the foot of the bed, and giving IV fluids if necessary. Reflex tachycardia can be managed by increasing doses of a beta blocker. (Nitroglycerin should not be mixed in a plastic bottle because it is absorbed by polyvinylchloride.) When the pain has resolved and while the nitroglycerin infusion is being tapered, treatment with oral medications should be furthered. The addition of aspirin, 325 mg daily, as an antiplatelet agent is recommended.

If patients fail to respond to nitroglycerin infusion and other pharmacologic interventions, then arteriography, with consideration of mechanical intervention, is recommended. The use of the intra-aortic balloon pump in refractory cases may be a temporizing measure while arranging for angiography and subsequent surgery or angioplasty. For those patients who responded to pharmacologic interventions, stratification and early cardiac angiography is recommended in the high-risk group. The decision for mechanical intervention should be individualized and based on symptoms and laboratory data.

c. **Thrombolytic Agents in Unstable Angina.** Given the pathophysiology of unstable angina, several multicenter trials (urokinase in unstable angina [UK for USA], TIMI 3) are in progress to learn if thrombolytic therapy when given alone or in combination with standard treatment decreases morbidity and mortality from unstable angina. Preliminary studies thus far have demonstrated no differences.

3. **SILENT MYOCARDIAL ISCHEMIA**

a. **Clinical Findings.** Myocardial ischemia is "silent" when objective evidence of its presence is demonstrated by ischemic changes during exercise testing or Holter monitoring in otherwise asymptomatic patients. Three subsets of these patients have been classified by Cohn: **Type I:** Patients with coronary artery disease who have never experienced symptoms. **Type II:** Patients who have had an MI and subsequently exhibit painless ischemia on exercise testing. **Type III:** Patients with angina pectoris who have intermittent episodes of silent ischemia.

The full clinical implications of silent ischemia are not known. However, several studies suggest that patients with known coronary artery disease and documented silent ischemia have a worse prognosis than patients without silent ischemia. The diagnosis is based on ECG or scintigraphic evidence of transient ischemia. Ischemia can occur with or without evidence of increased myocardial O_2 demand (increased product of heart rate and blood pressure).

b. **Treatment.** There have been few studies to evaluate whether pharmacologic intervention in silent ischemia has the same effect as seen in patients who manifest symptoms. It appears that the same principles apply, however, and that all 3 classes of antiangina drugs may be beneficial. Because vasoconstriction may be an important pathophysiologic component, a calcium channel blocker is recommended as first-line therapy. Beta blockers may also be used. Nitrates are not recommended as standard therapy chiefly because tolerance develops. They may be used intermittently to achieve maximal anti-ischemic effects. Whereas silent myocardial ischemia alone is not currently an indication for surgery or angioplasty, it requires close follow-up.

4. **VARIANT ANGINA (CORNOARY ARTERY SPASM, PRINZMETAL'S ANGINA)**

a. **Clinical Findings.** The pain associated with coronary artery spasm is similar to that of other forms of angina pectoris and responds to nitroglycerin. A major difference is that the pain is spontaneous. It occurs predominantly at rest, especially in the early hours of the morning. The pain is usually not provoked by exertion.

Coronary artery spasm should be suspected on the basis of the patient's history. Patients sometimes note that beta blockers exacerbate symptoms. Transient elevation of the ST segment on the ECG with an episode of pain is highly suggestive of spasm. Provocation of spasm with IV ergonovine is the most effective method of diagnosis; however, acetylcholine, an endothelial cell–dependent agent, currently is frequently used to demonstrate endothelial cell vasoreactivity. Provocation with ergonovine or acetylcholine is not recommended in patients with significant fixed obstructive coronary artery disease.

b. Treatment. Calcium channel blockers are the treatment of choice. Usually a single agent is sufficient; in resistant cases, combination therapy with diltiazem and nifedipine, or verapamil and nifedipine around the clock, is useful. Continuous nitrate therapy is not recommended because of problems with tolerance, but targeted nitrates may be helpful in patients with a predictable pattern of pain. Beta blockers are contraindicated.

The natural history of spasm is one of periods of worsening symptoms followed by periods of relative quiescence. If a patient has been without symptoms for 6–12 months on therapy, withdrawal of therapy can be tried. Patients with spasm who do not have significant fixed coronary stenoses are not candidates for mechanical intervention.

5. ANGINA WITH NORMAL CORONARY ARTERIES (SYNDROME X)

a. Clinical Findings. A diagnosis of angina with normal coronary arteries is suspected when there is a convincing history of anginal chest pain (with or without documented reversible ischemic ECG changes) and when angiography fails to demonstrate either obstruction of major coronary vessels or spasm. Other causes of chest pain (esophageal spasm, acid reflux with esophagitis, gallbladder disease, cervical radiculopathy, Tietz's syndrome, and costochondritis) should be ruled out.

The etiology of syndrome X is still not fully understood, although studies show that some patients have an abnormal vasodilating response of the small or resistance vessels (diminished coronary reserve), whereas others apparently have a low pain threshold or some other noncardiac causes of pain. The natural history of the disorder is variable. Many patients' symptoms resolve with time, but some may experience exacerbation. Even in patients with persistent symptoms, syndrome X does not appear to be a risk factor for MI or sudden death.

b. Treatment. Therapy is empiric for this poorly understood condition. Calcium channel antagonists are often successful, and other antianginal drugs also can be useful. Patient reassurance is an important part of therapy.

Braunwald E: Heart Disease: A Textbook of Cardiovascular Medicine, 4th ed. Philadelphia, WB Saunders Co., 1992.
Opie LH: Drugs for the Heart, 3rd ed. Philadelphia, WB Saunders Co., 1991.
Braunwald E: Symposium: Calcium antagonists, emerging clinical opportunities. Am J Cardiol (suppl B) 59:1B–187B, 1987.
Braunwald E: Mechanism of action of calcium-channel blocking agents. N Engl J Med 307:1618–1627, 1982.

Nabel EG, Barry J, Rocco MB: Effects of dosing intervals on the development of tolerance to high-dose transdermal nitroglycerin. Am J Cardiol 63:663–669, 1989.

Singh BN: Silent Myocardial Ischemia and Angina. New York, Pergamon Press, 1988.

Cohn PF: Asymptomatic coronary artery disease. Mod Conc Cardiovasc Dis 50:55–60, 1981.

Opherk D, Zebe H, Weihe E, et al: Reduced coronary dilating capacity and intrastructural changes of the myocardium in patients with angina pectoris but normal angiograms. Circulation 65:817, 1981.

II. MYOCARDIAL INFARCTION (MI)

A. General Management of Acute Myocardial Infarction. Management of acute myocardial infarction (AMI) has changed considerably in recent years. Of major interest has been thrombolytic therapy and angioplasty to re-establish arterial patency and limit infarct size. Figure 4–1 shows an approach to the **triage** of patients with acute infarction. The most crucial aspect of intervention management is preserving the myocardium and re-establishing coronary flow within a short time frame. Studies

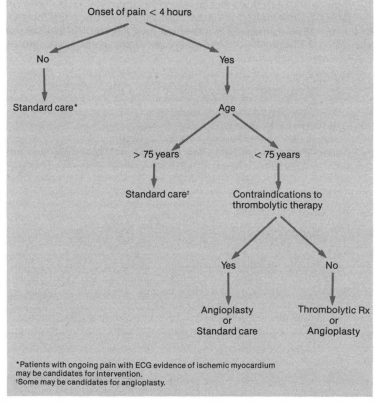

Figure 4–1. History suggesting acute myocardial infarction and electrocardiographic (ECG) changes with ST elevation: Triage strategy.

indicate that lytic therapy initiated within 4–6 hours after onset of symptoms is effective in reducing mortality.

General **contraindications to lytic therapy** include recent surgery or head trauma, active internal bleeding, suspected aortic dissection, pregnancy, diabetic hemorrhagic retinopathy, severe hypertension, history of cerebral vascular accident, and previous allergic reaction to the thrombolytic agent. As of this writing there are no clear guidelines for how to treat patients who are elderly ($\geq$75) or who present more than 6 hours after the onset of symptoms. Several ongoing trials are looking at the latter. Decisions about thrombolytic therapy must be made on a case-by-case basis in these patients (see below).

1. **PAIN RELIEF. Morphine, 2 to 6 mg IV,** should be given every 5–30 minutes. Many patients require large doses, and a total of up to 15–20 mg may be needed. Caution must be used in elderly patients and patients with COPD. Nitroglycerin (NTG) paste or infusion is used if ischemia continues. NTG both reduces systemic vascular resistance and pulmonary capillary wedge pressure and increases collateral coronary blood flow to the subendocardium, thereby protecting ischemic myocardium. Routine use of NTG is not recommended owing to a paradoxic response that may exacerbate the ischemia. When NTG is administered, adequate coronary perfusion pressure should be maintained.

2. **OXYGEN THERAPY** at 2–3 L/min via nasal prongs and **sedation** are given as required. Patients should be on a light diet during the first 24 hours.

3. **ARRHYTHMIA PREVENTION**
There is no demonstrated survival advantage for patients given prophylactic antiarrhythmic therapy after admission to a monitored unit. Arrhythmias should be promptly diagnosed and treated to prevent further deterioration related to increased myocardial O_2 demands, decreased cardiac output, or electrical instability.

4. **BETA-ADRENERGIC BLOCKERS**
For many years the use of beta blockers in the early phase of AMI was controversial. Today, early use of IV beta blockers is increasing. Several studies (ISIS, Goteborg, TIMI 2) have demonstrated beneficial effects, including limitation of infarct size and reduction of ventricular fibrillation. Use caution when administering beta blockers because of their occasional unpredictable hemodynamic effects. Propranolol (Inderal) (0.5 mg increments IV up to a total of 0.1 mg/kg) and metoprolol (Lopressor) (5 mg every 5 minutes to a total of 15 mg IV) are the most commonly used beta blockers as of this writing.

5. **CALCIUM CHANNEL BLOCKERS**
Calcium channel blockers are effective in acute and chronic stable angina, but there have been conflicting reports about their effectiveness in AMI. Patients with continued post-MI ischemia caused by coronary vasospasm may benefit from a calcium channel blocker. Diltiazem, in both long- and short-term studies, has demonstrated

beneficial effects (prevention of reinfarction and reduction in mortality) following non–Q-wave MI in patients without CHF.

B. Acute Transmural Myocardial Infarction

1. PATHOPHYSIOLOGY

The pathophysiology of AMI has been controversial since Hippocrates first postulated that heart disease can cause sudden death. The causes of MI can be divided into those that *decrease* myocardial O_2 supply and those that *increase* myocardial O_2 demand. **Atherosclerotic plaque** is the most common cause for reduction of coronary blood flow, thereby reducing oxygen supply. These plaques reduce the cross-sectional area of coronary artery lumen, thus reducing coronary perfusion pressure. When a critical stenosis develops, coronary blood flow is adequate at rest but cannot increase to meet metabolic demand. The subendocardium blood reserve becomes much more limited than that of the subepicardium. Disruptions of atherosclerotic plaques are commonly observed post mortem in patients who died following AMI. A disrupted plaque may serve as a nidus for formation of a thrombus that may occlude the infarct-related vessel. A thrombus, if present, usually contains platelet aggregates and substances from the plaque. Platelet aggregates are more common in the coronary arteries of patients who die suddenly from coronary artery disease than in those with coronary artery disease who die of noncardiac causes.

2. SYMPTOMS

Classically, AMI is diagnosed as a constellation of symptoms: chest pressure associated with nausea and/or diaphoresis. The chest pressure or ache may radiate to the arm, elbow, jaw, or neck. Any combination of these symptoms may occur. Chest discomfort in AMI may be atypical; it even is absent in 15–30% of AMI cases (silent AMI).

3. LABORATORY FINDINGS

The initial ECG shows ST elevation in the leads reflecting the area of the myocardium involved. As the ECG changes evolve, the associated T waves may be tall and peaked. Within hours, the T waves usually become inverted, and Q waves develop. In most cases, the ST segment returns to the baseline unless an aneurysm develops (then ST elevation persists). Cardiac enzymes (creatinine phosphokinase, CPK-MB) become elevated within 4–6 hours and peak around 18–24 hours.

4. REPERFUSION IN AMI

Approaches to the management of AMI have changed significantly in the past decade with better understanding of the pathophysiologic mechanism. Since the advent of the CCU, the extent of myocardial dysfunction determines both early and late mortality and morbidity. Interventions to limit myocardial damage have become standard (i.e., thrombolytic therapy).

a. **Thrombolytic Therapy.** Both endogenous and exogenous throm-bolytic agents reduce mortality and morbidity from AMI by achieving vascular reperfusion. Thrombolytic agents directly or indirectly activate plasminogen. Table 4–6 describes their charac-teristics.

Streptokinase (SK) is given as a 1-hr IV infusion of 1.5 MU. Aspirin, 324 mg, is also given at this stage. Allergic reactions may be treated with corticosteroids and diphenhydramine. Streptoki-nase opens vessels in 50–60% of cases when given within 6 hours of onset of symptoms. As with any agent that is effective in restabilizing blood flow to ischemic or infarcted myocardium, reperfusion arrhythmias such as ventricular tachycardia, frequent ventricular ectopy, and various degrees of heart block may occur.

Following streptokinase therapy, **IV heparin** is started to main-tain the activated partial thromboplastin time (PTT) at a level of 1.5–2 times the control value. Heparin therapy is continued for about 48 hours.

Anisoylated plasminogen-streptokinase activator complex (AP-SAC), a substance derived from modification of the streptokinase molecule, is administered over 2–5 minutes by IV infusion of 30 mg. Plasma half-life is 95 minutes. The reperfusion rate is time-dependent and is similar to that of streptokinase. IV heparin is started after infusion of APSAC.

Urokinase has the advantage over SK of not causing an allergic reaction. It is more expensive than streptokinase but less costly than tissue plasminogen activator (t-PA). The IV dosage is 3 MU over 45–60 minutes (not yet FDA-approved use). Therapy is followed by heparinization. Urokinase is used as an alternative to SK in patients who are allergic to or who have recently received SK.

Single-chain urokinase plasminogen activator (scu-PA) is the precursor of urokinase. Preliminary studies have shown that scu-PA in a dose range of 30–50 mg has a low performance rate and has taken a long time to reperfuse. More recent evidence suggests augmentation of its efficacy when used in combination with uro-kinase or t-PA.

Tissue plasminogen activator (t-PA) is an endogenous plas-minogen activator secreted by the vascular endothelium. It has a high affinity for specific binding sites. The current recommended dose is 100 mg (60 mg over 1 hour, 40 mg over the next 2 hours). Major bleeding is an infrequent but serious side effect. After use of t-PA, heparinization followed by aspirin is recommended. The cost of t-PA is several times that of SK. Though t-PA has been demonstrated to produce a higher patency rate acutely than does SK, SK patency rate eventually equals that of t-PA. No difference in clinical outcomes in patients treated with SK or t-PA has been demonstrated. The choice of thrombolytic agent must be made on a case-by-case basis.

Ever since Meyer described the successful application of per-cutaneous transluminal coronary angioplasty (PTCA) for AMI in

TABLE 4-6. CHARACTERISTICS OF THROMBOLYTIC AGENTS

	SK	APSAC	t-PA	scu-PA	UK
Fibrin selective	No	No	Yes	Yes	Yes
Plasminogen binding	Indirect	Indirect	Direct	Direct	Direct
Duration of infusion (min)	60	2–5	90–180	90–180	5–15
Half-life (min)	23	90	8	7	16
Fibrinogen breakdown	4+	3+	1–2+	2+	3+
Early heparin required	No	No	Yes	No	Yes
Hypotension	Yes	Yes	No	No	No
Allergic reactions	Yes	Yes	No	No	No
Approximate cost/dose	$200/1.5 MU	$1200/30 U	$2200/100 mg	High	$2200/3 MU
Patency at 90 min	53–65	55–65	69–79	71	66
Patency at 24 hours	81–88	88–92	78–85	85	73

Abbreviations: APSAC, anisoylated plasminogen streptokinase activator complex (anistreplase); SK, streptokinase; t-PA, tissue plasminogen activator; UK, urokinase; scu-PA, single-chain urokinase (pro-urokinase) plasminogen activator; MU, million units; U, units.

1982, the combination of thrombolysis and PTCA in treating AMI seemed attractive. First, no thrombolytic agent has allowed reperfusion rates greater than 75–80%. Identification of the 25% of patients in whom thrombolytic therapy has failed may provide the select group of patients who would benefit from treatment by PTCA. Second, thrombolytic therapy does little to alter the underlying pathology responsible for initiating the acute infarction. Third, the combination of thrombolysis followed by PTCA should reduce the flow-limiting stenosis left by thrombolysis alone. Although this approach was attractive in theory, the predicted benefit of PTCA was not established in early studies.

The feasibility of PTCA as **primary treatment for AMI** has been reported in 1 study. Other studies, however, did not show the same success. An unusually high rate of early reocclusion was noted and an increase in mortality and bleeding complications observed. Angioplasty is generally reserved for patients who are not candidates for thrombolytic therapy, patients who are in cardiogenic shock, or those in whom thrombolytic therapy fails, with demonstrable ongoing ischemia (rescue PTCA).

The **combination of IV thrombolysis and PTCA** has been the subject of several major clinical trials. The optimal timing of coronary angioplasty following IV thrombolysis has important implications for management of AMI patients. Strategies for determining the optimal time for coronary angioplasty include deferring it for 18 to 48 hours, up to 10 days, or indefinitely if stress testing shows no evidence of ischemia.

Three large randomized trials investigated the above strategies. Although different in design, they arrived at the same conclusions:

1. Immediate PTCA offered no advantage over an elective strategy which reserves PTCA for those with clinical indications;
2. In-hospital mortality was higher with the immediate PTCA group;
3. Emergency coronary artery bypass graft surgery was required more frequently in the immediate PTCA group;
4. There was a substantially higher incidence of thrombolytic complications in the immediate PTCA group.

These studies support a more conservative approach to mechanical reperfusion except in patients who demonstrate recurrent ischemia or show evidence of provocable ischemia on predischarge exercise tolerance test.

C. Acute Nontransmural MI. Patients with nontransmural infarction may present with **symptoms similar to those with transmural infarction,** though they are more likely to have a "**stuttering**" **course** like patients with unstable angina. The ECG changes are usually ST depression or T-wave inversions, which may persist or worsen over the first 24–48 hours. The diagnosis is made on the basis of clinical history, ECG changes, and the characteristic enzyme pattern (similar to that of transmural infarct, though usually with a lower peak CK). The pathophysiology is probably more like that of unstable angina than transmural infarction: occlusive thrombus is uncommon, but some combination of plaque disruption, change in vasomotor tone, and subocclusive thrombus is the underlying cause. Many of these patients have diffuse coronary artery disease, and may go on to have unstable courses (hence the concept of "incomplete" infarction). The efficacy of thrombolytic agents in this condition has not been proved. **Care should be similar to that for transmural infarction.** Some authors believe that there should be a lower threshold for angiography and invasive therapy because of the high incidence of recurrent ischemia and subsequent infarction. Others think that the clinical course and the usual stratification strategies are sufficient to select patients for more aggressive therapy. Studies are still needed to define optimal diagnostic and therapeutic strategies in patients with nontransmural MI.

D. **Complications of Q-Wave and Non–Q-Wave MI.** Regardless of the type and mechanism of infarction, all patients post-MI must be carefully monitored and managed because of the risk of complications in their course.

1. ACUTE COMPLICATIONS

   a. **Electrical Disturbances.** Electrical disturbances are the most frequent complication associated with AMI and vary from premature atrial and ventricular beats to ventricular fibrillation (Table 4–7).

   b. **Conduction Disturbances.** Ischemic injury can produce conduction disturbances at any level of the atrioventricular or intraventricular conduction system. **First degree AV block and Mobitz type I block** generally occur in the AV node and are commonly seen in patients with acute inferior MI (IMI). Both are usually transient. **Mobitz type II AV block** is usually associated with anterior MI. It often progresses suddenly to complete atrioventricular block (CHB). Treatment requires insertion of a temporary pacemaker electrode. **Complete AV block** may occur with IMI. In this circumstance, the block progresses from first to second to complete AV block; it is usually transient and may resolve within days. Complete AV block associated with acute anterior MI is generally sudden. Treatment is with a temporary pacemaker and later a permanent transvenous pacemaker if indicated, depending on the patient's subsequent course.

   c. **Intraventricular Blocks.** Isolated left anterior fascicular block (LAFB) and left posterior fascicular block (LPFB) rarely progress to CHB. The combination of right bundle branch block (RBBB) with LAFB, LPFB, or first degree AV block (if new) has a high risk of progressing to CHB and constitutes an indication for the insertion of a temporary pacemaker. Similarly a new LBBB in the setting of an AMI is an indication for a temporary pacemaker. Usually the infarct is anterior and extensive and is associated with a high mortality rate.

   d. **Volume Depletion.** Volume depletion as the cause of hypotension should be suspected in patients with hypotension and clear lungs on exam and x-ray. It is particularly common in IMIs. If the patient does not respond promptly to aggressive volume expansion,

TABLE 4-7. ARRHYTHMIAS ASSOCIATED WITH ACUTE MYOCARDIAL INFARCTION

ARRHYTHMIA	PRIMARY THERAPY	SECONDARY THERAPY	OTHER
Ventricular fibrillation	Cardioversion, 200–400 Wsec; CPR	Bretylium IV, 5 mg/kg	
Ventricular tachycardia	Lidocaine IV, 75–100 mg, precordial thump, cardioversion	Lidocaine IV, 75–100 mg Procainamide IV, 0.5–1 gm loading dose should be given	
Ventricular premature beats (≥6/min, 1–3 mg/min R on T, coupling, multifocal)	Lidocaine IV, 75–100 mg bolus, then 1–3 mg/min infusion	Procainamide IV, 0.5–1 gm loading dose; 2–6 mg/min infusion oral quinidine	Exclude other causes, such as low K^+ or Mg^{2+}, digitalis intoxication
Ventricular asystole	CPR Intracardiac epinephrine	Transthoracic or transvenous pacing	
Accelerated idioventricular rhythm			
Symptomatic	Lidocaine IV, 75–100 mg; pacing if heart block or inappropriate bradycardia is underlying only		
Asymptomatic	None		
Accelerated junctional rhythm	None, unless appropriate	Pacing	R/O digitalis toxicity
Sinus tachycardia	None	None	Seek underlying cause; reflects underlying heart failure requiring treatment; also R/O fever, anemia, hypovolemia

Condition			
Sinus bradycardia			
Symptomatic	Atropine IV, 0.5–1 mg	Temporary transvenous pacemaker	
Asymptomatic	Atropine		
Atrial premature beats	None		
Paroxysmal supraventricular tachycardia	Carotid sinus massage; Digoxin IV, 0.25 mg	Propranolol IV, 0.5–2 mg Verapamil IV, 5–10 mg Cardioversion	
Atrial fibrillation	Digoxin IV, 0.25 mg	Propranolol IV, 0.5–2 mg Verapamil IV, 5–10 mg diltiazem IV 20–25 mg bolus, then 5–15 mg/min infusion; Cardioversion (synchronized)	May indicate early left ventricular failure
Atrial flutter	Digoxin IV, 0.25 mg	Propranolol IV, 0.5–2 mg Verapamil IV, 5–10 mg diltiazem IV 20–25 mg bolus, then 5–15 mg/min infusion; Cardioversion (synchronized)	May indicate early left ventricular failure
First degree	None		
Mobitz type I			
Asymptomatic	None		
Symptomatic	Atropine, temporary transvenous pacing		
Mobitz type II			
Asymptomatic	Temporary pacing		
Symptomatic	Temporary transvenous pacing		
Complete heart block	Temporary transvenous	Atropine IV, 0.5–1 mg isoproterenol IV, infusion 1–2 μg/min	

the diagnosis requires documentation of low filling pressures and low cardiac output by a Swan-Ganz catheter to rule out other causes and guide volume replacement.

e. Right Ventricular Infarction. Hypoperfusion caused by right ventricular (RV) infarction may be confused with that caused by hypovolemia, since both are associated with low, or normal, PCWP. RV infarction also usually occurs in the setting of inferior wall MI. Vigorous fluid therapy that raises both left and right ventricular filling pressures to an appropriate level is indicated. Patients may require RA pressures in the range of 15 to 20 in order to adequately fill the left ventricle.

f. Infarct Extension. Infarct extension occurs in 10–30% of patients with AMI. It is diagnosed by re-elevation of plasma CPK. New chest pain and new persistent ECG changes frequently but not universally develop. Infarct extension has been reported to occur more frequently in nontransmural myocardial infarction, suggesting a higher prevalence of subtotal coronary occlusion. Since infarct extension results in further left ventricular dysfunction, aggressive management of post-MI ischemia is essential.

g. Post-MI Ischemia. Post-MI ischemia may occur early or late after AMI. It is evidence that additional myocardium is at risk and may represent an incomplete or nontransmural myocardial infarction (non–Q-wave); this may also represent myocardial ischemia at a distance due to critical narrowing of a second coronary artery. Diagnosis may be made by the recurrence of classic angina pectoris with or without ECG changes after a pain-free period. Frequent bouts of CHF secondary to worsening left ventricular function or papillary muscle ischemia may be the only evidence that post-MI ischemia is occurring. In addition to pharmacologic intervention for treatment of ischemia and heart failure, coronary angiography and possible mechanical intervention should be undertaken.

h. Left Ventricular Failure. Left ventricular function is restricted by the extent of myocardial necrosis; this determines both short-term and long-term prognosis. To establish the prognosis of patients with AMI, Killip categorized patients into 4 hemodynamic subsets based on admission physical findings. The Cedars-Sinai Hemodynamic characterization is based on hemodynamic features.

KILLIP CLASS

Class I:	No signs of left ventricular failure
Class II:	S_3 gallop and/or pulmonary congestion limited to basal lung segments
Class III:	Acute pulmonary edema
Class IV:	Shock syndrome

CEDARS-SINAI HEMODYNAMIC CLASS

Class I:	PCW≤ 18; CI> 2.2
Class II:	PCW> 18; CI> 2.2
Class III:	PCW≤ 18; CI≤ 2.2
Class IV:	PCW> 18; CI≤ 2.2

---

i. **Management of Pump Failure.** Invasive monitoring is essential in the management of patients with moderate to severe left ventricular dysfunction in the setting of AMI. This will enable hemodynamic differentiation of the causes of pump failure.

Maintenance of adequate gas exchange requires careful attention; hypoxemia can precipitate postinfarction ischemia. Supplemental O_2, intubation, or positive end-expiratory pressure (PEEP) may be required.

Patients with AMI complicated by mild to moderate heart failure usually respond well to **diuretics.** This results in reduced pulmonary capillary wedge pressure (PCWP) and left ventricular end diastolic pressure (LVEDP), which, in turn, enhance myocardial O_2 perfusion. However, most patients are not total body volume overloaded. Since the systolic and diastolic dysfunction accompanying MI necessitates relatively high filling pressures to maintain cardiac output, one must be careful not to induce hypovolemic hypotension through excess diuretics.

Vasodilators are used in moderate to severe pump failure or in heart failure unresponsive to diuretics (patients with severe mitral regurgitation and ventricular septal defect). These drugs decrease afterload and left ventricular filling pressures, thereby increasing stroke volume and cardiac output. Since vasodilators have a propensity to induce systemic hypotension and decrease coronary perfusion, it is essential that left ventricular filling pressures be maintained at 18–20 mm Hg. IV and short-acting agents are recommended during the early stages of therapy (see Table 4–13). After stabilization, long-acting agents may be used.

Administration of **digitalis** to patients with AMI has always been controversial. Digitalis is presently reserved for the treatment of patients with atrial fibrillation or atrial flutter and those with heart failure that persists beyond the acute management phase.

j. **Cardiogenic Shock.** Cardiogenic shock is characterized by prolonged tissue hypoperfusion, low arterial blood pressure, markedly reduced cardiac output, and oliguria. The prognosis is extremely poor, with an in-hospital mortality of 80–100% in patients who are not candidates for acute mechanical intervention. The cause of cardiogenic shock must be determined in order to plan appropriate intervention. The diagnosis of acute mitral regurgitation, secondary to papillary muscle rupture, versus ventricular septal defect (VSD) is made by cardiac catheterization and echocardiography. Urgent surgical intervention, usually with intra-aortic balloon support, is required. Cardiogenic shock due to pure left ventricular dysfunction may be treated with pharmacologic agents or intra-aortic balloon counterpulsation (IABP). If there is an element of ongoing ischemia some of these patients may be candidates for acute revascularization; therefore, in appropriate patients, acute angiography should be performed.

2. **LATE IN-HOSPITAL COMPLICATIONS OF AMI**
Late in-hospital complications include ventricular arrhythmias, CHF, pericarditis, and mural thrombi.

a. **Ventricular arrhythmias** are generally seen in the early phase of AMI. The arrhythmia carries a poor prognosis if observed 4–7 days after the event. Long-term antiarrhythmic therapy is often necessary, and electrophysiologic studies may be required to guide therapy.

b. **Congestive Heart Failure.** Moderate to severe pump failure is usually recognized in the acute phase. However, mild to moderate CHF in some patients is not recognized until the rehabilitation phase. Treatment may only be a diuretic. Digitalization is indicated if cardiomegaly and S3 gallop persist. Initiation of afterload reduction with an ACE inhibitor not only may improve symptoms but also may improve ventricular geometry and long-term ventricular function.

c. **Pericarditis and Dressler's Syndrome.** Acute pericarditis is a frequent complication of AMI occurring within 1–4 days afterward. A friction rub can be heard in many cases; it is potentiated by the supine position. One must distinguish acute pericarditis pain from that of recurrent ischemia. This pain may be treated with aspirin.

A delayed form of pericarditis called *Dressler's syndrome* may occur 1 week to several months post-AMI. It is thought to be secondary to an immunologic or autoimmune mechanism. A clinical picture of fever, malaise, anorexia, and arthralgia is often seen. Pleural effusion and even pulmonary infiltration may occur. Treatment is with aspirin or other anti-inflammatory drugs.

d. **Mural thrombi** tend to occur in patients with an acute anterior wall MI with or without aneurysm formation as early as 36 hours after infarction. Systemic embolization is infrequent. Diagnosis may be made by 2-dimensional echocardiography. Immediate anticoagulation with heparin followed by warfarin for 3–6 months is indicated if there are no contraindications. In the absence of contraindications, prophylactic anticoagulation should be considered in all patients with large anterior MI, even in the absence of intramural thrombus on 2-D echo. This strategy has not been subjected to prospective randomized study, however.

e. **Ventricular rupture** generally occurs between 5 and 7 days after transmural AMI in approximately 1% of patients. It is usually catastrophic and is associated with electromechanical dissociation. Rarely do patients survive.

E. **Rehabilitation.** Rehabilitation of the AMI patient occurs in 2 phases.

1. **PHASE I (IN-HOSPITAL)**
Patients with uncomplicated AMI should stay approximately 2–3 days in a CCU. They should begin leg exercise immediately and progressive ambulation within 5–7 days. Progressive increase in activity is aimed at return to a normal lifestyle.

Before discharge, most patients should have a *low-level exercise test* for risk stratification. Such testing may show evidence of ischemia, arrhythmia, or hypotension that might not have been observed otherwise. Depending on the data obtained, early invasive intervention may be indicated before discharge. Before leaving the hospital all patients should be started on aspirin and a beta blocker (if there are no contraindications). Several studies have shown a decrease in mortality when patients with AMI are treated with a beta blocker.

2. PHASE II (POST-HOSPITAL)
This phase of rehabilitation is aimed at conditioning and return to normal function within 2 months and should include an organized program of walking. Later this should be advanced to jogging or running as appropriate under supervised conditions. For long-term rehabilitation, a patient may enroll in an individual program. Advancement within rehabilitation depends on individual capabilities. Over the past decade, several studies have shown that lifestyle intervention programs can have a significant impact on morbidity and mortality post-AMI. Finally, the psychologic effects of AMI on patient and family alike can be crippling. Fear of death and hesitation in resuming social and sexual activities are best handled by the physician and family together.

F. Prevention

1. RISK FACTORS FOR ATHEROSCLEROSIS
Remediable risk factors are hypercholesterolemia, high blood pressure, and cigarette smoking. Age and male gender are also powerful risk factors. Others include diabetes mellitus, stress, family history of coronary artery disease, obesity, and sedentary lifestyle. Obesity has not been proved to be an independent risk factor of coronary artery disease; however, it is associated with hypertension, diabetes, and hypercholesterolemia.

    a. Hypercholesterolemia. In general, a cholesterol level less than 200 mg/dL is desirable. It is difficult to designate a limit for cholesterol: elevated serum cholesterol is multifactorial. Serum cholesterol varies from population to population. Atherosclerosis primarily correlates with elevated low-density lipoprotein (LDL) cholesterol. In addition, growing evidence supports the hypothesis that lipoprotein(a) (Lpa) and homocysteine may be a marker for the development of atherosclerosis. Elevation of high-density lipoprotein (HDL) correlates negatively with atherosclerosis. A favorable ratio of LDL to HDL is ≤4:1.

    b. Hypertension. The role of hypertension in coronary artery disease is twofold: it is a predisposing factor for atherosclerosis and it increases myocardial O_2 demands in patients with coronary artery disease.

    c. Cigarette Smoking. Cigarette smoking is related to the development of coronary thrombosis, AMI, and sudden death.

2. PRIMARY PREVENTION
Since atherosclerosis is a result of multiple risk factors, it is important to control several risk factors simultaneously (multiple risk factor intervention). The Oslo Study Group Intervention Trial demonstrated a significant reduction in incidence of first-time MI and sudden cardiac death in the trial group. The Multiple Risk Factor Intervention Trial

(MRFIT) demonstrated a significantly lower overall mortality in the treatment group when multiple risk factors were addressed simultaneously in the subjects taking aspirin. **Aspirin** is presently used in primary prevention because it inhibits platelet aggregation, thus limiting thrombus formation in atherosclerotic plaques. Several studies have shown a reduction in MI.

3. SECONDARY PREVENTION
Secondary prevention is aimed at reducing the risk of complications, recurrence of AMI, or progression of disease in patients who have already had a complication from coronary artery disease. Many studies have confirmed the importance of drugs and lifestyle changes in reducing the consequences of coronary artery disease. Measures such as the administration of aspirin or beta blockers reduce mortality following an AMI. Modification of factors predisposing to atherosclerosis also influence its progression. In addition, not only may lowering serum cholesterol retard the **progression** of atherosclerosis, but **regression** may occur in some patients. Secondary prevention trials have demonstrated also that exercise reduces weight, modifies lipoprotein profile, and reduces mortality and morbidity from AMI.

Gruppo Italiano per lo Studio Della Streptokinasi nell' Infarto Miocardio (GISSI): Effectiveness of intravenous thrombolytic treatment in acute myocardial infarction. Lancet 1:397, 1986.

Topol EJ, Califf RM, George BS, et al.: A randomized trial of immediate versus delayed elective angioplasty after intravenous tissue plasminogen activator in acute myocardial infarction. N Engl J Med 317:581, 1987.

Topol EJ, O'Neil WW, Lanburd AB, et al.: A randomized, placebo controlled trial of intravenous recombinant tissue-type plasminogen activator and emergency coronary angioplasty in patients with acute myocardial infarction. Circulation 75:420, 1987.

TIMI Research Group: Immediate versus delayed catheterization and coronary angioplasty following thrombotic therapy for acute myocardial infarction: TIMI IIA results. JAMA 260:2849–2858, 1988.

The TIMI Research Group: Comparison of invasive and conservative strategies after treatment with intravenous tissue plasminogen activator in acute myocardial infarction: Results of the thrombolysis in myocardial infarction (TIMI) phase II trial. N Engl J Med 320:618–627, 1989.

Simoons ML, Betriu A, Col J: Thrombolysis with tissue plasminogen activator in acute myocardial infarction: No additional benefit from immediate coronary angioplasty. Lancet 1:197–203, 1988.

ISIS-2 Collaborative Group: Randomized trial of intravenous streptokinase, oral aspirin, both, or neither among 17,187 cases of suspected acute myocardial infarction: ISIS-2. Lancet 2:349–360, 1988.

AIMS Trial Study Group: Long-term effects of intravenous anistreplase in acute myocardial infarction: Final report of the AIMS study. Lancet 335:427–431, 1990.

Norwegian Multicenter Study Group: Timolol induced reduction in mortality and reinfarction in patients surviving acute myocardial infarction. N Engl J Med 304:801, 1981.

Beta-blocker Heart Attack Trial Research Group: A randomized trial of propranolol in patients with acute myocardial infarction. 1. Mortality results. JAMA 247:1707–1714, 1982.

Gibson RS, Boden WE, Theroux P: Diltiazem and reinfarction in patients with non Q-wave myocardial infarction: Results of a double-blind, randomized multicenter trial. N Engl J Med 3156:423–429, 1986.

Oberman A: Exercise and the primary prevention of cardiovascular disease. Am J Cardiol 55:10–D, 1985.

Hjermann I, Holme I, Byre K, and Leren P: Effects of diet and smoking on the incidence of coronary heart disease: Report from the Oslo Study Group of a randomized trial in healthy men. Lancet 2:1303, 1981.

Multiple-Risk Factor Intervention Trial Research Group: Multiple-Risk Factor Intervention Trial: Risk factor changes in mortality results. JAMA 248:1465, 1982.

III. CONGESTIVE HEART FAILURE (CHF)

A. Clinical Manifestations. CHF is a clinical state of increased left atrial and/or right atrial pressure. This discussion will focus on CHF caused by decreased left ventricular contractility, which is its most common cause. CHF secondary to decreased contractility results in increased left atrial pressure and left ventricular end-diastolic pressure, decreased stroke volume, and therefore decreased cardiac output. As a result, a number of reflex mechanisms are activated, including the sympathetic nervous system and the renin-angiotensin-aldosterone system. The resulting vasoconstriction and fluid retention lead to increased afterload and preload.

It is important, when planning therapy for patients with heart failure, to exclude potentially reversible causes and to identify surgically correctable lesions (valvular disease, ventricular aneurysm, and constrictive pericarditis). Echocardiography is useful to help screen for valvular disease. Coronary artery disease and consequent MI constitute the most common cause of depressed ventricular function in our society. Other causes for cardiomyopathy are listed in Table 4–8. In some patients presenting with heart failure without an obvious cause, detailed cardiovascular evaluation, including catheterization and endomyocardial biopsy, may be appropriate.

The New York Heart Association classification (Table 4–9) is a useful way to stratify patients into a functional class according to the severity

TABLE 4–8. COMMON CAUSES OF CARDIOMYOPATHY OTHER THAN CAD

INFECTIVE	TOXIC
Viral	Alcohol
Coxsackie B	Bleomycin
Coxsackie A	Adriamycin
ECHO	Lead
AIDS	Corticosteroids
Parasitic	Cocaine
Bacterial	
Spirochetal	**INFILTRATIVE**
	Amyloidosis
METABOLIC	Hemochromatosis
Thiamine deficiency	Sarcoidosis
Acromegaly	Neoplastic
Myxedema	Glycogen storage disorders
Thyrotoxicosis	
Diabetes mellitus	**OTHERS**
Uremia	Endocardial fibroelastosis
Cushing's disease	Sickle cell anemia
Kwashiorkor	Neuromuscular disorders
Scurvy	Postpartum disorders
	Hypertrophic cardiomyopathy

TABLE 4–9. NEW YORK HEART ASSOCIATION CLASSIFICATION FOR SEVERITY OF HEART FAILURE

Class I	Ordinary physical activity does not cause undue dyspnea or fatigue.
Class II	Comfort is present at rest, but ordinary physical activity results in dyspnea or fatigue.
Class III	Comfort is present at rest, but less than ordinary physical activity results in dyspnea or fatigue.
Class IV	Dyspnea or fatigue may be present at rest and is made worse by any physical effort.

of their symptoms. Formal exercise stress testing provides additional functional evaluation. Studies have shown that the survival of patients can be predicted by functional classification and exercise performance.

The clinical manifestations of heart failure vary depending on the chamber involved. Right heart failure results primarily in systemic venous congestion, whereas left heart failure causes primarily pulmonary vascular congestion. Biventricular failure leads to both pulmonary and systemic venous congestion.

B. Treatment of Heart Failure. Treatment of a syndrome as variable as CHF must be tailored to the patient. The aim of therapy in CHF is to reduce both preload and afterload, to relieve symptoms of atrial hypertension, and to improve cardiac output. Cardiac glycosides directly affect the myocardium to improve contractility and are useful short-term, but may have less benefit in long-term therapy. Diuretics benefit patients with mild failure (Tables 4–10 and 4–11), but in patients with moderate or severe failure, diuretics alone are insufficient.

In Table 4–12, vasoactive agents that can be used orally are listed. ACE inhibitors have been the mainstay of therapy for long-term use.

Among the drugs that can be used parenterally, direct-acting vasodilators are the mainstay (Table 4–13). Sympathomimetic drugs to improve inotropy and support blood pressure may be necessary in the severely ill patient but may pose a high risk for inducing arrhythmias, myocardial ischemia, or peripheral vasoconstriction. It is sometimes appropriate to use **combination therapy,** such as dopamine and nitroprusside. The phosphodiesterase inhibitors (PDE), such as amrinone, can be combined with the sympathomimetic drugs. A potential concern about use of phosphodiesterase drugs is the risk of ischemia, arrhythmias, and apparent deterioration in cardiac function when the drugs are discontinued.

1. ACUTE THERAPY

The approach depends on the severity of the failure. Often patients will be hypoxic, needing supplemental O_2 via nasal prongs, 3–4 L/ min. In severe hypoxia and marked respiratory difficulty, intubation and mechanical ventilation may be necessary. In severe failure, particularly with AMI, Swan-Ganz catheter monitoring will help optimize pharmacologic therapy.

Text continued on page 161

TABLE 4–10. THIAZIDE DIURETICS: DOSES AND DURATION OF ACTION

GENERIC NAME	TRADE NAME	DOSAGE*	DURATION OF ACTION (HR)
Hydrochlorothiazide	HydroDIURIL, Esidrix, Thiuretic	12.5–25 mg (BP) 25–100 mg (CHF)	6–12
Hydroflumethazide	Saluron, Diucardin	12.5–25 mg (BP) 25–200 mg (CHF)	6–12
Chlorthalidone	Hygroton, Thalitone	12.5–50 mg	48–72
Metolazone	Zaroxolyn, Diulo	1–5 mg (BP) 5–20 mg (CHF)	18–25
Bendrofluazide	Naturetin	1.25–2.5 mg (BP) 10 mg (CHF)	6–12
Bendroflumethiazide			
Polythiazide	Renese	1–2 mg (BP)	24–48
Chlorothiazide	Diuril	250–1000 mg	6–12
Cyclothiazide	Anhydron	1–2 mg	6–12
Trichlormethazide	Metahydrin, Naqua	1–4 mg	About 24
Indapamide	Lozol	2.5 mg (BP)	16–36

*BP, use for blood pressure lowering; CHF, use for congestive heart failure.

157

TABLE 4–11. DIURETICS

DRUG	DOSAGE	ADMINISTRATION	DURATION OF ACTION	SIDE EFFECTS
Potassium-Depleting Agents				
Furosemide	20–240 mg/day or 20–120 mg bid	Oral IV	6–8 hr 2 hr	Hypokalemia, hypotension, hyperuricemia, skin rash, abnormal liver function
Bumetanide	0.5–2 mg/day	Oral IV	24 hr 24 hr	Muscle cramps, hypotension, dizziness, encephalopathy in patients with liver disease
Ethacrynic acid	50–100 mg/day	Oral IV	24 hr 4–6 hr	Hypotension, hypokalemia
Potassium-Sparing Agents				
Amiloride	5–15 mg/day	Oral	24 hr	Hyperkalemia
Triamterene	100–200 mg/day	Oral	24 hr	Hyperkalemia, nausea
Spironolactone	50–200 mg/day	Oral	24 hr	Hyperkalemia, gynecomastia

TABLE 4–12. NONPARENTERAL DRUGS FOR CONGESTIVE HEART FAILURE

CLASS	DOSAGE	VENODILATOR	ARTERIAL DILATOR	BP	CO	SVR	RAP
Direct-Acting Vasodilators							
Hydralazine	50–200 mg q 6–8 hr	+/0	+ + +	0/—	+ +	—	0
Isosorbide dinitrate	20–60 mg q 4–6 hr	+ + +	+	0/—	+	0/—	—
Nitroglycerin ointment	1.5–2.0 inches q 6 hr	+ + +	+				
Nitroglycerin patches	5–30 cm² q 12 hr	+	+				
Alpha-Receptor Blockade							
Prazosin q 8 hr	1–5 mg	+	+ +	—	+	—	—
Converting Enzyme Inhibitors							
Captopril	6.25–37.5 mg q 6–8 hr	+	+ + +	—	+	—	—
Enalapril	2.5–10 mg daily or bid	+	+ + +				

BP = blood pressure; CO = cardiac output; SVR = systemic vascular resistance; RAP = right atrial pressure.
Key: + = increase; 0 = no effect; 0/— = moderate decrease; — = no effect to moderate decrease; — = marked decrease.

TABLE 4–13. PARENTERAL DRUGS FOR CONGESTIVE HEART FAILURE

CLASS	DOSAGE	VENODILATOR	ARTERIAL DILATOR	INOTROPIC EFFECT
Direct-Acting Vasodilators				
Nitroprusside	0.5–10 μg/kg/min	+	+++	0
Nitroglycerin	10–200 μg/min	+++	++	0
Sympathomimetic Agents				
Dopamine	1–10 μg/kg/min	0	+	+++
Dobutamine	2.5–20 μg/kg/min	0	0	+++
Phosphodiesterase Inhibitors				
Bipyridine Derivatives				
Amrinone	0.5 mg/kg bolus × 2, 40 μg/kg/min infusion	0	0	+++
Milrinone	12.5–75 μg/kg (given as 10-mg boluses)	0	++	+++
Imidazolone Derivatives				
Enoximone	0.5–5 mg/kg/day, intermittent boluses 3–6 hr, not to exceed 12.5 mg/min	0	+	+++

+ = increase; 0 = no effect

a. **Mild Failure.** Patients with mild failure can be treated with **diuretics** (Table 4–11) and **digoxin, 0.125–0.25 mg/day,** depending on the patient's size, age, and renal function. Digoxin is particularly effective for a patient with atrial fibrillation with a rapid ventricular response. Digoxin toxicity may be exacerbated by hypokalemia.

b. **Moderate-to-Severe Failure.** In this setting, **IV diuretics** are supplemented by afterload- and preload-reducing agents. **IV nitroglycerin** offers both preload and afterload reduction and is the agent of choice in acute myocardial ischemia. **Nitroprusside** is also effective, especially as an afterload-reducing agent; it is the agent of choice if severe hypertension is present. If patients are not responding adequately, the addition of a sympathomimetic agent (dopamine or dobutamine) is appropriate. Inotropic agents increase cardiac output but differ widely on their effects on peripheral vascular resistance. As noted, these agents may induce myocardial ischemia. Therefore a more desirable agent may be necessary (such as a vasodilator). A vasodilator may induce hypotension by decreasing arterial pressure, thereby exacerbating cardiac ischemia. All agents must be used with caution in patients with ischemic heart disease and hypotension. General measures should include bed rest, diet control, and oxygen. Usually Swan-Ganz catheter monitoring at this stage is necessary. If failure persists, phosphodiesterase inhibitors (administered IV) may be added.

2. CHRONIC THERAPY

Mild failure is treated with **diuretics.** A long-acting diuretic is favored because of once-a-day administration. A digitalis agent is usually added. There is now evidence that afterload reduction will improve not only symptoms but also survival. A **converting enzyme inhibitor** is recommended for patients with moderate to severe failure who require afterload reduction. These drugs are favored because they have fewer side effects than nitrates or hydralazine. More important, development of **tolerance** is much less frequent. Tolerance is a universal finding with chronic nitrate therapy.

Another factor that should be considered in treating patients with dilated cardiomyopathy is the role of **anticoagulation** in preventing systemic emboli. Patients with evidence of myocarditis on biopsy may benefit from steroids and possibly immunosuppressive drugs; however, this has not been proved in prospective randomized studies.

In suitable candidates with refractory failure and severe impairment of cardiac capacity, cardiac transplantation should be considered (see Cardiac Transplantation).

C. Other Causes of Heart Failure

1. CARDIOMYOPATHY ASSOCIATED WITH HYPERTENSION

Some patients with longstanding hypertension develop marked left ventricular hypertrophy and present with pulmonary edema secondary to impaired left ventricular relaxation (left ventricular diastolic dysfunction). Evaluation of function with echocardiography or radio-nuclide scanning usually indicates preserved systolic function, but diastolic abnormalities can be detected. In this situation, **calcium channel blockers (verapamil, slow-release capsule, 240–360 mg/day; diltiazem, 90 mg qid; or nifedipine, 20–30 mg tid)** may lower blood pressure and increase compliance, thus allowing more rapid filling during diastole and reducing wedge pressure. The most important issues in management are careful blood pressure control and careful monitoring of the patient's volume status as the hypertrophic ventricle is sensitive to hyper- and hypovolemic states.

2. HYPERTROPHIC CARDIOMYOPATHY

Hypertrophic cardiomyopathy may occur with or without probable LV outflow obstruction. Patients are at risk of sudden death. Doppler echocardiography is the most useful diagnostic test. Estimates of the left ventricular outflow tract pressure difference can also be made using Doppler echocardiography.

Strenuous physical activity should be avoided. Administration of **beta blockers (propranolol, 80–120 mg qid) or verapamil, 240–480 mg/day,** can lessen symptoms. Diuretics should be avoided. If atrial fibrillation develops, digoxin should be used to control the ventricular response, and patients should receive **anticoagulation** to prevent emboli.

Surgical therapy (myomectomy with or without mitral valve replacement) should be considered for patients who have significant outflow tract pressure differences and whose conditions are refractory to medical treatment. Recent data suggest that sudden death in hypertrophic cardiomyopathy is often due to ventricular arrhythmia or, less commonly, bradyarrhythmias. Therefore, Holter monitoring and electrophysiologic (EP) studies are indicated in patients with syncope or documented life-threatening arrhythmias.

The VHEFT study: Effects of vasodilator therapy on mortality in congestive heart failure: Results of a Veterans Administration Cooperative Study. N Engl J Med 314:1547, 1986.

The Consensus Trial Study Group: Effects of enalapril on mortality in severe congestive heart failure: Results of the Cooperative North Scandinavian Enalapril Survival Study. N Engl J Med 316:1429, 1987.

Packer M: Therapeutic options in the management of chronic heart failure: Is there a drug of first choice? Circulation 79:198, 1989.

IV. VALVULAR HEART DISEASE

A. General Principles of Treatment. Regardless of severity, all patients with valvular heart disease should receive antibiotic prophylaxis for endocarditis (see Ch. 3). In general, valve surgery is not recommended for asymptomatic patients. However, formal evaluation of cardiac function and exercise capacity is recommended in most.

B. Approach to Specific Conditions

1. AORTIC STENOSIS

Aortic stenosis (AS) may be due to rheumatic heart disease (RHD), congenital bicuspid valve, or senile calcific changes. AS frequently occurs as a mixed lesion, with some degree of aortic insufficiency.

Valve replacement is recommended for patients with symptoms of angina, syncope, or CHF who have severe AS (aortic valve area <1.0 cm^2). Medical management of symptomatic patients with AS is fraught with difficulty because of the high risk of inducing hypotension, potassium shifts, myocardial ischemia, and worsening LV function with agents usually employed to treat angina or CHF. Echocardiography with Doppler is an excellent screening test for severe AS, but most patients will require cardiac catheterization before valve replacement. Percutaneous transluminal valvuloplasty may be a temporizing measure in severely symptomatic patients who could not tolerate surgery. Although the long-term results of this procedure are not known, studies do indicate a 30–50% restenosis rate by 6–12 months.

2. Aortic Regurgitation

Aortic insufficiency (AI) may be due to RHD, arteritis, endocarditis, aortic dissection, or collagen vascular disease. Acute AI (as with endocarditis) is tolerated poorly and often leads promptly to CHF. Chronic AI may be well tolerated for long periods in spite of impressive peripheral manifestations of acute runoff.

Chronic aortic regurgitation can lead to irreversible left ventricular dysfunction; therefore, valve replacement is advised when the first symptoms of CHF develop. In the asymptomatic individual with severe regurgitation who demonstrates deterioration of ventricular function in serial noninvasive studies (echocardiograms, gated blood pool studies, or exercise tolerance test), valve replacement may also be recommended.

3. Mitral Stenosis

Mitral stenosis (MS) is almost always due to RHD. Less common causes include prosthetic valve dysfunction, left atrial thrombus, and left atrial myxoma.

Mildly symptomatic patients can be improved by **diuretics** and controlling the ventricular response (if they are in atrial fibrillation) with **digoxin or a beta blocker.** Patients with atrial fibrillation should receive **anticoagulation therapy** to prevent systemic emboli. **Surgery** is indicated for symptomatic patients (NYHA class III–IV) who do not respond to a simple drug regimen or who show signs of progressive pulmonary hypertension (valve area ≤ 1.0 cm^2) or systemic emboli. The symptomatic state of MS tends to progress slowly, so intervention is rarely urgent. Mitral valve balloon valvuloplasty may be performed, but long-term results are not known. Initial reports indicate better long-term results with mitral valvuloplasty than with aortic valvuloplasty.

4. Mitral Regurgitation

Mitral regurgitation (MR) may be due to RHD, myxomatous mitral valve, endocarditis, dilated cardiomyopathy, or coronary artery disease. The most common cause today is coronary artery disease with papillary muscle dysfunction.

Surgery is recommended when symptoms develop and the regurgitation is moderate to severe. Chronic MR is generally well tolerated for long periods, but acute or subacute MR (secondary to MI, papillary muscle rupture, chordae tendineae rupture, or endocarditis) may be associated with more acute deterioration. If left ventricular function is severely compromised (ejection fraction <30%), surgery carries an increased risk and may result in little improvement in symptoms. Surgery is also a higher risk in patients with concomitant coronary artery disease, and in general a decision must be made about revascularizing the patient at the same time.

5. MITRAL VALVE PROLAPSE

Mitral valve prolapse (MVP) is a myxomatous degenerative change of the valve leaflets and chordae tendineae that results in displacement (prolapse) of the valve leaflet(s) into the left atrium. Though it is a feature of many connective tissue disorders, it frequently occurs in the absence of any systemic illness. Symptoms include atypical chest pain, dyspnea, palpitation, and dizziness. Common physical signs include a mid-to-late systolic click or systolic murmur or both. Diagnosis is made by 2-D echocardiography (systolic displacement of a leaflet beyond the mitral annulus into the left atrium). For most patients this is a benign disorder. In a few patients serious complications may occur, including cardiac arrhythmias, infectious endocarditis, systemic emboli, sudden death, and chordae rupture with flail leaflet and severe mitral regurgitation.

6. TRICUSPID STENOSIS AND REGURGITATION

Tricuspid regurgitation usually develops in association with pulmonary hypertension or other causes of a dilated RV. TR may also result from RHD or endocarditis.

Tricuspid stenosis is rare, but when present it is nearly always rheumatic in origin. In these cases, the left-sided valves are always involved by the rheumatic process. Methysergide may also cause tricuspid stenosis.

7. PROSTHETIC VALVES

The major complications of prosthetic valves are endocarditis, thromboembolism, and valve dysfunction. Endocarditis is the most serious complication. Clinical manifestations of prosthetic valve endocarditis (PVE) can be subtle: changing murmur, fever, failure to thrive, and heart failure are the most common findings. The mortality rate associated with medically treated PVE is extremely high; therefore, the timing of surgical intervention is crucial.

Thromboembolism remains an important complication of prosthetic valves. Most of the clinically detected emboli are cerebral. Patients with mechanical prosthetic valves must receive anticoagulation. Bioprosthetic valves without anticoagulation have a thrombotic rate equal to that of mechanical valves with anticoagulation. Major drawbacks of bioprosthetic valves are early degeneration, cusp tear, perforation, and flail leaflets. Mechanical valves are much more durable.

V. CARDIAC ARRHYTHMIAS

A. **Normal Cardiac Physiology.** In the normal heart, the sinus node has the fastest intrinsic rate of depolarization and consequently serves as the pacemaker site. Depolarization spreads across the atria (the P wave on the surface ECG represents this event). The wave of depolarization reaches the specialized conduction tissue in the lower part of the interatrial septum, the atrioventricular (AV) node. Conduction through the AV node is slowed to allow adequate ventricular filling following atrial contraction and to protect the ventricle from too rapid a rate. The bundle of His originates in the AV node and is responsible for conducting the impulse into the ventricle. These events are not seen on the surface ECG and occur during the P-R interval. The wave of depolarization is propagated into the ventricles via 3 branches of the bundle of His (right, left anterior, and left posterior fascicles). The fascicles branch into an extensive network of fibers, transmitting impulses to the ventricular myocardium (QRS on the surface ECG). Repolarization of the ventricle is represented by the T wave. Repolarization of the atria is usually not seen on the surface ECG.

In the resting state, there is a large electrical gradient between the inside and the outside of the cells (range of -60 to -90 mV). The gradient is maintained because of the difference between intracellular and extracellular potassium concentrations. During depolarization, the gradient becomes less negative owing to the influx of sodium and calcium ions. The initial phase of depolarization is rapid due to the influx of sodium through fast channels. The plateau phase of depolarization lasts much longer and is due primarily to the influx of calcium through the calcium slow channels. After depolarization, cells remain in a refractory state for a variable period of time. During this refractory state, further stimulation will not result in depolarization. **Repolarization** occurs as an active process in which sodium and calcium are exchanged for potassium via an active transport mechanism.

A feature possessed by some of the heart cells is **automaticity.** Cells that have this property are found in the sinus node, atria, AV node, and His-Purkinje system. Automaticity refers to a slow depolarization during electrical diastole. When the membrane potential reaches a threshold level that varies from site to site, an action potential results. In the normal situation, the sinus node has the fastest intrinsic rate of spontaneous depolarization. Consequently, it becomes the pacemaker site for normal sinus rhythm. However, in certain pathologic conditions (i.e., if the sinus node is malfunctioning) other areas may take over the pacemaker function, usually at a slower rate.

B. **Tachyarrhythmias.** Tachyarrhythmias are rhythms with ventricular rates of more than 100 bpm and can be regular or irregular with a narrow or wide QRS. There are 2 basic mechanisms for the development of tachyarrhythmias: (1) enhanced automaticity and (2) re-entrant arrhythmias.

Enhanced automaticity is due to an increased rate of diastolic depolarization. A variety of potentially reversible causes increase automaticity. These include ischemia, hypoxia, electrolyte abnormalities (hypokalemia or hypomagnesemia), digitalis toxicity, and use of beta agonists.

Re-entrant arrhythmias require the presence of 2 pathways that have the potential for conduction. In general, there must be a difference in the speed of conduction and refractoriness of the 2 pathways for tachycardia to develop so that an impulse will encounter a unidirectional block in one of the pathways. By the time the other pathway has conducted the impulse, the pathway that was initially blocked will then conduct the impulse in the reverse direction and thus maintain the circuit to conduct the tachycardia.

1. REGULAR TACHYARRHYTHMIAS WITH NARROW QRS COMPLEXES
The differential diagnosis of regular tachyarrhythmias with a narrow QRS includes sinus tachycardia, paroxysmal supraventricular tachycardia, atrial flutter, and nonparoxysmal junctional tachycardia. All originate above the bifurcation of the His bundle—thus the name *supraventricular arrhythmia.*

a. **Sinus Tachycardia.** Sinus tachycardia is an acceleration of the normal depolarization of the sinus node. The heart rate rarely exceeds 150 bpm except in infants and adults during exercise.

Treatment is usually directed at the underlying cause. Common causes include fever, sepsis, CHF, hypovolemia, anemia, thyrotoxicosis, pulmonary embolism, and anxiety. If the patient has unstable angina or AMI, direct therapy to lower the heart rate may be indicated.

b. **Paroxysmal Supraventricular Tachyarrhythmias (PSVTs).** PSVT may be secondary to a re-entrant arrhythmia or, less commonly, enhanced automaticity (ectopic tachycardias). The heart rate is usually 150–200 bpm but may occasionally be faster. Diagnosis is usually made by the history of abrupt onset and termination. In general those due to re-entry are more responsive to therapy than are the ectopic tachycardias.

Initial **treatment** includes measures to increase vagal tone, such as carotid sinus massage and Valsalva maneuver. If vagal maneuvers are unsuccessful, pharmacologic agents are used to alter conduction and interrupt a re-entry circuit.

Verapamil is the drug of choice, **IV 0.075–0.15 mg/kg (5–10 mg)** given over 2–3 minutes. Peak effects occur in 10 minutes. A repeat dose may be given in 30 minutes. Verapamil should be used with caution in the presence of hypotension, severely compromised left ventricular function, or known conduction system disease.

Beta blockers are also used to treat PSVTs. They should be used with caution in patients with hypotension, severe left ventricular dysfunction, and bronchospastic pulmonary disease. Propranolol is administered in increments of 1 mg every 5 minutes until either the rate is controlled or a total of 0.1 mg/kg (5–10 mg) is administered. Labetalol may be administered as 1–2 mg/kg and metoprolol as a 5–15 mg bolus.

Adenosine, a Class IV agent with multiple cellular effects, is approved by the FDA for the treatment of PSVT. It has an extremely short half-life of 10–30 seconds. Side effects include dyspnea, flushing, and chest pain. Adenosine is given as an initial IV bolus of 6 mg; if no effects occur within 1–2 minutes, a 12 mg bolus is given and may be repeated. Contraindications are asthma, second or third degree AV block, and sick sinus syndrome.

IV **digitalis glycosides** are also effective agents but have a longer time course of action.

Once normal sinus rhythm (NSR) is achieved, an **antiarrhythmic agent** should be prescribed to prevent recurrence. Digoxin or a beta blocker, particularly propranolol, is most commonly used. Patients should be cautioned about the role that stimulants such as caffeine may play in the initiation of paroxysmal supraventricular tachycardia.

If pharmacologic agents are unsuccessful, either synchronized direct-current countershock or rapid atrial stimulation may be successful. These should be used urgently if the patient is hemodynamically unstable or is having ongoing ischemia.

c. **Atrial Flutter.** Atrial flutter is commonly seen in patients with valvular heart disease or other structural heart disease. It is due to rapid atrial depolarization at a regular rate of 250–300 bpm. Because the AV node cannot conduct atrial impulses at this rate, a 2:1 AV block develops producing a regular ventricular response of one-half the atrial rate. Any regular narrow complex tachycardia at 150 bpm should be assumed to be atrial flutter until proven otherwise. Carotid sinus massage will usually increase the degree of AV block (2:1–4:1) without a change in the atrial depolarization rate. Diagnosis is made by observing atrial depolarization appearing as a "sawtooth" deflection in the inferior leads.

Digoxin, verapamil, diltiazem, or a **beta blocker** alone or in combination remains the mainstay of therapy for atrial flutter. Verapamil and beta blockers are given as above for more rapid control of the ventricular response. IV beta blockers should be given with caution if IV calcium channel blockers have been given. Digoxin may be given as an initial 0.25 mg dose IV.

Cardioversion should be performed if the patient is symptomatic (hypotension, angina, pulmonary congestion) from the arrhythmia. Atrial flutter is usually terminated by low-level energy (20–50 joules). Cardioversion is safe with small amounts of digitalis glycoside, but it is not recommended when large amounts must be given. Patients may convert to atrial fibrillation or NSR. Rapid atrial pacing is commonly used in the post-coronary artery bypass patients and in patients resistant to drug therapy.

d. **Nonparoxysmal Junction Tachycardia.** This occurs most commonly with digitalis toxicity, after cardiac operation (particularly mitral valve replacement), and in patients with inflammation close to or involving the AV node. The rate rarely exceeds 140–150 bpm. The electrocardiographic morphology reveals regular QRS complexes, and retrograde atrial activity can sometimes be seen. This arrhythmia is generally well tolerated by the patient. Correction of any electrolyte imbalance or withholding digoxin is usually the only intervention required.

2. **REGULAR TACHYCARDIA WITH WIDE QRS COMPLEXES**
This is one of the most difficult arrhythmias to diagnose. The differential diagnosis is SVT with aberrant conduction or ventricular tachycardia (VT).

a. **SVT with Aberrant Conduction.** The QRS is usually wide, notched, and has a bizarre complex. The abnormal QRS complex may be due to existing bundle branch block. In some instances the aberration is present only in association with the arrhythmia. Diagnosis of SVT with aberration vs. ventricular tachycardia is made by additional features:

1. Evidence of AV dissociation favors ventricular tachycardia
2. A bundle branch block before or after the tachycardia with identical QRS morphology during the tachycardia favors SVT with aberrancy.
3. A QRS duration of greater than 0.14 favors VT. Although the Wellens criteria for ventricular tachycardia serve as a guideline for the diagnosis of VT, they are not absolute.

Patients with SVT with aberration are usually more stable than a patient with VT at a similar rate, but this does not reliably distinguish the cause. If one is confident of the diagnosis of SVT with aberration, **therapy** should be initiated as described above for SVT. In any patient with structural heart disease, a wide-complex tachycardia should be assumed to be VT, and therapy for presumed VT should be initiated.

b. **Ventricular Tachycardia (VT). Cardioversion** is the treatment of choice in the presence of hemodynamic compromise. Cardioversion of ventricular tachycardia is usually accomplished with low energy (50–100 joules). A thump to the precordium is successful in some patients in converting VT. **Lidocaine** is usually the drug of choice for VT via an initial bolus of 1 mg/kg. A maintenance dose of 1–4 mg/min or 20–55 μg/kg/min is administered to suppress further ventricular activity. Another medication that may be given if lidocaine is ineffective is **procainamide.** An initial bolus of 100 mg over 2 minutes up to 25 mg/minute to 1 gm in the first hour is followed by an infusion of 20–40 μg/kg/min (1–4 mg/min). **Quinidine** may also be used to suppress recurrent VT. Therapeutic blood levels of quinidine are achieved with doses of 300–600 mg oral or IM every 6 hours. IV quinidine produces severe hypotension and should be avoided. There are several other second-line agents that may be useful in treating or preventing recurrent VT. **Disopyramide** has electrophysiologic properties similar to quinidine and may be used orally (100–300 μg q 6 hr). **Tocainide** (300–600 mg orally q 8 hr) and **mexiletine** (250–300 mg orally q 8 hr) are lidocaine analogs. They have the advantage over procainamide and quinidine of not prolonging the QT interval.

Phenytoin is effective in digitalis-toxic arrhythmias. The IV dose is 10–15 mg/kg over 1 hour followed by oral maintenance of 400–600 mg/day.

Moricizine (Ethmozine) is effective in treating both supraventricular and ventricular tachycardia. The usual dose is 200–300 mg orally q 8 hr.

Bretylium tosylate is used to treat recurrent or resistant ventricular tachycardia. It may be given as an IV bolus of 5–10 mg/kg over 10 minutes followed by a 1–2 mg/min infusion. The major side effect is hypotension from peripheral vasodilation. However, initial sympathomimetic effects may occur.

c. **Torsades de Pointes.** This is a form of ventricular tachycardia usually associated with prolongation of the QT interval and caused by pharmacologic agents such as quinidine, procainamide, or disopyramide and by electrolyte abnormalities. Cardioversion is often necessary, but the tachycardia may recur. Correcting the precipitating factor and in some cases overdrive pacing and isoproterenol infusion (2–8 μg/min) to shorten the QT interval may be successful in preventing recurrences.

d. **Ventricular Flutter and Fibrillation.** Both are medical emergencies and require immediate cardioversion.

3. **IRREGULAR TACHYCARDIA WITH NARROW OR WIDE COMPLEXES**
The differential diagnosis of irregular tachycardia with narrow or wide complex is among atrial fibrillation (AF), multifocal atrial tachycardia (MAT), SVT with varying degrees of AV block, and multiple premature beats originating from the atrium, junction, or ventricle.

a. **Atrial fibrillation** is usually recognized by its irregularly irregular ventricular response and a baseline with no organized atrial activity. "Fine atrial fibrillation" and "coarse atrial fibrillation" refer to the amplitude of the fibrillatory waves and have no therapeutic significance. Carotid sinus pressure usually results in slowing of the ventricular response.

The most common underlying heart diseases in patients with AF are atherosclerosis, hypertension, rheumatic heart disease (particularly mitral stenosis), pericarditis, and cardiomyopathy. Noncardiac causes include thyrotoxicosis, COPD, pneumonia, and pulmonary embolism. Elderly patients may have atrial fibrillation as a manifestation of degenerative changes in the conduction system and may have no underlying structural heart disease (see Sick Sinus Syndrome below).

Digitalis glycosides are the drugs of choice for treating atrial fibrillation. An initial IV loading dose of **0.25–0.5 mg of digoxin** may be given to the patient who has not been receiving digoxin. The loading dose is governed by the lean body weight. IV digoxin begins to exert its effect in 15–30 minutes. Additional digoxin may be administered every 2–4 hours in increments of 0.125 or 0.25 mg as needed for rate control to a total of 1.0–1.25 mg in 24 hours.

Verapamil is the drug of choice if rapid control of ventricular response is necessary. The effect is exerted solely on the AV node. Verapamil is administered IV at a dose of 5–10 mg over 1 minute and repeated in 30 minutes if necessary. Effects are seen in 10 minutes. Caution should be used when administering this drug to an elderly patient or when sick sinus syndrome is suspected. IV beta blockers may also be used for rapid control of the ventricular response. Patients who are hemodynamically unstable with a rapid ventricular response may require emergency cardioversion. Elective conversion to NSR may be performed in stable patients. It is recommended that patients be given anticoagulants for 2–3 weeks before elective cardioversion. Long-term anticoagulation is recommended in patients with chronic or recurrent AF. If the time of onset of atrial fibrillation can be determined accurately to be less than 3–5 days, anticoagulation before cardioversion is not necessary.

b. **Multifocal Atrial Tachycardia.** This arrhythmia is easily confused with atrial fibrillation because it usually has a similar ventricular rate and the rhythm is irregularly irregular. The diagnosis is made by the presence of organized P waves with 3 or more different morphologies, varying P-P intervals, and varying P-R intervals. The rhythm is generally not responsive to carotid sinus massage. It occurs most frequently in patients with chronic pulmonary disease.

The arrhythmia is **best treated** by correcting the underlying respiratory or metabolic disorder if present. If rate control is necessary, the **treatment of choice is verapamil 5–10 mg** IV, though this is not uniformly successful.

c. **Atrial or Junction Premature Beats.** Multiple atrial or junction premature beats produce an irregular rhythm. The QRS complex of the premature beat may be similar to or slightly different from the normal sinus beat. If a P wave precedes the QRS complex, it is usually atrial in origin; if a P wave follows the QRS complex, the beat is usually junctional. Atrial and junctional premature beats are benign, and no treatment is required. They sometimes may be harbingers of other atrial arrhythmias.

d. **Ventricular Premature Beats.** Ventricular premature beats usually produce bizarre QRS complexes, which are usually followed by a compensatory pause. Occasionally there is no compensatory pause, and the premature beat is said to be "interpolated." The morphology of the premature beat varies depending on the site of origin. Premature beats originating from the left ventricle have a RBBB morphology and those originating from the right ventricle have a LBBB morphology. Treatment depends on the presence or absence of symptoms, the setting, and the frequency. When treatment is indicated on symptomatic grounds, the agents of choice are the same as those used in VT.

C. **Bradyarrhythmias.** Bradyarrhythmias are rhythms with heart rates of less than 60 bpm and usually indicate pathology of the sinus or AV nodes.

1. SINUS BRADYCARDIA
   The presence of sinus bradycardia may indicate pathology of the sinus node, may be a normal physiologic response especially in well-trained athletes, or may be the result of pharmacologic agents such as beta blockers or calcium channel blockers. Sinus bradycardia may also be seen in patients with a diagnosis of hypothyroidism.

2. SINUS ARREST AND SINUS EXIT BLOCK
   In sinus arrest the sinus node stops depolarization instantaneously. In sinus exit block the sinus node depolarizes normally but the impulse cannot exit the sinus node. Therefore in both arrhythmias P waves are usually absent or intermittent.
   a. **Treatment.** Treatment of either type of block is indicated if the rate is associated with symptoms (hypotension, dizziness, syncope, CHF). Negative chronotropic drugs should be discontinued. Immediate therapy of choice is atropine 0.5–1.0 mg IV or Isuprel 1–2 μg/min IV. Insertion of a permanent transvenous pacemaker is indicated only if the rhythm is refractory to these measures and the patient remains symptomatic.

D. AV Block

1. DIAGNOSIS

   a. **First Degree AV Block.** This is present if the P-R interval is greater than 0.20 second and all P waves are followed by a QRS complex.
   b. **Second Degree AV Block.** In second degree AV block all P waves are not followed by a QRS complex. There are 2 types of second degree AV block: Wenckebach (or Mobitz type I) is diagnosed by observing progressive prolongation of the P-R interval for each conducted beat until a P wave is not followed by a QRS (blocked beat). The classic features of **Wenckebach periodicity** are not always present on the ECG ("atypical Wenckebach"). Typically, the first P-R interval of each group is constant and is the shortest interval. The increments in the P-R interval progressively decrease; thus the R-R interval progressively shortens until the pause. Type I block usually implies disease in the AV node.
   c. **Mobitz Type II.** Blocked beats, P waves, occur without progressive prolongation of the P-R interval. Type II block implies disease in the distal His-Purkinje system, making it a more serious arrhythmia than type I because the risk of sudden asystole is greater.
   d. **Third Degree AV Block.** In contrast to first and second degree AV block, there is no relationship between the P waves and the QRS complexes in third degree AV block. The P-P and R-R intervals are usually regular and the P waves may precede or follow the QRS or may be found within the QRS complex. The QRS complex may be of junctional or ventricular origin.
   e. **Syncope (Adams-Stokes Attacks).** These are usually due to profound bradycardia or asystole. The treatment of choice is permanent transvenous ventricular pacing.

2. TREATMENT

Mobitz type I AV block is usually transient and commonly occurs in the setting of acute inferior wall MI. It is most likely to respond to atropine or isoproterenol if any therapy is needed. **Digitalis toxicity** should always be considered in patients with Mobitz type I AV block who are receiving digoxin therapy. Patients with Mobitz type II have a more serious AV block that is more likely to progress to complete heart block. Patients should be evaluated for a permanent transvenous pacemaker. The treatment of choice for third degree heart block is a **permanent transvenous pacemaker,** unless it occurs in a clearly reversible disorder such as digitalis toxicity or an acute IMI.

E. Arrhythmia in Special Circumstances

1. WOLFF-PARKINSON-WHITE SYNDROME (WPW)

Patients with this syndrome have another bypass tract in addition to conducting via the A-V node. When conduction occurs via the bypass tract it produces a short P-R interval, a delta wave, and a wide QRS complex. During bypass tract conduction, the QRS complex may be similar to that seen in AMI. The two most common arrhythmias that occur in patients with WPW are paroxysmal SVT and atrial fibrillation. Most cases of PSVT involve a narrow complex (antegrade conduction is through the AV node and retrograde via the bypass track). Treatment of paroxysmal SVT is the same as previously described. Atrial fibrillation may be conducted quite rapidly through the bypass track with wide QRS complexes and rates approaching 300 bpm. Both digoxin and verapamil are contraindicated for control of ventricular response in atrial fibrillation occurring in WPW syndrome as they may paradoxically accelerate the ventricular response. Patients may require cardioversion and treatment with quinidine or procainamide to prevent recurrence of AF.

2. SICK SINUS SYNDROME (TACHY-BRADY SYNDROME)

This syndrome is a constellation of arrhythmias. It occurs most frequently in the elderly. Patients with sick sinus syndrome (SSS) may have periods of sinus bradycardia, sinus arrest, PSVT, atrial flutter, and atrial fibrillation with either rapid or slow ventricular response. In patients with SSS who have atrial tachyarrhythmia, treatment of the tachyarrhythmia may result in symptomatic bradycardia. Therefore some patients may require a transvenous permanent pacemaker as part of their treatment regimen. Care must be taken during cardioversion as there is a high likelihood that there may be no spontaneous sinus activity after cardioversion or that the patient may have an extremely slow sinus node response.

F. Classification of Antiarrhythmic Drugs.

A useful classification (Vaughn-Williams) based on electrophysiologic properties is shown in Table 4–14. The pharmacologic and electrophysiogic properties of various intravenous and oral antiarrhythmic agents are shown in Tables 4–14 and 4–15. Table 4–16 shows drug interactions.

Wilkins EW: Emergency Medicine, 3rd ed. Baltimore, Williams & Wilkins, 1989.

Mandel WJ: Cardiac Arrhythmias, Their Mechanism, Diagnosis and Management, 2nd ed. Philadelphia, JB Lippincott Co., 1987.

TABLE 4–14. ANTIARRHYTHMIC DRUGS USED IN THERAPY OF VENTRICULAR ARRHYTHMIAS

AGENT	DOSAGE	PHARMACOKINETICS	SIDE EFFECTS AND CONTRAINDICATIONS
Quinidine (Class IA)	1.2–1.6 gm/day PO in divided doses, 4–12 hourly, depending on preparation. Not IV; risk of hypotension	$T_{1/2}$ 7–9 hr. Level 2.3–5 μg/ml; hepatic metabolism; reduce dose in liver disease	Diarrhea, nausea; torsades de pointes and hypotension
Procainamide (Class IA)	IV 100 mg bolus over 2 min, up to 25 mg/min to 1 gm in 1st hr; then 2–6 mg/min; oral 1 gm, then up to 1000 mg q 6 hr	$T_{1/2}$ 3.5 hr. Level 4–10 μg/ml; renal elimination	Hypotension with IV dose, induce lupus, torsades de points rare
Disopyramide (Class IA)	Oral dose 100–200 mg q 6 hr; loading dose 300 mg (less if CHF)	$T_{1/2}$ 8 hr. Level 3–6 μg/ml, toxic > 7 μg/ml; hepatic metabolism (50%), unchanged urinary excretion (50%)	Hypotension, QRS or QT prolongation; torsades, negative inotropic effects
Lidocaine (Class IB)	IV 100–200 mg; then 2–4 mg/min for 24–30 hr	Effect of single bolus lasts only few min, then $T_{1/2}$ about 2 hr, hepatic metabolism. Level 1.4–5 μg/ml; toxic > 9 μg/ml	Reduce dose by half if liver blood flow low (shock, β-blockade, cirrhosis, cimetidine, severe heart failure). High-dose CNS effects
Tocainide (Class IB)	Oral loading 400–800 mg; then 400–800 mg/po, then 2–3 × daily	$T_{1/2}$ 13.5 hr. Level 4–10 μg/ml; unchanged renal excretion (50%)	CNS, GI side effects. Sometimes immune-based problems (lung fibrosis, blood dyscrasias)
Mexiletine (Class IB)	Oral 100–400 mg PO q 8 hr; loading dose 400 mg	$T_{1/2}$ 10–17 hr. Level 1–2 μg/ml; hepatic metabolism, inactive metabolites	CNS, GI side effects. Bradycardia, hypotension especially during co-therapy
Phenytoin (Class IB)	IV 10–15 mg/kg over 1 hr; oral 1 gm; 500 mg for 2 days; 400–600 mg daily	$T_{1/2}$ 24 hr. Level 10–18 μg/ml; hepatic metabolism; hepatic or renal disease requires reduced doses	Hypotension, vertigo, dysarthria, lethargy, gingivitis, macrocytic anemia, lupus, pulmonary infiltrates

Table continued on following page

TABLE 4-14. ANTIARRHYTHMIC DRUGS USED IN THERAPY OF VENTRICULAR ARRHYTHMIAS *Continued*

AGENT	DOSAGE	PHARMACOKINETICS	SIDE EFFECTS AND CONTRAINDICATIONS
Flecainide (Class IC)	100–400 po mg 2 × daily; hospitalize	$T_{1/2}$ 13–19 hr. Hepatic metabolism (⅔); ⅓ renal excretion, unchanged; 1.0 µg/ml	QRS prolongation. Pro-arrhythmia; depressed LV function. CNS side effects. Increased incidence of of death post-infarct
Encainide (Class IC)	25–75 mg 3 × daily po; hospitalize	$T_{1/2}$ 1–2 hr. No levels. Hepatic normal phenotype produces long-acting metabolites (3–12 hr)	QRS prolongation. CNS side effects; pro-arrhythmia. Increased incidence of death post-infarct
Propafenone (Class IC)	Oral 150–300 mg po 3 × daily	$T_{1/2}$ variable 2–10 hr, up to 32 hr in nonmetabolizers. Level 0.2–3.0 µg/ml. Variable hepatic metabolism (P-450 deficiency slows)	QRS prolongation. Modest negative inotropic effect. GI side effects; pro-arrhythmia
Sotalol (Class III)	160–640 mg daily, occasionally higher, may divide doses. Not approved in use	Not metabolized. Renal loss	Myocardial depression, sinus bradycardia, AV block. Torsades especially if hypokalemic or if dose too high
Amiodarone (Class III)	Oral loading dose 1200–1600 mg daily; maintenance 200–400 mg daily, sometimes less	$T_{1/2}$ 25–110 days; level 1.0–2.5 µg/ml; hepatic metabolism. Lipid soluble with extensive distribution in body. Excretion by skin, biliary tract, lacrimal glands	Pulmonary fibrosis. QT-prolongation
Bretylium (Class III)	IV 5–10 mg/kg, lifting arm, repeat to max 30 mg/kg, then IV 1–2 mg/min or IM 5–10 mg/min or IM 5–10 mg/kg q 8 hr at varying sites (local necrosis)	$T_{1/2}$ 7–9 hr. Level 0.5–1.0 µg/ml	IV: hypotension. Initial sympathomimetic effects

$T_{1/2}$ = plasma half-life
Modified from Opie L.H.: Drugs for the Heart, 3rd ed. Philadelphia, W. B. Saunders Co., 1991.

TABLE 4–15. EFFECTS AND SIDE EFFECTS OF SOME ANTIARRHYTHMIC AGENTS ON ELECTROPHYSIOLOGY AND HEMODYNAMICS

AGENT	SINUS NODE	A-HIS	PR	H-P	QRS	QT	RISK OF TORSADES	RISK OF MONO-MORPHIC VT
Lidocaine	0	0/↓	0	0	0	0	0?	0?
Quinidine	→	0	0/→	→	↑	↑	++	0,+
Procainamide	0	0/↓	0/→	0/↓	0/→	↑	+	0,+
Disopyramide	→	0	0/→	→	↑	↑	+	0,+
Phenytoin	0	←/0	0	0	0	↓	0,+	0,+
Mexiletine	0	←/0	0	→/0	0/→	0	0,+	0,+
Tocainamide	0	→/0	0	→	0	0	0,+	0,+
Flecainide	0/↓	→↑	↑	→	↑	↑ (via QRS)	0	+++
Encainide	0/↓	↓↑	↑	↓	↑	↑ (via QRS)	0	+++
Sotalol	→↑	→	0/→	0	0	↑	++	0,+
Amiodarone	→	→	0/→	0/↓	0	↑	+	0,+
Bretylium	→↑	→	←↑	→	0	−	0,+	0,+
Verapamil	→	→	↑↑	→	0	0	0	0

A-His = atria-His conduction; H-P = His-Purkinje conduction; LV = left ventricle; R = retrograde; A = antegrade; BBB = bundle branch block; IV = intravenous; ↓ = depresses; ↑ = increases; → = prolongs; ← = shortens.

Modified from Opie L.H.: Drugs for the Heart, 3rd ed. Philadelphia, W. B. Saunders Co., 1991.

TABLE 4–16. INTERACTION OF ANTIARRYTHMIC DRUGS

DRUG	INTERACTION WITH	RESULT
Quinidine	Digoxin	Increased digoxin level
	Beta-blockers, verapamil	Enhanced hypotension, negative inotropic effect
	Amiodarone, sotalol	Increased risk of torsades
	Diuretics	If hypokalemia, risk of torsades
	Verapamil	Increased quinidine level
	Nifedipine	Decreased quinidine level
	Warfarin	Enhanced anticoagulation
	Cimetidine	Increased blood levels
	Enzyme inducers	Decreased blood levels
Procainamide	Cimetidine	Decreased renal clearance
Disopyramide	Amiodarone, sotalol, beta blockers, verapamil	Torsades Enhanced hypotension, negative inotropic effect
Lidocaine	Beta blockers, cimetidine, Halothane	Reduced liver blood flow (increased blood levels)
Mexiletine	Theophylline	Theophylline levels increased
Flecainide	Added SA or AV node inhibition (beta blockers, verapamil, diltiazem, digoxin)	SA and AV nodal depression; depressed myocardium; conduction delay
Encainide	See flecainide	See flecainide
Propafenone	As for flecainide, digoxin, warfarin	Enhanced SA, AV, and myocardial depression; digoxin level increased; anticoagulant effect enhanced
Sotalol	Diuretics, class IA agents, amiodarone, phenothiazines	Risk of torsades
Amiodarone	As for sotalol, digoxin, flecainide, warfarin	Risk of torsades; digoxin and flecainide levels increase
Verapamil	Beta blockers, excess digoxin	Increased myocardial or nodal depression

Enzyme inducers: hepatic enzyme inducers, i.e., barbiturates, phenytoin, rifampin.
Modified from Opie L.H.: Drugs for the Heart, 3rd ed. Philadelphia, W. B. Saunders Co., 1991.

VI. SELECTION AND MANAGEMENT OF HEART TRANSPLANT PATIENTS

Cardiac transplantation is performed to improve quality of life and prolong survival. Most people who undergo heart transplantation have a diagnosis of ischemic or idiopathic cardiomyopathy. Other less common diagnoses are postpartum cardiomyopathy and congenital heart disease. The most common indicator for heart transplantation is Class IV heart failure.

A. **Patient Selection.** Patients selected for cardiac transplantation have a poor prognosis and an expected 6- to 12-month survival of less than 50%. Patients deemed appropriate for transplantation on the basis of their prognosis must meet the following selection criteria:

1. AGE
55 years has been the preferred cut-off age, although there have been no significant differences in incidence of rejection and 1-year survival among younger patients age 19–54 versus older patients age 55–60. Recently some transplant centers have liberalized this age limit.

2. PULMONARY VASCULAR RESISTANCE
Early data suggest that patients with pulmonary hypertension do poorly after cardiac transplantation.

3. COMORBID DISEASE
Patients who are candidates for transplantation must be free of other diseases. Diseases that preclude transplantation are malignancy, peripheral vascular disease, collagen vascular disease, renal dysfunction beyond that expected from severe CHF, hepatic dysfunction, diabetes mellitus—presently a relative contraindication, peptic ulcer disease–related contraindication, concurrent infection, marked obesity, and cachexia.

4. PSYCHOSOCIAL BEHAVIOR
Since the stress and demands placed on patients after cardiac transplant are intense, it is imperative that they be emotionally stable. Patients are excluded if there is a history of active drug or alcohol abuse. In addition, mental illness is an absolute contraindication for transplantation.

B. **Management of the Post Cardiac Transplant Patient.** Postoperative immunosuppression therapy has become the mainstay of cardiac transplantation. Immunosuppressive therapy may be divided into 3 phases. **Early rejection prophylaxis** occurs 2–3 weeks after transplantation. **Chronic maintenance therapy** is given chronically throughout the duration of the transplant. Rejection is usually diagnosed by endomyocardial biopsy. Treatment of acute allograft rejection varies in part due to variation in chronic maintenance regimens.

C. **Prognosis.** Currently, the 1-year survival for cardiac transplant patients is 85 to 90%; the 5-year survival for cardiac transplant patients is 85 to 90%; the 5-year survival is approximately 70%. The majority of surviving patients lead active lives with few or no cardiac symptoms.

Kannel WB, Sorlie P, McNamara PM: Prognosis after initial myocardial infarction: The Framingham Study. Am J Cardiol 44:53, 1979.
Copeland JG, Emery RW, Levinson MM, et al: Selection of patients for cardiac transplantation. Circulation 75:1, 1987.
Macoviack JA: Selection and management of heart transplant patients. Cardiol Clin North Am 8:1, 1990

555555555555555

HYPERTENSION

MARGARET THORNTON
DAVID C. DUGDALE

5555555555555555

I. GENERAL PRINCIPLES

Excess morbidity and mortality rises in proportion to blood pressure elevation, and even mild hypertension adds to the risk of atherosclerotic disease. Prospective studies show that lowering blood pressure prevents or delays:

1. **Cardiac disease** (CHF, left ventricular hypertrophy, aortic dissection, and ischemic heart disease);
2. **Cerebrovascular disease** (stroke and transient ischemic attack);
3. **Progressive renal insufficiency;**
4. **Accelerated hypertension.**

Benefits are greatest among patients with severe hypertension. Long-term studies of preventing hypertensive complications have primarily utilized thiazides, propranolol, metoprolol, hydralazine, alpha-methyl-dopa, and reserpine. Newer agents have been tested for efficacy of blood pressure control. The presence of other independent risk factors for atherosclerosis enhances the detrimental effect of hypertension and may affect decisions on the benefits of treatment.

Treatment should be considered if blood pressures above 140/90 mm Hg have been documented on at least 3 occasions. The measurements should be done after 5 minutes of rest, and at least 30 minutes after caffeine or cigarette use. The blood pressure cuff should have a rubber bladder that encircles at least two thirds of the arm. Patients should be questioned about use of medications that may raise blood pressure, including nonsteroidal anti-inflammatory drugs (NSAIDs), oral contraceptives, tricyclic antidepressants, decongestants or appetite suppressants, and monoamine oxidase (MAO) inhibitors.

A. Nonpharmacologic approaches are appropriate initial treatment of uncomplicated, mild hypertension (Ann Intern Med 102:359–373, 1985; Arch Intern Med 149:661–665, 1989). **Weight reduction** may cause a fall of up to 2 mm Hg/kg that is independent of reduced sodium intake (Arch Intern Med 44:1581–1584, 1984). **Halving of dietary sodium intake** may lower diastolic blood pressure by up to 7 mm Hg, though it is effective in only 50–60% of patients (Lancet 1:227–230, 1978). Low sodium intake may also decrease diuretic-induced kaliuresis. A reasonable goal is a daily intake of 4–5 gm NaCl.

Regular aerobic exercise (walking, swimming, cycling) should be prescribed within the cardiovascular limits of the patient. Relaxation techniques may help some patients (Ann Intern Med 102:709–715, 1985).

Alcohol intake should be limited to no more than 1 ounce of ethanol daily (Ann Intern Med 105:124–125, 1986).

B. Pharmacologic Treatment. The best initial pharmacologic treatment of essential hypertension remains controversial, as does the blood pressure level at which pharmacologic treatment is begun.

The once-common stepped care approach (a diuretic, followed by a beta blocker, followed by a centrally active sympatholytic or vasodilator) has become less popular, primarily because of concern about the metabolic side effects of the thiazides and acknowledged failure to demonstrate clear benefit of diuretics in preventing coronary artery disease. Many antihypertensives affect serum lipoprotein levels adversely (Table 5–1). Studies of these effects have been relatively short-term, and their clinical importance is not yet clear (J Hypertension 3:297–306, 1985).

In 1988, the Joint National Committee on High Blood Pressure recommended an "individualized stepped care approach." The initial drug is chosen on the basis of expected response to therapy, expected side effect profile, and treatment of co-morbid conditions. Older patients and blacks usually respond better to diuretics and calcium channel blockers. Younger patients and whites respond better to beta blockers and angiotensin-converting enzyme (ACE) inhibitors.

If monotherapy is not effective, a second and then a third drug selected from different drug classes may be added or substituted. Monotherapy with most agents is effective in 40–50% of patients. The condition in 80–90% can be controlled with 2 drugs.

TABLE 5–1. LIPID EFFECTS OF ANTIHYPERTENSIVES

DRUG	EFFECT ON CHOLESTEROL	EFFECT ON TRIGLYCERIDES
Thiazides	Increase by 5–7%; Increase LDL chol	Increase
Loop diuretics	Increase	Increase
Prazosin and terazosin	Reduce LDL chol and increase HDL chol	Reduce
Sympatholytics		
clonidine	Neutral	Neutral
alpha-methyldopa	Slight decrease HDL chol	Slight increase
guanabenz	Lowers chol by 20 mg/dl	Reduces
ACE inhibitors	Neutral	Neutral
Calcium channel blockers	Neutral	Neutral
Beta blockers	Reduce HDL chol by 5–15%	Increase by 10–30%

Comments: Labetalol and acebutolol are lipid neutral. In general, effect of nonselective agents > effect of selective agents > effect of agents with ISA.

II. SPECIFIC MEDICATIONS

A. Diuretics (Table 5–2)

1. **THIAZIDES**
Among the diuretics, thiazides remain the cornerstone of antihypertensive therapy. Their metabolic side effects include hypokalemia, hyperuricemia, hyperglycemia, and hyperlipidemia. The consequences of mild hypokalemia are uncertain. Adverse effects of hypokalemia are more likely for patients with ischemic heart disease, arrhythmias, hepatic insufficiency, diabetes mellitus, and concomitant use of corticosteroids or cardiac glycosides (Am J Med 77:1–4, 1984).

In patients without edema, thiazides are more effective than loop diuretics, may be given once daily, and are less likely to cause hypokalemia. The antihypertensive effect may require 2–4 weeks to develop. Indapamide or metolazone should be used when the serum creatinine is above 2.0 mg/dL.

2. **THE LOOP DIURETICS**, more potent than the thiazides, are useful in patients with renal insufficiency and in combination with sodium-retaining antihypertensives, such as minoxidil. They should be used twice daily for blood pressure control.

3. **POTASSIUM-SPARING DIURETICS** are usually used in combination with a thiazide and minimize hypokalemia due to the potassium-wasting diuretics. They should be used with caution in patients with renal disease or at risk for hyperkalemia. **Spironolactone** is as potent as hydrochlorothiazide but has a higher incidence of side effects, particularly at doses above 100 mg per day. **Triamterene** and **amiloride** are not, by themselves, useful antihypertensive agents.

B. Beta-adrenergic Blockers (Table 5–3).
These drugs are effective in the treatment of hypertension and in prevention or delay of hypertensive complications. **Metoprolol** is significantly more effective than diuretics in primary prevention of coronary heart disease among hypertensive men (JAMA 259:1976–1982, 1988). **Propranolol, metoprolol, atenolol, and timolol** reduce the rates of reinfarction and cardiovascular death after MI. Properly titrated, the agents in this class are equally effective in blood pressure reduction.

The adverse effects of the beta blockers differ.

Beta$_1$-selective agents vary in the relative degree of beta$_1$ inhibition. Their selectivity is less at higher doses but may be an important theoretical consideration in choosing therapy for patients with obstructive pulmonary disease, diabetes, and peripheral vascular disease. **Beta$_2$ blockade** may trigger adverse effects such as bronchospasm, dampened manifestations of hypoglycemia, and loss of beta$_2$-mediated peripheral vasodilation.

Intrinsic sympathomimetic activity (ISA) occurs with **pindolol** and **acebutolol**, which are mild sympathetic agonists that block access of more potent circulating catecholamines to beta-adrenergic receptors. They are less likely to affect resting cardiac function than are beta blockers lacking ISA. However, they cause a comparable decrement in maximal heart rate response to exercise.

Labetalol is unique in its ability to block both alpha and beta receptors.

TABLE 5–2. DIURETICS

AGENT	ADULT DOSE (MG)	DURATION (HR)	COMMENT
Thiazides and Related Agents			Effect may be blunted by probenecid; absorption decreased by bile acid binders; may decrease lithium clearance; associated with photosensitivity, pancreatitis, and interstitial nephritis
Chlorothiazide (Diuril)	125–500 qd	6–12	Available for IV use, usually 500 mg q 12–24h
Chlorthalidone (Hygroton)	12.5–50 qd	24–72	
Hydrochlorothiazide (Esidrix, Oretic, HydroDIURIL)	12.5–50 qd	6–12	In combination therapy, 12.5–25 mg qd may be sufficient; least expensive diuretic
Indapamide (Lozol)	2.5–5 qd	24–36	Daily dose above 2.5 mg has no added antihypertensive effect but may decrease edema; may be used for renal insufficiency
Metolazone (Diulo, Zaroxolyn)	2.5–20 qd	12–24	Daily dose above 5 mg has no added antihypertensive effect but may decrease edema; may be used for renal insufficiency
Loop Diuretics			Agents are chemically dissimilar, but cleared hepatically and renally; all cause urinary loss of K, Ca, and Mg and effect glucose tolerance less than do thiazides; ototoxicity may occur at high doses; decrease the effect of probenecid and decrease lithium clearance; may cause hyperuricemia; onset of action in 5 min with IV
Ethacrynic acid (Edecrin)	25–100 po qd–bid 50 IV	6–8 (po) 2 (IV)	Usually used twice daily; maximum daily dose 400 mg; may potentiate warfarin
Furosemide (Lasix)	20–160 po bid 10–40 IV or IM	6–8 (po) 2 (IV)	Should be used twice daily for hypertension; maximum daily dose 600 mg; least expensive of loop diuretics
Potassium-Sparing Diuretics			All may cause hyperkalemia (see text); may decrease lithium clearance; all available as fixed-dose combination medication with HCTZ
Amiloride (Midamor, Moduretic)	5–10 qd	Used qd	Least expensive of K+-sparing diuretics
Spironolactone (Aldactone, Aldactazide)	25–100 qd	Used qd–bid	Interferes with digoxin immunoassay; may cause gynecomastia, menstrual irregularity; least expensive of this class
Triamterene (Dyrenium, Dyazide, Maxide)	50–150 qd	Used qd–bid	Has little intrinsic antihypertensive effect; may promote nephrolithiasis with stones containing triamterene.

TABLE 5-3. BETA-ADRENERGIC BLOCKERS

All are cleared by the liver except nadolol and atenolol, which are cleared renally. For the hepatically metabolized drugs, enzyme inducers (e.g., rifampin, barbiturates) may decrease level while cimetidine may increase it. Beta blockers may reduce plasma clearance of drugs metabolized by the liver (e.g., lidocaine, warfarin) and should be used cautiously with calcium channel blockers.

AGENT	USUAL ADULT DOSE (MG) (MAXIMUM DAILY DOSE)	PLASMA T$_{1/2}$ (HR)	BETA$_1$ SELECTIVE	ISA	COMMENT
Acebutolol (Sectral)	200–400 qd–bid (1200)	3	+	1+	Reduce dose in renal insufficiency due to active metabolite
Atenolol (Tenormin)	50–100 qd (150)	6–8	+	–	Excreted unchanged in urine
Betaxolol (Kerlone)	10–20 qd (40)	14–16	+	–	
Labetalol (Normodyne, Trandate)	100–600 bid (1800)	4–6	–	–	Has alpha blocking activity; available for IV
Metoprolol (Lopressor)	50–100 qd–bid (200)	3–4	+	–	Loses beta₁ selectivity above daily doses of 200 mg; should be taken with meals; available for IV
Nadolol (Corgard)	40–320 qd (640)	14–18	–	–	Excreted unchanged in urine
Penbutolol (Levatol)	20–80 qd	5	–	1+	
Pindolol (Visken)	5–20 bid (60)	3–4	–	3+	Decrease dose in renal insufficiency; may cause insomnia, nervousness
Propranolol (Inderal, Inderal-LA)	40–160 bid (640)	3–5	–	–	Used qid for angina pectoris; available for IV; may increase plasma level of theophylline and lidocaine; bile acid and aluminum binding agents may decrease level; least expensive beta blocker
Timolol (Blocadren)	10–20 bid (80)	4	–	–	

183

The most common **side effects** of the beta blockers are fatigue, depression, and impotence. They are contraindicated in patients with severe cardiac conduction defects (greater than first degree AV nodal block) or in those using MAO inhibitors. Beta blockers must be used carefully in patients with bronchospastic pulmonary disease, diabetes, peripheral vascular disease, and CHF. After abrupt discontinuation, a withdrawal syndrome including hypertension and cardiac ischemia may occur (Circulation 59:1158–1164, 1979).

C. **ACE Inhibitors** (Table 5–4). These agents decrease levels of circulating angiotensin II and aldosterone. They are a reasonable "first step" in treating mild to moderate hypertension. In hypertensive patients with diabetic nephropathy, the proteinuria and progression of renal disease may be slowed. Although particularly effective in treating renovascular hypertension, ACE inhibitors may cause reversible acute renal failure in such patients, especially those with bilateral renal artery stenosis or a stenotic artery to a solitary kidney.

ACE inhibitors do not precipitate changes in glucose, lipid, or uric acid levels. They can cause hyperkalemia, especially in patients with diabetes, renal disease, or CHF, and should not be given concomitantly with potassium-sparing diuretics, potassium supplements, or NSAIDs. Adverse effects are rash, dysgeusia, angioedema, and cough. Early reports of neutropenia due to captopril were generally in patients with renal insufficiency or collagen vascular disease during treatment with relatively high doses.

D. **Calcium Channel Blockers** (Table 5–5). These drugs share a common mechanism, but their chemical structures and typical effects vary considerably. **Verapamil** has negative inotropic and chronotropic effects, and cardiotoxicity is likely with concurrent use of beta blockers. Constipation is the most common side effect. Verapamil is less likely than nifedipine to cause peripheral edema and reflex tachycardia. The vasodilatory effect of **nifedipine** occurs well before cardiotoxic levels develop, so careful concurrent use with beta blockers is reasonable. Headache and flushing are other common side effects. Some patients treated with **nicardipine** experience an aggravation of angina; the mechanism is unknown.

E. **Peripheral Alpha-Adrenergic Receptor Blockers** (Table 5–6). **Prazosin** and, to a lesser extent, **terazosin** may cause severe postural hypotension with the first dose, typically 30–90 minutes after administration. This effect may be minimized by giving 1 mg at bedtime as the initial dose. It may recur with retreatment after a hiatus of a few days. It is more common in volume-depleted or elderly patients.

F. **Centrally Acting Sympatholytics** (Table 5–6). **Clonidine, guanabenz,** and **alpha-methyldopa** have central alpha$_2$ agonist properties. Sedation, dry mouth, and postural symptoms are common side effects of all 3 drugs. Clonidine has the most rapid effect and is used in oral treatment of "hypertensive urgencies." A demonstrated lack of adverse fetal effects allows alpha-methyldopa to be used in pregnant patients. 10–20% of patients treated with alpha-methyldopa develop a positive direct Coombs test, but clinically apparent hemolysis is unusual.

TABLE 5–4. ANGIOTENSIN-CONVERTING ENZYME (ACE) INHIBITORS

May cause acute hypotensive response in the elderly and patients taking diuretics. Monitor renal function in patients with congestive heart failure or possible renovascular hypertension. Decrease dose for patients with renal insufficiency. May cause hyperkalemia.

AGENT	USUAL ADULT DOSE (MG) (MAXIMUM DAILY DOSE)	TIME TO PEAK EFFECT (HR)	COMMENT
Captopril (Capoten)	12.5–50 bid–tid (300)	1–2	Food leads to decreased bioavailability; dysgeusia may occur in 2–3% of recipients, may resolve with continued use
Enalapril (Vasotec)	2.5–20 qd–bid (40)	4–6	A "prodrug," metabolized to active agent; may be given once daily at doses above 5 mg
Enalaprilat (Vasotec IV)	1.25–2.5 q 6 hrs (20)	Onset 15 min; peak 1–4 hrs	Only parenteral ACE inhibitor
Lisinopril (Prinivil, Zestril)	5–40 qd (40)	6	No taste alterations; least expensive of ACE inhibitors

TABLE 5–5. CALCIUM CHANNEL BLOCKERS

Cleared by the liver; cimetidine may increase effect. Used as antianginal drugs. May increase serum digoxin level or cause edema, headache, and constipation. All agents available as slow-release preparations except nicardipine.

AGENT	USUAL ADULT DOSE (MG) (MAXIMUM DAILY DOSE)	TIME TO PEAK EFFECT (HR)	COMMENT
Diltiazem (Cardizem)	30–90 tid–qid (360)	3–6	Less cardiac depressant effect than verapamil
Nicardipine (Cardene)	20–30 tid (120)	1–2	Some patients report worsening of angina
Nifedipine (Procardia, Adalat)	10–30 tid–qid (180)	1–3 (po) onset in 5–15 min	Edema and flushing occur in 10% of recipients; reflex tachycardia may occur; may increase warfarin effect and decrease quinidine level
Verapamil (Calan, Isoptin, Verelan)	80–120 tid (480)	2–5	May increase plasma levels of quinidine, carbamazepine, and theophylline, decrease plasma levels of lithium

G. Direct Vasodilators (Table 5–7). These drugs act primarily on arteriolar smooth muscle, may lead to reflex tachycardia, and are often combined with beta blockers. **Hydralazine** is often used in pregnant patients and in those with pregnancy-induced hypertension (preeclampsia). It is associated with a lupus-like syndrome that is rare unless the total daily dose is greater than 200 mg. **Minoxidil** is a potent drug usually used only in patients with severe hypertension. It causes significant sodium retention and usually must be given with furosemide, 20–40 mg twice daily. Abrupt withdrawal may cause rebound hypertension.

H. Cost Considerations. Because hypertension is so common, the cost of an antihypertensive regimen should be considered carefully. Important variables to consider in addition to the cost of the drug are dosing interval, drug potency, and the need for laboratory monitoring. Hydrochlorothiazide is the least expensive single agent. However, if potassium supplements are required, combination with a potassium-sparing diuretic or a different class of drug may be less expensive. Hydralazine is also inexpensive; if beta blockers must be added, the cost is raised considerably.

Because propranolol may be used twice per day, it is usually the cheapest beta blocker. However, drugs given once daily, while more expensive per dose, may have lower daily cost. Many fixed-dose drug combinations are available but are generally inappropriate as initial therapy. They often may impede individualization of drug regimens.

TABLE 5–6. ANTIADRENERGIC AGENTS

AGENT	ADULT DOSE (MG)	TIME TO PEAK EFFECT (HR)	COMMENT
Peripheral Alpha Antagonists	Cleared by liver and kidneys; 1st-dose postural hypotension; less tachycardia than direct vasodilators		
Prazosin (Minipress)	1–5 bid–tid	1–3	Marginal benefit of doses above 10 mg per day
Terazosin (Hytrin)	1–10 qd–bid	2–3	Maximum daily dose of 20 mg; less postural effect than prazosin
Central Alpha Agonists	All agents may cause sedation, dry mouth, sexual dysfunction; rebound hypertension may occur with abrupt withdrawal		
Alpha-methyldopa (Aldomet)	250–1000 bid–tid max 2000 daily 250–500 q 6h IV	4–6	Increase risk of toxicity of lithium and haloperidol; May give entire dose at hs; may cause chronic active hepatitis
Clonidine (Catapres)	0.1–0.6 bid	1–3	Withdrawal syndrome uncommon if daily dose less than 0.6 mg; least expensive of this class; available in transdermal form, administered weekly
Guanabenz (Wytensin)	4–32 bid	2–4	Main route of clearance is hepatic
Other Agents			
Reserpine (Serapsil)	0.1–0.25 qd, may give 0.5 qd for 1st week	24, full effect requires 1–3 weeks	Contraindicated in patients with depression, history of depression, or peptic ulcer disease; weight gain and nasal congestion common; increases risk of quinidine, digoxin toxicity; induces supersensitivity to sympathomimetics
Guanethidine (Ismelin)	10–150 qd	1 week	Increases pressor effect of nonprescription directly acting sympathomimetics; low rate of CNS side effects; effect antagonized by TCAs, chlorpromazine; prolonged effect after drug discontinued

TABLE 5–7. DIRECT VASODILATORS

Commonly cause reflex tachycardia, edema, and headache. May precipitate angina in patients with coronary artery disease.

AGENT	USUAL ADULT DOSE (MG) (MAXIMUM DAILY DOSE)	TIME TO PEAK EFFECT (HR)	COMMENT
Hydralazine (Apresoline)	25–100 bid po (300) 10–40 IM or IV q3–6 h	0.5–2 (po) 10–20 min IM/IV; lasts 2–4 h	Traditionally drug of choice for pregnancy-induced hypertension; ingestion with food increases bioavailability; may increase plasma levels of hepatically cleared beta blockers; least expensive vasodilator
Minoxidil (Loniten)	2.5–20 qd–bid (100)	2–3	Effect may last 2–3 days; reduce dose in patients with renal insufficiency; may cause pleural or pericardial effusions; causes hypertrichosis in 80% of recipients

III. RENOVASCULAR HYPERTENSION

A. **General Considerations.** 1% of patients with hypertension have reno-vascular hypertension, the most common type of secondary hypertension. It should be suspected in patients with blood pressure that is difficult to control, particularly if a patient is relatively young or has renal insufficiency.

Renovascular hypertension results from macrovascular stenosis leading to excess renin production and high plasma aldosterone and angiotensin levels. The most common causes are fibromuscular dysplasia (younger patients, mainly female, 25% of cases) and atherosclerotic disease (75%).

The best sequence of diagnostic testing for renovascular hypertension is controversial. **Noninvasive screening** may be done with **peripheral renin determinations** before and after captopril stimulation and **duplex ultrasonic study** of the renal arteries. Confirmation requires **renal angiography** followed by selective renal vein renin testing during captopril stimulation. Renin-suppressing drugs (beta blockers, sympatholytics) should be discontinued before testing.

B. **Management.** The most logical treatment is anatomic: either translu-minal angioplasty or surgical revascularization. Percutaneous **translumi-nal angioplasty** is successful in two thirds of patients with atherosclerotic lesions (though those of the renal artery ostium respond poorly) and

90% of those with fibromuscular dysplasia. Resolution or improvement of hypertension occurs in 85% of patients, but the annual restenosis rate is 15%.

The rate of cure or improvement is similar for **surgical revascularization,** but it should be considered only when angioplasty is impossible or has failed.

Treatment with an ACE inhibitor, beta blocker, and/or diuretic is the regimen of choice for nonoperable disease. Acute renal failure may result from ACE inhibitor therapy in patients with bilateral renal artery stenosis or renal artery stenosis in a solitary kidney. Regardless of the medical regimen, renal function (creatinine clearance) and size (ultrasound) should be followed, as renal damage can progress even with apparently satisfactory blood pressure control.

IV. HYPERTENSIVE CRISIS

The most common cause of hypertensive crisis is an abrupt change in the blood pressure control of a chronic hypertensive. Sympathomimetic ingestion or dietary indiscretion by a patient taking an MAO inhibitor may be occult causes. Most patients have a diastolic blood pressure (DBP) greater than 120–130 mm Hg, though children and pregnant women may have lower blood pressures.

Patients with **acute end-organ damage** (cardiopulmonary symptoms/ signs, ECG changes, new retinopathy, azotemia, hematuria, or microangiopathic hemolytic anemia) are considered medical emergencies. The cases of patients without these findings are considered urgent and often may be managed with oral therapy and close outpatient follow-up ("next day").

Most patients are already volume-depleted, and diuretics should not be used (except in pulmonary edema). Particularly in cases of cerebral ischemia, overzealous therapy can be hazardous, worsening the ischemia. The goal should not be normalization of the blood pressure, but either a 20% reduction or a DBP of 100 mm Hg, whichever is higher. In patients with myocardial ischemia or aortic dissection, the DBP should be rapidly reduced to 100 mm Hg unless organ perfusion is compromised.

A. Drug Therapy (Tables 5–8 and 5–9). The most rapidly effective agent is continuous IV nitroprusside, though close monitoring is required. It should be avoided in pregnancy-induced hypertension owing to the risk

TABLE 5–8. DRUGS FOR HYPERTENSIVE URGENCIES

DRUG	DOSE (MG)	FREQUENCY	ONSET	DURATION
Clonidine	0.1–0.2	q 1 h	30–60 min	8–12 h
Nifedipine	10	q 15–30 min	5–10 min (sl) 10–20 min (po)	3–6 h

TABLE 5–9. DRUGS FOR HYPERTENSIVE EMERGENCIES

DRUG	ROUTE	ONSET (MIN)	DURATION	DOSE	COMMENT
Sodium nitroprusside	IV infusion	Immediate	2–3 min	0.5–10 µg/kg/min	Risk of thiocyanate toxicity, especially with renal insufficiency; may cause reflex tachycardia; may decrease oxygen saturation
Labetalol	IV bolus	5–10	3–6 hr	20 mg q 5–10 min up to 300 mg	Risk of heart block, congestive heart failure, bronchospasm; may have paradoxic pressor response; may be given continuously IV
Nitroglycerin	IV infusion	1–2	3–5 min	5–100 µg/min	May cause headache
Hydralazine	IV bolus	10–20	3–6 hr	5–10 mg q 20 min	May cause tachycardia, local phlebitis; if not effective after 20 mg, choose different drug; may also be given IM
Phentolamine	IV bolus	1–2	3–10 min	5–10 mg q 5–15 min	May cause paradoxic pressor response

of thiocyanate toxicity. IV nitroglycerin is the drug of choice when cardiac ischemia is present. Treatment may be initiated topically or sublingually while IV access is being established.

Oral or sublingual nifedipine or oral clonidine may be used for the "hypertensive urgency."

B. Special Circumstances. These include:

1. AORTIC DISSECTION

Blood pressure reduction and decrease of shear forces are the goal. Thus, beta blockers (given first) are combined with vasodilators (usually nitroprusside) (JAMA 264:2537–2541, 1990). Labetalol may also be used alone.

2. PREGNANCY-INDUCED HYPERTENSION

Hydralazine is the drug of choice. Labetalol and nifedipine are alternatives.

3. PHEOCHROMOCYTOMA

Phentolamine, given in intermittent IV boluses, is the drug of choice. Labetalol is an alternative (because it has both alpha and beta blockade); simple beta blockers should be avoided.

4. HYPERTENSIVE CRISIS OF PROGRESSIVE SYSTEMIC SCLEROSIS

ACE inhibitors are the drugs of choice (Ann Intern Med 113:352–357, 1990).

The 1988 Report of the Joint National Committee on Detection, Evaluation, and Treatment of High Blood Pressure. Arch Intern Med 148:1023–1038, 1988.

Hollenberg NK: The treatment of renovascular hypertension: Surgery, angioplasty, and medical therapy with converting enzyme inhibitors. Am J Kidney Dis 10(suppl):52, 1987.

Calhoun DA, Oparil S: Treatment of hypertensive crisis. N Engl J Med 323:1177–1183, 1990.

Houston MC: Treatment of hypertensive emergencies and urgencies with oral clonidine loading and titration: A review. Arch Intern Med 146:586–589, 1986.

Houston MC: The comparative effects of clonidine hydrochloride and nifedipine in the treatment of hypertensive crises. Am Heart J 115:152–159, 1988.

Kaplan NM: Maximally reducing cardiovascular risk in the treatment of hypertension. Ann Intern Med 109:36–40, 1988.

Oberman A, Wassertheil-Smoller S, Langford HG, et al: Pharmacologic and nutritional treatment of mild hypertension: Changes in cardiovascular risk status. Ann Intern Med 112:89–95, 1990.

Littenberg B, Garber AM, Sox HC: Screening for hypertension. Ann Intern Med 112:192–202, 1990.

Mejia AD, Egan BM, Schork NJ, Zweifler AJ: Artefacts in measurement of blood pressure and lack of target organ involvement in the assessment of patients with treatment-resistant hypertension. Ann Intern Med 112:270–277, 1990.

Williams GH: Converting-enzyme inhibitors in the treatment of hypertension. N Engl J Med 319:1517–1525, 1988.

Kaplan NM: Calcium entry blockers in the treatment of hypertension: Current status and future prospects. JAMA 262:817–823, 1989.

666666666666666

RENAL DISEASES

LESLIE S. T. FANG

666666666666666666

I. MANAGEMENT OF PATIENTS WITH ACUTE RENAL FAILURE

A. General Principles. Although the causes of acute renal failure (ARF) are diverse, the complications are similar, and general guidelines are applicable to all patients with acute progressive deterioration of renal function. About 70% of patients with ARF have an oliguric phase; the remainder have nonoliguric renal failure. A number of complications can arise during acute renal insufficiency, and patient management depends on the complications.

B. Management During the Oliguric Phase

1. **FLUID MANAGEMENT**
   The major goal is to avoid fluid overload and excessive fluid depletion. The patient should be weighed daily, with a weight loss goal of about ¼ pound each day. Intake and output should be carefully monitored, and the patient's fluids should be restricted so that the total intake matches the urine output plus insensible losses. In patients with intractable volume overload and congestive heart failure (CHF), peritoneal dialysis or hemodialysis may be necessary.

2. **MANAGEMENT OF ACIDOSIS**
   Patients with metabolic acidosis should be given **sodium bicarbonate,** starting with oral doses of 600 mg bid, increasing to 1.2 gm qid, as necessary. The goal is to give enough sodium bicarbonate to maintain serum bicarbonate levels between 16 and 20 mEq/L. The considerable sodium load will limit sodium bicarbonate use if volume overload is a concern. Hypocalcemia can also limit the use of sodium bicarbonate. Rapid reversal of acidosis may worsen hypocalcemia and induce tetany and seizures.

3. **ELECTROLYTE MANAGEMENT**
   The primary concern is the management of hyperkalemia (Table 6–1). Cardiac monitoring is indicated until the serum potassium level has been stabilized. In an acute situation, the serum potassium level can be rapidly lowered by the use of glucose and insulin. Sodium bicarbonate can also shift potassium from the extracellular to the intracellular space on an acute basis. **Sodium polystyrene sulfonate** (Kayexalate), 30 to 50 gm in a sorbitol solution, can be given either po or as an enema for long-term management. This resin exchanges sodium for potassium, calcium, and magnesium. Protracted use may result in sodium overload, hypocalcemia, or hypomagnesemia. In patients with refractory hyperkalemia, peritoneal dialysis or hemodialysis may be necessary.

TABLE 6–1. TREATMENT OF HYPERKALEMIA

ACUTE MANAGEMENT	
Sodium bicarbonate	50 mEq IV
$D_{50}W$	1 ampule
Insulin	10 U regular insulin
Calcium gluconate	1 ampule
CHRONIC MANAGEMENT	
Low-potassium diet	
Sodium polystyrene sulfonate	50 gm po or pr
Dialysis	

4. MANAGEMENT OF UREMIA
To minimize the degree of uremia, patients should receive adequate caloric intake and a low-protein diet. Usually protein intake should be restricted to 0.5 gm/kg/day. Adequate caloric intake should be maintained to minimize catabolism. Maximize the use of high-quality protein, essential amino acids, or alpha-keto analogues of essential amino acids in the diet. Prospective randomized studies have suggested that patients in the postsurgical period who develop ARF and require dialysis have improved survival when given **renal failure fluid,** a glucose solution containing essential amino acids.

5. MANAGEMENT OF CALCIUM AND PHOSPHATE HOMEOSTASIS
Hyperphosphatemia should be corrected before aggressive correction of serum calcium to minimize metastatic calcification. Correction of hyperphosphatemia can most easily be done with **aluminum hydroxide** preparations. Amphojel or Basaljel, 30–120 mL po qid, can be given. The goal is to bring the serum phosphate to a level less than 5 mg/dL. After optimal adjustment of the serum phosphate level, hypocalcemia can be corrected with calcium supplement and vitamin D. Calcium carbonate also has been shown to be an effective phosphate binder and is often the preferred agent since it would avoid aluminum overload. A reasonable starting dose of calcium would be 500 mg of Os-Cal tid. A reasonable starting dose of vitamin D would be 0.25 mg of 1,25-dihydroxycholecaliferol daily. Serum calcium values should be monitored closely to avoid hypercalcemia.

6. MANAGEMENT OF DRUGS THAT ARE EXCRETED RENALLY
In patients with oliguric renal failure, all medications should be reviewed and doses of renally excreted drugs should be adjusted. Drugs containing magnesium should be avoided, since seemingly innocuous drugs such as milk of magnesia or Mylanta can result in magnesium accumulation, which can lead to CNS toxicity. Life-threatening drug toxicity can be avoided if a careful review of drugs has been carried out.

7. MANAGEMENT OF CARDIOVASCULAR COMPLICATIONS
Careful attention should be focused on fluid management to minimize the likelihood of fluid overload, hypertension, and CHF. Uremic pericarditis, however, is usually an indication that there has been

considerable accumulation of uremic toxins and may force initiation of dialysis.

8. **MANAGEMENT OF NEUROLOGIC COMPLICATIONS**
Dialysis is indicated if conservative management fails to control CNS symptoms.

9. **MANAGEMENT OF HEMATOLOGIC COMPLICATIONS**
The role of **erythropoietin** in the management of anemia of ARF remains under investigation. Preliminary indications suggest that erythropoietin is less effective in the acutely ill patient. Prolongation of bleeding time should be addressed, particularly if a patient has clinically evident bleeding or if a surgical procedure is planned. Trials should be made with **desmopressin** (DDAVP) (0.4 μg/kg IV about 4 hours before a contemplated procedure) and *cryoprecipitate* (10 units) to see if the bleeding time can be reversed. Premarin has also been shown to be effective in correcting bleeding time. However, the effect of Premarin is usually apparent only after 3–7 days of therapy. Prolonged bleeding time can also be corrected by dialysis, which should be considered in a patient with significant bleeding and uremia.

C. **Management During the Diuretic Phase.** After volume overload is corrected, intake should be adjusted to match urine output until renal function is at a reasonable level, with a BUN value less than 40 mg/dL and a serum creatinine value less than 2.5 mg/dL. This goal may require supplementation with 0.45% normal saline with 20 mEq/L potassium chloride. As renal function approaches normal, fluid infusion should be progressively decreased and discontinued. This step will minimize the likelihood of overdiuresis during the diuretic phase, which occurs occasionally. During the diuretic phase, medication doses must be readjusted as the patient's renal function improves.

D. **Indications for Dialysis.** Dialysis is indicated in patients for whom conservative management has failed. Specific indications include the following:

1. Intractable volume overload, causing hypertension and congestive heart failure,
2. Progressive CNS symptoms,
3. Clinically significant bleeding in severely azotemic patients not responding to DDAVP or cryoprecipitate,
4. Uremic pericarditis,
5. Life-threatening drug toxicity,
6. Intractable hyperkalemia unresponsive to conservative management,
7. Intractable acidosis.

In practice, intractable volume overload and progressive uremic symptoms are the most likely reasons for initiation of dialysis.

E. **Selected Issues.** Several issues that arise in the management of patients with ARF remain controversial.

1. **ROLE OF LOOP DIURETICS**
Although **furosemide** given early in its course may convert oliguric renal failure to nonoliguric renal failure in about 25–75% of cases, this effect may not be associated with improved renal or patient outcome. However, since the patient with nonoliguric renal failure is much easier to manage, attempts should be made to see if loop diuretics are beneficial. Before a loop diuretic is used, volume status should be carefully adjusted. Diuresis in a patient with prerenal azotemia can markedly aggravate the problem. If the patient is euvolemic or volume overloaded, furosemide can be used in increasing doses for diuresis. The starting dose should be 40 mg IV; increasing doses can be given at hourly intervals to see if diuresis ensues. In general, the dose should not exceed 400 mg in any 24-hour period to avoid ototoxicity. Some authors advocate progressive increase of furosemide to doses of 3600 mg daily, but this program can lead to furosemide accumulation and resultant ototoxicity.

2. **ROLE OF MANNITOL**
Mannitol is an osmotic diuretic that some believe will convert oliguric to nonoliguric renal failure. However, mannitol can result in volume overload in the oliguric patient and should be used cautiously.

3. **CONTINUOUS INFUSION OF FUROSEMIDE-MANNITOL SOLUTION**
Combination therapy utilizing a continuous infusion of furosemide and mannitol has gained popularity in some institutions. 1 gm furosemide is mixed in 500 mL of 20% mannitol and infused at a rate of 10 mL/hour. Usually an effect is observed about 6 hours after initiation of infusion. Since both furosemide and mannitol are infused at a fairly low rate, the toxicity of such an infusion is limited, but hyponatremia can still occur. In general, the continuous infusion should be stopped if no significant diuresis is seen within 12 hours of the initiation of therapy. Again, although continuous infusion of furosemide and mannitol has been associated with conversion of oliguric renal failure to nonoliguric renal failure, such therapy may not affect renal recovery or mortality.

4. **ROLE OF LOW-DOSE DOPAMINE**
Dopamine, given in low doses (less than 5 μg/kg/min), has been shown to enhance diuresis, natriuresis, and kaliuresis. Therefore, low-dose dopamine may be of benefit in patients with oliguric ARF. Unfortunately there are few clinical studies to substantiate the benefit of low-dose dopamine. Again, in selected patients, low-dose dopamine can convert oliguric renal failure to nonoliguric renal failure, but it is not clear that the therapy actually improves renal recovery or outcome.

5. **ROLE OF EARLY, AGGRESSIVE DIALYSIS**
Early, aggressive dialysis has been advocated by some as beneficial in ARF. However, only minimal, conflicting clinical information attempting to address this issue is available. In most instances, dialysis should be reserved for the patient in whom conservative measures have failed.

Hakim RM, Lazarus JM: Hemodialysis in acute renal failure. *In* Brenner BM, Lazarus JM (eds): Acute Renal Failure. 2nd ed. New York, Churchill Livingstone, 1988, pp 767–808.

Levinsky NG, Bernard DB: Mannitol and loop diuretics in acute renal failure. *In* Brenner BM, Lazarus JM (eds): Acute Renal Failure. 2nd ed. New York, Churchill Livingstone, 1988, pp 841–856.

Nolph KD, Sorkin MI: Peritoneal dialysis in acute renal failure. *In* Brenner BM, Lazarus JM (eds): Acute Renal Failure. 2nd ed. New York, Churchill Livingstone, 1988, pp 809–840.

II. THERAPY FOR SPECIFIC FORMS OF ACUTE RENAL FAILURE

A. Ischemic ARF (Acute Tubular Necrosis). Ischemic ARF, often called **acute tubular necrosis,** is the result of prolonged compromise in renal perfusion. It is believed that the blood supply to normal kidneys can be interrupted for up to 30 minutes without damage. However, in critically ill patients with sustained hemodynamic compromise, progressive renal dysfunction that is unresponsive to correction of blood volume and cardiac output can develop even with shorter intervals of compromise in renal blood flow. Ischemic ARF is likely to occur in a number of clinical settings (Table 6–2).

Clinically, acute oliguria and progressive deterioration in renal function coincide with the acute ischemic event. Usually an oliguric phase lasts hours to 10 days, followed by a diuretic phase. Examination of the urinary sediment reveals cellular debris with many cellular and granular casts. Urinary indices show low urine osmolality, and the urinary osmolality seldom exceeds the serum osmolality by greater than 100 mOsm/kg. The urinary sodium level tends to be high in these patients, and the fractional excretion of sodium is usually greater than 1%. The ratio of urinary creatinine to plasma creatinine is usually less than 20:1. Urinary findings are important in the differentiation of acute tubular necrosis and prerenal azotemia (Table 6–3).

1. CONTRAST AGENT–INDUCED ARF

   a. Clinical Course. After antibiotics, contrast media are the most common causes of nephrotoxic acute renal failure. Clinically, osmotic diuresis occurs during the first 10–18 hours after admin-

TABLE 6–2. COMMON CAUSES OF ISCHEMIC ACUTE TUBULAR NECROSIS

After cardiac surgery, particularly in patients with low cardiac output
After vascular surgery, particularly in procedures with cross-clamping of aorta above renal arteries
Loss of intravascular volume by massive hemorrhage
Crush injury
Sepsis, particularly gram-negative
Pancreatitis
Gastroenteritis
Postpartum hemorrhage
Rhabdomyolysis with myoglobinuria
Transfusion reaction

TABLE 6–3. RENAL INDICES IN ACUTE TUBULAR NECROSIS AND IN PRERENAL AZOTEMIA

INDEX	ACUTE TUBULAR NECROSIS	PRERENAL AZOTEMIA
Urinary sediment	Cellular debris Granular and cellular casts	Benign sediment
Blood urea nitrogen/ creatinine ratio	About 10:1	>10:1
Urinary osmolality	About 300 mOsm/kg	>350 mOsm/kg
Urinary Na	>40 mEq/L	<20 mEq/L
Urinary creatinine/plasma creatinine ratio	<20:1	>40:1
Fractional excretion of Na	>1%	<1%

istration of contrast medium, since most available contrast agents are hyperosmolar. In susceptible patients, oliguric, and occasionally anuric, renal failure occurs about 24 hours after the contrast study. In these patients, renal function deterioration occurs over 4–10 days. Diuresis begins after the oliguric phase, and renal function recovery begins about 1–3 days after the beginning of the diuresis. During the oliguric phase, the urinalysis may be benign, with only an occasional granular cast. The patient often has isosthenuria. The urinary sodium level and fractional excretion of sodium are unusually low during the oliguric phase of contrast medium–induced ARF. This is important, since the clinical syndrome can be mistaken for volume depletion and prerenal azotemia. Fluid challenge in these instances can lead to volume overload. Most patients recover the level of renal function that existed before the contrast study. Some patients may have renal insufficiency severe enough to require dialysis. Rarely, patients fail to recover renal function. Diabetics with preexisting renal dysfunction are at highest risk of developing irreversible renal failure. A number of conditions predispose patients to contrast medium–induced ARF (Table 6–4).

TABLE 6–4. PREDISPOSING FACTORS TO CONTRAST MEDIUM–INDUCED ACUTE RENAL FAILURE

MAJOR PREDISPOSING FACTORS
Preexisting renal insufficiency
Diabetes mellitus
MINOR PREDISPOSING FACTORS
Dehydration
Amount of contrast administered
Cardiac output
OTHER PREDISPOSING FACTORS
Multiple myeloma
Advanced age
Previous episodes of contrast medium–induced ARF

b. **Management.** Patients at risk for contrast agent–induced renal failure should be **hydrated,** as their clinical status permits, before the contrast study (Table 6–5), and the **amount of contrast medium should be minimized.** Several newer contrast agents have recently been introduced (nonionic or low–osmolarity contrast agents). Although some data in animals indicate less nephrotoxicity, the information in humans is less clear. A randomized, prospective study failed to reveal any advantages of the nonionic contrast agents over conventional contrast agents. There is increasing evidence that **furosemide** or **mannitol** (or both) given shortly after the contrast study minimizes the likelihood of contrast agent–induced ARF in susceptible patients. Usually, 12.5–25.0 gm of mannitol and 40 mg of furosemide can be infused at the end of the contrast study. When mannitol or furosemide is used, it is important to monitor the intake and output rigidly and match output with intake for about 24 to 48 hours after the study. In some patients, contrast agent–induced ARF may develop either because of failure to identify the risk factor (or factors) or in spite of all appropriate precautions. In these patients, fluids, electrolytes, and acid-base balance should be managed carefully. During the oliguric phase of ARF, fluid challenge, use of diuretics, and mannitol infusion have all been shown to be ineffective. Since most patients will experience spontaneous recovery within 7–10 days, dialysis can usually be avoided with meticulous conservative management. In a few patients, peritoneal dialysis or hemodialysis may be necessary.

2. MYOGLOBINURIC ACUTE RENAL FAILURE

a. **Clinical Course.** Rhabdomyolysis with associated myoglobinuric ARF has been described in a number of clinical settings. The manifestations and therapeutic options are sufficiently distinctive to warrant special consideration. Myriad clinical settings can result in myoglobinuria and ARF (Table 6–6). Although trauma and crush injury remain the leading causes of rhabdomyolysis, 50% of cases of rhabdomyolysis are nontraumatic. Some clinical settings can potentiate rhabdomyolysis: dehydration, hypokalemia, hypophosphatemia, and acidosis predispose the patient to myoglobinuric ARF. The clinical history should alert physicians to the

TABLE 6–5. MANAGEMENT OF CONTRAST MEDIUM–INDUCED ACUTE RENAL FAILURE

BEFORE CONTRAST STUDY
Identify patients at risk for contrast medium–induced ARF
Hydrate before contrast study, as patient's clinical status permits
DURING CONTRAST STUDY
Minimize amount of contrast administered
AFTER CONTRAST STUDY
Give furosemide (40 mg IV) and mannitol (12.5–25.0 gm IV) at study end
Match output with intake for next 24–48 hr

TABLE 6–6. CAUSES OF MYOGLOBINURIA

Trauma
Exertional rhabdomyolysis
Seizures
Drug-related rhabdomyolysis
  Heroin and barbiturates
  Amphetamine, succinylcholine, amphotericin B
Ischemic injury to muscles
Heat stroke and heat cramps
Malignant hyperthermia
Electrical burns
Infections (influenza, leptospirosis, *Clostridium* and *Shigella* species)
Myopathy
  Hereditary (McArdle's disease, Tarui disease)
  Acquired (alcoholic myopathy, polymyositis, dermatomyositis)
Toxins (sea snake bite, spider bite, hornet bite)

possibility of myoglobinuria. Patients have dark amber urine, and electrophoresis or radioimmunoassay will confirm the presence of myoglobin. Marked elevation of serum potassium, phosphate, creatinine (out of proportion to the elevation of BUN), and uric acid levels can occur. Severe hypocalcemia, secondary to hyperphosphatemia as well as deposition of calcium on damaged muscle surfaces, is also common. The patient may become markedly oliguric, with progressive deterioration of renal function. A diuretic phase occurs 5–10 days later, with gradual recovery. During the recovery phase, severe hypercalcemia has been noted and is thought to be secondary to remobilization of calcium from damaged muscles.

b. Management. After careful assessment to rule out the possibility of volume overload, **initial management should be directed at inducing diuresis. Mannitol** (12.5–25.0 gm) can be given IV to induce osmotic diuresis. **Saline** should be infused, together with IV administration of a **loop diuretic,** such as furosemide, bumetanide, or ethacrynic acid. **Alkalinization of urine with sodium bicarbonate** should be attempted only after careful assessment of the patient's volume and calcium status. The patient should be carefully monitored to avoid volume overload. When muscle compartmentalization is a problem, the situation should be promptly corrected by fasciotomy.

If the initial attempts at inducing diuresis with optimization of volume status and diuretics fail, the patient should be managed in the same fashion as other patients with oliguric renal failure. However, special attention should be paid to the patient's potassium, calcium, and phosphate levels and acid-base balance. **Peritoneal dialysis** or **hemodialysis** may be necessary in cases of severe myoglobinuric renal failure. Most patients who develop ARF from myoglobinuria will eventually recover, with normalization of renal function.

B. Obstructive Uropathy

1. CLINICAL COURSE

Obstruction of the urinary tract is a common and potentially reversible cause of acute and chronic renal failure. Obstructive uropathy occurs whenever flow of urine is obstructed at any level from the renal calyces to the urethral meatus (Table 6–7). With significant and persistent obstruction, the renal pelvis and calyces may become abnormally dilated, resulting in hydronephrosis.

2. MANAGEMENT

Therapeutically the obstruction must be relieved. In instances of bladder outlet obstruction, the placement of a Foley catheter will allow optimization of metabolic parameters prior to surgical correction of obstruction. When the ureters are obstructed at the ureteropelvic junction, either retrograde or antegrade urography can be used for the placement of a stent or nephrostomy tube for temporary relief. The patient should have surgical correction of the obstruction, if necessary. During the postobstructive phase, brisk diuresis is often noted. This is due in part to fluid overload during the oliguric period and in part to the accumulation of osmotically active products. The patient should be monitored carefully, and adequate hydration should

TABLE 6–7. CAUSES OF URINARY TRACT OBSTRUCTION

URETHRA AND BLADDER NECK
 Benign prostatic hypertrophy
 Urethral stricture
 Urethral valves
 Meatal stenosis
 Phimosis
BLADDER
 Neurogenic bladder
 Blood clot
 Calculus
 Carcinoma of bladder
URETER
 Intrinsic obstruction (calculus, blood clot, renal papilla,
  carcinoma of ureter)
 Extrinsic obstruction (Retroperitoneal or pelvic tumors,
  strictures, retroperitoneal fibrosis, uterine prolapse, ureterocele)
 Reflux (vesicoureteral reflux, megaloureter)
URETEROPELVIC JUNCTION
 Intrinsic obstruction (calculus, blood clot, renal papilla)
 Extrinsic obstruction (stricture, aberrant vessels, fibrous band)
RENAL PELVIS
 Calculus
 Blood clot
 Papilla
 Carcinoma of renal pelvis
 Carcinoma of kidney
 Tuberculosis

be maintained until renal function returns to a reasonable level (a serum creatinine value of less than 2.5 mg/dL). Half-normal saline with 20 mEq/L of potassium chloride is an appropriate replacement solution. During the postobstructive phase, patients often have an acidifying defect mimicking distal renal tubular acidosis. The degree of recovery depends on the nature and duration of obstruction, and some degree of renal recovery is expected if the duration of obstruction is less than 6 months.

C. **Acute Interstitial Nephritis.** In patients with ARF, acute interstitial nephritis induced by drugs should be considered because prompt recognition and intervention can prevent the morbidity associated with prolonged renal insufficiency. A number of drugs have been implicated (Table 6–8). Some patients with acute interstitial nephritis may have symptoms of hypersensitivity, such as fever, rash, or arthralgias. On examination of the urine, red cells, white cells, low-grade proteinuria (1 +), and white cell casts may be noted. Urinary eosinophils, when present, are particularly helpful in confirming the diagnosis. Peripheral eosinophilia and elevated immunoglobulin E (IgE) levels are sometimes present. Gallium 67 scans may also be useful. Patients often have nonoliguric renal failure, with gradual deterioration of renal function. Nephrotoxicity appears not to be dose related. The deterioration usually reverses with discontinuation of the offending drug. Reexposure to the drug will result in recurrence of nephrotoxicity. In some instances, renal failure may be irreversible, particularly in older patients.

The offending agent should be stopped immediately upon recognition of the problem. Some investigators believe that steroids are helpful in hastening renal recovery and in optimizing the return of renal function to baseline levels.

D. **Nephrotoxicity and Acute Renal Failure.** Nephrotoxins have become increasingly important causes of ARF, especially in critically ill patients. Some drugs cause acute renal deterioration on the basis of allergic interstitial nephritis. Others cause acute renal insufficiency by direct nephrotoxicity. In the latter category of agents, antibiotics (particularly aminoglycosides), heavy metals, organic solvents, and some antineoplastic agents are the usual toxins.

TABLE 6–8. DRUGS COMMONLY ASSOCIATED WITH ACUTE INTERSTITIAL NEPHRITIS

ANTIBIOTICS	NONSTEROIDAL ANTIINFLAMMATORY DRUGS
Penicillins	**Diuretics**
Cephalosporins	Thiazides
Sulfonamides	Furosemide
Trimethoprim-sulfamethoxazole	Chlorthalidone
Rifampin	**Miscellaneous**
	Allopurinol
	Phenytoin
	Phenylbutazone

1. AMINOGLYCOSIDES

Aminoglycoside nephrotoxicity is encountered in about 7–20% of patients receiving aminoglycosides. Different aminoglycosides appear to be associated with slightly different risks of nephrotoxicity. Neomycin is the most nephrotoxic and is therefore not used IV. Limited absorption of neomycin from the GI tract can occur, however, and may result in nephrotoxicity in susceptible patients. Gentamicin is less nephrotoxic than neomycin and is a commonly used drug for gram–negative systemic infections. In comparative studies, tobramycin, kanamycin, amikacin, and streptomycin appear to be slightly less nephrotoxic than gentamicin. Aminoglycoside nephrotoxicity is more likely to occur in elderly patients with evidence of preexisting renal dysfunction in whom there is volume contraction. Patients with hepatic dysfunction are particularly susceptible to aminoglycoside nephrotoxicity. Concurrent administration of other nephrotoxins may enhance nephrotoxicity. These patients have nonoliguric ARF. The onset of deterioration of renal function is insidious, usually beginning 5–14 days after initiation of aminoglycoside therapy. Renal function may continue to deteriorate for 3–10 days after cessation of aminoglycoside therapy. Recovery is slow, and the patient may not return to a baseline level of renal function for several months. Some patients may require dialysis. Preventive measures are important. If clinically feasible, aminoglycosides should be avoided, particularly in elderly patients, those with hepatic dysfunction, and those with preexisting renal insufficiency. In patients with renal insufficiency, the dose interval of aminoglycoside administration should be carefully adjusted. In those receiving aminoglycosides, volume depletion and the concurrent use of other nephrotoxic drugs should be avoided. Renal function and serum levels of aminoglycosides (peak and trough levels) should be monitored closely. If acute renal failure develops, aminoglycosides should be stopped immediately if acceptable alternative antibiotics are available, and management should be conservative. Dialysis may be necessary if conservative measures fail.

2. ANTINEOPLASTIC AGENTS

a. *Cis*-**Platinum.** *Cis*-platinum is excreted renally and can cause nephrotoxicity, which becomes clinically apparent 5–7 days after administration of the agent. Patients have nonoliguric renal insufficiency, with gradual deterioration of renal function. The renal dysfunction may persist.

Cis-platinum nephrotoxicity is more common in elderly patients, in those with preexisting renal insufficiency, and in those with volume contraction and acidosis. Nephrotoxicity can be largely avoided if care is taken to assess renal function before administration of the drug. The patient should be prehydrated and acidosis should be corrected prior to *cis*-platinum therapy. Urine should be alkalinized with sodium bicarbonate infusion. Diuresis should be sustained with the use of saline hydration and loop diuretics for 24–48 hours after *cis*-platinum administration.

b. Methotrexate. Methotrexate, particularly in high doses, is nephrotoxic. Clinically evident deterioration of renal function may occur within 24–48 hours after administration. When administering high-dose methotrexate, renal function should be carefully assessed and the dose of methotrexate adjusted according to the level of renal dysfunction. Toxicity can be prevented by vigorous hydration with saline and alkalinization of the patient's urine prior to administration of the agent. Saline diuresis, alkalinization, and use of a loop diuretic to maintain diuresis should be continued for 48 hours after administration of high-dose methotrexate to minimize toxicity. With preexisting renal dysfunction, diuresis and rescue therapy with citrovorum factor should be continued until the serum level of methotrexate is less than 10^{-7} mmol.

3. **HEAVY METALS**
Lead, arsenic, gold, mercury, bismuth, uranium, and cadmium are associated with nephrotoxicity. Nephrotoxicity usually occurs following attempted suicide or accidental or industrial exposure. Some metals, such as gold, are used therapeutically. Affected patients develop ARF with clinical evidence of tubular necrosis. In some instances, diverse syndromes, ranging from the nephrotic syndrome to Fanconi's syndrome, have been reported. Dimercaprol sometimes can be used to remove the heavy metal load.

4. **ORGANIC SOLVENTS**
Organic solvents, including carbon tetrachloride (used in cleaning agents, industrial solvents, antihelmintics, and some fire extinguishers), trichloroethylene (spot remover), tetrachloroethylene (dry cleaning), and other chlorinated hydrocarbon compounds have been associated with nephrotoxicity. Patients who have been exposed to these solvents (accidentally, in an industrial setting, or as the result of a suicide attempt) can develop oliguric renal failure and abnormal results of liver function tests about a week after exposure. Urinalysis reveals proteinuria, hematuria, pyuria, and granular casts. The usual cause of death is acute hepatic failure. Treatment is primarily supportive.

5. **MISCELLANEOUS AGENTS**

a. Ethylene Glycol. Ethylene glycol (antifreeze) is extremely toxic when ingested; 50–100 ml can be lethal. During the first 12 hours after ingestion, patients have GI and CNS symptoms: nausea, vomiting, lethargy, and coma. Between 12 and 24 hours after ingestion, the cardiopulmonary symptoms of hypotension and pulmonary edema can be seen. After 24 hours, evidence of oliguric renal failure is apparent, and severe metabolic acidosis with an increased anion gap may develop. Measured serum osmolality is higher than calculated serum osmolality because of the presence of ethylene glycol in the serum.

The patient should first be stabilized hemodynamically. Metabolic acidosis should be corrected with sodium bicarbonate infusion. Alcohol should be infused to prevent the metabolism of ethylene glycol (100 mL of 10% ethanol initially and 100 mL/hour of continuous infusion, with the intention of keeping the serum ethanol level at around 100 mg/dL). Saline diuresis, if feasible, should be sustained. Thiamine and pyridoxine administration may be helpful. Peritoneal dialysis and hemodialysis may be important for the removal of ethylene glycol and for the correction of metabolic abnormalities of ARF.

  b. Methoxyflurane and Enflurane (Ethrane). These commonly used anesthetic agents have rarely been associated with ARF. Patients develop slowly progressive renal insufficiency after exposure. The diagnosis is made usually by the exclusion of all other possible causes. Patients should be treated conservatively, with the expectation of slow recovery of renal function.

E. Glomerular Diseases. Diseases affecting the glomeruli and the small vessels can first become evident as acute progressive renal deterioration. Most are associated with systemic diseases, discussed further in "Renal Manifestations of Systemic Diseases."

Prompt recognition of the disease processes is important because a number of the diseases may respond to treatment. A brief description of the various management options is given in Table 6–9.

F. Vascular Diseases. Rarely, occlusion of both renal arteries or both renal veins can result in renal insufficiency. Since the processes are

TABLE 6–9. THERAPEUTIC INTERVENTIONS IN DISEASES OF THE GLOMERULI AND SMALL BLOOD VESSELS

DISEASE	THERAPEUTIC OPTIONS
Poststreptococcal glomerulonephritis	Conservative management
Malignant hypertension	Control of hypertension
Systemic lupus erythematosus	Steroids; cytotoxic drugs, particularly cyclophosphamide given IV in pulse doses; ?plasmapheresis
Subacute bacterial endocarditis	Antibiotics for underlying infection
Wegener's granulomatosis	Cyclophosphamide; steroids, plasmapheresis in severe cases
Goodpasture's syndrome	Steroids; cyclophosphamide, plasmapheresis
Thrombotic thrombocytopenic purpura	Plasmapheresis—Fresh frozen plasma; possibly antiplatelet agents, possibly cytotoxic agents
Polyarteritis nodosa	Steroids; cyclophosphamide
Rapidly progressive glomerulonephritis	Steroids; cyclophosphamide, plasmapheresis
Serum sickness	Steroids
Drug-induced vasculitis	Stop offending agent; steroids

potentially reversible, it is important to include large-vessel disease in the differential diagnosis of progressive renal function deterioration.

1. ARTERIAL OCCLUSION

The most common reason for arterial occlusion is progression of renal artery stenosis, either from atherosclerotic renal artery stenosis or from fibromuscular hyperplasia. Arterial occlusion can also result from emboli to the renal arteries. Necrotizing angiitis secondary to IV drug abuse is a rare cause of renal artery occlusion.

Renal artery occlusion should be suspected in patients with abrupt onset of flank pain and oliguric, progressive deterioration of renal function. Examination of the urine reveals hematuria and cellular casts. The diagnosis can be confirmed by renal scan, IV pyelography, or renal arteriography, which demonstrate the absence of flow. Once renal artery occlusion is documented, vascular reconstruction should be promptly done if clinically feasible.

2. CHOLESTEROL EMBOLI

Cholesterol emboli can cause progressive deterioration of renal function. Cholesterol emboli are seen in 3 clinical settings: (1) abdominal aortography and angiography performed with catheters passing through the abdominal aorta can result in embolization; (2) resection of an abdominal aortic aneurysm, manipulation of the abdominal aorta during vascular surgery, repair of a thoracic aneurysm, and aortic valve replacement have been associated with cholesterol embolization; and (3) severe ulcerated atherosclerotic disease of the aorta can result in spontaneous cholesterol emboli.

Patients with cholesterol emboli usually have nonoliguric renal failure, although oliguric renal failure can occur in patients with severe disease. Deterioration of renal function begins immediately after the injury and is usually slow. Renal function may gradually improve; however, renal deterioration progressing to end–stage renal disease may occur. The diagnosis should be suspected in patients with nonspecific GI symptoms, anorexia, nausea, vomiting, crampy abdominal pain, and diarrhea. There are often cutaneous signs of cholesterol emboli, particularly in the toes and in the soles of the feet. Some may have evidence of pancreatitis or rhabdomyolysis. Examination of the urine shows red cells, white cells, white cell casts, and eosinophils. Peripheral eosinophilia has been reported. No specific therapy is available.

G. Hepatorenal Syndrome

1. CLINICAL COURSE

The hepatorenal syndrome consists of progressive failure of renal function of unknown etiology in patients with severe liver disease. Factors associated with the precipitation of hepatorenal syndrome include excessive use of diuretics, paracentesis, infection, and GI hemorrhage. Hepatorenal syndrome carries an extremely poor prognosis, with a reported survival rate of less than 5%. Patients experience oliguric renal failure with slow, progressive renal deterioration. Despite compromises in renal function, these patients usually die of complications from hepatic insufficiency; GI bleeding and infection are the most common causes of death. The urinary sediment is normal in these patients despite progressive renal deterioration. The urinary sodium concentration is invariably less than 10 mEq/L, and the fractional excretion of sodium is usally less than 1%. The urinary osmolality is usually only slightly above the serum osmolality. The diagnosis of hepatorenal syndrome has to be one of exclusion, and care should be taken to rule out prerenal azotemia.

2. MANAGEMENT

Therapy for the hepatorenal syndrome has been unsatisfactory. Numerous pharmacologic agents have proved unsuccessful in reversing the functional abnormalities in the syndrome. In certain instances, several surgical procedures, such as orthotopic liver transplantation, have been reported to be successful in reversal of the hepatorenal syndrome. Peritoneojugular shunts (LeVeen's shunts) also have been beneficial in some cases. Dialysis and hemoperfusion have been employed; but, in general, these have merely delayed the inevitable outcome.

Coggins CH, Fang LSF: Acute renal failure associated with antibiotic, anesthetic agents and radiographic contrast agents. *In* Brenner BM, Lazarus JM (eds): Acute Renal Failure. 2nd ed. New York, Churchill Livingstone, 1988, pp 295–352.

Knochel JP: Rhabdomyolysis. West J Med 125:312, 1976.

Madias NE, Donohue JF, Harrington JT: Postischemic acute renal failure. *In* Brenner BM, Lazarus JM (eds): Acute Renal Failure. 2nd ed. New York, Churchill Livingstone, 1988, pp 251–278.

Papper S: Hepatorenal syndrome. Contrib Nephrol 23:55, 1980.

III. MANAGEMENT OF PATIENTS WITH CHRONIC RENAL FAILURE (CRF)

The goal of managing the patient with CRF is to optimize the clinical and metabolic status by conservative measures. When these measures fail, dialysis and transplantation should be considered.

A. Management of Fluid Balance. In patients with moderate renal insufficiency there is loss in concentrating ability, and they develop polyuria and polydipsia. They depend on adequate intake for excretion of the solute load, and thus they should not have fluid restriction. Fluid restriction can result in intravascular volume depletion, decreased renal perfusion, and worsening of renal function. For these reasons, diuretics should be used judiciously. With severe renal insufficiency, patients may be oliguric and have symptoms of fluid overload. Fluid restriction and diuretics may be necessary in these patients.

B. Management of Sodium Balance. In some instances, patients with a moderate degree of renal dysfunction may have salt-losing nephropathy. These patients should be encouraged to take in salt, and sodium replacement may be required under certain circumstances. In most patients with CRF, however, there is difficulty in excreting salt, and they have problems with sodium overload. In these patients, salt restriction and diuretics may be necessary.

C. **Management of Potassium Balance.** Hyperkalemia is the most important electrolyte abnormality to correct in patients with CRF. Rare patients may have potassium-losing nephropathy, and their hypokalemia can be treated with cautious potassium replacement.

D. **Management of Calcium and Phosphate Balances.** Hyperphosphatemia should be corrected first with the use of phosphate binders, such as Amphojel, Basaljel, Dialume, or Alu-Cap (starting at 30 mL tid). Recently, calcium carbonate has been used to optimize calcium and phosphate balance and has been shown to be an effective phosphate binder. Calcium carbonate is now the preferred long-term phosphate binding agent because it avoids aluminum overload. Phosphate binders should be given shortly before meals to optimize phosphate binding. When the serum phosphate level is less than 5 mg/dL, the hypocalcemia should be corrected with calcium supplements and vitamin D preparations. A reasonable starting dose of calcium carbonate is 500 mg po tid. Dihydrotachysterol can be given in doses ranging from 0.1–0.4 mg/day, and 1,25-dihydroxycholecalciferol (Rocaltrol) can be given in doses of 0.25–0.50 μg/day.

E. **Management of Acidosis.** Metabolic acidosis should be managed with sodium bicarbonate, starting at 600 mg po tid. The doses of bicarbonate should be increased until the serum bicarbonate level is between 16 and 20 mEq/L. Hypertension or CHF may limit the ability to use sodium bicarbonate.

F. **Management of Nitrogen Balance.** Restriction to 0.5 gm of protein/kg/day usually allows sufficient amounts for daily requirements while reducing increases in azotemia. With use of a diet high in essential amino acids, some investigators have been able to restrict protein intake to 0.3 gm/kg/day. Alpha-keto analogues of essential amino acids have been shown to spare nitrogen even more than essential amino acids do, but they are costly and unpalatable. In all instances, it is important to maintain adequate caloric intake to prevent catabolism and muscle breakdown (30–50 Kcal/kg/day, more in critically ill patients).

G. **Management of Hematologic Abnormalities.** Anemia can be managed by replacement of iron and folate in patients shown to have deficiencies. Blood drawing should be minimized. Drugs that can cause hemolysis should be avoided, since a defect in the hexose monophosphate shunt function can be demonstrated in 10–25% of uremic patients. *Erythropoietin* appears to be the solution in the future and is effective for many patients when given 3 times per week. Transfusions may be necessary for patients with severe and symptomatic anemia. Patients with CRF have abnormal results on platelet function tests and prolonged bleeding time. Antiplatelet drugs, such as aspirin and dipyridamole (Persantine), should be avoided. In patients with clinically evident bleeding, cryoprecipitate (10 units) and DDAVP (0.4 μg/kg) can be given IV to reverse platelet function abnormalities. Premarin has also been shown to be effective in correcting bleeding time. However, the effect of Premarin usually is apparent only after 3–7 days of therapy.

H. Management of Renal Osteodystrophy. Persistent hypocalcemia can result in secondary hyperparathyroidism, which leads to bone demineralization. Attention has been increasingly directed at the role of aluminum in the bone disease associated with chronic renal insufficiency. The difficulty is in part related to excessive ingestion of aluminum products and in part to decreased aluminum clearance. It is therefore important to use aluminum hydroxide compounds judiciously to avoid problems with bone disease. In patients with mild hyperparathyroidism, vitamin D and calcium therapy may be beneficial in the suppression of parathyroid activity. These have to be used judiciously to avoid hypercalcemia. In addition to management of calcium and phosphate balances, aluminum excesses should be addressed. Deferoxamine therapy is useful in the removal of aluminum deposited in bone.

I. Management of Cutaneous Symptoms. Severe pruritus can cause significant morbidity in the patient with CRF. Itching may respond to menthol or phenol lotions applied locally and can be treated with antihistamines. Ultraviolet light is also helpful in some patients.

J. Management of Cardiovascular Complications. Patients with CRF can develop CHF, coronary ischemia, and uremic pericarditis. CHF can be managed with fluid and sodium restriction and cautious use of loop diuretics. Transfusions may be required in anemic patients with coronary ischemia. In patients with uremic pericarditis, dialysis should be considered. Instillation of nonabsorbable steroids such as triamcinolone, 100 mg given intrapericardially via a pericardial catheter every 6 hours, appears to be effective in preventing recurrence of pericardial effusions. In patients with recurrent and refractory pericardial effusions, pericardiectomy may be necessary.

K. Management of Hypertension. It is important to control hypertension in the patient with CRF to avoid further renal damage. However, it is equally important not to overtreat and cause renal hypoperfusion. Since volume overload is present in many patients, a diuretic is a reasonable first-line drug to use. Many diuretics are ineffective in patients with severe renal failure. Others are associated with possible hyperkalemia and should be avoided. Some commonly used diuretics include furosemide, bumetanide, ethacrynic acid, and metolazone. Converting enzyme inhibitors and calcium channel blockers are acceptable drugs to use. In both instances, renal function should be monitored carefully, since there is a chance of acute renal function deterioration with these drugs in patients with preexisting renal insufficiency. Beta blockers, particularly in combination with vasodilators, are often effective. Calcium channel blockers such as nifedipine, diltiazem, and verapamil are all reasonably effective. Vasodilators, including hydralazine, prazosin, and minoxidil, are also effective in CRF. Other drugs that can be used include methyldopa, clonidine, reserpine, and guanethidine.

L. Management of Drug Therapy. Drugs that are potentially nephrotoxic should be avoided, and drugs that are excreted renally must be adjusted. Conservative management is directed toward prolongation of a symptom-free period. When conservative therapy becomes ineffective, dialysis or transplantation must be considered.

IV. HEMODIALYSIS

With progressive deterioration, renal performance may be so compromised that mechanical assistance becomes necessary. Hemodialysis is useful in patients with ARF or CRF. The procedure involves the passage of blood across a semipermeable membrane. On the other side of the membrane is a specially prepared dialysate designed to correct the metabolic derangements commonly associated with renal failure. The dialysate is usually made hypertonic with the addition of glucose, which allows correction of fluid overload. Acidosis is corrected by the use of bicarbonate or acetate in the dialysate. Calcium is added for correction of hypocalcemia, and the potassium content of the dialysate can be adjusted for correction of hyperkalemia. Nitrogenous wastes are removed along a concentration gradient.

For hemodialysis to be effective, a vascular access is required that permits a rate of blood flow of 200 to 300 mL/minute into the dialyzer. In addition, an anticoagulant is needed to avert clotting in the dialyzer.

A. **Indications and Contraindications for Hemodialysis.** Uremic symptoms (particularly changes in mental status), refractory volume overload, bleeding secondary to uremic effects on platelet adhesiveness, uremic pericarditis in a patient with progressive renal insufficiency, hyperkalemia or acidosis refractory to conservative measures, and life-threatening overdose of a dialyzable toxin are the most common indications for dialysis. Progressive uremic neuropathy, progressive malnutrition and physical deterioration, and emotional considerations may also lead one to initiate dialysis.

The major contraindications to hemodialysis include concern over the risk of heparinization, hemodynamic instability, and other systemic illnesses with grave prognoses that may preclude the initiation of hemodialysis. Patients with active GI bleeding, intracranial hemorrhage, subdural hematoma, hypotension, and unstable angina should be considered for other methods of dialysis.

B. **Medical Therapy for Patients on Hemodialysis.** Most patients require 4–5 hours of hemodialysis 3 times weekly. Other measures are necessary to avoid significant metabolic derangements. Patients are usually restricted to 60–80 gm of protein intake each day. Salt and potassium intake is also restricted, usually to 2 gm/day each. Fluid restriction may be necessary to avoid overload. Phosphate binders are generally needed to prevent hyperphosphatemia. Vitamin D or analogues and calcium supplements may be necessary to correct hypocalcemia and to prevent renal osteodystrophy. Water-soluble vitamins and folic acid are dialyzable and need to be supplemented.

C. **Complications of Hemodialysis.**

1. MECHANICAL COMPLICATIONS
   In rare instances, leaking of blood from the dialyzer or from the lines can create substantial blood loss. Dialyzers can clot because of

inadequate heparinization. Rarely, air entering the dialyzer or lines can cause air embolism.

2. COMPLICATIONS RELATED TO VASCULAR ACCESSES

Arteriovenous shunts are prone to infection, clotting, bleeding, and erosion of skin around the insertion sites of the shunts. Arteriovenous fistulas are less prone to infections than shunts, but they may fail to mature adequately for dialysis. The fistulas are also prone to thrombosis or stenosis and may create problems with ischemia of an extremity secondary to a steal syndrome. On occasion, aneurysms can develop, particularly at the sites of repeated punctures. An arteriovenous fistula may also result in high-output failure in susceptible patients. Subclavian or internal jugular catheters are used for temporary access to the bloodstream. These are prone to infections and clotting and should not be expected to be functional for more than 6–8 weeks.

3. HEMODYNAMIC COMPLICATIONS

The most common problem during hemodialysis is hypotension, due in part to excessive volume removal and in part to compromised cardiac contractility during the procedure, presumably resulting from the cardiosuppressant effect of the dialysate. During dialysis, angina, arrhythmia, and, rarely, cardiac tamponade can complicate the procedure.

4. PULMONARY COMPLICATIONS

During the initial 30–45 minutes of dialysis, transient hypoxemia is seen, caused partly by diffusion of CO_2 across the dialyzing membrane resulting in hypoventilation, and partly by microembolization of aggregates of white cells formed as a result of complement activation as the blood passes through the dialyzer. On rare occasions, air embolism can complicate dialysis.

5. NEUROLOGIC COMPLICATIONS

A dysequilibrium syndrome, with headache, nausea, vomiting, lethargy, and seizures, can complicate dialysis. This syndrome is of particular concern when there is rapid shifting of fluids and solute. The syndrome can be ameliorated by slower dialyses and by the use of the mannitol procedure. A more worrisome neurologic complication is dialysis dementia. Patients have intermittent symptoms of dysarthria, myoclonus, and apraxia. The symptoms subsequently become persistent, and the condition progressively deteriorates until patients are in a mute, vegetative state. Patients usually die within a year of diagnosis. The syndrome is thought to be related to aluminum excess, with deposition in the brain. With deionization of the water used in dialysis and more judicious use of phosphate binders, the syndrome is now uncommon. Deferoxamine and renal transplantation have been reported to be beneficial in anecdotal instances.

6. MUSCULAR COMPLICATIONS

Cramping can occur during dialysis, particularly with rapid fluid shifts, and can be treated with hypertonic saline infusion.

7. Metabolic Complications

Rapid fluid and electrolyte shifts and rapid correction of acidosis can create symptoms, particularly in a patient prone to arrhythmias. Hypercholesterolemia and hypertriglyceridemia are common in uremic patients undergoing dialysis. Hyperglycemia is occasionally seen.

8. Hematologic Complications

Patients with CRF who are undergoing dialysis are more prone to infectious complications because of compromised antibody production and compromised cellular immunity. Septicemia from vascular accesses and infections at skin sites, usually with gram-positive organisms, can be treated readily with vancomycin. Since the drug is excreted renally and is not dialyzable, 1 gm of vancomycin given at dialysis weekly would usually be adequate therapy. Patients undergoing hemodialysis, because of the increased transfusion requirement, are at higher risk for non-A, non-B hepatitis and for cytomegalovirus (CMV) and human immunodeficiency virus (HIV) infections.

Even with meticulous care and marked improvement in technical aspects, the annual mortality is estimated at 7–13%. Coronary artery disease and sepsis are the major causes of death. Hemodialysis can dramatically improve the well-being of the patient and prolong life, but the physician should be aware of its many possible complications.

V. ACUTE PERITONEAL DIALYSIS

Peritoneal dialysis can be used in the management of patients with ARF or CRF. In patients with ARF, a percutaneously placed peritoneal catheter is generally used. Peritoneal dialysis is preferred when the heparinization needed for hemodialysis is contraindicated. It is also preferred in patients with hemodynamic instability. Otherwise, the indications for initiation of peritoneal dialysis are the same as those for hemodialysis.

A. Percutaneous Placement of the Peritoneal Dialysis Catheter. The percutaneous placement of a peritoneal dialysis catheter is contraindicated in the patient with ileus, multiple adhesions secondary to previous surgery, or severe bleeding diatheses. In these instances, surgical placement of the catheter under direct visualization is preferred.

The patient should be able to lie flat for at least 20 minutes during the placement and should be asked to void immediately before the procedure to avoid perforation of the bladder. The abdomen should be carefully examined: Evidence of ileus and lower midabdominal surgical scars are relative contraindications to the placement of a catheter, since the likelihood of bowel perforation is increased in these instances. The lower abdomen should be percussed to be sure that the bladder is empty. If the bladder is full and the patient cannot empty the bladder voluntarily, a Foley catheter should be inserted prior to placement of a peritoneal catheter.

For placement of the peritoneal dialysis catheter, the patient should be supine; the lower abdominal wall should be cleaned with iodine and alcohol solutions, and a sterile field should be created. A point about midway between the umbilicus and the suprapubic notch in the midline is usually the ideal site for placement of the catheter. If lower midabdominal scars necessitate selection of a different site, either the right or the left lower quadrant may be used instead.

The skin should be anesthetized with 1 or 2% lidocaine and a small incision made with a number 11 blade. The stylet is placed in the catheter, and the pointed tip of the stylet should be exposed at the end of the catheter. The stylet should be grasped firmly with one hand, and the end of the catheter is held with the thumb and index finger of the other hand. The catheter is inserted into the peritoneal cavity through the small previously made incision in the skin, using firm pressure and a twisting motion. As soon as the catheter penetrates the peritoneal cavity, the stylet is withdrawn about 1 inch so that the pointed tip of the stylet is now sheathed within the soft catheter. The catheter should now be advanced gradually into either the right or the left lower gutter of the pelvic space. When the catheter is in the desired position, the retaining device can be slid over the catheter until it rests against the abdominal wall. The extension set with the L-shaped connector is attached and connected to the tubings from the dialysate bag. Dialysate solution is infused to assess the adequacy of flow through the catheter. The dialysate solution should flow in and out of the peritoneal cavity in a steady, pencil-sized stream. The catheter should be repositioned if either the inflow or the outflow of the dialysate solution is inadequate. The catheter can be sutured to the abdominal wall with 3-0 or 4-0 silk sutures to prevent accidental dislodging.

B. Care of the Peritoneal Dialysis Catheter. The site of insertion of the peritoneal catheter should be treated with aseptic techniques at all times to avoid infection. Abdominal dressings should be changed daily. The tubings used to administer the dialysate should be changed every 72 hours to minimize the possibility of peritonitis.

C. Dialysis Exchanges. Commercially available dialysate solutions are generally used. Available solutions include 1.50, 2.50, and 4.25% solutions. The more hypertonic solution should be used in the patient with fluid overload. Potassium must be added to the dialysate, because most dialysates are potassium free. Small amounts of heparin (250–500 U) may be added to the dialysate to minimize fibrin deposition and clotting of the catheter. The dialysate should be warmed to body temperature and should be infused into the peritoneal cavity over a 10-minute period. The dialysate is then allowed to remain in the peritoneal cavity for varying periods (at least 20 minutes) to allow for exchange. The dialysate is permitted to drain until dry over a 30-minute period. Intake and output should be carefully monitored hourly, and blood chemistry studies, including determination of potassium, BUN, creatinine, and glucose levels, should be performed every 8 hours. The dialysate should be examined and cultured periodically.

D. Complications of Peritoneal Dialysis. Bleeding is a rare complication of peritoneal dialysis. The dialysate may be slightly blood tinged during the first few exchanges. Bleeding is usually from small veins lining the peritoneal cavity, and the bleeding should decrease after the first few exchanges. If it persists, the dialysis catheter should be removed and replaced. Another rare complication of the percutaneously placed catheter is **perforation of a viscus.** This can be avoided if surgical placement is used in the presence of ileus or adhesions from prior lower abdominal surgery. If a viscus is perforated, the catheter should be left in place, and surgical exploration for repair of the viscus should be undertaken as soon as possible. The most common problem with peritoneal dialysis is **fluid drainage.** If difficulties occur with either the infusion or the drainage of dialysis solutions, the patient should be placed in a different body position to determine if the flow can be improved. In general, poor drainage is due to trapping of the catheter in the mesentery, and changing body position can improve flow. If problems with adequate flow persist, the catheter can be flushed with about 50 ml of heparinized saline to dislodge possible fibrin clots from the end of the catheter. If dialysate flow is still inadequate, the catheter should be removed and replaced. No attempt should be made to reposition the dialysis catheter, except at the time of the initial placement, since this procedure markedly increases the possibility of peritonitis. **Leakage** may occur around the insertion site. Small amounts of drainage can be managed with more frequent dressing changes. At times it may be possible to decrease the amount of leakage by placement of a pursestring suture at the skin. With leakage, the likelihood of wound infection and peritonitis is markedly increased. If leakage is not stopped by a pursestring suture, the dialysis catheter should be removed and replaced. During peritoneal dialysis, the **fluid and electrolyte balance** should be monitored closely. It is important to assess the blood glucose level frequently, particularly if the 4.25% dialysate is used. In general, avoid using 4.25% dialysate solely, but instead alternate 4.25% with 2.50% dialysate in patients with fluid overload.

TABLE 6–10. ANTIBIOTICS USED INTRAPERITONEALLY FOR TREATMENT OF PERITONITIS

ANTIBIOTICS	DOSE (MG) ADDED TO EACH 2-L DIALYSATE BAG
Penicillins	
Ampicillin	100
Methicillin	100
Carbenicillin	400
Cephalosporin	
Cephapirin (Cefadyl)	200
Aminoglycosides	
Gentamicin	8–10
Tobramycin	8–10
Clindamycin	20
Vancomycin*	30
Amphotericin*	4

*May cause some peritoneal irritation.

The major problem with peritoneal dialysis is **peritonitis.** The dialysate should be monitored periodically (every other day) in patients undergoing acute peritoneal dialysis. The dialysate should be closely examined, and cultures should be done whenever patients show clinical signs of peritonitis or if the dialysate is cloudy. The presence of significant numbers of white cells, of organisms detected under microscopic examination, or of bacterial growth mandates treatment with antibiotics. The most common pathogen in dialysis-related peritonitis is *Staphylococcus* (either *S. aureus* or *S. epidermidis*). Cephalosporins can be added to the dialysate for these infections, although *S. epidermidis* may be resistant to penicillins and cephalosporins. For peritonitis caused by gram-negative organisms, an antibiotic (e.g., gentamicin, tobramycin) can be used. The antibiotics and doses most commonly used are listed in Table 6–10. Persistent infection in the presence of appropriate therapy requires removal of the peritoneal dialysis catheter.

VI. CONTINUOUS AMBULATORY PERITONEAL DIALYSIS (CAPD)

To manage patients with chronic renal disease with CAPD, the catheters must be placed surgically, and patients should be instructed how to perform peritoneal dialysis on a continuous outpatient basis. The procedure first came into clinical use in the early 1970s and is gaining popularity because of the convenience and the ease with which it can be mastered.

A. **Patient Selection.** Because CAPD is designed for patients who can manage the exchanges themselves, it is important to select individuals who are motivated, have reasonable eyesight, and have good manual dexterity. Sometimes family members can be trained to perform the procedure.

B. **Placement of the Dialysis Catheter.** The catheter for long-term use should be placed surgically at least 2 weeks before the planned initiation of dialysis. A double-cuffed catheter is usually used, and the patient will need a period of catheter training. 500 mL of heparinized dialysate is infused into the peritoneal cavity and drained immediately every 6 hours for approximately a 72-hour period to minimize the likelihood of fibrin deposition in the catheter. The catheter should then be filled with heparinized solution and capped and not be used for the ensuing 2 weeks to ensure sealing of the peritoneum and the tunnel. Premature use of the peritoneal dialysis catheter usually results in leakage and the need for catheter replacement.

C. **Principles.** Since the peritoneal membrane is a rather ineffective exchange membrane, CAPD calls for the continuous use of the membrane to maximize clearances. The patient would usually do 4 exchanges a day. The dialysate is infused into the peritoneal cavity and is left there for 4–6 hours and drained at the next exchange. The drained dialysate is discarded, and a new dialysate bag is used for the new exchange. The last exchange of the day occurs at bedtime, and the dialysate is allowed to remain in the peritoneal cavity overnight. With the continuous process, excellent fluid, salt, and metabolic control can be achieved.

D. **Advantages.** Outpatient CAPD can be performed without the use of machines and thus allows for greater flexibility and mobility. Blood pressure control is usually excellent with CAPD because of the ease with which fluid and salt can be removed throughout the procedure. Therefore, fluid, salt, and potassium restriction may be less stringent for the patient using CAPD. Because there is continuous loss of protein throughout the dialyzing process, dietary protein restriction is also relaxed, and most patients are permitted an intake of 80 gm of protein each day. Uremia is ordinarily under adequate control, and anemia is usually less of a problem because of decreased blood loss. Since the procedure proceeds relatively slowly, patients are less likely to experience the dysequilibrium syndrome.

E. **Complications.** The major problem with CAPD is peritonitis. Patients are taught to monitor the fluid carefully, to obtain fluid for analysis and cultures, and to begin antibiotics on an empiric basis with an intraperitoneal infusion of cephalosporin if they have signs of peritonitis or if a cloudy dialysate is seen. If infection is confirmed, the intraperitoneal administration of antibiotic is continued for 14 days. Follow-up cultures are done a week after the termination of therapy to ensure clearance of the infection. If infection is persistent despite adequate therapy, the peritoneal catheter should be removed. Hemodialysis for a short period is necessary before another peritoneal catheter can be placed. Removal of the catheter is particularly important in patients with fungal peritonitis, since the infection is rarely cleared without catheter replacement. Excessive weight gain can be a problem because of the continuous glucose infusion. Glucose intolerance can also result. Patients also often have hypercholesterolemia and hypertriglyceridemia.

Eschbach JW, Ergic JC, Downing MR, et al: Correction of the anemia of end-stage renal disease with recombinant human erythropoietin: Results of a combined phase I and II clinical trial. N Engl J Med 316:73, 1987.

Fine LG: The uremic syndrome: Adaptive mechanisms and therapy. Hosp Pract 22:63, 1987.

Friedman EA: Outcome and complications of hemodialysis. *In* Schrier RW, Gottschalk CW (eds): Diseases of the Kidney. 4th ed. Boston, Little, Brown, 1988, pp 3323–3346.

Mion CM: Chronic ambulatory peritoneal dialysis (CAPD) and chronic cycling peritoneal dialysis. *In* Schrier RW, Gottschalk CW (eds): Diseases of the Kidney. 4th ed. Boston, Little, Brown, 1988, pp 3235–3280.

VII. DRUG THERAPY IN PATIENTS WITH RENAL INSUFFICIENCY

One of the most important aspects of patient care with either acute or chronic renal insufficiency is the appropriate management of drug therapy, including avoiding certain drugs (Table 6–11). Drugs and drug metabolites may accumulate in these patients, causing toxicity. In renal insufficiency, drug binding may be altered either because of decreased protein available for binding (particularly in patients with the nephrotic syndrome) or because of displacement of the drug from binding sites by uremic toxins. Although a variety of nomograms have

TABLE 6–11. DRUGS TO AVOID IN RENAL INSUFFICIENCY

DRUG	REASON FOR AVOIDING DRUG
Antibiotics	
Tetracycline	Antianabolic and may raise BUN; may potentiate acidosis; nephrotoxic
Nitrofurantoin	Accumulates in renal insufficiency; ineffective for UTI;* peripheral neuropathy
Methenamine mandelate	Ineffective for UTI
Nalidixic acid	Metabolic acidosis
Cardiovascular agents	
Acetazolamide	Potentiates metabolic acidosis; ineffective in renal failure
Mercurials	Accumulates in renal insufficiency; nephrotoxic
Spironolactone	Hyperkalemia
Triamterene	Hyperkalemia
Amiloride	Hyperkalemia
Analgesics and narcotics	
Aspirin	Antiplatelet effect
	Gastrointestinal irritation
Nonsteroidal anti-inflammatory drugs	Antiplatelet effect; gastrointestinal irritation; nephrotoxic
Phenazopyridine	Ineffective in renal failure
Sedatives, hypnotics, and tranquilizers	
Lithium carbonate	Nephrogenic diabetes insipidus; lithium toxicity
	Possible nephrotoxicity
Antineoplastic agents	
Cis-platinum	Nephrotoxic
Miscellaneous agents	
Phenylbutazone	Gastrointestinal irritation; nephrotoxic
Gold	Accumulates in renal insufficiency
	Nephrotoxic
Magnesium compounds	Accumulates in renal insufficiency; CNS side effects
Aminosalicylic acid	Potentiates acidosis; GI irritation

*Urinary tract infection.

been constructed for the commonly used drugs, only careful monitoring of drug levels permits dose adjustments to ensure therapeutic levels. Sometimes drug levels may have to be reinterpreted. For example, the therapeutic level of phenytoin is between 4 and 8 µg/dL in patients with advanced renal insufficiency because of enhanced metabolic rate, compared with 10–20 µg/dL in patients with normal renal function. In patients undergoing hemodialysis or peritoneal dialysis, it is important to know whether a drug is cleared by dialysis to be able to adjust doses.

A. Drugs That Require Dose Adjustment. Drugs (or their metabolites) that are renally excreted require dose adjustment (Table 6–12). In most instances, the loading dose of medication does not need to be altered

TABLE 6-12. DRUGS REQUIRING DOSE ADJUSTMENT IN RENAL FAILURE

DRUG	ADJUSTMENT FACTOR	DRUG	ADJUSTMENT FACTOR
Antimicrobial Agents		**Cardiovascular Agents**	
Penicillins		Antiarrhythmics	
Penicillin G	2	Procainamide	4
Ampicillin, amoxicillin	2	Disopyramide	4
Carbenicillin, ticarcillin	2	Flecainide	4
Methicillin	2	Encainide	4
Imipenem	2	Mexilitene	2
Aminoglycosides		Antihypertensive agents	
Gentamicin, tobramycin	4–6	Methyldopa	2
Kanamycin, amikacin	4–6	Guanethidine	2
Streptomycin	4–8	Cardiac glycosides	
Cephalosporins		Digoxin	3–4
Cephalexin, cephalothin, cefazolin, cephapirin	1–2	Digitoxin	1.5–2.0
Cephradine	4	**Analgesics and Narcotics**	
Cefamandole, cefoxitin	1–2	Acetaminophen	2
Cefuroxime	1–2	Meperidine	2
Cefotaxime	1–2	Methadone	2
Ceftriaxone	1–2	**Sedatives, Hypnotics, and Tranquilizers**	
Ceftazadime	1–2	Phenobarbital	2
Sulfonamides		Meprobamate	2
Sulfisoxazole	2	**Antineoplastic and Immunosuppressive Agents**	
Trimethoprim-sulfamethoxazole	2	Bleomycin	2
Minocycline	2	Cyclophosphamide	2
Antifungal agents		**Miscellaneous**	
Amphotericin	1.5	Hypoglycemic agents	
5-Flucytosine	4–8	Insulin	2
Fluconazole	1–2	Acetohexamide	2
Antituberculous drugs		Chlorpropamide	2
Ethambutol	2	Glyburide	2
Others		Others	
Vancomycin	10	Cimetidine	2
Metronidazole	3	Ranitidine	2
Pentamidine	2	Propylthiouracil	2
		Clofibrate	4
		Neostigmine	2

even in severe renal failure. Subsequent doses for maintenance therapy require adjustments. Coggins, Bennett, and Singer advocate the use of an **adjustment factor** in severe renal insufficiency (creatinine clearance of less than 20 mL/minute). The adjustment factor can be used either to reduce the dose of medication administered or to increase the intervals between doses. For example, tobramycin has an adjustment factor of 4: In a patient with severe renal failure, the dose of tobramycin can be reduced by a factor of 4 given at normal intervals; alternatively, the patient can be given a normal dose of tobramycin at a dose interval that has been increased by a factor of 4 (i.e., given at 32-hour intervals instead of 8-hour intervals). The adjustment factor applies to patients with severe renal insufficiency. Patients with moderate or mild renal insufficiency should have intermediate dose adjustments. It should be stressed that the *exact doses should be governed by clinical responses and serum levels and not rigidly by these approximations.*

B. **Drugs That Do Not Require Dose Adjustment.** Some drugs can be used in patients with renal insufficiency without dose adjustment (Table 6–13). These drugs are not excreted renally and do not aggravate uremic symptoms. Consequently, whenever feasible, these drugs are preferred to drugs that require dose adjustments.

C. **Drugs That Are Dialyzable by Peritoneal Dialysis.** Drugs that can be dialyzed by peritoneal dialysis are listed in Table 6–14. The list is partial because the dialyzability of many drugs has not been investigated. Patients who are receiving peritoneal dialysis should have these medications adjusted. Patients with severe overdoses of these medications can be treated with peritoneal dialysis. The clinical responses and the serum levels of these drugs should be monitored closely to ensure therapeutic levels.

D. **Drugs That Are Dialyzable by Hemodialysis.** Drugs that can be dialyzed by hemodialysis are listed in Table 6–15. The list is partial because the dialyzability of many drugs has not been investigated. In general, patients receiving hemodialysis who require these medications should have supplementation of them at the completion of dialysis. Patients with severe overdoses of these medications can benefit from hemodialysis.

Anderson RD: Drug prescribing for patients in renal failure. Hosp Pract 18:145, 1983.
Bennett WM, Aronoff GR, Morrison G, et al: Drug prescribing in renal failure: Dosing guidelines for adults. Am J Kidney Dis 3:155, 1983.
Bennett WM, Blythe WB: Use of drugs in patients with renal failure. *In* Schrier RW, Gottschalk CW (eds): Diseases of the Kidney. 4th ed. Boston, Little, Brown, 1988, pp 3437–3506.

VIII. NEPHROLITHIASIS

The incidence of nephrolithiasis appears to be increasing, and recent studies have estimated that 10–25% of the population may have symptomatic nephrolithiasis. Most stones (over 60%) contain calcium. Magnesium ammonium phosphate stones account for 15%. Uric acid, cystine, and other stones are less frequent (Table 6–16). Physicochemical factors increasing urinary concentration of stone constituents are

TABLE 6–13. DRUGS NOT REQUIRING DOSE ADJUSTMENT IN RENAL INSUFFICIENCY

ANTIMICROBIAL AGENTS
Penicillins
 Cloxacillin, dicloxacillin
 Nafcillin
 Oxacillin
Chloramphenicol
Clindamycin
Erythromycin
Chloroquine
Antituberculous drugs
 Isoniazid
 Rifampin

CARDIOVASCULAR AGENTS
Antiarrhythmics
 Lidocaine
 Propranolol
 Quinidine
Antihypertensive agents
 Clonidine
 Captopril and enalapril
 Lisinopril
 Diazoxide
 Diltiazem, nifedipine, verapamil
 Hydralazine and prazosin
 Minoxidil
 Nitroprusside
 Reserpine
Diuretics
 Bumetanide, ethacrynic acid,
  furosemide
 Thiazides
 Metolazone
Anticoagulants
 Heparin
 Warfarin

ANALGESICS AND NARCOTICS
Codeine
Morphine
Naloxone
Pentazocine
Propoxyphene

SEDATIVES, HYPNOTICS, AND TRANQUILIZERS
Barbiturates
 Phenobarbital
 Secobarbital
Benzodiazepines
 Chlordiazepoxide
 Diazepam
 Flurazepam
 Triazolam
Tricyclic antidepressants
 Amitriptyline
 Desipramine
 Imipramine
 Nortriptyline
Fluoxetine
Haloperidol
Glutethimide
Ethchlorvynol
Methaqualone

ANTINEOPLASTIC AND IMMUNOSUPPRESSIVE AGENTS
Adriamycin
Azathioprine
Cytosine arabinoside
5-Fluorouracil
Methotrexate
Vincristine

MISCELLANEOUS
Steroids
Tolbutamide
Theophylline
Tubocurarine
Succinylcholine

TABLE 6–14. DRUGS CLEARED BY PERITONEAL DIALYSIS

ANTIMICROBIAL AGENTS
Penicillin
  Ticarcillin
Imipenem
Cephalosporins
  Cephalexin
  Cephalothin
  Cephradine
  Ceftriaxone
  Cefuroxime
  Cefotaxime
  Ceftazadime
  Cefoxitin
  Cefamandole
Aminoglycosides
Sulfonamides
  Sulfisoxazole
  Trimethoprim-sulfamethoxazole
Antifungal agents
  Flucytosine
Antituberculous drugs
  Ethambutol
  Isoniazid

CARDIOVASCULAR AGENTS
Antiarrhythmics
  Quinidine
  Procainamide
Antihypertensive agents
  Methyldopa
  Diazoxide
  Nitroprusside
SEDATIVES, HYPNOTICS, AND TRANQUILIZERS
  Phenobarbital
  Ethchlorvynol
  Lithium carbonate
  Meprobamate
MISCELLANEOUS
  Phenytoin

thought to be the cause of stone formation. An acidic pH favors the formation of uric acid, cystine, and xanthine stones. An alkaline pH favors the formation of magnesium ammonium phosphate stones (struvite).

Increased urinary excretion of calcium or oxalate can enhance stone formation in a number of instances. Increased calcium excretion can occur in patients with hyperparathyroidism, vitamin D excess, excessive dietary calcium intake, or idiopathic hypercalciuria. Increased excretion of urinary oxalate can be observed in patients with primary hyperoxaluria or enteric hyperoxaluria. Increased uric acid excretion can result from either greater uric acid production or greater renal uric acid excretion. Cystine stones are formed exclusively in patients with an inherited disorder involving abnormal intestinal and renal transport of cystine, ornithine, lysine, and arginine. Xanthine stones are usually seen in patients with a genetic deficiency of xanthine oxidase, resulting in abnormalities in purine metabolism. Rarely, patients taking xanthine oxidase inhibitors for the treatment of uric acid disorders have xanthine stones.

Patients with distal renal tubular acidosis have increased urinary concentration of calcium and phosphate and are prone to stone formation. Infection in the upper tract with urea-splitting organisms can result in persistently alkaline urine, potentiating formation of magnesium ammonium phosphate stones. A number of substances appear to inhibit stone formation, and these include magnesium,

TABLE 6–15. DRUGS CLEARED BY HEMODIALYSIS

ANTIMICROBIAL AGENTS
Pencillins
  Penicillin G
  Ampicillin, amoxicillin
  Carbenicillin, ticarcillin
Imipenem
Cephalosporins
  Cephalexin
  Cephalothin
  Cefazolin
  Cephapirin
  Cefoxitin
  Cefotaxime
  Ceftazadime
  Cefamandole
  Cefuroxime
  Ceftriaxone
  Cephradine
Aminoglycosides
Sulfonamides
  Sulfisoxazole
  Trimethoprim-sulfamethoxazole
Chloramphenicol
Antifungal drugs
  Flucytosine
Antituberculous drugs
  Isoniazid
  Ethambutol
Metronidazole
Quinine

CARDIOVASCULAR AGENTS
Antiarrhythmics
  Procainamide
  Quinidine
Antihypertensive agents
  Methyldopa
  Diazoxide
  Nitroprusside
ANALGESICS AND NARCOTICS
Acetaminophen
Pentazocine
SEDATIVES, HYPNOTICS, AND TRANQUILIZERS
Lithium carbonate
Meprobamate
Methaqualone
Phenobarbital
Ethchlorvynol
ANTINEOPLASTIC AND IMMUNOSUPPRESSIVE AGENTS
Azathioprine
Cyclophosphamide
5-Fluorouracil
MISCELLANEOUS
Primidone

citrate, pyrophosphate, and certain protein peptides. Other factors appear to potentiate stone formation; these include much protein matrix and scar tissue in the kidney.

A. **General Treatment Principles.** In general, in a patient with acute renal colic, relief should come with generous use of analgesics. Fluids should be forced to ensure diuresis over the entire 24-hour period. If possible, patients can be managed on an outpatient basis. Patients in severe pain and those who are unable to maintain adequate oral intake because of

TABLE 6–16. INCIDENCE OF DIFFERENT TYPES OF STONES

Calcium stones	
Calcium oxalate	33%
Calcium oxalate and phosphate	34%
Calcium phosphate	6%
Magnesium ammonium phosphate	15%
Uric acid	8%
Cystine	2%
Others	1%

vomiting may need to be hospitalized for IV hydration and analgesia. Stone passage may take hours to weeks. The patient should be given a strainer and should attempt to retrieve the excreted stone. Knowledge of the stone composition may be critical for appropriate medical management. Surgical intervention should be considered only if conservative measures fail.

Patients with fever, chills, and symptoms of renal colic require hospitalization and prompt intervention. If the presence of an infection behind an obstructed ureter is indeed confirmed, antibiotic coverage and surgical decompression are mandatory.

24-hour urine collection should be done after the acute episode, at a time when the patient is back to his or her routine activity and diet. The urine should be sent to a laboratory for analysis of calcium, uric acid, and creatinine content.

B. Treatment for Specific Kinds of Stones

1. CALCIUM STONES

The dietary intake of calcium should be modestly restricted. Severe restriction may be counterproductive because of increases in urinary oxalate levels. **Hydrochlorothiazide** ([HCTZ] 50–100 mg/day), together with a mild degree of salt restriction, is useful, since thiazide inhibits distal tubular sodium reabsorption and causes a mild degree of volume contraction and enhanced proximal reabsorption of sodium, calcium, and uric acid. Prior to initiation of HCTZ therapy, it is important to rule out hyperparathyroidism as the cause of the hypercalciuria, since HCTZ can result in hypercalcemia. Although HCTZ can potentially lead to hypercalcemia in patients with absorptive hypercalciuria, this is not borne out clinically. **Allopurinol** is useful in some patients with calcium stones, since sodium hydrogen urate crystals may form heterogeneous nuclei for calcium oxalate crystal growth. Allopurinol is customarily used in dosages ranging from 100–300 mg/day and is particularly useful in patients demonstrated to have increased urinary uric acid excretion. **Orthophosphate** may be used, as either neutral or acidic sodium or potassium phosphate, in dosages of elemental phosphorus, 1.5–2.0 gm/day. Orthophosphate can cause significant GI side effects, and its dosage may have to be adjusted. **Cellulose phosphate** has been used to bind calcium in the GI tract. It is, however, bulky and expensive, and efficacy has not been established.

2. URIC ACID STONES

In patients known to form uric acid stones, an attempt should be made to alkalinize the urine, since uric acid has higher solubility in alkaline urine. Allopurinol, in dosages of 100–300 mg/day, should be prescribed for patients demonstrated to have recurrent uric acid stones.

3. STRUVITE (MAGNESIUM AMMONIUM PHOSPHATE)

Struvites are formed primarily in alkaline urine and are usually the result of upper urinary tract infections with a urea-splitting organism. It is therefore important to eradicate the infection. Since the majority of struvites are in the form of staghorn calculi, surgical intervention may be necessary to remove the stone.

4. CYSTINE STONES
A vigorous attempt should be made to alkalinize the urine with oral administration of sodium bicarbonate. Dosages of 2.4 gm tid may be necessary to accomplish the alkalinization. D-Penicillamine has been shown to be effective in selected patients.

5. XANTHINE STONES
The dietary intake of purines should be limited, and a vigorous attempt should be made to alkalinize the urine. In addition to these measures, several less well evaluated modes of therapy have been advocated. Administration of magnesium oxide may improve the solubility of urinary oxalate. It has been suggested that methylene blue is an effective inhibitor of calcium oxalate stone formation. In an uncontrolled study, the administration of potassium citrate, an inhibitor of calcium stone formation, was associated with a very low incidence of new stone formation.

In recent years, surgical intervention for nephrolithiasis has changed with the introduction of lithotripsy techniques. The stone is shattered by subjecting it to focused ultrasonic shock waves. Extracorporeal shock-wave lithotripsy is quickly becoming the treatment of choice for fragmentation and removal of simple stones in the kidney and upper ureters. Its low complication rate and high efficacy are rapidly eliminating the need for surgical lithotomy in centers where the lithotriptor is available.

American Urological Association: Report of American Urological Association Ad Hoc Committee to study the safety and clinical efficacy of current technology of percutaneous lithotripsy and non-invasive lithotripsy, May 16. 1985, pp 1–26.

Arnold EP: Advances in management of renal stones. NZ Med J 99:947, 1986.

Smith LH: Urolithiasis. *In* Schrier RW, Gottschalk CW (eds): Diseases of the Kidney. 4th ed. Boston, Little, Brown, 1988, pp 785–814.

IX. THE NEPHROTIC SYNDROME

Heavy proteinuria can lead to progressive decline in the serum albumin level, lower plasma oncotic pressure, and formation of edema. When more than 3.5 gm of protein are excreted in the urine each day and the serum albumin level falls to less than 3.0 gm/dL, the nephrotic syndrome is said to be present. The serum cholesterol level is often increased, and lipiduria is common. Heavy proteinuria leading to the nephrotic syndrome is usually the result of glomerular disease, but can occasionally occur with severe tubular diseases. Intrinsic glomerular diseases account for 75% of the conditions causing the nephrotic syndrome. Among these, membranous nephropathy and focal segmental sclerosis are the most common causes of the nephrotic syndrome in the adult. In children, the nephrotic syndrome is due to minimal-change disease more than 95% of the time. In the remaining 25% of adult

TABLE 6–17. CAUSES OF THE NEPHROTIC SYNDROME

GLOMERULAR DISEASES CAUSING NEPHROTIC SYNDROME
Membranous nephropathy
Focal glomerular sclerosis
Minimal-change disease
Focal and diffuse proliferative glomerulonephritis
Membranoproliferative glomerulonephritis
SYSTEMIC DISEASES CAUSING NEPHROTIC SYNDROME
Diabetes mellitus
Systemic lupus erythematosus
Amyloidosis
LESS COMMON CAUSES OF NEPHROTIC SYNDROME
Infection (subacute bacterial endocarditis, shunt infection, malaria, syphilis, hepatitis, schistosomiasis)
Toxins (heroin, mercury, gold, penicillamine, bismuth)
UNCOMMON CAUSES OF NEPHROTIC SYNDROME
Allergens (bee stings, serum sickness)
Mechanical causes: constrictive pericarditis, renal vein thrombosis, obstruction of the inferior vena cava)
Malignant disease (Hodgkin's disease, lymphoma, and other malignant diseases)
Pregnancy
Congenital disorders (Fabry's disease, nail-patella syndrome, Alport's syndrome)

cases, the nephrotic syndrome is associated with systemic illnesses that can produce glomerular pathology (Table 6–17). Among these illnesses, diabetes mellitus, SLE, and amyloidosis are the most commonly encountered disorders.

A. General Management Principles

1. **RENAL FUNCTION**
The major goal of managing the nephrotic syndrome is to keep the patient reasonably comfortable without compromising the renal function by excessive diuresis. A moderate amount of edema should be tolerated, and aggressive diuretic therapy should be reserved for those with symptomatic edema, particularly if skin breakdown or infection becomes a factor. Fluid and salt restriction should invariably be the first step in treating the patient with fluid retention and symptomatic edema. Fluid restriction to 1000 and 2000 mL is usually well tolerated. Sodium should be limited to 2 gm/day.

2. **DIET**
Because of the continuing losses of protein throughout the urinary tract, patients should be instructed to take in a diet rich in high-quality protein. Adequate caloric intake should be maintained to minimize catabolism. Protein should be limited when uremia accompanies the nephrotic syndrome.

3. **DIURETICS** should be used judiciously. Patients with hypoalbuminemia have intravascular contraction, and aggressive diuresis can accentuate prerenal azotemia by further contraction of the vascular space. In general, thiazides should be tried first, although they are

usually of marginal efficacy. A loop diuretic (furosemide, bumetanide, or ethacrynic acid) is usually necessary. The loop diuretic regimen can be gradually escalated to a three-times-a-day schedule. If diuresis is still suboptimal, metolazone, starting at 5 mg each day, can be added. The combination of a loop diuretic with metolazone is usually effective in promoting diuresis in patients with intractable edema.

B. Specific Therapy. Specific therapy is directed at the underlying glomerular lesion.

1. MINIMAL-CHANGE DISEASE IN ADULTS
Minimal-change disease in the adult is reasonably steroid sensitive, although the incidence of steroid resistance is much higher than that in children with minimal-change disease. Patients should be managed with fluid and salt restriction and a defined course of steroids (daily or alternate-day steroids). For symptomatic patients whose condition is refractory to steroid therapy, cytotoxic agents (cyclophosphamide) may be of help. Minimal-change disease in the adult, particularly the elderly, may be associated with a lymphoproliferative disorder, and the possibility of associated malignant disease should be evaluated in the elderly patient with the nephrotic syndrome.

2. FOCAL GLOMERULAR SCLEROSIS
Unfortunately, no therapeutic interventions have been proved effective in changing the clinical course of focal glomerular sclerosis. Management should therefore focus on conservative measures.

3. MEMBRANOUS DISEASE
Young males with high-grade proteinuria due to membranous disease appear to be most prone to renal function deterioration. These patients should be considered for aggressive therapy. A multicenter prospective randomized study suggests that alternate-day steroids in doses of 125 mg of prednisone every other day, are effective in minimizing renal difficulties in patients with membranous nephropathy. A more recent randomized prospective trial suggests that combinations of pulse doses of IV steroids and chlorambucil are effective in preventing renal function deterioration in patients with membranous nephropathy.

4. FOCAL AND DIFFUSE PROLIFERATIVE DISEASE
There are few studies examining the efficacy of therapy, but treatment with steroids and treatment with cyclophosphamide appear to be of help.

5. MEMBRANOPROLIFERATIVE GLOMERULONEPHRITIS
Few studies have been done on effectiveness of therapy in this condition, but steroid therapy and cyclophosphamide therapy seem to be of some benefit.

Cameron JS: The nephrotic syndrome and its complications. Am J Kidney Dis 10:157, 1987.
Glassock RJ: Clinical aspects of glomerular diseases. Am J Kidney Dis 10:181, 1987.

X. RENAL MANIFESTATIONS OF SYSTEMIC DISEASES

A number of systemic illnesses have significant renal manifestations, and careful attention to the renal issues is critical for successful management.

A. Diabetic Nephropathy

1. CLINICAL COURSE

50% of patients with juvenile-onset diabetes and 6–10% of patients with adult-onset diabetes eventually develop end-stage renal disease requiring dialysis or transplantation. Currently, 25% of all new uremic patients with end-stage renal disease have diabetic nephropathy. Patients with juvenile-onset diabetic nephropathy usually follow a predictable course. Careful measurements have revealed that early in the disease patients actually have increased glomerular filtration rate. Renal size is correspondingly increased. Urinalysis reveals no abnormal findings, with no proteinuria. About 10–12 years into the illness, intermittent proteinuria is noted, but the patient continues to have normal renal function. However, the presence of intermittent proteinuria identifies a group who will eventually develop significant renal disease. About 15–17 years after the onset of diabetes, patients may develop the nephrotic syndrome. The onset is often abrupt and is associated with a grave prognosis, with progression to end-stage renal disease usually within 2–5 years. With the onset of renal dysfunction, hypertension and CHF become significant problems, and retinopathy is often more difficult to control. Renal function classically deteriorates rapidly.

2. MANAGEMENT

Three maneuvers have been instituted early in the course of the disease in an attempt to decrease the rate of renal deterioration. Rigid **control of both blood sugar and blood pressure** has been shown to be of benefit. A number of studies are now examining the efficacy of **restricting dietary protein** in controlling the rate of declining renal function. In appropriate patients, such dietary restriction should be tried.

For the diabetic patient with end-stage renal disease, **hemodialysis, CAPD, renal transplantation,** and simultaneous transplantation of kidney and pancreas are all options. The outlook for diabetic patients receiving hemodialysis has improved substantially. However, mortality in diabetic patients receiving dialysis is still greater than that in the nondiabetic, although the gap is narrowing. Hemodialysis is associated with a first-year mortality of 15–30%. By the fifth year, the survival rate of patients is often down to 30–50% (Table 6–18). Morbidity is also high for diabetic patients on hemodialysis.

CAPD is a reasonable treatment for diabetics. Since heparinization is not necessary for the procedures and since hemodynamic fluctuations are less drastic than those in hemodialysis, retinopathy is less of a problem in patients undergoing CAPD. Similarly, the problems with construction of vascular accesses are obviated. Nonetheless,

TABLE 6–18. SURVIVAL OF DIABETIC PATIENTS RECEIVING HEMODIALYSIS

INVESTIGATOR	NO. PATIENTS	SURVIVAL (%)			
		1 yr	2 yr	3 yr	4 yr
Rothschild	17	85	66	—	—
Soricelli	25	—	62	—	—
Slifkin	97	78	65	55	50
Totten	27	—	75	—	—
Ma	18	85	85	—	—
Shapiro	198	70	50	45	30

cardiovascular and infectious complications continue to be significant in these patients. Peritonitis is of particular concern. The mortality figures are similar for hemodialysis and CAPD, with a mortality of 15–20%/year.

Transplantation, in the appropriate candidate, appears to be the most reasonable option for diabetics with end-stage renal disease (Table 6–19). Graft survival probably is similar to that in nondiabetic patients. The major cause of death after transplantation is MI, accounting for about 40% of deaths. Infectious complications account for 20–30%. Peripheral vascular disease remains a problem, but neuropathy and retinopathy are improved by transplantation. Vision is stabilized or improved in 75–80% of those with transplants. The rehabilitation potential is far superior to that associated with either hemodialysis or CAPD. In selected patients, the simultaneous transplantation of pancreas and kidneys has been attempted with reasonable success rates. The procedure is still considered experimental and should be reserved only for carefully selected patients. In general, a fistula should be constructed when the serum creatinine level in the diabetic patient has reached 4 mg/dL, and transplantation should be

TABLE 6–19. SURVIVAL OF DIABETIC PATIENTS RECEIVING TRANSPLANTATION

SERIES	NO. PATIENTS	SURVIVAL (%)			
		1 yr	2 yr	3 yr	4 yr
Living-related donors					
Minnesota	196				
HLA-identical		90	90	88	80
Non-HLA identical		85	75	68	60
Mayo Clinic	39	80	80	80	80
Scandinavian	25	85	85	66	65
Cadaveric donors					
Minnesota	109	75	70	60	60
Mayo Clinic	22	64	52	52	52
Scandinavian	121	60	50	40	35

planned. At a serum creatinine level of 6 mg/dL, transplantation should be considered, and patients without a living related donor should be placed on a cadaveric transplant list.

B. Systemic Lupus Erythematosus (SLE)

1. CLINICAL COURSE

Renal failure is the leading cause of death in patients with SLE. Clinical manifestations of renal disease are usually seen during the first 3 years after diagnosis. Such clinical evidence of renal involvement is observed in 60–75% of patients. If renal biopsy is performed, light microscopic examination of the biopsy specimen reveals changes in about 90% of patients, and electron microscopic examination demonstrates abnormalities in virtually 100%. The biopsy findings of renal involvement in an overwhelming majority of patients, as well as the discrepancy between the clinical and pathologic findings, complicate decisions with regard to the selection of appropriate candidates for biopsy and therapy. The clinical presentation and the prognosis differ, depending, in part, on the underlying pathology. Patients with mesangial proliferative and focal proliferative glomerulonephritis usually have a better prognosis than patients with diffuse proliferative glomerulonephritis. A small number of patients may have membranous glomerulonephritis or interstitial nephritis.

2. THERAPY

In general, therapy is reserved for patients with biopsy evidence of diffuse proliferative glomerulonephritis and for patients with either deterioration of renal function or an increase in the activity of urinary sediment. **Steroids** are often the first agents used for patients with lupus nephritis. Unfortunately, a prospective, randomized study comparing steroids with placebo is lacking. Uncontrolled, nonrandomized studies suggest that high-dose steroids are more beneficial than low-dose steroids. The recommended starting dosage is 60–100 mg/day, with tapering as the disease activity permits. **Pulse therapy with steroids,** using methylprednisone, 1 gm IV daily for 3–5 days, has been advocated. Alternate-day steroid therapy has low toxicity, but its efficacy has not been uniformly demonstrated. A number of prospective controlled randomized studies have shown benefit from using **cyclophosphamide.** IV pulse therapy using cyclophosphamide every third month has been demonstrated to have low toxicity and high efficacy. 5 prospective, controlled, randomized trials also indicate that **azathioprine,** though of marginal benefit, may allow faster tapering of steroids. Anecdotal reports suggest that patients with elevated levels of circulating immune complexes may respond to **plasmapheresis,** whereas those without these elevated levels do not respond. Further studies are needed to confirm efficacy. **Transplantation** has been successful in patients with end-stage renal disease secondary to lupus nephritis. Recurrence of lupus nephritis has been reported in the transplanted kidney. In general, it is important to be sure that lupus is clinically and serologically quiescent before transplantation to minimize the likelihood of recurrence in the transplanted kidney.

C. Wegener's Granulomatosis

1. CLINICAL COURSE

In a patient with progressive renal failure and respiratory tract symptoms, Wegener's granulomatosis is an important disease to be included in the differential diagnosis. If the disease remains untreated, rapid renal deterioration terminates in death within months. Prompt therapy with cytotoxic drugs, on the other hand, usually results in stabilization and gradual improvement in renal function. The mean age of patients at the onset of the disease is 40 years, and there is a 2:1 male-female ratio. The clinical triad of Wegener's granulomatosis includes: (1) necrotizing granulomatous vasculitis of the upper and lower respiratory tracts, (2) necrotizing glomerulonephritis, and (3) varying degrees of disseminated small-vessel vasculitis. Recently, determination of antineutrophil cytoplasmic antibody (ANCA) has allowed for easier diagnosis of Wegener's granulomatosis. The ANCA assay appears to have a high degree of sensitivity and specificity. Spontaneous remission of renal disease is not known to occur. Before the availability of cytotoxic agents, most patients with Wegener's granulomatosis succumbed to renal disease. Without therapy, the mean survival has been 5 months from the onset of clinically evident renal involvement. As noted before, cytotoxic drug therapy generally results in stabilization and gradual improvement of renal function.

2. THERAPY

Cyclophosphamide is now generally regarded as the mainstay of therapy. In clinically toxic states, cyclophosphamide, 2–3 mg/kg/day, can be given IV for several days. This can be followed by oral administration of cyclophosphamide in a dosage of 1–2 mg/kg/day. In less toxic situations, the oral regimen can be started from the outset. The total duration of cyclophosphamide therapy required is unclear, but a course of at least 6–12 months is recommended unless severe drug toxicity complicates therapy. The disease can recur after the termination of therapy, but recurrences can be treated successfully.

Temporary remissions, especially of the extrarenal disease manifestations, can be seen with the administration of **steroids** alone. However, the renal disease often progresses despite corticosteroid therapy. Steroids can therefore be used only to ameliorate symptoms in toxic states in patients with Wegener's granulomatosis. Prednisone should be started at a dosage of 60–100 mg/day, with rapid tapering as the clinical situation permits.

Some studies have demonstrated that **plasmapheresis,** in combination with steroids and cyclophosphamide, can be helpful, particularly in the patient with advanced renal involvement. A number of patients undergoing dialysis have responded to the combination therapy enough to discontinue dialysis. Further studies are necessary to determine the effectiveness of this therapy.

D. Goodpasture's Syndrome and Antiglomerular Basement Membrane Nephritis

1. CLINICAL COURSE

Patients may have progressive renal insufficiency resulting from antibodies directed against the glomerular basement membrane. The disease may occur with renal involvement alone (antiglomerular basement membrane nephritis), or it may occur in association with pulmonary involvement (Goodpasture's syndrome). Prompt recognition is vital to treatment. The disease usually affects men between the ages of 20 and 30, and many patients have antecedent upper respiratory tract symptoms. There may be an association of the disease with exposure to hydrocarbons. In patients with Goodpasture's syndrome, pulmonary symptoms may range from cough, dyspnea, and mild blood-tinged sputum to massive pulmonary hemorrhage. Pulmonary symptoms precede or are coincidental with renal manifestations in 70% of cases. In some instances, patients may have symptoms of renal insufficiency and may show no evidence of pulmonary involvement. These patients are said to have antiglomerular basement membrane disease. Classically, renal insufficiency progresses rapidly, and end–stage renal disease may result within weeks to months. The diagnosis can be established by renal or lung biopsy, with the finding of antiglomerular basement membrane antibodies.

2. THERAPY

Plasmapheresis has been demonstrated to be of benefit in patients with antiglomerular basement membrane disease, presumably by removing circulating antibodies. Plasmapheresis leads to prompt cessation of pulmonary hemorrhage and reversal of renal insufficiency. It is important to note that plasmapheresis is of limited benefit in patients with oliguria and severe renal insufficiency (a serum creatinine level greater than 6.8 mg/dL) at the initiation of therapy. Steroids and cyclophosphamide are usually employed also. In instances of life-threatening pulmonary hemorrhage, **bilateral nephrectomy** has been reported to be effective. In all instances, plasmapheresis should be attempted before consideration of bilateral nephrectomy. **Dialysis** can be used for support of patients who have antiglomerular basement membrane disease with renal insufficiency. Dialysis does not remove the antibodies and is of no use in the control of pulmonary hemorrhage. **Renal transplantation** has been successful in patients with end-stage renal disease. However, recurrence of disease in the transplanted kidney has been reported, and it is important to wait until antiglomerular basement membrane antibody titers are undetectable before transplantation is considered.

E. Multiple Myeloma

1. CLINICAL COURSE

Renal insufficiency is the second most common cause of death, after infection, in patients with multiple myeloma. Renal involvement may occur as a direct result of the disease or may be secondary to complications arising during the course of the disease. Clinically evident renal involvement occurs in about half of the patients with multiple myeloma and is associated with a markedly worse prognosis. In the majority of patients with renal involvement, deterioration of renal function is insidious, with slow progression over months to years. Few patients have ARF. The most important factor contributing to renal dysfunction is the presence of Bence Jones proteinuria. Approximately half of the patients with multiple myeloma have Bence Jones proteins (light-chain immunoglobulins) in the urine. The presence and amount of Bence Jones proteins appear to correlate roughly with degree of renal dysfunction. However, some patients with heavy proteinuria may have no evidence of renal dysfunction, and some may have renal insufficiency with no demonstrable Bence Jones proteinuria. Bence Jones proteins may be directly nephrotoxic or may cause tubular obstruction by precipitation in the distal tubules. Renal insufficiency may be the result of amyloidosis, found in about 10% of patients with multiple myeloma. In these cases, a light-chain immunoglobulin, or a fragment thereof, is the major constituent of the amyloid fibrils deposited. Patients with renal amyloidosis usually have hypertension, the nephrotic syndrome, and progressive renal insufficiency. Hypercalcemia is another important contributing factor in the development of renal insufficiency in patients with multiple myeloma. Hypercalcemia can cause compromises in renal concentrating ability, volume contraction, nephrocalcinosis, and nephrolithiasis. Hypercalcemia may also have direct nephrotoxic effects.

Other factors that can contribute to the development of renal failure include infections, particularly pyelonephritis; plasma cell invasion of the renal parenchyma; and the hyperviscosity syndrome, with compromises in renal blood flow. Patients with multiple myeloma are also more prone to contrast agent–induced ARF. Although the exact incidence is not known, patients with multiple myeloma should not be exposed to contrast media unless there is an absolute indication for the study.

2. MANAGEMENT

Preventive measures are as important as treatment measures in patients with multiple myeloma. The state of **hydration** should be optimized at all times to prevent dehydration and possible precipitation of Bence Jones proteins in the renal tubules. Use of **contrast agents should be avoided** unless there are absolute indications for contrast studies. If use of these agents is necessary, the patient should be vigorously hydrated before the study, and furosemide and mannitol should be given immediately after. The urine, renal function, serum globulin and viscosity, serum calcium level, and uric acid concentration should all be serially monitored. Hypercalcemia should be aggressively treated. Prolonged immobilization should be avoided to minimize the chance that hypercalcemia will develop. This measure is particularly important for patients with bone pain, in whom aggressive radiation therapy and liberal analgesia may be necessary. **Before the initiation of chemotherapy, prophylactic allopurinol, al-**

kalinization, and saline diuresis should be used. Unnecessary instrumentation of the genitourinary tract should be avoided to reduce the likelihood of infection. Potentially nephrotoxic drugs should not be used.

F. Progressive Systemic Sclerosis (Scleroderma)

1. CLINICAL COURSE

Approximately 40–50% of patients with progressive systemic sclerosis have clinically evident renal involvement, which becomes manifest about 2–3 years after diagnosis. Patients have proteinuria, hypertension, or renal insufficiency. There are two forms of renal involvement. An "indolent" form is insidious, with mild proteinuria, hypertension, and azotemia. Physiologic studies indicate decreased renal blood flow. Even patients with indolent renal involvement have a worse prognosis than those without renal involvement, and the mortality rate is 6 times that in patients with no renal involvement. Patients with "malignant" renal scleroderma have rapid and dramatic deterioration of renal function in the setting of malignant hypertension. Progressive renal insufficiency requires intervention within weeks to months.

2. MANAGEMENT

Malignant renal scleroderma constitutes a medical emergency, since patients often have malignant hypertension and rapid deterioration of renal function. The **control of blood pressure** with converting enzyme inhibitors (captopril, enalapril) has been shown to reverse progressive renal deterioration in a number of cases and should be tried. **Malignant hypertension** should be aggressively treated with IV **nitroprusside.** Malignant hypertension and progressive renal deterioration unresponsive to converting enzyme inhibitors have been successfully managed with bilateral nephrectomy in a number of instances. **Dialysis** and **transplantation** have also been successful in patients with renal scleroderma. Steroids, D-penicillamine, and anticoagulation therapy have been tried but have not been shown to be helpful.

G. Henoch-Schönlein Purpura

1. CLINICAL COURSE

Renal involvement is an important complication in patients with Henoch-Schönlein purpura. The syndrome occurs primarily in young children, with 75% of cases occurring in children under the age of 7. There appears to be some seasonal variation in the occurrence of the disease, with spring and fall being the most common seasons. The salient features of the syndrome include (1) skin manifestation of nonthrombocytopenic purpura, (2) joint manifestation of arthralgia, (3) GI manifestations of abdominal pain and hemorrhage, and (4) renal involvement. Clinical evidence of renal involvement is reported in 30–70% of patients with Henoch-Schönlein purpura. Some patients with no signs of renal disease have been reported to have pathologic changes on renal biopsy. Fortunately, fewer than 10% of patients have progressive renal failure. Renal involvement is potentially the most life-threatening complication in Henoch-Schönlein purpura and is of important prognostic value. Renal presentations include hematuria, proteinuria (including the nephrotic syndrome), and renal insufficiency. Pathologically, either focal or diffuse proliferative glomerulonephritis can be seen. Immunoglobulin A (IgA) deposition in the mesangium is classically observed.

2. MANAGEMENT
Several therapeutic measures have been tried, but with limited efficacy.
   a. **Conservative Measures.** Supportive care should be undertaken, and drugs such as aspirin should be avoided.
   b. **Steroids.** No controlled trials examining the efficacy of steroids in the management of renal complications are available. Joint and GI complications seem to respond to steroid therapy. However, steroids do not appear to affect skin lesions, duration of illness, or development of renal complications.
   c. **Cytotoxic Agents.** There are no available controlled trials investigating the effectiveness of cytotoxic agents, although there are suggestions that the prognosis may be improved in some patients with severe renal disease.
   d. **Plasmapheresis.** No controlled trials have examined the use of plasmapheresis in the management of renal involvement in Henoch-Schönlein purpura.

H. Hemolytic Uremic Syndrome

1. CLINICAL COURSE
The hemolytic uremic syndrome primarily affects young children and infants and is characterized by microangiopathic hemolytic anemia, thrombocytopenia, and ARF. Recently a strong association between *Escherichia coli* 0157:H7 infection and the hemolytic uremic syndrome has been established. There is no specific treatment for the bloody diarrhea induced by *E. coli* 0157:H7, which is associated with the hemolytic uremic syndrome. Treatment with antibiotics is not indicated.
   Rarely the syndrome can be seen in adults. Most patients have abdominal pain, vomiting, and bloody diarrhea as a prodromal syndrome. Some patients may have an upper respiratory prodrome. The major morbidity arises from ARF and bleeding complications. On renal biopsy, vasculitic changes and focal segmental proliferative glomerulonephritis are seen.

2. MANAGEMENT
No specific therapeutic interventions have been demonstrated to be of benefit. Trials with heparin, steroids, streptokinase, antiplatelet drugs, and plasmapheresis have been reported to be variably effective. Early intervention with dialysis appears to be beneficial. Some patients may develop malignant hypertension and should be aggressively treated. Many patients with the hemolytic uremic syndrome will recover normal renal function.

I. Thrombotic Thrombocytopenic Purpura

1. CLINICAL COURSE

Thrombotic thrombocytopenic purpura is a disease of unknown etiology characterized by the clinical triad of hemolytic anemia, thrombocytopenia, and abnormal mental status. In many patients, fever and renal failure are also present. The syndrome occurs predominantly in patients 10–40 years of age, with a slight increase in prevalence among females. Many patients have prodromes of nonspecific symptoms, such as arthralgia, pleuritis, and Raynaud's phenomenon. Neurologic symptoms range from paresthesia and changes in mental status to seizures and coma. ARF occurs in approximately 50%. These patients have hematuria, pyuria, active urinary sediment (including red cell casts), and abnormal renal function.

2 forms of the disease have been identified. In the chronic form, symptoms may wax and wane over a period of months. In its acute form, symptoms begin abruptly and follow a fulminant course, with progressive neurologic and renal disorders, often culminating in death. Patients who have the fulminant type often die within 90 days. Thrombotic thrombocytopenic purpura, like the hemolytic uremic syndrome, has recently been associated with *E. coli* 0157:H7 in some acute cases.

2. MANAGEMENT

Controlled studies on therapy are lacking owing to the paucity of cases and the fulminant nature of the presentation. **Fresh frozen plasma** has been effective in the treatment of patients with thrombotic thrombocytopenic purpura. In critically ill patients, **plasmapheresis** has produced dramatic successes.

Balon JE, Austin HA, Tsokos GC, et al: Lupus nephritis. Ann Intern Med 106:79, 1987.
Balon JE, Fauci AS: Vasculitic diseases of the kidney. *In* Schrier RW, Gottschalk CW (eds): Diseases of the Kidney. 4th ed. Boston, Little, Brown, 1988, pp 2335–2361.
De Fronzo RA, Cooke JR, Wright JR, et al: Renal failure in patients with multiple myeloma. Medicine 57:51, 1978.
Rees Al, Lockwood CM: Antiglomerular basement membrane antibody-mediated nephritis. *In* Schrier RW, Gottschalk CW (eds): Diseases of the Kidney. 4th ed. Boston, Little, Brown, 1988, pp 2091–2126.
Wardle EN: Diabetic nephropathy. Nephron 45:177, 1987.

XI. RENAL TRANSPLANTATION

Considerable advances have been made in transplantation and immunology over the past 25 years to make renal transplantation a safe and logical choice in end-stage renal disease. Transplantation, however, should not be regarded as a panacea, since considerable morbidity and mortality are still associated with it. A number of options are possible for the patient considering renal transplantation: The kidney can come from a cadaver, from a living related donor, and, in very selected instances, from a living unrelated donor. Patients receiving kidneys from a living donor have slightly better graft survival, and the amount of immunosuppression required is usually less. However, with the use of cyclosporine, graft survival, even in cadaveric transplants, is reasonable (Table 6–20). It is important to be familiar with the immunosuppressive agents commonly used for transplantation and to be aware of the possible complications related to the procedure.

TABLE 6–20. GRAFT AND PATIENT SURVIVAL AT 1 YEAR WITH CYCLOSPORINE

DONOR TYPE	GRAFT SURVIVAL (%)	PATIENT SURVIVAL (%)
Living-related donors		
HLA-identical	92	95
Non-HLA-identical	85	92
Cadaveric donor	80	86
Living-unrelated donor	85	90

A. Maintenance Immunosuppressive Agents

1. STEROIDS

Steroids are still an important part of immunosuppressive therapy. With the advent of cyclosporine, steroid doses can be tapered much more rapidly, thereby avoiding some of the complications of steroid therapy. Steroids are often used in relatively high doses immediately after transplantation and tapered rapidly as the clinical setting permits. During the first few days after transplantation, 60–100 mg of prednisone is often necessary. The doses are tapered over the course of the next 6–12 weeks to a maintenance dosage of usually 15 mg/day.

2. AZATHIOPRINE

Azathioprine is an important immunosuppressant with limited side effects. It is usually given in dosages ranging from 50–150 mg/day, depending on the patient's bone marrow reserve. Its major side effect is bone marrow suppression, making the patient more prone to infections. Anemia and thrombocytopenia can also occur. Rarely, azathiopine may cause liver function abnormalities.

3. CYCLOPHOSPHAMIDE

Cyclophosphamide is sometimes used in place of azathioprine. The dosage is similar (50–150 mg/day). Its major side effect is bone marrow suppression.

4. CYCLOSPORINE

Cyclosporine has been an important addition to the group of immunosuppressive agents. It has little suppressive effect on bone marrow and has permitted faster tapering of steroid doses during the post-transplant period. However, cyclosporine has a number of side effects, including nephrotoxicity, particularly when excessive cyclosporine doses are employed. The nephrotoxic effect of cyclosporine has complicated treatment, since it is often difficult to differentiate between rejection and cyclosporine nephrotoxicity. Serum cyclosporine levels are of marginal help, because toxicity may not correlate with serum levels. Other side effects are hyperkalemia, hypertension, and hirsutism. With long-term immunosuppression, malignant disease increases, and unusual tumors such as CNS lymphoma can be seen in these patients. It is therefore desirable to use the lowest possible maintenance doses of immunosuppressants that can prevent graft rejection.

B. Treatment of Acute Rejection. Several options are available. Prompt recognition and treatment are essential to prevent loss of the graft.

1. STEROIDS
Pulse administration of steroids, with a concomitant increase in steroid dose, is effective in rejection. This measure is often all that is necessary for mild rejection. However, repeated pulse administration of steroids and prolonged treatment with high doses of steroids should be avoided because of the morbidity involved.

2. ANTILYMPHOCYTE GLOBULIN
Antilymphocyte globulin (ALG) is an immunoglobulin directed against human lymphocytes that is produced usually in horses and is effective for the treatment of rejection. Side effects include hypersensitivity reactions, particularly with the initial doses; production of antibodies against ALG, thereby precluding a repeat course; and excessive immunosuppression, leading to infectious complications. ALG has to be administered in a large volume of solution, which may be a problem if volume overload is present.

3. OKT3
A monoclonal antibody directed against a selected population of T cells appears to be an extremely powerful agent in the treatment of rejection. More than 95% of patients treated have responded to a course of OKT3, although some of these patients subsequently had another episode of rejection. OKT3 can be given in small volumes and will not aggravate problems with volume overload. Patients may have a hypersensitivity reaction to initial doses and can form antibodies to the drug, thereby precluding a repeated course. OKT3 can also cause infectious complications by excessive immunosuppression but appears safer than repeated pulse administration of steroids.

4. ACTINOMYCIN D
Actinomycin D is usually reserved for patients with chronic rejection in whom the other therapeutic interventions have failed. Its effectiveness appears to be limited.

5. RADIATION
Radiation, similarly, is reserved for patients with chronic rejection in whom the other treatments have failed. It, too, is of limited efficacy.

Bach FH, Sachs DH: Current concepts—immunology: Transplantation immunology. N Engl J Med 317:489, 1987.
Morris PJ: Outcome and complications of transplantation. *In* Schrier RW, Gottschalk CW (eds): Diseases of the Kidney. 4th ed. Boston, Little, Brown, 1988, pp 3211–3234.

7777777777777

PULMONARY CONDITIONS

TERRY J. MENGERT
RICHARD K. ALBERT

I. PULMONARY TESTS: STRUCTURE AND FUNCTION

Accurate diagnosis of pulmonary disease requires an adequate database, including both a thorough review of the patient's symptoms and any history of exposure to environmental risks that affect pulmonary function. The **physical examination** must include vital signs, skin, nails, accessory muscle use, percussion and auscultation of the lungs, thorough cardiac examination, and evaluation of the other organ systems. Many pulmonary tests are available to add to this database.

A. Arterial Blood Gas. The preferred site for drawing blood for arterial blood gas (ABG) studies is the radial artery; the brachial and femoral arteries are other possibilities. One must be careful to eliminate excess heparin from the syringe, evacuate air bubbles, immediately place the sample in ice, record the temperature of the patient, record the Fio_2, and analyze the specimen promptly.

    1. INDICATIONS

    ABG studies are indicated in the critically ill patient and the patient with a potentially serious O_2, CO_2, or acid-base abnormality. The test is also indicated in chronically or critically ill patients with a change in clinical status or ventilator settings. ABG should **not** be routinely determined in patients with acute asthma (unless clinical status or pulmonary function tests [PFTs] indicate severe obstruction), stable patients in the ICU, or patients receiving prophylactic low-flow oxygen (Ann Intern Med 105:390–398, 1986).

    2. NORMAL VALUES

    Normal ABG values are as follows: pH 7.35–7.45 and Pco_2 35–45 mm Hg. Hypoxia is defined as Po_2 less than 80 mm Hg. Normal Po_2 does decline with age. The equation $Po_2 = 109 - 0.43 \times age$ (in years) may be used to predict the expected Po_2 at sea level in the older patient.

B. Oximetry. Oximeters determine the concentration of oxyhemoglobin in the blood by means of a spectrophotometer that measures the absorbance of light due to oxyhemoglobin. Advantages over traditional ABG studies include continuous monitoring of O_2 saturation and the noninvasive nature of the test. Disadvantages include lack of Pco_2 and pH determinations and measurement errors secondary to jaundice, carboxyhemoglobin levels over 3%, or poor blood flow. Continuous O_2 saturation monitoring is used in the operating room and ICU during cardiopulmonary resuscitation, during bronchoscopy, in exercise studies, and in evaluation of sleep apnea.

C. Spirometry. Spirometry measures volumes of inspired and/or expired gas. The test is used to

    (1) detect early lung disease;

    (2) quantitate current pulmonary dysfunction;

(3) assist with differential diagnosis of dyspnea, cough, and wheezing;
(4) follow the course of pulmonary disease;
(5) monitor patient response to therapy;
(6) screen for possible toxic injury.

The measured volumes may be presented as a resting spirogram (Fig. 7–1), flow-volume loops (Fig. 7–2), or forced spirometry (Fig. 7–3).

1. **MAXIMAL VOLUNTARY VENTILATION**
Maximal voluntary ventilation (MVV) is the greatest volume of air the patient can move per minute. It is a composite measurement that depends on the cooperation, strength, and endurance of the patient as well as the intrinsic mechanical properties of the lung. It can be estimated by forced expiratory volume in 1 second (FEV_1) × 35.

2. **INTERPRETATION OF SPIROMETRY** (Table 7–1)

a. **Obstructive Lung Disease.** This is indicated spirometrically by an FEV_1/forced vital capacity (VC) of less than 70–75%. Patients with air-flow obstruction are seldom limited in normal activity if FEV_1 is greater than 2 L. They are symptomatic if FEV_1 is less than 1 L, and conversation can be limited at FEV_1 less than 500 mL.

In normal individuals, FEV_1 declines with age. In patients who have smoked more than 10 cigarettes/day, the decline in FEV_1 is greater, especially in men, particularly in those between 50 and 70. In patients younger than 35, smoking cessation is associated

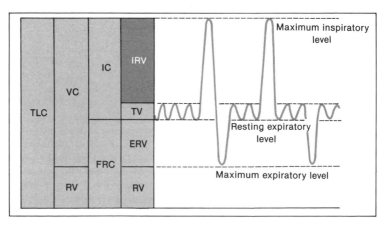

Figure 7–1. Static lung volumes are derived from standard spirometry and from a measurement of functional residual capacity either by body plethysmography or by gas dilution. Total lung capacity (TLC), vital capacity (VC), residual volume (RV), functional residual capacity (FRC), tidal volume (TV), inspiratory reserve volume (IRV), expiratory reserve volume (ERV), inspiratory capacity (IC). (From Forster RE II, et al: The Lung: Physiologic Basis of Pulmonary Function Tests. 3rd ed. Chicago, Year Book Medical Publishers, Inc., 1986.)

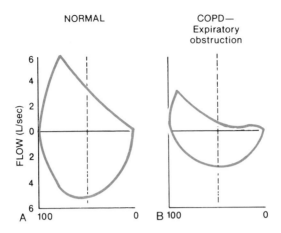

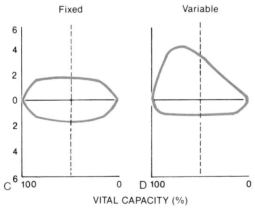

Figure 7–2. Flow-volume curves (loops) of maximal forced expiration (upper) and maximal inspiration (lower). Expiratory and inspiratory flow is plotted against lung volume expressed as a percentage of vital capacity. The dashed line can be used to compare flow rates at 50% of the vital capacity, at which point inspiratory flow rates normally exceed expiratory flow rates. *A,* Normal flow-volume curves. *B,* Flow-volume curves illustrating expiratory airflow obstruction showing decreased flow rates at all points in lung volume throughout maximal expiration. *C,* Fixed extrathoracic airway obstruction (cancer or fracture of the larynx). *D,* Variable extrathoracic obstruction (vocal cord paralysis) produces a pattern in which there is a decrease and flattening of maximal inspiratory flow-volume curves. (Modified from Hyatt RE, Black LF: The flow-volume curve: A current perspective. Am Rev Respir Dis 107:191, 1973.)

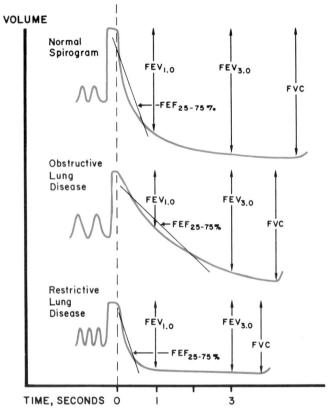

Figure 7–3. Simple spirometry usually allows differentiation of obstructive and restrictive patterns. Note that in both patterns the forced vital capacity (FVC) is reduced; however, flows are reduced in obstruction and are normal or "supernormal" in restriction. FEV, forced expiratory volume; FEF, forced expiratory flow. (From Slonim NB, Hamilton LH: Respiratory Physiology. 5th ed. St. Louis, C.V. Mosby, 1987.)

TABLE 7–1. INTERPRETATION OF SPIROMETRY*

STATUS	FVC† (%)	FEV₁† (%)	FEV₁/FVC (%)	DL_co† (%)
Normal	≥80	≥80	≥75	≥80
Mildly impaired (usually not related to decreased ability to work)	60–79	60–79	60–74	60–79
Moderately impaired (decreased ability to meet the physical demands of many jobs)	51–59	41–59	41–59	41–59
Severely impaired (unable to meet the physical demands of most jobs)	≤50	≤40	≤40	≤40

*% predicted.
†FVC = forced vital capacity; FEV₁ = forced expiratory volume in 1 sec; DL_CO = diffusing capacity of the lungs for carbon monoxide.
Adapted from American Thoracic Society: Evaluation of impairment/disability secondary to respiratory disorders. Am Rev Respir Dis 133:1205–1209, 1986.

with an increase in FEV_1. In men 50–70, smoking cessation results in a return to the normal age-related decline in FEV_1 (Am Rev Respir Dis 135:794–799, 1987).

  b. **Restrictive Lung Disease.** This disease may reduce the FEV_1, but in the absence of obstructive disease, the FEV_1/VC will still be greater than the 70–75% predicted. Normal VC rules out significant restrictive lung disease.

  c. **Bronchodilators.** The effectiveness of bronchodilators may be tested with spirometry. If after bronchodilator treatment the FEV_1 increases by at least 15% (or the VC by 10%), a significant response has occurred.

  d. **Postoperative Respiratory Failure.** Postoperative respiratory failure is increased in patients with chronic obstructive pulmonary disease (COPD). Pulmonary function abnormalities that suggest a higher risk of postoperative morbidity and mortality include maximal breathing capacity <50% predicted, FEV_1 <2 L, and P_{CO_2} >45 mm Hg (Am Rev Respir Dis 119:293–310, 1979).

  e. **Pulmonary Resection.** An MVV less than 50% predicted indicates that the patient is at risk for significant complications. Further assessment of regional lung function is then indicated, using radioisotopic lung scanning techniques. If postoperative FEV_1 is predicted to be less than 800 mL, pulmonary resection is contraindicated (Am Rev Respir Dis III:379–387, 1975). If the patient has pulmonary hypertension from primary vascular disease or has pulmonary hypertension more severe than would be predicted on the basis of COPD, measurement of unilateral pulmonary artery occlusion pressures may be necessary to estimate adequacy of the pulmonary vascular bed after resection.

D. **Diffusing Capacity.** Diffusing capacity of the lung (DL_{CO}) is a measure of its ability to transfer gas across its alveolar surface. The results of the DL_{CO} assessment depend on hemoglobin concentration, area of perfused alveolar membrane, and the resistance of that membrane to carbon monoxide. Diseases that obliterate the alveolocapillary membrane, that recruit or eliminate capillaries, or that change hemoglobin concentration will change the DL_{CO}. The DL_{CO} is decreased in emphysema, restrictive diseases like sarcoidosis, recurrent pulmonary emboli, diffuse interstitial fibrosis, and bleomycin toxicity. The DL_{CO} is increased in erythrocytosis or early CHF.

E. **Other Tests.** These may include CT of the thorax, esophageal pressure measurement, ventilatory drive assessment, inhalational challenges, scintiscans (including perfusion, ventilation, and gallium scans), pulmonary dead-space determinations, ultrasonography, bronchoalveolar lavage, and bronchoscopy.

American Thoracic Society: Standardization of spirometry—1987 update. Am Rev Respir Dis 136:1285–1298, 1987.

Burki NK, Albert RK: Noninvasive monitoring of arterial blood gases Chest 83:666–669, 1983.

Clawsen JL: Pulmonary function testing. *In* Bordow RA, Moser KM (eds): Manual of Clinical Problems in Pulmonary Medicine. 2nd ed. Boston, Little, Brown, 1985, pp 9–17.

Marini JJ: Respiratory Medicine and Intensive Care for the House Officer. Baltimore, Williams & Wilkins, 1987.

Raffin TA: Indications for arterial blood gas analysis. Ann Intern Med 105:390–398, 1986.

Tisi GM: Evaluation of pulmonary function before surgery. J Respir Dis, January 1984, pp 105–113.

II. OXYGEN THERAPY

Oxygen therapy is used to increase the oxygen delivered to the tissues to improve cellular, tissue, and organ function and thereby avert injury and death of the organism. Oxygen supplementation is justified in a variety of situations. Examples include (1) acute or chronic hypoxia from pulmonary disease, (2) acute myocardial infarction, (3) acute anemia, (4) postoperative care, and (5) CHF. In general, if tissue hypoxia is either suspected clinically or anticipated, it is reasonable to initiate empirically based O_2 supplementation. When O_2 supplementation is expected to exceed 24–48 hours, ABG should be measured to document continued need.

A. **Oxygen Delivery Systems.** The types of oxygen delivery systems, along with their advantages and disadvantages, are given in Table 7–2.

B. **Problems with Oxygen Supplementation.** Obvious disadvantages of O_2 therapy include cost, fire hazard, infection risk (e.g., from organisms that colonize humidifiers), and development of psychologic dependence on O_2 therapy. Additional problems are described below.

1. **WORSENED RESPIRATORY ACIDOSIS**
   Aggressive O_2 supplementation may blunt the hypoxic respiratory drive in COPD patients with chronic CO_2 retention, resulting in increased respiratory acidosis, deteriorating mental status, and worsening respiratory failure. Additional evidence, however, suggests that minute ventilation is only minimally decreased in patients with O_2 supplementation and that the cause of increased CO_2 retention is relaxation of hypoxia-induced vasoconstriction. Oxygen supplementation should always be used judiciously in chronic CO_2 retention.

Therapy should be initiated with 1.0–1.5 L O_2/minute via nasal prongs and the clinical status followed closely.

2. OXYGEN TOXICITY

High concentrations of Fio_2 over time can injure the lungs. Pulmonary damage depends on Fio_2 and duration of exposure. Opinions vary, but the threshold for clinically significant toxicity is an Fio_2 of about 0.60. It should be remembered that the goal of O_2 supplementation is to maintain Pao_2 above 55–60 mm Hg (90% hemoglobin O_2 saturation) and use the minimal Fio_2 necessary to achieve that level.

C. Indications for Long-Term Oxygen Supplementation. Some patients with hypoxia and chronic COPD, sleep apnea, and interstitial lung disease will benefit from long-term oxygen use. Benefits may include improved survival, better intellectual function, reduced pulmonary hypertension, and increased exercise tolerance. The following guidelines are suggested to determine who should receive "home oxygen":

1. Arterial hypoxemia should be documented (Pao_2 55 mm Hg or less when breathing room air);

2. If the patient has stable disease, hypoxemia should be present even though the patient's condition is stable and optimally treated (the decision to prescribe long-term O_2 therapy should not be based on results of ABG determinations obtained during an exacerbation);

3. Exercise-induced hypoxemia (Pao_2 <55 mm Hg) is an indication for O_2 supplementation if such supplementation improves exercise capacity, tolerance, or duration;

4. Sleep-induced hypoxemia is an indication for O_2 supplementation if there is evidence of induced organ dysfunction (pulmonary hypertension, cardiac dysrhythmia, or disturbed sleep pattern) and if nocturnal O_2 supplementation reduces the degree of hemoglobin desaturation.

D. Additional Concepts

1. Low-flow O_2 with nasal prongs at 1–3 L/minute is sufficient for most patients.

2. The goal is a Pao_2 necessary to maintain hemoglobin at 90% saturation (approximately 60 mm Hg).

3. If the patient is chronically hypoxemic, O_2 supplementation is of no benefit if used 12 hours or less/day; in the chronically hypoxemic patient, maximal benefit is realized with continuous therapy;

4. Once the supplementation is prescribed, the need for "home O_2," should be reevaluated 1, 6, and 12 months after its initiation. Thereafter, the need should be reassessed annually.

Findley LJ, Whelan DM, Moser KM: Long term oxygen therapy in COPD. Chest 83:671–674, 1983.

Fulner JD, Snider GL: ACCP–NHLBI National Conference on Oxygen Therapy. Chest 86:234–247, 1984.

III. COUGH

Cough is a frequent presenting complaint. The 5 most common causes of cough are acute respiratory tract infection, asthma, postnasal drip,

TABLE 7-2. OXYGEN DELIVERY SYSTEMS*

SYSTEM	ADVANTAGES	DISADVANTAGES	COMMENTS
Nasal cannula (prongs)	Simple; fairly comfortable; can be used during airway care, eating, and drinking	Limited FiO_2 capability; exact FiO_2 quite variable (dependent on inspiratory flow rate and minute ventilation); may dry or irritate mucous membranes	Each liter/minute raises FiO_2 about 3%; humidify if flow rate >4 liters/min (for two prongs); a water-soluble lubricant may help avoid mucous membrane irritation
Simple O_2 mask	Provides higher FiO_2 than nasal cannula	Uncomfortable and must be removed when eating, drinking, and expectorating; FiO_2 is variable, dependent on inspiratory flow and minute ventilation	FiO_2 of about 35% at 6 liters/min flow; FiO_2 about 55% at 10 liters/min flow; because of CO_2 entrapment, dead space may be increased (with increased work of breathing)
Nonrebreather reservoir mask (the reservoir is attached to the base of the mask, but a one-way valve prevents rebreathing of expired gas)	Provides highest FiO_2 short of intubation (approximately 90–95%)	See "Simple O_2 mask" above	The reservoir *must* remain filled; because of high FiO_2 absorption atelectasis and O_2 toxicity may occur; if reservoir bag collapse occurs, O_2 delivery will be insufficient to maintain adequate ventilation

Method			
Continuous positive airway pressure (CPAP) mask	Increases pulmonary volume, opens previously closed alveoli (reducing shunt); may improve V/Q mismatch	Uncomfortable; risk of aspiration if patient vomits	May improve PaO_2 in intrapulmonary arterialveno shunt for given FiO_2
Jet-mixing "Venturi" mask	Provides more exact FiO_2 than other methods described above	Uncomfortable; must be removed when eating, drinking, and so forth	Most accurate FiO_2 at 24% (flow of 4 liters/min) and 28% (flow of 6 liters/min); other FiO_2's available (31%, 35%, 40%, and 50%) are less accurate
Open face tent	May be better tolerated in some patients than nasal cannula or face masks; communication and expectoration not impeded	FiO_2 varies with flow rate and minute ventilation; eating impaired	May be able to provide FiO_2 as high as 70%
T tube	Exact FiO_2 possible up to 100%; humidification excellent	Requires endotracheal tube or tracheostomy	Maintain flow rate at least two times minute ventilation; humidification is mandatory because upper airway has been bypassed

*Medical gases do not contain water vapor. Humidification is appropriate at flow rates greater than 4 L/min. Humidification options include pass-over type, bubble, jet, and heated units. The last-named is the most efficient.

chronic bronchitis, and gastroesophageal reflux with aspiration. Additional possibilities include cardiac failure, bronchogenic or metastatic carcinoma, sarcoidosis, long uvula, nasal polyps, external auditory canal disorders, and psychogenic cough (J Respir Dis, March 1986, pp 21–30). Angiotensin-converting enzyme (ACE) inhibitor drugs (e.g., captopril, enalapril, and cilazapril) are well known to cause a chronic cough in some patients (Am J Med 85:887, 1988; Arch Intern Med 149:2701–2703, 1989).

Useful points to review in determining the cause of cough include cigarette use, exposure to environmental irritants, duration of cough, whether onset was acute or subacute, circumstances at onset, sputum production, aggravating situations like exercise or cold air exposure, other associated symptoms, and origin of the cough (e.g., pharynx or trachea) (J Respir Dis, January 1985, pp 97–107). See Table 7–3 for clues to the etiology of cough, as well as information about specific therapy. Cough is crucial to bronchial hygiene, and it is important to remember this before planning symptomatic therapy. A chronic cough may have associated morbidity: syncope, fractured ribs, costochondral inflammation, costochondral separations, respiratory muscle strain, and abdominal or inguinal hernia formation.

A. Symptomatic Therapy for Chronic Cough. Either of the following may be used for chronic cough: (1) dextromethorphan 15 mg q 6 hr or (2) codeine 15–30 mg q 4–6 hr.

Irwin RS, Pratter MR: Treatment of cough. Chest 82:662–663, 1982.

Irwin RS, Larro WM, Pratter MR: Chronic persistent cough in the adult: The spectrum and frequency of causes and successful outcome of specific therapy. Am Rev Respir Dis 123:413–417, 1981.

Irwin RS, Curley FJ, French CL: Chronic cough: The spectrum and frequency of causes, key components of the diagnostic evaluation, and outcome of specific therapy. Am Rev Respir Dis 141:640–647, 1990.

IV. DYSPNEA

Dyspnea is the subjective sensation of breathlessness. As a presenting complaint, dyspnea usually requires evaluation because it may be associated with life-threatening disorders.

A. Approach to the Patient. Immediate assessment is necessary to rule out life-threatening problems (e.g., upper airway obstruction, myocardial infarction, pulmonary embolism, tension pneumothorax, anaphylactic shock, asthma or COPD exacerbation, noncardiogenic pulmonary edema, and acute paralysis). If needed, establishing an adequate airway, ventilation, and circulatory support including oxygen treatment are the first priorities. Otherwise, evaluation may proceed more deliberately. When taking the history, one should place particular emphasis on abruptness of onset and duration of dyspnea and its severity (grade 1 = dyspnea when walking up stairs or hills; grade 2 = dyspnea when walking on level ground; grade 3 = dyspnea when walking on level ground ≤100 m; grade 4 = dyspnea with routine activities; grade 5 = dyspnea at rest).

TABLE 7–3. CLUES TO THE ETIOLOGY OF COUGH AND GUIDE TO SPECIFIC THERAPY

DIAGNOSIS	FINDINGS	THERAPY
Asthma	Cough with exercise, cold air exposure, environmental irritant, or wheezing; spirometry may reveal reversible obstruction; if spirometry is normal, then consider an inhalational challenge (with methacholine or carbachol)	Bronchodilators; consider corticosteroids if *no* improvement occurs with bronchodilator therapy after several weeks
Postnasal drip and/or sinusitis	Repeated throat clearing; sensation of secretions "dropping" down back of throat, especially at night; mucoid secretions may be seen in nares or posterior pharynx	Oral antihistamine or decongestants; avoid known precipitants; if sinusitis is a good possibility, then consider sinus films and empiric oral antibiotic therapy
Postinfection cough	Patient with recent (past 2 to 3 mo) upper respiratory tract infection; often no other cause will be apparent; *do not* perform inhalational challenge in recent upper respiratory tract infection because even normal patients will demonstrate airway hyperactivity	No specific treatment necessary; patient may be given symptomatic treatment; follow-up encouraged until cough resolves
Chronic bronchitis	Patient usually a cigarette smoker; cough accompanied by sputum production daily for 3 mo in 2 consecutive yr	*Strongly* recommend stopping cigarette use; bronchodilators reasonable; about 70% of smokers will be free of cough by 6 wk after stopping smoking
Gastroesophageal reflux	Dyspepsia symptoms, heartburn; consider further investigation with upper GI series, endoscopy, esophageal pH monitoring	Dietary change (avoid alcohol, caffeine, fats, and chocolate); elevate head of bed on 6-inch blocks; drug treatment may include antacids, histamine$_2$ (H$_2$) blockers, or metoclopramide
Malignancy	Chest radiograph may reveal mass or infiltrate; further evaluation may include sputum cytology and/or bronchoscopy	Depends on exact diagnosis and stage of disease
Interstitial lung disease (including sarcoidosis)	Chest film and pulmonary function testing reveal interstitial disease	Depends on final diagnosis

Adapted from Brown SE: What to do when patients complain of chronic cough. J Respir Dis 7(3):21-30. 1986.

B. Therapy. Treatment should always be **specific** to the disease causing dyspnea (described in appropriate sections of this manual). Only rarely can symptomatic treatment be considered (e.g., therapy with benzodiazepines or narcotics to reduce respiratory drive).

Wartak J, Sproule BJ, King GE: Algorithmic approach to evaluating dyspnea. J Respir Dis, September 1987, pp 71–84.
Wartak J, Sproule BJ, King GE: Dyspnea differential: Why the breathing difficulty? J Respir Dis, March 1988, pp 113–125.

V. HEMOPTYSIS

Hemoptysis should alert the physician to a possibly life-threatening disorder.

A. General Approach to the Patient. The goals of therapy are to prevent asphyxia, stop bleeding, and treat the cause of hemorrhage. The ABCs of resuscitation (**A**irway, **B**reathing, **C**irculation) always take priority. The cause of death in massive hemoptysis is **asphyxiation,** not exsanguination. Other sources of hemorrhage, including nasopharyngeal bleeding and GI bleeding (the latter characterized by dark red blood, clots with food particles, history of abdominal symptoms, and acid pH), should be excluded. In true hemoptysis the blood is frequently alkaline, frothy, and bright red. The quantity and rate of bleeding should be determined as accurately as possible. In most cases, hemoptysis is of short duration and the volume is small, but blood loss greater than 600 mL in 24–48 hours is a medical or surgical emergency. Thorough history and physical are important. Tests may include chest x-ray, CBC, PT, PTT, platelet count, ABG, Gram stain and culture of sputum, ECG, and bedside spirometry, if possible. A urinalysis is reasonable if Goodpasture's syndrome or other vasculitis is suspected. Bronchoscopy, rigid or fiberoptic, depending on bleeding rate, allows for examination of the larynx and lower respiratory tract.

If there is active bleeding, humidified oxygen should be given, large-bore IV access established, the bleeding lung placed dependent (may be difficult to determine), and emergent pulmonary, surgical, and anesthesiology consultations obtained. Airway management is crucial.

B. Treatment. Since hemoptysis usually is minor and transient, evaluation need not be emergent. Therapy depends on the specific diagnosis (based on Gram stain studies of sputum culture). Antibiotics are often helpful, since bronchitis is the major cause. In an emergent situation the guidelines presented above should be followed. While awaiting bronchoscopy, one should monitor the patient's status closely with frequent ABG determinations and chest radiographs. In one study, 6% of 123 patients died while awaiting bronchoscopy and definitive therapy (J Thorac Cardiovasc Surg 85:120–124, 1983). Fiberoptic bronchoscopy may be used to localize the bleeding site, although if bleeding is particularly active, rigid bronchoscopy will be necessary for adequate suctioning.

Specific treatment of an actively bleeding lesion may include Fogarty balloon catheter inflation proximal to the bleeding site and use of topical vasoconstrictors (epinephrine), or coagulants (Gelfoam) during bronchoscopy. Angiographic embolization of bleeding bronchial arteries may be effective, especially if the patient is not a surgical candidate (Diagn Radiol 122:33–37, 1977). Experimental modalities include radiation and laser therapy. Surgery is the treatment of choice for patients with rapid bleeding (600 mL or more/24 hours) who are surgical candidates when the bleeding site can be localized.

Clausen JL: Hemoptysis. *In* Bordow RA, Moser KM (eds): Manual of Clinical Problems in Pulmonary Medicine. 2nd ed. Boston, Little, Brown, 1985, pp 61–64.
Rudzinski JP, del Castillo J: Massive hemoptysis. Ann Emerg Med 16:561–564, 1987.
Varkey B, Kutty K: Pulmonary diseases. *In* Kochar MS (ed): Textbook of General Medicine. New York, John Wiley & Sons, 1983, pp 559–634.

VI. PLEURAL EFFUSIONS

Pleural effusion, although the most common clinical manifestation of pleural disease, may occur as a consequence of disease processes far removed from the pleura (e.g., nephrotic syndrome). Normally the pleural space contains only about 10 mL of transudate. This fluid is a result of the balance between hydrostatic and oncotic pressures. The normal flow of fluid is from the parietal to the visceral pleura. Pleural fluid accumulates abnormally when pleural lymphatic drainage is compromised, plasma or pleural space oncotic pressures are shifted, pleural hemodynamics are altered, vascular hydrostatic pressures change, and/or capillary permeability and surface area are affected by disease.

A. Diagnosis. About 300 mL of pleural fluid is necessary before costophrenic angle blunting occurs on a PA chest film, but a lateral decubitus radiograph will reveal as little as 150 mL of fluid. A subpulmonic effusion may mimic an elevated hemidiaphragm.

1. THORACENTESIS

Thoracentesis is indicated when the cause of the pleural effusion is uncertain or when the volume of fluid is large and is inducing such symptoms as dyspnea. In general, thoracentesis can proceed without difficulty if a fluid layer at least 10 mm thick is visualized on a lateral decubitus chest radiograph. Reexpansion pulmonary edema may occur after thoracentesis if too large a volume of pleural fluid is removed too rapidly. Traditionally, no more than 1500 ml of fluid should be removed at one time to avoid this complication.

Laboratory Evaluation. The first priority is to distinguish an exudate from a transudate, which can be done by determining pleural fluid lactate dehydrogenase (LDH) and protein levels. Additional fluid can be held in the laboratory pending results of these tests. A transudate generally does not require further evaluation; an exudate does. Clinical suspicion of the likely disease or diseases should then guide other tests ordered. Options include the following:

1. Cell count and differential yield useful information. Bloody fluid suggests cancer, pulmonary embolus, trauma, and tuberculosis. Leukocyte count and differential are helpful in distinguishing parapneumonic effusions from tuberculosis or cancer.

2. Gram stain and culture are useful in parapneumonic effusions, in which tuberculosis or other infections are possible.

3. The pH may be useful diagnostically when rheumatoid disease or cancer is suspected or in evaluation of parapneumonic effusions.

4. Glucose levels may be decreased in cancer, tuberculosis, parapneumonic effusion, and rheumatoid disease.

5. Cytology has variable diagnostic yield but is more useful in detecting malignancy if multiple specimens (from separate thoracenteses) are submitted (Arch Intern Med 132:854–860, 1973).

6. Amylase levels may be helpful in suspected pancreatitis or esophageal rupture.

7. Additional tests may include hematocrit, triglycerides, and rheumatoid factor.

2. TRANSUDATE VERSUS EXUDATE
Any one of the following is sufficient to label pleural fluid as exudative:

1. A pleural fluid/serum protein ratio greater than 0.5:1.0 (or absolute protein greater than or equal to 3.0 gm/dL),
2. A pleural fluid/serum LDH ratio greater than 0.6:1.0,
3. An absolute LDH value greater than 200 IU/L.

B. Specific Problems

1. PLEURAL EFFUSIONS IN CANCER PATIENTS
The patient with cancer may have fluid accumulation secondary to the disease, but other possibilities should also be considered: transudates from CHF, hypoalbuminemia, and venous outflow obstruction; and exudates from pulmonary embolism with infarction and from pneumonia. The most common malignant diseases associated with pleural effusion are lung cancer (25–40%), breast cancer (25%), and lymphoma (10–15%).

   a. **Pleural Fluid Characteristics.** Usually the fluid is exudative (5–10% may be transudates) and serosanguineous and has an LDH level of more than 500 IU/L. The leukocyte count is typically 1000–5000/L, with mononuclear cells predominating. Cytologic findings are positive 30–70% of the time, depending on the pleural tumor burden. Cytologic study and pleural biopsy together will increase the yield. Pleural fluid pH and glucose levels have prognostic significance: If the pH is less than 7.3 and the glucose level is less than 60 mg/dL in a patient having known pleural involvement with cancer, the mean survival is shorter and the response to tetracycline pleurodesis is poorer (Ann Intern Med 108:345–349, 1988).

   b. **Management.** When the diagnosis of malignant pleural fluid is confirmed, the rate of fluid reaccumulation will dictate the approach. If reaccumulation occurs over days to a few weeks, palliation should be considered.

c. **Palliation.** Chest tube drainage alone has about a 50% response rate. In the United States, tetracycline (500 mg in 50 mL of saline) is probably the agent of choice for pleurodesis, with reported response rates as high as 83% or more. Other treatments include intrapleural administration of chemotherapeutic agents, talc poudrage, and pleurectomy with pleural abrasion. Factors important in considering palliation include the patient's overall condition, symptoms, expected survival, and biochemical characteristics of the pleural fluid (pH and glucose) (Am Rev Respir Dis 138:184–234, 1988).

2. **BLOODY PLEURAL EFFUSIONS**
When the pleural fluid is grossly bloody, the effusion may be classified as serosanguineous (5000–100,000 RBC/mL), bloody (greater than 100,000 RBC/mL), and a hemothorax (hematocrit of the effusion exceeds 50% of the venous blood hematocrit). Exudative bloody effusions may result from malignant disease, trauma, infection, pulmonary embolism, collagen vascular disease (such as SLE) and contact with asbestos. Traumatic thoracentesis may have occurred: Usually the blood will clear during the course of the tap. Blood from a traumatic tap should also clot.
   Management. In hemothorax, chest tube thoracostomy is appropriate. If hemorrhage continues at the rate of 100–200 mL/hour, thoracotomy is indicated to ligate the bleeding vessels. If the bleeding has stopped but the hemothorax is incompletely drained, some question the need for thoracotomy. One approach is that if 30% of the hemithorax is occupied by undrained clot, then thoracotomy is reasonable (J Respir Dis, June 1986, pp 18–24).

3. **PLEURAL EFFUSIONS AND PNEUMONIA**
Effusions associated with pneumonia may be: **parapneumonic** (secondary to inflammation and increased permeability of the pleura); **complicated parapneumonic** (may or may not be infected but becomes fibrinopurulent and loculated); **empyema** (frank pus in the pleural space). A simple parapneumonic effusion will resolve without specific therapy, except that aimed at the pneumonia itself. A complicated parapneumonic effusion may require closed chest tube drainage. Empyema **always** requires chest tube drainage. Thoracentesis should be performed in pneumonia if layering of 10 mm of fluid or more is observed on a lateral decubitus film. If there is concern about the best location to tap the fluid, one should use ultrasound guidance. Pleural fluid should be sent for protein and LDH determinations, in addition to pH, glucose level, Gram stain and culture, and total white blood cell count (WBC) with differential. If the fluid is frank pus, however, the only studies necessary are Gram stain and culture. Even if there is no growth on culture, some authors suggest that an effusion with a pH <7.0 or a glucose level <40 mg/mL (in the setting of pneumonia) should be treated as empyema.
   Management. Empyemas require closed chest tube drainage in addition to the antibiotic appropriate for the pneumonia. As

mentioned, complicated pleural effusions with low pH and/or low glucose level probably should be treated like empyemas. If the pleural effusion has a pH of 7.00–7.20 and a glucose level >40 mg/dL, repeat thoracentesis in 12–24 hours may be useful. If the pleural fluid shows a decreasing glucose level and/or lowered pH, closed chest tube drainage may be appropriate. Otherwise, close observation and treatment of pneumonia should be continued.

Brody J.: Diseases of the pleura, mediastinum, diaphragm, and chest wall. *In* Wyngaarden JB, Smith LH Jr (eds): Cecil Textbook of Medicine. 18th ed. Philadelphia, WB Saunders Co, 1988, pp 466–473.
Jay SJ: Pleural effusions. Postgrad Med 80:164–191, 1986.
Light RW, Girard WM, Jenkinson SG, George RB: Parapneumonic effusions. Am J Med 69:507–512, 1980.
Sahn, SA: The pleura. Am Rev Resp Dis 138:184–234, 1988.

VII. SOLITARY PULMONARY NODULE

The solitary pulmonary nodule (SPN) is a fairly common problem. It is a lesion no more than 5–6 cm in diameter in the lung parenchyma, surrounded by aerated lung tissue. The percentage of pulmonary nodules that are malignant depends on the population base. When possible, resection of the malignant SPN is the treatment of choice. Benign lesions that may manifest as an SPN include hamartomas, granulomas (from tuberculosis or a variety of fungal infections), pulmonary infarction, and arteriovenous malformation.

A. **Approach to the Patient.** A lesion is more likely to be benign if the patient has no history of cigarette smoking or exposure to other carcinogens, is younger than 35, and/or has a history of tuberculosis, or exposure to *Coccidioides, Histoplasma,* or other fungi. Routine work-up should include CBC, electrolyte panel, calcium level, urinalysis, and stool Hemoccult. Routine searching for an extrapulmonary malignant lesion beyond the above is not indicated.

Chest x-rays should be reviewed thoroughly and old films obtained for comparison. Any of the following calcification patterns strongly suggests a benign lesion: diffuse, clustered or "popcorn," dense central nidus, and/or a concentric or laminated pattern. If diagnosis is still uncertain, chest CT may reveal calcifications and define the relationship of the SPN to nearby thoracic structures and other abnormalities (e.g., enlarged mediastinal lymph nodes). If work-up to this point leaves doubt about the potential malignancy of the lesion, a number of approaches may be reasonable.

1. PERCUTANEOUS NEEDLE ASPIRATION AND BIOPSY
This procedure is reasonable if clinically the lesion is unlikely to be malignant and if a tissue diagnosis will otherwise influence therapy (e.g., tuberculosis). Contraindications include patient uncooperativeness, a bleeding diathesis, pulmonary hypertension, markedly compromised pulmonary function (e.g., FEV_1 less than 1 L), or surrounding bullous disease. Complications include pneumothorax (11–30%) and hemoptysis (10 to 20%).

2. FIBEROPTIC BRONCHOSCOPY

Fiberoptic bronchoscopy has an accuracy of less than 30% in the tissue diagnosis of the SPN if the lesion is less than 2 cm in diameter, and a diagnostic accuracy of about 50–80% for lesions larger than 3 cm. The yield is also better for an endobronchial lesion and a more proximal lesion.

3. THORACOTOMY

This procedure should be performed when the lesion is growing, when other approaches have not revealed a benign process, or when malignancy is otherwise likely. The patient must be a surgical candidate. It is contraindicated in the patient with severe COPD, severe CHF, recent MI, or unstable angina. Complications include chest pain, bleeding, and infection. Mortality has been traditionally reported as 3–5%.

B. Therapy. A lesion "proven" to be benign on the basis of a stable appearance on the chest radiograph for 2 or more years, a benign calcification pattern, or a tissue diagnosis confirming granuloma or other nonneoplastic process should be followed. For a suspected malignant SPN, thoracotomy is the treatment of choice in the appropriate surgical candidate. If chest CT shows abnormal mediastinal lymph nodes or mediastinal tumor, mediastinoscopy should be undertaken before surgery. Mediastinoscopy is also appropriate before surgery when the SPN is located centrally, when it has a diameter of more than 3 cm, or when biopsy has revealed that it is a small-cell or undifferentiated large-cell carcinoma.

Cummings SR: Monitoring solitary pulmonary nodules. Am Rev Respir Dis 134:453–460, 1986.
Khouri NF: The solitary pulmonary nodule: Assessment, diagnosis, and management. Chest 91:128–133, 1987.
Miller KS: Prediction of pneumothorax rate in percutaneous needle aspiration of the lung. Chest 93:742–745, 1988.
Rohwedder JJ: The solitary pulmonary nodule: A new diagnostic agenda (editorial). Chest 93:1124–1125, 1988.

VIII. PHARMACOLOGY OF AIRWAY DISEASE

Airway abnormalities may include hyperactivity, inflammation, excessive mucus production, and plugging of the airways with mucus and inflammatory debris. Clinically the patient with airway dysfunction suffers from cough, sputum production, dyspnea, and wheezing. V/Q mismatch may result in hypoxia. Many therapeutic agents are available to combat these problems.

A. Sympathomimetics. The effects of these agents depend on the receptors they stimulate. Alpha receptors mediate vasoconstriction, beta$_1$ receptors mediate cardiac stimulation, and beta$_2$ receptors mediate bronchodilation, hyperglycemia, and muscle tremors.

1. PARENTERAL AGENTS

In some asthmatics, parenteral administration of sympathomimetics results in improved bronchodilation when compared with inhaled agents alone, presumably by delivering medication to airways so

constricted that effective delivery is not achieved by the inhaled route
(J Allergy Clin Immunol, 84:90–98, 1989).

   a. Epinephrine. Epinephrine has both alpha- and beta-agonist effects
and short action duration (15–30 minutes). It is available in a
nonprescription metered dose inhaler (MDI), injectable solution,
or inhaled racemic compound. Epinephrine is crucial in severe
allergic reactions, in which its alpha effects make it the drug of
choice. Epinephrine may be administered as follows: 0.3 mL of a
1:1000 solution SQ every 15–30 minutes, to a maximum of 3
doses. Epinephrine should not be used in the patient with recent
myocardial infarction, history of angina, or history of cardiac
dysrhythmia. Traditionally, epinephrine use has been avoided in
the patient over 40, but age alone should **not** be considered an
absolute contraindication (Ann Emerg Med 17:322–326, 1988).

   b. Terbutaline. Terbutaline is a $beta_2$ selective agent. It is available
in tablets, ampules for SQ administration, and MDI. It has a
longer duration of action than epinephrine and about twice the
bronchodilator effect. It also may be better tolerated in the adult
but should be used cautiously in the patient with known cardiac
disease. An SQ dose of terbutaline is 0.25 mg, which may be
repeated in 15–30 min (not to exceed 0.5 mg SQ every 4 hr).

2. **INHALED AGENTS**

   Inhaled agents include epinephrine (over the counter), isoproterenol,
isoetharine, metaproterenol, albuterol, terbutaline, and bitolterol. Of
these, the most $beta_2$ selective are metaproterenol (Alupent, Meta-
prel), albuterol (Proventil, Ventolin), terbutaline (Brethine), and
bitolterol (Tornalate). Table 7–4 summarizes available inhaled beta
agonists. Generally oral forms are less well tolerated because they
induce more systemic side effects. However, oral agents are added
to augment bronchodilation if symptoms remain poorly controlled.

   When prescribing an MDI to a patient, it is the physician's
responsibility to review the use of the inhaler with the patient (Table
7–5). As many as one third of patients use MDI incorrectly. For
patients who cannot master MDI technique, spacers are available to
improve delivery of the medication.

B. Methylxanthines. Methylxanthines have been reported to stimulate
respiratory drive, cause bronchodilation, improve cardiovascular function, increase the endurance and contractile function of the diaphragm,
and enhance mucociliary clearance. Their exact mechanism of action
remains uncertain. Recently the effectiveness of theophylline in the
treatment of acute asthma and COPD has been questioned. Several
studies have shown not only no improvement in bronchodilation (when
compared with the aggressive use of beta agonists alone) but an increased
incidence of side effects (Ann Intern Med 107:305–309, 1987; Am Rev
Respir Dis 132:283–286, 1985). These studies should not prejudice the
clinician against the value of theophylline in the long-term management
of the still symptomatic patient with stable asthma or COPD. Double-
blind, randomized, controlled studies have demonstrated that theophylline is effective in decreasing the frequency and severity of asthma

TABLE 7–4. THE INHALED BETA AGONISTS

DRUG	TRADE NAME	BETA SELECTIVITY	DRUG FORM	MDI* DOSE	NEBULIZED DOSE	RELATIVE BRONCHODILATOR EFFECT
Isoproterenol	Isuprel Mistometer Medihaler-Iso	Beta$_1$ and beta$_2$	MDI, nebulized solution	1–2 puffs, up to 5 doses per day	0.5 mL in 2.5 mL NS every 15–20 min up to 3 doses, then every 4 hr	Less effective than albuterol
Isoetharine	Bronkometer Bronkosol	Beta$_1$ and beta$_2$	MDI, nebulized solution	1–2 puffs q 4 hr	0.5–1.0 mL (5–10 mg) in 1.5 mL NS every 15–20 min for 3 doses, then every 4 hr	Less effective than albuterol
Metaproterenol	Alupent Metaprel	Beta$_2$	Tablets, syrup, MDI, nebulized solution	2–3 puffs q 3–4 hr	0.3–0.5 mL (15–25 mg) in 2.5 mL NS every 15–20 min up to 3 doses, then every 4 hr	4 puffs = 2 puffs of albuterol
Albuterol	Proventil Ventolin	Beta$_2$	Tablets, syrup, MDI, nebulized solution	2 puffs q 4–6 hr	0.5–1.0 mL in 2.0 ml NS every 20 min for 6 doses, then every 4–6 hr	Most effective pharmacologically of agents listed
Terbutaline	Brethine Bricanyl	Beta$_2$	SQ injection, tablets, MDI, nebulized solution	2 puffs q 4–6 hr	0.5 mL in 2.5 ml NS every 15–20 min up to 3 doses, then every 4–6 hr	3 puffs = 2 puffs of albuterol, but longer half-life
Bitolterol	Tornalate	Beta$_2$	MDI	2–3 puffs q 4–6 hr	—	3 puffs = 2 puffs of albuterol, but longer half-life

*MDI = metered dose inhaler; NS = normal saline. Adapted from Webb-Johnson DC, Chin B, Andrews JL: Bronchodilator therapy: Part 1. N Engl J Med 297:476–482, 1977.

TABLE 7–5. HOW TO USE A METERED DOSE INHALER

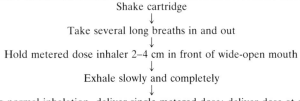

Shake cartridge
↓
Take several long breaths in and out
↓
Hold metered dose inhaler 2–4 cm in front of wide-open mouth
↓
Exhale slowly and completely
↓
During normal inhalation, deliver single metered dose; deliver dose at start of inhalation
↓
Hold breath for minimum of 5–10 sec (if possible)
↓
Wait 1–3 min before taking next puff in same manner
↓
Rinse mouth afterward to minimize systemic effects from medication
↓
Rinse mouthpiece daily with warm water

Adapted from West W: Update on drug therapy for your COPD patient. J Respir Dis, September 1985, pp 44–58.

symptoms when used on a long-term basis, compared with the effectiveness of cromolyn (Lancet 1:381–385, 1977), inhaled albuterol (J Allergy Clin Immunol 79:78–85, 1987), and oral metaproterenol (J Pediatr 101:281–287, 1982). Patients with severe but stable COPD have been shown to have significant improvement in dyspnea, pulmonary gas exchange, vital capacity, and respiratory muscle performance when treated with theophylline as compared to placebo (N Engl J Med 320:1521–1525, 1989).

1. **METHYLXANTHINE DOSING**
   To achieve optimal benefits from **theophylline** the plasma level should generally be between 10 and 20 μg/mL. In mild airway disease, some patients still derive benefit with lower serum concentrations. The dose required to produce a particular level varies widely, and numerous medications affect methylxanthine metabolism (Tables 7–6 and 7–7).
   Theophylline toxicity increases when the serum level exceeds 20 μg/mL. Symptoms of toxicity include anorexia, nausea, CNS irritability, tremor, seizures, and cardiac dysrhythmias.
   a. **IV Aminophylline Load. Aminophylline** is 80% anhydrous theophylline. An IV load of 5–7 mg/kg is based on the concept that every 1 mg/kg load will increase the serum level 2 μg/mL. If the patient has ingested theophylline in the past 12 hours, one should wait for determination of serum theophylline level. The IV load should be infused over 20 minutes. The blood level should subsequently be checked 1–2 hours after the beginning of maintenance infusion.

TABLE 7–6. CLINICAL SITUATIONS AND MEDICATIONS INFLUENCING METHYLXANTHINE METABOLISM

SERUM LEVELS INCREASED (METABOLISM DECREASED)
Infants <1 yr old
Elderly patients
Congestive heart failure
COPD
Hepatic dysfunction
Viral or bacterial illness with fever
Cimetidine
Oral contraceptives
Erythromycin
Ciprofloxacin
Allopurinol

SERUM LEVELS DECREASED (METABOLISM INCREASED)
Children
Cigarette and marijuana smokers
Phenytoin (Dilantin)
Carbamazepine
Barbiturates

Adapted from Hendeles L: Asthma therapy: State of the art, 1988. J Respir Dis, March 1988, pp 82–107.

TABLE 7–7. METHYLXANTHINE DOSING: INTRAVENOUS AND ORAL

	INTRAVENOUS	
Maintenance Infusion	**Aminophylline (mg/kg/hr)**	**Theophylline (mg/kg/hr)**
Nonsmokers	0.5–0.7	0.4–0.6
Smokers	0.9	0.75
Cimetidine use	0.3–0.4	0.25–0.30
Cor pulmonale	0.25–0.30	0.20–0.25
Hepatic insufficiency	0.20–0.25	0.18–0.20
	ORAL	
Eventual Oral Dose*	**Aminophylline (mg/day) (70-kg patient)**	**Theophylline (mg/day) (70-kg patient)**
Nonsmokers	900	800
Smokers	1300	1100
Cimetidine use	600	500
Cor pulmonale	500	400
Hepatic insufficiency	450	350

*Attained over a 9-day period to minimize side effects
Data from Garrity ER Jr, Gross NJ: Prompt management for status asthmaticus. J Respir Dis, May 1987, pp 21–32; Hendeles L: Asthma therapy: State of the art, 1988. J Respir Dis, March 1988, pp 82–107; Med Lett Drugs Ther 29:11–16, 1987.

   b. Oral Dosage. At the beginning of oral therapy in the patient in stable condition, the dosage should be titrated slowly over 9 days to achieve desired serum levels and minimize side effects. The initial dose should be about 400 mg/day (a lower starting dose should be considered in patients with hepatic dysfunction, CHF, or cor pulmonale or in those taking cimetidine). Serum levels should be checked after 3 days and the dose increased every 3 days until therapeutic serum levels are reached. Average eventual oral doses in patients weighing 70 kg are given in Table 7–7.
      NOTE: In patient able to take oral medication, there is no good evidence, even in an asthmatic or COPD exacerbation, that IV aminophylline or theophylline is more efficacious than oral delivery of the medication. Strongly consider orally loading the patient and avoiding IV use entirely.

C. Anticholinergic Drugs. Anticholinergic agents have become the drugs of first choice in the management of the stable patient with COPD because they produce bronchodilation as well as or better than beta agonists and have longer duration of action. In the asthmatic, however, they appear to be less potent bronchodilators than beta agonists, although in some asthmatics anticholinergics serve as useful adjunctive therapy. They **do not** provide impressive benefit to the patient in either an asthmatic or COPD crisis (Chest 98:295–297, 1990).

1. ATROPINE
Atropine is available in a nebulized solution, which may be administered in a dosage of 0.025 mg/kg qid. Side effects include dry mouth, dry skin, tachycardia, drying of respiratory secretions, urinary retention, and headache. It should not be used in patients with glaucoma, benign prostatic hypertrophy, or problems with urinary retention.

2. IPRATROPIUM BROMIDE
Ipratropium bromide is available as an MDI. The dosage is 2 puffs every 4–6 hours. Sensitivity to the drug is a contraindication to its use. It has a favorable side effect profile and is the preferred anticholinergic.

D. Corticosteroids. The mechanism by which these drugs improve limitation of air flow remains unknown. Potential beneficial mechanisms include stabilization of lysosomal membranes, reduced release of cellular mediators of inflammation, decreased mucus secretion, reduction in airway inflammation, and restored beta-receptor sensitivity. Corticosteroids have been documented to shorten the duration and severity of severe exacerbations in asthma and to prevent some hospitalizations. Several experts have concluded that the most important intervention that may prevent the several thousand deaths in this country per year from status asthmaticus is earlier and more aggressive use of corticosteroids. The prominent inflammatory component of asthma argues that more aggressive use of inhaled corticosteroids in asthma management is appropriate. Steroids can also play an important role in COPD management. In an acute exacerbation, their early use has been demonstrated to result in more rapid improvement in FEV_1. In chronic, stable COPD (Table 7–8), benefit is seen in relatively few patients (6–29%). When

TABLE 7–8. CLINICAL STEROID TRIAL IN THE PATIENT WITH CHRONIC, STABLE COPD BUT CONTINUED SEVERE SYMPTOMS

1. Obtain baseline PFTs while patient is optimally and maximally treated.
2. Repeat PFTs on one other occasion before beginning trial to ensure an adequate baseline.
3. Begin patient on 40 mg prednisone per day.
4. Trial should be a minimum of 2 wk and preferably 4 wk.
5. At the end of the trial, repeat PFTs. An increase of FEV_1 by 20% or more (some would use 15%) or a 20% increase in FVC is a significant change.
6. If there is *no improvement* in PFTs, the patient should be tapered slowly off steroids.
7. If the patient responds, attempt to get the patient on an alternate-day regimen or on the lowest dose that maintains functional and PFT improvement.

Adapted from Alberts WM, Corrigan KC: Corticosteroid therapy for chronic obstructive pulmonary disease: Is it worth the risks? Postgrad Med 81:131–137, 1987.

corticosteroids are given IV, some benefit is seen in as little as 1 hour, but the full effect is not reached for 6–8 hours. The preferred drug for IV use is methylprednisolone (Medrol). Hydrocortisone is more expensive than methylprednisolone at equipotent doses and has a greater mineralocorticoid effect. The IV dose should generally be followed by a tapering oral dose, as outlined in Table 7–9.

The side effects of corticosteroids are numerous, including weight gain, cataracts, osteoporosis, glucose intolerance, aseptic necrosis of femoral heads, capillary fragility, fluid retention, hypokalemia, cushingoid appearance, and suppression of the hypothalamic-pituitary axis. Reactivation of tuberculosis is of concern after a positive purified protein derivative (PPD) tuberculin skin test only if the patient is faced with a prolonged steroid course (months to years). In this circumstance, isoniazid prophylaxis is appropriate. In asthma, aerosol steroids can reduce airway inflammation and hyperreactivity and/or lower the dose of oral corticosteroid needed to maintain airway stability. Some consider inhaled steroids to be either first- or second-line agents in asthma management. Their role in the management of COPD is not well established, but their use is common. Although some minimal systemic absorption occurs when aerosol steroids are used as recommended, the risk of steroid side effects is reduced.

Aerosol steroids may be given as follows:

1. Beclomethasone MDI, 2 puffs tid or qid, up to 4 puffs 8 times/day;
2. Flunisolide MDI, 2 puffs bid, up to 4 puffs bid;
3. Triamcinolone MDI, 2 puffs tid to qid.

These agents should **not** be used to treat moderate to severe asthma exacerbation. Cough may be prevented by delivering a beta$_2$ agonist via MDI 10–15 minutes before use of the aerosol corticosteroid. To avoid oral candidiasis, the mouth and pharynx should be rinsed with water after use. If the voice becomes hoarse, the aerosol steroid should be

TABLE 7–9. USE OF CORTICOSTEROIDS IN ACUTE ASTHMA OR COPD EXACERBATION

ASTHMA

IV loading dose: Methylprednisolone 2 mg/kg or about 125 mg (1 vial) IV.
Subsequent doses should be 40–60 mg at least once a day for minimum of 48 hr or until patient is stable. (Optimal dose of corticosteroids is debated by many authors.)

Oral therapy: Keep dosing to 1 time/day or every other day; keep dose as small as necessary; keep treatment course as short as possible.

When patient's condition has stabilized, change IV dose to 40–60 mg prednisone a day or every other day. Steroid dose should be tapered off in 1 wk to 10 days if patient's clinical status allows.

Sample steroid taper (every-day regimen): 60 mg × 2 days, 40 mg × 2 days, 30 mg × 2 days, 20 mg × 2 days, 10 mg × 2 days.

COPD

IV loading dose: Methylprednisolone 0.5 mg/kg IV every 6 hr for 72 hr.

Oral therapy: if possible, corticosteroids should be discontinued after 72 hr of IV treatment; if not, begin 60 mg/day and taper as clinical status allows.

Additional General Concepts (Asthma or COPD)

1. Do not begin taper until patient's condition is stable with the initial starting prednisone dose.
2. Search carefully for exacerbating conditions: environmental irritants, suboptimally used medications, poorly tolerated medications (e.g., beta blockers for hypertension management or beta blocker eye drops for glaucoma).
3. Attempt to get patient on an alternate-day regimen (as dose is reduced on even days, add that dose to odd day, or start taper by tapering dose on even days only).
4. Use inhaled steroids to assist with taper or to help with switching patient to an alternate-day regimen (in the asthmatic).
5. In major stress or surgery, patient will need stress doses of corticosteroids (patient receiving oral steroids longer than 2 wk should be presumed to have hypothalamic-pituitary suppression).

discontinued for 3–5 days. Systemic steroids will generally be necessary during serious illness or surgery (because some suppression of the hypothalamic-pituitary axis still occurs with high-dose aerosol therapy).

E. Cromolyn. Disodium cromoglycate is thought to interfere with immunoglobulin E (IgE)–induced release of mediators from mast cells and basophils. It has no antiinflammatory or bronchodilator activity. Thus, it is an agent for airway hyperactivity prophylaxis. If administered during an asthma exacerbation or COPD flare, it may worsen existing bronchospasm. Cromolyn is available as an inhaled powder, a nebulized solution, and an MDI. Except for causing cough in some patients, it is nearly free of side effects. The use of a beta$_2$ agonist first may prevent cough. Cromolyn is especially effective in treating extrinsic asthma. It is given in a dosage of 2–4 puffs qid or 2 puffs 30 min before contact with an asthma-provoking stimulus. This drug should not be used if the patient is wheezing. Cromolyn should be tried for at least 4 weeks before being considered ineffective.

F. Miscellaneous Agents

1. METHOTREXATE

Experience is accumulating in the use of methotrexate as a steroid-sparing agent in the patient with asthma who is "steroid dependent." It should be used only when all other treatment options (e.g., maximal other drug therapy, optimal environmental control) have been exhausted and by pulmonary specialists familiar with its use. The starting dose is 15 mg/week. Multiple side effects include pulmonary fibrosis.

2. IODINATED GLYCEROL

In stable chronic obstructive bronchitis, iodinated glycerol (Organidin) has recently been shown to improve cough symptoms, patient well-being, and ease in bringing up sputum and to decrease the duration of acute disease exacerbations. The dose is 60 mg qid (Chest 97:75–83, 1990).

3. MAGNESIUM SULFATE

IV magnesium sulfate (1.2 gm over 20 min) has been shown to increase peak expiratory flow rate (PEFR) and decrease hospital admission in patients with asthma exacerbations who do not respond adequately to aggressive use of beta agonists. Consider using this agent in the patient who is "refractory" to acute and aggressive asthma management in the emergency department or clinic. Its exact mechanism of action or duration of action is not known (JAMA 262:1210–1213, 1989).

4. PARALYSIS AND SEDATION

In the **already intubated** asthmatic, paralysis and sedation are sometimes necessary. Patients with status asthmaticus who require intubation are frequently difficult to manage with the ventilator. When high peak airway pressures and respiratory acidosis continue to be difficult to control, sedation with a benzodiazepine (e.g., Lorazepam) and paralysis (e.g., Pavulon) are of assistance.

5. GENERAL INHALATION ANESTHESIA

All of the commonly used inhalation general anesthetics are powerful bronchodilators (avoid halothane because of arrhythmia risk). In the **intubated** asthmatic who is doing poorly despite maximal conventional bronchodilator management, aggressive sedation, paralysis, and general inhalation anesthesia should be considered.

Braun SR, McKenzie WN, Copeland C, et al: A comparison of the effect of ipratropium and albuterol in the treatment of chronic obstructive airway disease. Arch Intern Med 149:544–547, 1989.

Hendeles L: Asthma therapy: State of the art, 1988. J Respir Dis, March 1988, pp 82–107.

Mullarkey MF, Blumenstein BA, Andrade WP, et al: Methotrexate in the treatment of corticosteroid-dependent asthma: A double-blind crossover study. N Engl J Med 318:603–607, 1988.

Oates JA, Wood AJJ: Drug therapy: Ipratropium bromide. N Engl J Med 319:486–494, 1988.

Oates JA, Wood AJJ: A new approach to the treatment of asthma. N Engl J Med 321:1517–1527, 1989.

Paloucek FP, Rodvold VA, et al: Evaluation of theophylline overdoses and toxicities. Ann Emerg Med 17:135–144, 1988.

Shiner RJ, et al: Randomized, double-blind, placebo-controlled trial of methotrexate in steroid-dependent asthma. Lancet 336:137–140, 1990.

Stone RJ, Marvis RM, Parvin CA: Clinical predictions of theophylline blood levels in asthmatic patients. Ann Emerg Med 16:18–24, 1987.

IX. ASTHMA

The physiologic hallmarks of asthma are airway hyperreactivity and inflammation. Associated airway abnormalities include bronchial wall edema, desquamation of ciliated epithelium, and mucus plugging. The result is pulmonary hyperinflation, increased residual volume, increased functional residual capacity, elevated pulmonary artery pressure, V/Q imbalance, increased work of breathing, and hypoxia. Asthma affects as many as 5% of the US population and results in more than 28 million visits to physicians annually. The prevalence, morbidity, and mortality of asthma are increasing in the United States (MMWR 39:493–497, 1990).

Although asthma has been divided into intrinsic and extrinsic types on the basis of whether external agents induced the bronchospastic episodes, most asthmatics have manifestations of both intrinsic and extrinsic disease. Asthma should be considered a syndrome with intrinsic, extrinsic, and occupational aspects. Symptoms include dyspnea, wheezing, and cough. Some asthmatics may have only a chronic cough. Additional characteristics may be seasonal exacerbations, rhinitis, and the triad of chronic sinus disease, nasal polyps, and intolerance of aspirin and other NSAIDs. The differential diagnosis includes left ventricular dysfunction, vocal cord abnormalities, upper airway obstruction, cardiac ischemia, and obstructing endobronchial lesions. The results of the physical examination may be normal in patients with cough-variant asthma or in those who are between acute exacerbations. Patients with a severe asthma attack have tachycardia, tachypnea, diaphoresis, accessory muscle use, pulsus paradoxus (if greater than 18 mm Hg, the attack is life threatening), prolonged expiratory phase, and diffuse wheezing.

A. Laboratory Studies. Routine work-up may reveal peripheral blood eosinophilia and an elevated total IgE level.

1. **PULMONARY FUNCTION TESTS (PFTs)**
   Usually a reversible air-flow obstruction will be demonstrated. If results of the PFTs are normal, inhalational challenge to methacholine to reveal air-flow obstruction and airway hyperactivity may be necessary. Severe airway obstruction during an asthma attack is characterized by an FEV_1 of less than 0.8–1.0 L (less than 25% predicted) or a peak expiratory flow rate (PEFR) less than 100 L/minute (less than 20% predicted).

2. **CHEST X-RAYS**
   These should be obtained during the initial work-up for the new asthmatic. Routine films are not required for each asthma exacerbation unless pneumonia is suspected clinically.

3. **ARTERIAL BLOOD GAS**
   With a mild exacerbation, PaO_2 and $PaCO_2$ may be normal or only slightly decreased, but as air flow obstruction worsens, both hypoxia and hypocarbia occur (with resultant respiratory alkalosis). In a life-threatening attack, the work of breathing further increases, respiratory muscles fatigue, and the PCO_2 starts to rise again. When $PaCO_2$

reaches normal (the "crossover" point), a dangerous situation exists: Respiratory acidosis will soon follow, and respiratory arrest is imminent. Nowak and associates (JAMA 249:2043–2046, 1983) found that the measurement of Pao_2, Pco_2, and pH could not reliably distinguish patients requiring admission from those who could be discharged from the emergency room. Patients with an FEV_1 of less than 1 L (25% predicted) or a PEFR of less than 200 L/minute (30% predicted) were at risk for hypercarbia and marked hypoxia. It is in this group of patients that an ABG measurement is most important. Additional tests that may be useful include skin testing and inhalational challenge.

B. Therapy. There are 3 components in the treatment of asthma: environmental control, pharmacologic therapy for air flow obstruction and inflammation, and immunotherapy. The goal in treatment is to manage acute exacerbations aggressively, minimize the number of exacerbations, and minimize the number of medications the patient must take to achieve these ends. Comprehensive asthma treatment has proved successful in patient care (Ann Intern Med 112:864–871, 1990).

1. ENVIRONMENTAL CONTROL
   Possible precipitants include dust, exercise, chemicals, air pollution, occupational irritants, animal danders, environmental antigens (pollens, molds, and so on), and cigarette smoke. Environmental control is based on identifying precipitants and removing them, when possible, from the environment. Any patient who smokes should be strongly encouraged to stop.

2. PHARMACOTHERAPY
   See also the preceding section, "Pharmacology of Airway Disease."
   a. **Therapy in Acute Attacks.** An acute asthma exacerbation should be regarded as a medical emergency. Treatment depends on the severity of the attack. In a mild exacerbation, an inhaled beta agonist may be all that is necessary (in addition to O_2 supplementation and hydration). Table 7–10 presents emergency management of moderate to severe asthma exacerbations. Antibiotics are useful with fever, purulent sputum, or sinus infection. Choices include trimethoprim-sulfamethoxazole, amoxicillin, amoxicillin-clavulanate, tetracycline, and erythromycin. If the exacerbation requires steroid therapy and the patient has not been taking steroids, oral steroids should be given and the dosage tapered as rapidly as possible (ideally in less than 10 days).
   b. **Long-Term Therapy.** The approach should be "stepped care." Routine use of an inhaled corticosteroid with use of an inhaled beta agonist as needed for "breakthrough" symptoms should be the first-line treatment. Theophylline may also be considered as a second-line or third-line agent. Some patients may even do better with theophylline than with an inhaled beta agonist as a first-line drug. (Theophylline provides more constant 24-hour therapeutic efficacy than an inhaled beta agonist.) If symptoms are still poorly managed, the anticholinergic ipratropium bromide may be added. Cromolyn is an alternative agent to consider, especially in the case with a strong extrinsic component.

TABLE 7–10. EMERGENCY MANAGEMENT OF SEVERE ASTHMA EXACERBATION

Patient with moderate to severe wheezing, and/or marked dyspnea, air hunger, diaphoretic skin, accessory muscle use/sitting up and leaning forward/intercostal retractions/etc.

Administer O_2 (4–5 L/min via nasal prongs minimum) and cardiac monitor

Obtain vital signs, pulsus paradoxus, and FEV_1 (if possible). If FEV_1 less than 1.0 L (25% predicted) consider ABG. Determine theophylline level if patient is receiving theophylline.

Establish IV access

Beta agonist (first drug of choice):
    Albuterol 0.5–1.0 mL (2.5–5.0 mg) in 2.0 mL normal saline (NS) every 20 min, up to 6 doses (if necessary), then dose every 1–2 hr
OR

    Metaproterenol 0.3–0.5 mL (15–25 mg) in 2.5 mL NS every 15–20 min for 3–4 doses (if necessary), then dose every 1–2 hr
OR

    Terbutaline 0.5 mL in 2.5 mL NS every 15–20 min, up to 3 doses (if necessary), then dose every 1–2 hr

If attack is **moderate or severe,** administer 125 mg of methylprednisolone IV along with inhaled beta agonist.

Consider 0.25 mg terbutaline sq, repeating dose in 15–30 min (maximum dose 0.5 mg every 4 hr). Use terbutaline very cautiously in patients with a history of angina or heart disease.

If improvement: Watch serial PFTs and clinical status, and continue beta agonist TX

If no improvement then: Consider **aminophylline:** Loading dose (if patient not receiving theophylline): 5–7 mg/kg IV infused over 20 min (or oral theophylline 6 mg/kg if patient can take po medication). If patient has taken theophylline in past 12 hr, reduce loading dose by 50–75% or wait for theophylline level while using beta agonist aggressively.

ADDITIONAL CONCEPTS

1. In the **severe exacerbation,** begin O_2 and beta agonist therapy immediately while vital signs are being determined and blood work carried out and IV access is being established.
2. The patient **already receiving steroids** should be given **IV methylprednisolone bolus automatically.** In patient with asthma exacerbation who does not readily respond to beta agonist therapy, methylprednisolone should be given without significant delay. In **moderate to severe asthma** attack give **methylprednisolone immediately.**
3. In the patient who does not respond to aggressive beta agonist and corticosteroid treatment consider trying an inhaled anticholinergic agent (e.g., ipratropium bromide or atropine) or IV magnesium sulfate (1.2 gm IV over 20 min).
4. Obtain a **chest x-ray** if patient is febrile, has localizing signs, or does not respond to therapy.
5. Check **aminophylline level** 1–2 hr after maintenance infusion has started (if aminophylline/theophylline is being tried in the setting of beta agonist/methylprednisolone failure). Current evidence strongly suggests that aminophylline/theophylline is unlikely to help in emergent management of asthma exacerbation.
6. Be **prepared to intubate:** Especially worrisome findings include normal or rising P_{CO_2}, respiratory alternans (alternating rib cage and abdominal breathing), abdominal paradox (inward abdominal motion during inspiration), or apparent exhaustion of patient. The anesthesiologist should be called EARLY.
7. In patient who fails to respond despite maximal medical therapy as outlined above, particularly if fatigue is prominent, intubation is very likely. Do it electively rather than after respiratory arrest!
8. **Admission to hospital** is likely, based on recurrent failures of outpatient management, lack of subjective improvement, fatigue, failure of post-treatment FEV_1 to increase by greater than 500 mL or absolute FEV_1 remaining less than 60% predicted, change in mental status, poor social situation, pneumothorax, worrisome ABG findings, or other complicating factors (e.g., pregnancy or pneumonia).
9. **Do not** manage the patient with acute asthma for prolonged periods in the emergency department. If there is minimal improvement within 1–2 hr of arrival, then admit to hospital.

Oral corticosteroids may ultimately become necessary in the patient with persistent breakthrough symptoms who is taking an inhaled corticosteroid, beta agonist, therapeutic theophylline (as gauged by serum levels), or an inhaled anticholinergic and in whom a 4-week trial of cromolyn has failed. Alternate-day prednisone should be used for maintenance, if possible; the dose should be lowered as soon as possible; and trials of inhaled steroids should be used to achieve these ends. Methotrexate is reserved for the patient whose oral dose of corticosteroids cannot be tapered and who is suffering from steroid side effects.

3. IMMUNOTHERAPY
Immunotherapy should be considered in the asthmatic with significant symptoms who is allergic to specific inhaled allergens that cannot be removed from the environment and in whom pharmacotherapy does not provide good control. Immunotherapy is a possible treatment for allergic asthma caused by house dust, house dust mites, mold spores, and pollens from weeds, trees, and grasses.

Corre KA, Rothstein RJ: Assessing severity of adult asthma and need for hospitalization. Ann Emerg Med 10:45–52, 1985.

Dean NC, Brown JK: Status asthmaticus: Early institution of treatment. Postgrad Med 84:103–114, 1988.

Fanta CH: Glucocorticoids in acute asthma. Am J Med 74:845–851, 1983.

Garrity ER Jr, Gross NJ: Prompt management for status asthmaticus. J Respir Dis, May 1987, pp 21–32.

Grammer L: Immunotherapy for rhinitis and asthma: What's new? J Respir Dis, September 1985, pp 91–99.

Haskell RJ: A double blind randomized clinical trial of methylprednisolone in status asthmaticus. Arch Intern Med 143:1324–1327, 1983.

Hendeles L: Asthma therapy: State of the art, 1988. J Respir Dis, March 1988, pp 82–108.

Littenberg B, Gluck EH: A controlled trial of methylprednisolone in the emergency treatment of acute asthma. N Engl J Med 314:150–152, 1986.

X. CHRONIC OBSTRUCTIVE PULMONARY DISEASE (COPD)

In **chronic bronchitis** the patient suffers on most days from increased mucus production with chronic or recurrent productive cough that has persisted for at least 3 months/year for at least 2 successive years. **Emphysema** is a pathologic condition in which there are destructive changes in the alveolar walls, with air-space enlargement distal to the nonrespiratory bronchioles. Both disorders are grouped together under the term **chronic obstructive pulmonary disease (COPD)**. Since both disorders usually are present in the same patient, both result in expiratory flow obstruction, cause dyspnea on exertion, and may be complicated by bronchospasm. Smoking is the major risk factor. Additional etiologic agents include recurrent infection, inhaled irritants, environmental factors, and such genetic factors as alpha$_1$-antitrypsin deficiency (to be considered in the patient with a strong family history of emphysema, when COPD occurs at an early age, and/or if no other risk factors are identified).

A. Laboratory Studies. Chest x-rays are important initially but need be obtained again only if parenchymal infection, neoplasm, or a new cardiopulmonary disorder is suspected. PFTs are useful for diagnosis, prognosis, and assessing response to therapy (see "Pulmonary Tests: Structure and Function"). Spirometry reveals air-flow obstruction: FEV_1/FVC less than 75% predicted, reduced forced expiratory flow (FEF)25–75, increased FRC and RV, and normal or increased total lung capacity (TLC). The $D_{L_{CO}}$ is reduced in patients with emphysema and may be useful in predicting exercise-induced hypoxemia. Spirometry in COPD shows chronic persistent obstructive abnormalities.

B. Therapy. The goals of therapy are to alter the natural history of the disease, avoid complications, prevent and treat acute exacerbations, and teach patients to participate in their own management, with special emphasis on rehabilitation.

  1. GENERAL PRINCIPLES OF MANAGEMENT
  Cessation of smoking is important. Physicians should offer to work with patients, counsel them to select a "stop date," and make referrals as appropriate. Nicotine gum is sometimes successful; sometimes formal smoking cessation programs are effective. Exacerbating conditions should be identified in the home and work place. Coexisting problems, including sinusitis, esophageal reflux, and allergic phenomena, should be diagnosed and treated. Annual influenza vaccination is recommended (generally in the fall) because influenza is associated with greater morbidity and mortality in patients with COPD. Amantadine may be used as an adjuvant to late immunization or in the patient in whom immunization is contraindicated. Pneumococcal vaccine is clearly effective when tested in young immunocompetent patients with a high incidence of pneumococcal disease. In older patients with chronic disease, its usefulness is uncertain. Recent evidence suggests that in immunocompetent elderly patients it is still effective (Ann Intern Med 108:653–657, 1988), and some authors favor administering it routinely before age 55 (before development of immunodebilitating chronic diseases) (Ann Intern Med 108:757–759, 1988).
  Hydration has traditionally been encouraged to prevent the drying of secretions and inspissation of mucus. Excessive polypharmacy should be avoided by routine periodic review of the need for each of a patient's medications.
  Exercise will not improve pulmonary function, but it will increase cardiovascular fitness, improve skeletal muscle efficiency, increase exercise tolerance, and boost the patient's morale and sense of well-being. Routine and progressive exercise (generally walking 3–4 times a week) should be prescribed.
  The aggressive treatment of bacterial infections, especially pneumonia, is crucial. The role of antibiotics in a COPD exacerbation with purulent sputum but no frank pneumonia has been long debated (West J Med 149:347–351, 1988). Anthonisen and colleagues (Ann Intern Med 106:196–204, 1987) found antibiotic use beneficial (compared with placebo) for COPD exacerbation (as defined by increased dyspnea, sputum production, and sputum purulence). Treatment

choices (for 1–3 weeks) include ampicillin, amoxicillin, trimethoprim-sulfamethoxazole, doxycycline, tetracycline, and erythromycin.

The complete patient should be considered. Important issues include depression, dependence, impaired sexual function, and psychosocial dysfunction. The physician should be prepared to assist in their management. Oxygen is a drug, and the goal in its use is to maintain Pao_2 at 55 mm Hg or higher. See "Oxygen Therapy" for which patients with COPD are candidates for home oxygen treatment.

2. **MANAGEMENT OF ACUTE EXACERBATIONS OF CHRONIC OBSTRUCTIVE PULMONARY DISEASE**
   Acute exacerbations are characterized by increasing purulence of sputum, worsening of airway obstruction, and increased work of breathing. Causes include upper respiratory tract infection, sinusitis, pneumonia, irritant exposure, emotional upset, worsening environmental air, and medication noncompliance. Evaluation should proceed rapidly and include routine blood work, bedside spirometry, ABG determination, ECG, and probably chest x-rays. If the patient is taking theophylline, blood levels should be checked.

   a. **Aggressive Bronchodilation.** Beta agonists via nebulizer (metaproterenol, albuterol, and so on) are the drugs of choice initially in COPD exacerbation (see "Pharmacology of Airway Disease").

   b. **Oxygen Supplementation.** This is initiated cautiously, at 1–2 L/minute via nasal cannula. Further O_2 supplementation is based on ABG analysis, watching for worsening hypercarbia and respiratory failure.

   c. **Pharmacotherapy.** Although recent studies question the value of **theophylline** compared with beta agonists alone in COPD exacerbation, it is still reasonable to administer theophylline at therapeutic levels (10–20 $\mu g/mL$) to patients who do not respond quickly to beta agonist administration.

   Antibiotics may be helpful. **Corticosteroids** are appropriate if the patient is currently taking them, has recently discontinued them, or if the exacerbation is not immediately brought under control with aggressive use of a beta agonist and therapeutic theophylline (see "Pharmacology of Airway Disease" for dosage and Tables 7–4, 7–9, and 7–10). **Anticholinergics** are continued in patients already taking these agents. They may also be tried in other patients if standard therapy is not controlling the attack. Unlike the management of chronic stable COPD, in which anticholinergics are the drug of choice, they should **not** be considered the first-line drug in acute exacerbations.

   d. **Respiratory Failure.** Many patients with COPD have chronic respiratory failure. Progressive respiratory acidosis or worsening hypoxia, even with aggressive therapy, is an indication for ICU admission and possible endotracheal intubation.

3. **LONG-TERM MANAGEMENT OF CHRONIC OBSTRUCTIVE PULMONARY DISEASE**

   a. **Anticholinergics.** These drugs are the agents of choice in long-term management of the COPD patient. Ipratropium bromide is preferable to atropine because of a better side effect profile. Advantages over beta agonists include longer duration of action and no evidence for receptor tolerance.

   b. Beta Agonists. Long-acting and beta$_2$-selective agents are the second-line drugs to consider. Oral agents are less well tolerated than inhaled agents.

   c. Theophylline. This agent is only a second- or third-line drug, and the dosage should always be adjusted carefully. The patient must be instructed never to take the medication "as needed" for worsening dyspnea.

   d. Corticosteroids (see "Pharmacology of Airway Disease"). Some patients will achieve benefit from long-term corticosteroid use. A trial of steroids (2–4 weeks) should be considered in the patient whose symptoms and disease are not controlled by maximal doses of an anticholinergic, beta agonist, and theophylline dosed so as to achieve therapeutic levels. The risks of steroids should be reviewed with the patient. The role of inhaled corticosteroids in the care of the COPD patient is not certain. Steroid-induced osteoporosis may be slowed with calcium supplements, an appropriate exercise program, and estrogen in females.

   e. Antibiotics. Empiric antibiotic use may be reasonable for some patients when sputum becomes more purulent.

   f. Iodinated Glycerol (60 mg qid) has recently been shown effective in the management of stable patients with chronic obstructive bronchitis (see "Pharmacology of Airway Disease").

Centers for Disease Control: Recommendations for prevention and control of influenza. Ann Intern Med 105:399–404, 1986.

Francis PB: Chronic obstructive lung disease and acute respiratory failure. Postgrad Med 79:187–196, 1986.

Hughes JR, Gust SW, Keenan RM, et al: Nicotine versus placebo gum in general medical practice. JAMA 261:1300–1305, 1989.

XI. BRONCHIECTASIS

Abnormally dilated bronchi (bronchiectasis) are a consequence of severe damage to the bronchial wall. Several forms of bronchiectasis have been described. Cylindric bronchiectasis is the most common, is potentially reversible, and is characterized by failure of the bronchi to taper in diameter as they branch toward the periphery. Varicose bronchiectasis is a more advanced stage of the disease, with further dilation and distortion of the bronchi so that they resemble varicose veins. Saccular bronchiectasis is the worst and most advanced form of the disease: Actual outpouchings (sacs) form in the bronchial walls, and distal bronchi may even be larger than more proximal ones. Mucociliary clearance and cough are ultimately impaired. Once a common disease because of measles, pertussis, tuberculosis, and poorly treated bacterial pneumonias, bronchiectasis is now rare. Currently it is most often found in patients with cystic fibrosis, alpha$_1$-antitrypsin deficiency, complement deficiencies, neutrophil abnormalities, and immotile cilia syndrome.

A. Diagnosis. Bronchiectasis should be suspected in any patient with a chronic productive cough, especially when blood-streaked sputum and purulent sputum occur intermittently. Predisposing conditions or recurrent discrete pulmonary infections in the same lung zone or zones also should suggest the possibility of bronchiectasis. Childhood is the usual time of onset, with most cases diagnosed before the age of 20. Other symptoms may include sinusitis, dyspnea, and fatigue. The chest x-ray may be nondiagnostic, or display increased or crowded lung markings, honeycombing, atelectasis, or ringlike shadows. CT can be used to confirm the diagnosis. Bronchography is the definitive procedure, but should probably be reserved for surgical candidates only. Anatomic bronchiectasis is common, but symptomatic bronchiectasis is not. Therefore, bronchography should not be performed during an acute pulmonary infection or exacerbation. Bronchoscopy does **not** establish the diagnosis of bronchiectasis.

B. Therapy. All pulmonary irritants, especially cigarette smoking, should be avoided. An influenza vaccination should be provided yearly. In addition, postural drainage, adequate hydration, optimal nutrition, and bronchodilator therapy in bronchospasm are all important. Antibiotics are indicated for disease exacerbations (e.g., increased cough, purulent sputum, hemoptysis, malaise, and weight loss). Oral antibiotics include trimethoprim-sulfamethoxazole, amoxicillin, amoxicillin-clavulanate, tetracycline, and erythromycin. Choices can be guided by sputum culture. The duration of antibiotic therapy should be 1–3 weeks or longer.

Resectional surgery is indicated only in the setting of failed medical therapy, sharply localized bronchiectasis, and no other contraindications to lobectomy. Surgical treatment should not be considered if bronchiectasis is bilateral or involves multiple lobes.

Cystic Fibrosis

Mucoid infection with *Pseudomonas aeruginosa* is characteristic of cystic fibrosis (CF), diagnosable with a sweat chloride test. In the patient with CF and pulmonary infection, antibiotic choice must be culture-guided and aggressive (e.g., aminoglycoside and a third-generation cephalosporin or semisynthetic penicillin, or fluoroquinolone). Ciprofloxacin has been useful as an outpatient oral antibiotic after infection has been brought under control with an inpatient IV regimen. Yearly influenza vaccination, hydration, postural drainage, and chest percussion are also helpful.

Barker AF, Bardara EJ Jr: Bronchiectasis: Update of an orphan disease. Am Rev Respir Dis 137:969–978, 1988.
Newth CJL: Bronchiectasis. *In* Wyngaarden JB, Smith LN Jr (eds): Cecil Textbook of Medicine. 18th ed. Philadelphia, WB Saunders Co, 1988, pp 438–440.

XII. SLEEP APNEA

Sleep apnea may be defined as the cessation of respirations lasting 10 seconds (per apneic event) and occurring at least 5 times/hour during sleep. Episodes of hypopnea (ventilation persists, but tidal volume is less than 50% of the baseline) lasting 10 seconds or more are also significant. Oxygen desaturation occurs during the apneic/hypopneic episodes, with clinical consequences that include increased daytime sleepiness, sleep attacks, morning headaches, and psychosocial dysfunction.

A. **Types.** 3 types of sleep apnea are commonly described:

1. **Central apnea** (Ondine's curse) is rare. The apneic episodes are characterized by the lack of respiratory effort. Diseases that may be associated with central apnea include brain stem infarction, encephalitis, myasthenia gravis, bulbar poliomyelitis, and cervical cordotomy.

2. **Obstructive apnea** is manifested by occlusion of the upper airway in association with normal or augmented respiratory efforts.

3. **Mixed apnea** exists when episodes of central apnea and obstructive apnea occur together.

Sleep apnea is unusual in the otherwise normal patient. Typically there will be preexisting obesity, a narrowed upper airway, a neuromuscular disorder, or hypothyroidism. Causes of airway narrowing include nasal polyps, chronic rhinitis, macroglossia, and adenotonsillar hypertrophy. The differential diagnosis includes nocturnal myoclonus, narcolepsy, insomnia secondary to anxiety or depression, circadian rhythm disturbance, hypothyroidism, CHF, drug use and abuse (including alcohol), nocturnal asthma, esophageal reflux and aspiration, fibrositis, and inappropriate sleep habits.

B. **Diagnosis.** A complete sleep history, medical history, and interview with the partner should be obtained, and a physical examination should be performed. An otorhinolaryngologic evaluation is useful for oropharyngeal abnormalities. Sleep laboratory studies may be relatively simple and involve only nighttime recording of respirations and O_2 saturation (using finger or ear oximetry). More complicated sleep studies include continuous ECG monitoring, measurement of respiratory effort, and complete polysomnographic evaluation (with EEG, electro-oculogram, and submental electromyogram). The diagnosis requires the documentation of apneic or hypopneic episodes and their clinical consequences.

C. **Therapy.** Treatment is dependent on the severity of the disease, the type of apnea, and the patient's daytime symptoms.

1. OBSTRUCTIVE APNEA

Treatment of underlying medical conditions (CHF, COPD, hypertension, and hypothyroidism) and weight reduction are important, but results of voluntary weight reduction are frequently disappointing. Among drugs, alcohol often contributes to the symptomatology of sleep apnea. Additional agents to avoid include barbiturates, narcotics, sedative-hypnotics, and sedating analgesics. Other pharmacologic agents that may complicate the problem are propranolol (decreases the ventilatory response to CO_2), corticosteroids (weight gain), and diuretics (metabolic alkalosis).

Pharmacologic treatment may be useful in mild cases, but effectiveness is limited, and no studies have shown long-term benefit. Options include protriptyline (increases muscle tone and decreases rapid eye movement [REM] sleep), medroxyprogesterone (increases ventilatory drive), and acetazolamide (increases ventilatory drive and corrects metabolic alkalosis). **O_2 supplementation** may prolong apnea episodes, but some patients will benefit. The demonstration of decreased oxygen desaturation during a sleep study with O_2 supplementation is grounds for initiating oxygen therapy. Certain nonpharmacologic treatments may be effective:

1. **Nasal continuous positive airway pressure** will prevent upper airway collapse and has surpassed tracheostomy as the preferred treatment of moderate and severe apnea. Drawbacks, however, include discomfort and noncompliance.

2. **Nocturnal nasopharyngeal airway** produces inconsistent results because the lateral and posterior pharyngeal walls may still collapse and cause obstruction.

3. **Uvulopalatopharyngoplasty** enlarges the pharyngeal space. Only about 50% of patients who undergo the procedure will benefit, and in some patients the condition worsens after surgery.

4. **Tracheostomy** clearly bypasses upper airway obstruction. Drawbacks include the need for an invasive procedure, esthetic considerations, operative morbidity, and postoperative complications.

2. CENTRAL APNEA
Pharmacologic treatment is as described under "Obstructive Apnea," but effectiveness is limited. Severe central apnea with associated central alveolar hypoventilation may require aggressive intervention: tracheostomy with nocturnal mechanical ventilation, negative-pressure ventilation, or a diaphragmatic pacer.

Bradley TD: Diagnosing and assessing obstructive sleep apnea. J Respir Dis, March 1988, pp 32–56.
Kales A: Sleep disorders: Sleep apnea and narcolepsy. Ann Intern Med 106:434–443, 1987.
Kaplan J, Staats BA: Obstructive sleep apnea syndrome. Mayo Clin Proc 65:1087–1094, 1990.
Phillips BA, Shmitt FA, et al: A preliminary report comparing nasal CPAP to nasal oxygen in patients with mild obstructive sleep apnea. Chest 98:325–330, 1990.

XIII. SARCOIDOSIS

Sarcoidosis is a multisystem disease of unknown cause. Its hallmark is noncaseating granuloma. The lung is most frequently involved. Its clinical course is quite variable: 65% of patients have spontaneous resolution with no permanent loss of pulmonary function, while 35% experience tissue destruction and pulmonary fibrosis. Sarcoidosis usually occurs between the ages of 20 and 40 and is 10 times more frequent in American blacks than whites. The estimated incidence is 60 cases per 100,000 population, with 2–3 million Americans developing the disease during their lifetime.

A. Clinical Presentation. The disease is often first detected in an asymptomatic patient with an abnormal chest x-ray. These abnormalities are seen in 85–90% of patients with this disease. Pulmonary symptoms include cough, wheezing, and dyspnea on exertion. Extrathoracic manifestations are shown in Table 7–11.

Evaluation includes a complete history and physical examination, chest x-rays, PFTs, baseline ABG determination, PPD and control skin tests, CBC, and determination of calcium, globulin, and alkaline phosphatase levels. Ophthalmology consultation may be useful. Biopsy of

TABLE 7–11. EXTRATHORACIC MANIFESTATIONS OF SARCOIDOSIS

EXTRATHORACIC LOCATION	APPROXIMATE FREQUENCY	MANIFESTATION
Epidermal	20%	Erythema nodosum, plaquelike lesions of trunk and extremities, periorbital or paranasal vesicular lesions or violaceous plaques
Ocular	>20%	Granulomatous uveitis, enlarged lacrimal glands, nodular conjunctiva, retinal involvement (may lead to blindness)
Nasal	1–4%	Severe nasal obstruction, nasal polyps, occasionally destructive lesions of nasal bones and sinuses
Musculoskeletal	5–15%	Arthralgias, arthritis, myopathy, cystic changes of phalanges, osteoporosis
Cardiac	25% (but often clinically silent)	Ventricular ectopy, first-degree heart block, supraventricular tachycardia, angina, congestive heart failure; sudden death may occur
Neural	5%	Cranial and peripheral neuropathies, headaches, focal abnormalities, seizures, personality changes
Hepatic	Granulomas are seen in 80%, but clinical manifestations of same in only 5–10%	May be asymptomatic or may include abnormal liver function tests, hepatomegaly, right upper quadrant pain, fever, jaundice
Splenic	Palpable splenomegaly in 3–5%	Splenomegaly, thrombocytopenia
Gastric	Rare	Symptoms of sprue or picture mimicking tuberculous peritonitis; sometimes pancreatitis
Genitourinary	<1%	Renal granulomas are usually asymptomatic; when renal failure occurs, look for another cause; epididymitis, hypercalcemia, and nephrolithiasis may occur

Adapted from Israel HL: Recognizing sarcoidosis outside the lungs. J Respir Dis, September 1985, pp 69–87.

easily available extrapulmonary tissue involved in the disease or trans-bronchial biopsy allows tissue diagnosis. Yield from the latter is 60% when the chest film is normal and 85–90% if radiographic abnormalities are apparent. Additional studies sometimes helpful in gauging disease activity include bronchoalveolar lavage, serum angiotensin–converting enzyme levels, and gallium lung scans. Chest x-rays are graded as follows:

Radiographic abnormality grades:

0:	Normal chest radiographs
1:	Lymph node involvement, but no parenchymal abnormalities
2A:	Lymph node and diffuse parenchymal disease
2B:	Diffuse parenchymal disease with no lymph node involvement
3:	Chronic disease with pulmonary fibrosis (e.g., honeycombing)

The **activity** of sarcoidosis may be gauged by the clinical features of the disease, the patient's symptoms, worsening radiographic appearance, and declining values on PFTs. Elevated serum angiotensin–converting enzyme levels, positive results on gallium scanning, and bronchoalveolar lavage abnormalities also reflect disease activity. **Prognosis** is highly variable. The following factors favor a better outlook for the patient: white race; age under 40; normocalcemia; no extrathoracic involvement, erythema nodosum, or arthralgia; improvement since the initial diagnosis; radiographic stage 1; and anterior uveitis (as opposed to posterior uveitis).

B. Therapy. Prednisone is the drug of choice for sarcoidosis even though it does not increase the chance of remission. The goal is to reduce symptoms, alleviate organ dysfunction, and lessen the chance of pulmonary fibrosis. One of many recommended treatment strategies follows (J Respir Dis, December 1985, pp 18–22; April 1986, pp 50–58):

Stage 1 disease: Asymptomatic patients should not be treated (but should be reevaluated in 1 year). If the patient is symptomatic, drug therapy or closer observation (3–4 times/year) should be considered.

Stage 2 disease: Asymptomatic patients should be treated if there is radiographic evidence of disease progression or if the x-ray appearance does not improve after 1 year and there are no relative or absolute contraindications to corticosteroid therapy. The symptomatic patient should be treated.

Stage 3 disease: If active alveolitis is present, this stage of the disease should be treated whether the patient is symptomatic or not.

Initial prednisone dosage is 40–80 mg every other day. Daily therapy should be started if breakthrough symptoms occur on the off day or if inflammation of extrathoracic organs needs immediate attention. The response to therapy is evaluated by amelioration of symptoms, change in chest x-ray, improvement in PFT values, decrease in elevated serum angiotensin–converting enzyme levels, and/or improved appearance on gallium scans. The dose of prednisone may be increased to as much as 120 mg every other day if the response to 80 mg every other day is unsatisfactory. If there is no response in 6 months, the drug dose should be tapered and the drug discontinued. If response has occurred, the dose should be tapered to the lowest level that continues to suppress granulomatous alveolitis. Every 6–8 months, the need for continued prednisone therapy should be reassessed by decreasing the dose while monitoring for increased disease activity.

Fanburg BC: Sarcoidosis. *In* Wyngaarden JB, Smith LH Jr (eds): Cecil Textbook of Medicine. 18th ed. Philadelphia, WB Saunders Co, 1988, pp 451–457.
Israel HL: Recognizing sarcoidosis outside the lungs. J Respir Dis, September 1985, pp 69–87.
Rohatgi PK, Goldstein RA: Does your patient with sarcoidosis require treatment? J Respir Dis, December 1985, pp 18–22.
Rohatgi PK, Goldstein RA: Sarcoidosis: Treat or leave well enough alone? J Respir Dis, April 1986, pp 50–58.

XIV. PULMONARY THROMBOEMBOLISM

Pulmonary embolism (PE) involves pulmonary vascular obstruction by a displaced thrombus, air bubble, or other particulate matter. The most common precipitant is deep venous thrombosis (DVT). PE is responsible for about 10–20% of all hospital deaths, including up to 15% of postoperative deaths, and is the leading cause of pregnancy-related maternal mortality in the United States. The 3 major risk factors linked with DVT are blood stasis, endothelial injury, and hypercoagulable states. Patients at increased risk for DVT and PE include those with CHF, trauma, surgery (especially hip, knee, and prostate surgery), age over 50, previous history of thromboembolism, malignant disease, infection, inactivity or obesity, pregnancy, and oral contraceptive use. Hypercoagulable states may be seen with anti-thrombin III deficiency, protein C deficiency, protein S deficiency, defective fibrinolysis, or abnormal levels of plasminogen and/or plasminogen activator.

A. **Deep Venous Thrombosis.** Signs and symptoms include tenderness, leg pain, swelling (a difference in leg circumference of 1.4 cm in men and 1.2 cm in women is significant), and warmth. One also may see a positive Homans' sign, subcutaneous venous distention, discoloration, a palpable cord, and/or pain upon placement of a blood pressure cuff around the calf (considerable pain with the cuff inflated to 160–180 mm Hg). Unfortunately, at least one half of the cases of DVT are asymptomatic, and in up to 30% of patients with clinical evidence of DVT, no DVT is demonstrable.

1. DIAGNOSIS
   The choice of diagnostic tests depends on the location of the suspected DVT and local experience and expertise.

a. **Contrast Venography.** The diagnostic "gold standard." Complications, however, include induced thrombosis in up to 3–4% of patients. The postvenographic syndrome (leg pain, swelling, and tenderness) occurs in as many as 24% of patients.

b. **Doppler Ultrasound.** In this operator-dependent study, proximal venous thrombi are detected with an accuracy of about 90%, but venous thrombi in the calf are detected only 50% of the time. False-negative studies may occur with nonocclusive proximal thrombi.

c. **Real-Time Ultrasound.** Also an operator-dependent study, preliminary data indicate that it is excellent in detecting femoral and popliteal DVTs (mean sensitivity of 96% and mean specificity of 99%). It can also diagnose conditions that may mimic DVT (e.g., Baker's cyst and calf hematoma). It may miss calf DVTs and iliac vein DVTs (Arch Intern Med 149:1731–1734, 1989).

d. **Radioiodinated Fibrinogen.** Diagnostic accuracy as high as 92%, effective in detecting DVTs in the calf. It is not reliable in detecting pelvic DVTs. The test takes 1–2 days to perform.

e. **Impedance Plethysmography.** Sensitivity as high as 94% for proximal thrombi with specificity as high as 98%. The accuracy for calf thrombi is only about 30%.

f. **Additional Studies.** These include thermography (high sensitivity but low specificity) and radionuclide venography (good sensitivity but poor specificity, and fair effectiveness in detecting calf thrombi).

2. **THERAPY**

a. **Heparin.** This remains the treatment of choice in acute DVT. It prevents further propagation of the thrombus but does not reduce the immediate embolic risk or enhance clot lysis. The therapy for DVT with heparin and warfarin (Coumadin) is described in Table 7–12. Contraindications to heparin include active internal bleeding, intracranial bleeding, and intracranial lesions predisposed to bleeding.

b. **Inferior Vena Caval Barriers.** These are useful if anticoagulation is contraindicated. Possibilities include filters placed by internal jugular or femoral approach (with fluoroscopic guidance) and actual surgical interruption. The former are preferred. The left ovarian or testicular vein enters the left renal vein, so ligation is necessary if pelvic thrombosis is present.

c. **Thrombolytic Therapy.** Another viable option for DVT, this therapy can produce more rapid and complete clot lysis and may reduce the risk of venous hypertension and the post-thrombotic syndrome. This treatment should be considered when DVT is confirmed, the clot is less than 7 days old, and there are no contraindications to lytic therapy. Streptokinase, urokinase, or tissue plasminogen activator may be used. See "Pulmonary Embolism" below for dosages and contraindications.

B. **Pulmonary Embolism.** Signs and symptoms are nonspecific. Dyspnea, pleuritic chest pain, and cough are most common (seen in 81%, 73%,

TABLE 7–12. THERAPY FOR DEEP VENOUS THROMBOSIS WITH HEPARIN AND WARFARIN (COUMADIN)

Obtain baseline prothrombin time (PT), partial thromboplastin time (PTT), hematocrit, and platelet count
↓
Loading dose of *heparin* (5000 U) IV, followed by maintenance infusion of approximately 1200 U/hr
↓
Recheck PTT after 4–6 hr and as necessary thereafter (at least once per day); adjust heparin dose to maintain the PTT 1.5–2.0 × control (usual heparin dose is 800–1200 U/hr, but some patients may need 2000 U/hr)
↓
Warfarin (Coumadin) should be started simultaneously with heparin therapy; begin with 4–10 mg/day; the PT must be checked daily, and the goal is a PT 1.2–1.5 × control (total PT, 14–17 sec) or INR 2.0–3.0
↓
Even when the PT is "therapeutic," full anticoagulation effect from warfarin will not be achieved for 3–5 more days; heparin, therefore, should not be stopped until 4–5 days of *joint therapy* have been completed
↓
Warfarin should be continued for about 3 mo or until risk factors have been eliminated

Additional key therapeutic points
1. The patient should not ambulate for the first 7 days of treatment to avoid dislodgment of nonadherent clots.
2. Platelet count should be checked periodically while patient is receiving heparin because about 10% of patients will suffer heparin-induced thrombocytopenia.
3. Multiple drugs can interact with warfarin. All over-the-counter medications and prescription drugs should be checked for a possible interaction before being used.
4. Intermittent sq *calcium heparin* every 12 hr can be used instead of continuous IV heparin. Again, PTT should be maintained at 1.5–2.0 × control.

Data from Linn BJ, Mazza JJ, Friedenberg WR: Treatment of venous thromboembolic disease. Postgrad Med 79:171–180, 1986; Senior RM: Pulmonary embolism. *In* Wyngaarden JB, Smith LH Jr (eds.): Cecil Textbook of Medicine. 18th ed. Philadelphia, W. B. Saunders Co., 1988, pp 442–450.

and 60% of patients, respectively). The patient may also suffer from hemoptysis, apprehension, tachypnea (80% of patients), and fever (temperature as high as 39.5°C). As many as one half of patients have no readily apparent predisposing condition.

1. DIAGNOSIS

a. Arterial Blood Gas. Although ABG determination is routine, blood gas abnormalities are nonspecific. As many as 13% of patients with confirmed PE will have a Pao$_2$ greater than 80 mm Hg. Respiratory alkalosis will be seen in more than 80% of patients, and the alveolar–arterial oxygen gradient (A-a gradient) may be helpful. In the normal young person without pulmonary disease, the A-a gradient is 5–10 mm Hg. If PE is suspected, a normal A-a gradient makes the diagnosis highly unlikely (Chest 95:48–51, 1989).

b. **Electrocardiogram.** ECG findings are also nonspecific. About 75% of patients with PE will have sinus tachycardia. Other findings include right-sided strain, right-axis deviation, right bundle branch block (RBBB), and atrial arrhythmias.

c. **Pulmonary Scintigraphy.** The most useful screening test. A normal or near normal V/Q scan makes the diagnosis of PE unlikely.

d. **Pulmonary Angiography.** The definitive test in the diagnosis of pulmonary thromboembolism. With refinements in use and technique of this test, morbidity is low and mortality is 0.25%. Pulmonary angiography is indicated when anticoagulation has failed and surgical therapy is being considered; in patients with noninvasive studies suggestive of PE but who are not anticoagulation candidates; in patients with a high clinical likelihood for PE but a non–high probability V/Q scan; when lytic therapy is being considered.

e. **Additional Concept.** With V/Q scans of low or intermediate probability, sometimes one can demonstrate a DVT noninvasively before resorting to pulmonary angiography. Approximately 70% of patients with pulmonary thromboembolism will have coexisting thrombi of the deep veins of the thighs or pelvis. The treatment of both DVT and PE is essentially the same: anticoagulation.

2. **THERAPY**

a. **Heparin.** The classic treatment of choice in the acute phase of DVT or PE. Approach is outlined in Table 7–12. For an acute PE, some recommend a larger initial bolus of heparin (10,000–20,000 U in an IV bolus) followed 2 hours later by continuous heparin infusion.

b. **Inferior Vena Caval Barriers.** These should be considered (1) when the diagnosis of PE is confirmed but anticoagulation therapy is contraindicated or has failed or (2) when the patient has already suffered a massive, life-threatening PE. With devices such as the Greenfield filter, the recurrence rate for PE may be reduced to as low as 5%.

c. **Surgical Embolectomy** has a controversial role in the treatment of PE. Mortality is at least 25%.

d. **Thrombolytic Therapy.** Hemodynamically unstable patients improve more rapidly with lytic therapy than with heparin. One study demonstrated that capillary blood volume and DL_{CO} were more nearly normal at 2 weeks and at 1 year with thrombolytic therapy than with heparin (mortality was not different between the 2 groups). Thrombolytic therapy should be strongly considered in confirmed PE with hemodynamic instability.

(1). **Streptokinase.** Streptokinase is given in an IV load of 250,000 U over 30 min, followed by a maintenance infusion of 100,000 U/hr for 24 hours. Side effects include hemorrhage requiring transfusion in about 4% of patients, oozing from puncture wounds, fever in 20%, and marked allergic reactions in 6%. Some recommend giving 100 mg hydrocortisone IV to minimize allergic phenomena.

(2). Urokinase. Urokinase may be given in an IV load of 4400 U/kg over 10 min, followed by a maintenance infusion of 4400 U/kg/hour for 12 hours. Side effects include about the same hemorrhage rate as seen with streptokinase, but allergic reactions are rare.

(3). Tissue Plasminogen Activator. Dose: 100 mg infused through a peripheral vein over 2 hours (50 mg/hr).

(4). Laboratory Monitoring. With lytic therapy, a bleeding time, thrombin time (TT), PTT, and PT should be checked before the start of treatment. 4 hours after the initial bolus, TT should be obtained to confirm the attainment of a lytic state (TT does not need to be checked if tissue plasminogen activator [TPA] is used). All lytic therapy should be followed by administration of a heparin bolus and continuous infusion (pushing the PTT to 1.5–2.0 times the control value).

(5). Contraindications. Absolute contraindications include active internal bleeding, severe cerebrovascular disease, stroke, intracranial surgery, eye surgery, or head injury within the preceding 2 months. Relative contraindications apply to those patients who are within 10 days of major surgery; those who have had trauma, organ biopsy, cardiopulmonary resuscitation with rib fractures, or an invasive diagnostic procedure; or those who are pregnant or have severe hypertension or a prior coagulopathy.

e. Prevention of DVT and PE. Given the mortality of PE and the difficulties involved in its clinical diagnosis, prevention of DVT and PE is crucial. Fully one third of patients over age 40 who have major surgery or an acute MI will suffer DVT, and this number is even higher following hip, knee, or prostate surgery. Pulmonary thromboembolism occurs in 5–10% of patients who have undergone orthopedic procedures of the hip or knee.

(1). Heparin. Heparin is the most common and popular agent for prophylaxis. The usual dose is 5000 U SQ every 8–12 hours. Heparin is effective in patients undergoing general surgery who are at high risk for DVT or PE and patients with MI or CHF. For general surgery patients, heparin administration should be started 2 days before the operation. Despite fears regarding this practice, clinically or statistically significant increased bleeding is not seen. This heparin regimen may not be effective in patients with urologic or gynecologic cancer or traumatic hip fracture or in those undergoing hip surgery or prostatectomy. Adjusted-dose heparin should be considered in the patient undergoing elective total hip replacement. Heparin should be started 2 days before the operation, and the PTT should be pushed to the upper limit of normal. Apparently this practice still does not significantly increase the bleeding risk, and it is effective. Heparin should not be used for DVT or PE prophylaxis in patients with a high risk of hemorrhage during general surgery, in patients undergoing intracranial or eye surgery, or in patients with spinal cord trauma.

(2). Dextran. Probably effective but associated with a fairly high risk of inducing pulmonary edema in the elderly, allergic reactions, and excessive bruising. Dextran 40 is administered IV, 500 mL preoperatively and then every other day until the patient is ambulatory. Candidates for dextran therapy include patients undergoing surgery for a fractured hip and those having elective total hip replacement.

(3). Two-Step Warfarin. Oral warfarin should be given 10 days before the planned procedure, prolonging the PT by 1.5–3.5 seconds. After surgery, the warfarin dose is increased until the PT is 1.3–1.5 times the control value. Candidates include patients undergoing a general surgical procedure who have known malignant disease or a history of prior DVT. Two-step warfarin is also reasonable in patients scheduled for elective total hip replacement and in those with a fractured hip for which surgery is planned.

(4). Pneumatic Calf Compression. It should be begun before surgery and continued until the patient is fully ambulatory. It is the prophylaxis of choice in patients undergoing total hip replacement, major knee surgery, prostate surgery, and neurosurgery, and in women undergoing cesarean section. Gradient elastic stockings may be used in conjunction with pneumatic calf compression. Ineffective methods of prophylaxis include use of aspirin and simple compressive stockings. When prophylaxis is contraindicated, it is appropriate to screen high-risk patients to detect subclinical DVT early. Screening may include impedance plethysmography, Doppler ultrasound, or radiolabeled fibrinogen scanning.

Doyle DJ, Turpie AG, Hirsh J, et al: Adjusted subcutaneous heparin or continuous intravenous heparin in patients with acute deep venous thrombosis. Ann Intern Med 107:441–445, 1987.

Hull RD, et al: Effectiveness of intermittent pneumatic leg compression for preventing deep vein thrombosis after total hip replacement. JAMA 263:2313–2317, 1990.

Hull RD, et al: Serial impedance plethysmography in pregnant patients with clinically suspected deep-vein thrombosis: Clinical validity of negative findings. Ann Intern Med 112:663–667, 1990.

Kahn D, Bushnell DL, et al: Clinical outcome of patients with a "low probability" of pulmonary embolism on ventilation-perfusion lung scan. Arch Intern Med 149:377–379, 1989.

Levine MN: Hemorrhagic complications of long-term anticoagulant therapy. Chest 89:165–255, 1986.

Linn BJ, Mazza JJ, Friedenberg WR: Treatment of venous thromboembolic disease. Postgrad Med 79:171–180, 1986.

PIOPED Investigators: Value of the ventilation/perfusion scan in acute pulmonary embolism: Results of the Prospective Investigation of Pulmonary Embolism Diagnosis (PIOPED). JAMA 263:2794–2795, 1990.

Valenzuela TD: Pulmonary embolism. Ann Emerg Med 17:209–213, 1988.

XV. ADULT RESPIRATORY DISTRESS SYNDROME

The adult respiratory distress syndrome (ARDS) is a clinical diagnosis based on: (1) history of a preceding associated event (pulmonary or nonpulmonary) with rapid onset of respiratory failure; (2) diffuse bilateral pulmonary infiltrates on the chest x-ray; (3) no elevation of pulmonary capillary wedge pressure (noncardiogenic pulmonary edema); and (4) decreased Pao_2 refractory to O_2 supplementation (typically, the Pao_2 is less than 50 mm Hg, with an Fio_2 greater than 0.6). ARDS is the end point of a variety of disease processes, including physical trauma, sepsis, aspiration of gastric contents having low pH, drug or toxin exposure, diffuse pneumonia, oxygen toxicity, CNS disease, smoke and irritant gas inhalation, fat embolism, pancreatitis, uremia, burns, cardiopulmonary bypass, and multiple transfusions. ARDS has an average mortality of 65%. If ARDS is secondary to sepsis or a neoplastic process, the mortality may be as high as 85–90%. In the elderly nearly 100% mortality is the rule.

A. Management. The goals of therapy are to correct hypoxia, to identify and treat the cause of the syndrome, and to prevent complications.

1. **CORRECTION OF HYPOXIA**
   Because of the large shunt fraction, hypoxia is refractory to simple oxygen supplementation in ARDS. Every attempt should be made to maintain the Pao_2 >55 mm Hg (90% oxyhemoglobin saturation) while keeping the Fio_2 < 0.6–0.7. At the same time, an adequate cardiac output (>2.2 L/min/m²) is essential. To achieve these ends, endotracheal intubation, mechanical ventilation, and positive end-expiratory pressure (PEEP) are usually necessary.
   To avoid **barotrauma**, the minimal level of PEEP that allows an Fio_2 less than 0.6–0.7 and maintains cardiac output should be used. A decrease in cardiac output of >15–20% from baseline is probably unacceptable. Initial ventilator settings should allow for a tidal volume to help prevent atelectasis and worsening shunt (10 ml/kg is a good starting tidal volume). **Pulmonary barotrauma** is a frequent complication. Risk factors include high tidal volumes, high inflation and inspiratory airway pressures with low lung or chest wall compliance, and probably PEEP. The lowest level of PEEP necessary to provide adequate tissue oxygenation should be used; with poor pulmonary compliance, inspiratory pressures should be kept below 50 cm H_2O if possible (peak inspiratory pressure is less important as a cause of barotrauma in patients with marked airway obstruction) (Am Rev Respir Dis 137:1463–1493, 1988).
   Aggressive sedation (and possibly pharmacologic paralysis) may be needed to optimize mechanical ventilation, reduce airway pressures, and minimize oxygen consumption by the patient. Optimal **volume management** keeps the patient relatively volume depleted without compromising cardiac output, cerebral perfusion, or renal function.

2. **SEARCH FOR THE CAUSE OF ARDS**
   One cause of ARDS does not rule out a second or third cause (e.g., the patient with acute pancreatitis, pneumonia, or sepsis). Left ventricular dysfunction as a cause of pulmonary edema and diffuse pulmonary infection should be excluded. Once the cause or causes of ARDS have been determined, specific therapy for each should be implemented.

3. PREVENTION OF COMPLICATIONS

The patient with ARDS may have an ICU course that lasts 4–6 weeks or longer. During this time, mortality is usually not directly due to ARDS and hypoxia per se, but is secondary to sepsis or other complications. The following guidelines may be helpful in preventing complications:

a. **Infection** risk may be reduced by careful hand-washing, respiratory equipment care, regular IV access changes, and early use of antibiotics when required.

b. **GI hemorrhage** may be reduced by using sucralfate. Some authors have suggested that raising the gastric pH (with histamine$_2$ [H$_2$] blockers or antacids) may increase the risk of nosocomial pneumonia (N Engl J Med 317:1376–1382, 1987).

c. **Renal failure** risk can be reduced by careful selection and monitoring of drugs (e.g., aminoglycosides), optimal fluid management, and maintenance of adequate oxygenation.

d. **Prophylaxis of PE** should be implemented.

e. **Exercise** is important in boosting the patient's morale and in minimizing deconditioning. Regular physical therapy, isometrics, and even assisted walking should probably be used when possible.

f. **Nutrition** requirements may be high, but supplementation also is associated with complications (Am Rev Respir Dis 137:1463–1493, 1988). When possible, enteral feeding is the method of choice. If carbohydrate intake is too high, however, increased CO$_2$ production may complicate ventilation and respiratory management. If this becomes a problem, an increasing proportion of fat caloric intake should be provided.

g. **Emotional support** is crucial. This should be provided not only by family, friends, social workers, and chaplains but also by medical and nursing staff.

h. **Sleep** should be encouraged. A 6-hour period of nighttime rest is necessary. (One may consider using short-acting sedatives, minimizing interruptions, turning down lights, and providing eye shades and ear plugs.)

4. PROGNOSIS

The course of the patient with ARDS is usually prolonged and plagued by frequent setbacks (e.g., infection, renal dysfunction, and barotrauma). Of the patients who survive, however, as many as 85% may have nearly normal pulmonary function 1 year later.

Pingleton SK: Complications of acute respiratory failure. Am Rev Respir Dis 137:1463–1493, 1988.

Raffin TA: ARDS: Mechanisms and management. Hosp Pract 22:65–80, 1987.

Ward PA, Johnson KJ, Till G: Current concepts regarding adult respiratory distress syndrome. Ann Emerg Med 14:724–728, 1985.

XVI. ACUTE RESPIRATORY FAILURE AND MECHANICAL VENTILATION

Acute respiratory failure (ARF) is characterized by the inability to achieve adequate oxygenation or ventilation or both: Pao$_2$ less than

50 mm Hg or $Paco_2$ greater than 50 mm Hg are criteria frequently used to define respiratory failure.

Dysfunction of any component of the ventilatory system may result in respiratory failure: brain, spinal cord, neurovascular system, thorax, pleura, upper airway, cardiovascular system, lower airway, and alveoli. Diseases that may account for respiratory failure include bulbar poliomyelitis, drug overdose, cerebrovascular accident, Guillain Barré syndrome, spinal cord trauma, multiple sclerosis, myasthenia gravis, pneumothorax, trauma, flail chest, epiglottitis, laryngeal edema, tracheal obstruction from tumor or foreign body, pulmonary contusion, CHF, ARDS, COPD, asthma, pneumonia, and interstitial lung disease.

A. **Approach to Treatment** depends on the underlying pathophysiology. There are 5 basic mechanisms:

1. **DECREASED** Fio_2 may occur with exposure to high altitude or suicide attempts.

2. **INTRAPULMONARY ARTERIOVENOUS SHUNT** occurs with perfusion of nonventilated alveoli. The Pao_2 is decreased; if the shunt is large, even great increases in supplemental O_2 will not correct the hypoxia (e.g., as seen in ARDS).

3. **ALVEOLAR HYPOVENTILATION** will occur in the setting of decreased tidal volume and/or increased VD/VT. The Pao_2 is decreased, the $Paco_2$ is increased, and the A-a gradient is normal.

4. **DIFFUSION IMPAIRMENT** as a cause of hypoxemia is unusual. It may be important, however, if the Fio_2 is decreased (e.g., at high altitude) or following extreme physical exertion (e.g., a patient with interstitial lung disease during exercise). The calculated A-a gradient will be abnormal.

5. **V/Q IMBALANCE** is the most common cause of arterial hypoxemia. V/Q imbalance may be divided into low V/Q and high V/Q regions. Low V/Q regions are similar to intrapulmonary arterial-venous shunting, and high V/Q regions are similar to alveolar hypoventilation. Low V/Q abnormalities result in arterial hypoxemia, and the calculated A-a gradient will be increased.

An important method of determining whether respiratory failure is ventilatory (hypoventilation) or nonventilatory (disease of the lung parenchyma) is the alveolar air equation (Table 7–13). Other useful equations are also given.

B. **Clinical Manifestations** of respiratory failure depend on the etiology of the disease, on the duration and progression of the failure, and on the degree of concomitant hypoxemia and hypercarbia.

1. **HYPOXEMIA**

Acute symptoms are usually secondary to CNS dysfunction and include dyspnea, disorientation, confusion, delirium, and finally coma

TABLE 7–13. USEFUL EQUATIONS IN PULMONARY MEDICINE

Alveolar air equation

$$PA_{O_2} = FiO_2 (P_B - 47) - PaCO_2/0.8$$

where PA_{O_2} = the alveolar pressure of O_2
 FiO_2 = the fraction inspired concentration of O_2 (0.21–1.00)
 47 = the pressure of water vapor in mm Hg at 100% saturation
 P_B = the atmospheric pressure (at sea level = 760 mm Hg).
With this equation, the A-a gradient can be determined ($PA_{O_2} - Pa_{O_2}$). In the normal individual who is young to middle aged, the A-a gradient should be 5–15 mm Hg. With age, the gradient increases.

Dead space equation

$$V_D/V_T \text{ (the fraction of each breath wasted in "dead" space)}$$
$$= (PaCO_2 - PECO_2)/PaCO_2$$

where $PECO_2$ = pressure of CO_2 in mixed exhaled gas. Normally, the V_D/V_T is equal to 24.6 + 0.17 (age in years).

Shunt equation

$$Q_S/Q_T = \text{the percentage of blood flow being shunted}$$
$$= (Cc_{O_2} - Ca_{O_2})/(Cc_{O_2} - Cv_{O_2}) \times 100$$

where C denotes content of O_2 in blood and c, a, and v denote capillary, arterial, and venous, respectively. End-capillary PO_2 is estimated by calculated alveolar O_2 (as in the alveolar air equation). The normal shunt fraction is less than 7%. If the Pa_{O_2} is greater than 150 mm Hg, a shunt of less than 25% can be approximated when the patient is breathing pure O_2 by dividing the A-a O_2 difference by 20.

Oxygen content equation

$$Ca_{O_2} = 0.139 \text{ (Hgb) (\% sat)} + 0.003 (Pa_{O_2})$$

where Hgb = grams of hemoglobin per 100 ml of blood and
 % sat = per cent of hemoglobin saturation.

Compliance equations

Dynamic compliance = tidal volume/(peak airway pressure − positive end-expiratory pressure [PEEP])

Peak airway pressure is determined from the ventilator by looking at the maximal airway pressure attained during a ventilated breath. The normal dynamic "compliance" of a mechanically ventilated patient is 50–80 ml/cm H_2O.

Static compliance = tidal volume/(static pressure − PEEP)

Static pressure is determined by momentarily occluding the exhalation tubing of the ventilator before the patient exhales and looking at the airway pressure monitor. Normal static compliance in a mechanically ventilated patient is 60–100 ml/cm H_2O.

and death. Patients may become irritable and restless before loss of consciousness. Signs of hypoxemia include diaphoresis, tachypnea, tachycardia, cyanosis (if severe hypoxemia is present), and cardiac dysrhythmias.

2. HYPERCARBIA
Acute symptoms include headache, somnolence, dizziness, and eventually coma. Signs include diaphoresis, hyperventilation or hypoventilation, muscular twitching, tachycardia, and, in some cases, papilledema.

C. Management

1. GOALS OF TREATMENT

1. Restore adequate gas exchange (maintain the Pa_{O_2} >55 mm Hg, with at least 90% hemoglobin saturation);
2. Achieve the lowest Fi_{O_2} necessary for sufficient oxygenation (keep $Fi_{O_2} \leq 0.50$);
3. Correct the pH;
4. Treat the primary disorder responsible for the respiratory failure;
5. Prevent complications.

The Pa_{O_2} should be normalized only in the patient with a usually normal Pa_{CO_2}. The individual with chronic CO_2 retention and chronic lung disease should be allowed to maintain his or her usual Pa_{CO_2}.
The use of O_2 supplementation, adequate hydration, and bronchodilators, as well as the treatment of the primary problem (e.g., pneumonia, COPD exacerbation, and CHF), has been presented elsewhere in this manual. Criteria for intubation are shown in Table 7–14.

2. MECHANICAL VENTILATION
Mechanical ventilation provides the "bellows" function of the respiratory system while the primary disease process is being treated. Most presently in use are positive pressure systems.

TABLE 7–14. CRITERIA FOR ENDOTRACHEAL INTUBATION

Apnea

Inability to clear secretions (intubation may allow for more aggressive and frequent airway suctioning)

Progressive hypoventilation and worsening respiratory acidosis despite aggressive medical management ($Pa_{CO_2} > 50$ mm Hg with a pH < 7.3)

Inability to maintain $Pa_{O_2} \geq 55$ mm Hg despite an $Fi_{O_2} > 0.5$–0.6

Loss of airway protective mechanisms (e.g., absent gag reflex)

When heavy sedation or paralysis of the patient is necessary for treatment (e.g., general surgery) or diagnosis (e.g., pelvic examination performed with the patient under general anesthesia)

When respiratory failure is imminent (patient fatigued or exhausted, respiratory rate >30–40/min, inspiratory pressure <25 cm H_2O)

a. **Types of Positive-Pressure Ventilators**
    (1). Pressure-Cycled. Gas flows into the patient until a predetermined airway pressure is reached. Tidal volume, therefore, is not constant.
    (2). Time-Cycled. Gas flows for a certain percentage of time during the ventilatory cycle.
    (3). Volume-Cycled. The most common ventilators in use today. The tidal volume is determined, and a fixed tidal volume is delivered with each breath. The discussion below is limited to volume-cycled ventilators.
b. **Ventilator Modes.** Many are used; some of the most common are:
    (1). Controlled. The machine delivers a breath at a fixed rate irrespective of the patient's effort or demands.
    (2). Assist-Controlled. The machine senses a patient's efforts to breathe and delivers a fixed tidal volume with each effort, in addition to providing a predetermined "back-up" rate if the patient's inspiratory efforts are infrequent.
    (3). Intermittent Mandatory Ventilation (IMV). Breaths are delivered by the machine, but the patient may also breathe (without machine assistance) spontaneously.
    (4). Pressure Support. The patient breathes spontaneously and determines ventilator rate; a positive pressure effect is maintained by the ventilator (to compensate for endotracheal tube resistance). Therefore, tidal volume will be determined by "inflation" pressure and the patient's lung-thorax compliance.
c. **Ventilator Settings**
    (1). Tidal Volume. Tidal volume is the volume of gas delivered with each machine-powered breath. The value set on the machine is greater than the volume of gas the patient actually receives because of the distention of plastic tubing with each breath. A reasonable initial setting is 10–15 ml/kg. In the patient with COPD, 10 ml/kg is preferred to avoid hyperinflation and the risk of barotrauma.
    (2). Sighs are not used frequently because of the large tidal volumes used (a tidal volume of 10–15 ml/kg is about twice a person's "normal" tidal volume). If a small tidal volume is used (less than 8 ml/kg), then a sigh should be set at 1.5–2.0 times the tidal volume every 5–10 minutes to prevent atelectasis.
    (3). Respiratory Rate. Respiratory rate is the guaranteed rate the machine will deliver if the patient is completely apneic. A typical rate is 12–16 breaths/minute. Changes in the respiratory rate may be guided by the following equation:

New respiratory rate = old rate × (old Pa_{CO_2}/desired Pa_{CO_2})

    (4). Flow Rates. Flow rates should be set so that expiratory time exceeds inspiratory time, and a good rule of thumb is to give

the patient twice as much time to exhale as to inhale. In the setting of marked air flow obstruction, exhalation time should be increased more. Usually, flow rates between 40 and 80 L/minute will be adequate.

(5). *Sensitivity*. This is the amount of negative pressure the patient must generate before the machine will deliver an assisted breath in the assist-controlled mode. The usual initial setting is 2–3 cm H_2O.

(6). *Oxygen Concentration*. Adjustments to Fio_2 should be guided by blood gas analysis. The Fio_2 should be the lowest necessary to achieve adequate oxygenation. When mechanical ventilation is first instituted, however, 100% O_2 is often administered (unless it is known that a lower Fio_2 will be sufficient).

(7). *Humidifiers*. Gas delivered by the endotracheal route should be 100% humidified.

(8). *Monitors and Alarms*. Two of the most important include pressure limit (usually set about 5–10 cm H_2O above the pressure necessary to deliver the desired tidal volume) and exhaled tidal volume (to detect decreased tidal volumes being delivered to the patient because of ventilator malfunction or leaks in the circuit). Additional alarms include those that sound with electrical failure or because of inadequate oxygen line pressure.

(9). *PEEP* may be necessary in refractory hypoxemia despite oxygen supplementation. It increases end-expiratory and mean pressure across the walls of airways and alveoli, reexpanding collapsed alveoli and allowing them to participate in gas exchange. The chief disadvantage is decreased cardiac output. Additional potential problems include barotrauma (especially at PEEP > or = 25 cm H_2O), increased intracranial pressure, decreased renal function from renal vein back pressure, passive hepatic congestion, and exacerbation of intracardiac shunts. PEEP should be considered in the patient with refractory hypoxemia (Pao_2 less than 55 mm Hg despite an Fio_2 > or = 0.55) and a *diffuse* pulmonary process. The application of PEEP and additional concepts in its application are presented in Table 7–15. The PEEP weaning process is presented in Table 7–16.

d. Weaning the Patient from Mechanical Ventilation (Tables 7–17 and 7–18). Weaning can be a challenging process in certain patients. The physician must deal aggressively with all factors and the disease process responsible for respiratory failure in the first place before the ventilator wean is considered. In particular, the patient should be in optimal electrolyte (including potassium and phosphate) balance, should have a normal pH, and should be in ideal fluid balance (with appropriate management of heart failure and renal or iatrogenic fluid overload).

D. Complications of Respiratory Failure. The complications of respiratory failure were briefly described under "Adult Respiratory Distress

TABLE 7–15. THE USE OF PEEP

1. Routine monitors include pulse, blood pressure (BP), respiratory rate (RR), mean arterial pressure, peak inflation pressure, corrected tidal volume, and ABGs.
2. If PEEP is to be increased beyond 10 cm H_2O or patient's volume status is uncertain or patient has known left ventricular dysfunction, pulmonary artery (PA) catheter should be inserted. With PA catheter, additional variables to be monitored include wedge pressure, cardiac output, and mixed venous blood gases (optional).
3. Increments in PEEP should be made at 2.5–5.0 cm H_2O at a time.
4. Risk of significant complications is markedly increased at level of PEEP > or = 25 cm H_2O.
5. Goal of PEEP is to improve O_2 delivery to tissues, not simply to improve Pao_2. Thus, cardiac output, in addition to Pao_2, must be monitored. O_2 delivery may be calculated by Pao_2 × cardiac output. Additional factors to consider include risk of barotrauma, change in lung compliance, development of lactic acidosis, and change in mixed venous O_2.
6. Further benefits from PEEP ("late" PEEP response) may be seen hours after a particular level of PEEP has been achieved.
7. Patient with diffuse pulmonary infiltrates is most likely to benefit from PEEP. If pulmonary process is localized, PEEP may make oxygenation worse by shunting blood away from more compliant (and hence more easily expanded alveoli) lung to less compliant and more diseased lung.

Adapted from Marini JJ: Respiratory Medicine and Intensive Care for the House Officer. Baltimore, Williams & Wilkins, 1981, pp. 151–160.

TABLE 7–16. WEANING THE PATIENT FROM PEEP

1. PEEP reduction should be considered when underlying pulmonary disorder has improved in patients who were responsive to PEEP. If patient is unstable, requires an Fio_2 greater than 0.4–0.5 for adequate oxygenation, or is clinically deteriorating, PEEP withdrawal is unlikely to be successful. Keep in mind that abrupt withdrawal of PEEP may cause deterioration in oxygenation that will not be correctable by returning to previous level of PEEP.
2. Obtain baseline hemodynamic and respiratory parameters, as outlined in Table 4–19.
3. Reduce PEEP by no more than 2.5–5.0 cm H_2O at single step.
4. After 3 min at new level of PEEP, determine ABG and return patient to his or her previous PEEP level.
5. Compare new ABG with previous ABG to determine if patient will tolerate new level. Keep in mind that deterioration in ABG seen at 3 min will probably be amplified over the next 1–6 hr.
6. Perform PEEP reduction no faster than one step every 6–12 hr, as ABG results allow.
7. Monitor patient (including ABGs) several times over the 6–12 hr at the new level of PEEP before a change to the next lower level is contemplated.

Adapted from Marini JJ: Respiratory Medicine and Intensive Care for the House Officer. Baltimore, Williams & Wilkins, 1981, pp 151–160.

TABLE 7-17. GENERAL WEANING PARAMETERS

1. Vital capacity of 15 mL/kg
2. Inspiratory force more negative than 25 cm H_2O
3. Respiratory rate less than 24 breaths/min
4. Minute ventilation between 5 and 10 L/min
5. Patient awake and alert, with normal pH, appropriate electrolyte abnormalities (hypokalemia, hypophosphatemia, primary metabolic alkalosis) corrected, and volume status optimal
6. Maximal voluntary ventilation 2 $\times$ minute ventilation

TABLE 7-18. THE T-PIECE TRIAL

1. Perform trial early in day, with patient alert.
2. Explain procedure to patient.
3. Suction airway and oropharynx.
4. If Pa_{O_2} is marginal, increase the Fi_{O_2} by at least 10%.
5. Have patient sitting or at least semiupright to maximize functional residual capacity (FRC).
6. Place patient on T piece and monitor closely (pulse, BP, RR) every 5 min. Obtain ABG at 20 min. If the patient is tolerating trial well, extubate. If at any time the patient experiences intolerable dyspnea, the RR increases by more than 10/min, the pulse changes by more than 30/min, the BP (diastolic) changes by more than 20 mm Hg, mental status declines, arrhythmias develop, or the ABG is unacceptable, then terminate T-piece trial.

Adapted from Marini JJ: Respiratory Medicine and Intensive Care for the House Officer. Baltimore, Williams & Wilkins, 1981, pp 146–147.

Syndrome." The clinician must keep in mind that the patient with respiratory failure seldom succumbs because of inability to oxygenate, but rather because of the development of a complication while in the ICU. Multiple possibilities include the following: nosocomial infection with sepsis, laryngotracheal injury due to endotracheal intubation, GI hemorrhage, renal impairment or failure, pulmonary thromboembolism, pulmonary barotrauma, and cardiovascular complications.

Balter M, Morganroth ML: Managing acute respiratory failure in the patient with COPD. J Respir Dis, November 1987, pp 21–32.

Haake R, Schlichtig R, Ulstad DR, Henschen RR: Barotrauma: Pathophysiology, risk factors, and prevention. Chest 91:608–613, 1987.

Pingleton SK: Complications of acute respiratory failure. Am Rev Respir Dis 137:1463–1493, 1988.

Popovich J Jr: Mechanical ventilation: Treating arterial hypoxemia. J Respir Dis, February 1984, pp 69–79.

Popovich J Jr: Mechanical ventilation: Keeping all systems go. J Respir Dis, January 1985, pp 69–83.

XVII. PULMONARY HYPERTENSION

Pulmonary hypertension is a prolonged increase in the pressure of the main pulmonary artery (mean pressure >25 mm Hg). Potential causes are outlined in Table 7–19. Signs and symptoms include exertional dyspnea, chest pain, tachypnea, lightheadedness, syncope, and hemoptysis.

TABLE 7–19. THE CAUSES OF PULMONARY HYPERTENSION

PRECAPILLARY
Occlusive pulmonary vascular disease (pulmonary thomboemboli, foreign material [talc, cotton fibers in IV drug abusers], parasites)
Respiratory disease (obstructive and restrictive lung disease, sleep apnea and hypoventilation syndromes)
Congenital heart disease (intracardiac septal defects with resultant left-to-right shunt, peripheral pulmonic stenosis)
Pulmonary vasculitis
Primary pulmonary hypertension
POSTCAPILLARY
Valvular heart disease (including mitral and aortic valves)
Left atrial myxoma or thrombus
Left-sided cardiac failure
Pulmonary veno-occlusive disease
Mediastinal fibrosis
Anomalous pulmonary vein

Data from Rubin LJ: Pulmonary hypertension and cor pulmonale. *In* Kelley WN (ed): Textbook of Internal Medicine. Philadelphia, JB Lippincott, 1990, vol 1; Laor T, DeLuca SA. Pulmonary hypertension. Am Fam Physician, November 1989, pp 195–198.

A. Diagnosis. Physical examination may reveal the likely cause (e.g., mitral stenosis murmur). Findings associated with pulmonary hypertension may include a loud pulmonic component of the second heart sound, left parasternal fourth heart sound, tricuspid insufficiency, pulmonic insufficiency, and/or findings of right-sided heart failure.

Laboratory studies include ECG, ABG, pulmonary function tests (including DL_{CO}), and PA and lateral chest x-rays. Additional studies (echocardiography to evaluate chamber size, wall motion, and valvular abnormalities, ventilation-perfusion lung scanning to evaluate for recurrent or unresolved pulmonary thromboemboli, right-heart catheterization, and pulmonary arteriography) may be helpful. Open lung biopsy in the diagnosis of pulmonary hypertension is controversial.

B. Therapy. Management of pulmonary hypertension begins with the search for the underlying cause and disease-specific therapy, if possible. Additional considerations include:

1. Oxygen supplementation if Pao_2 is less than 60 mm Hg (less than 90% hemoglobin saturation) or if patient has improved nocturnal desaturation or exercise capacity with supplemental O_2.

2. Treatment of right-sided heart failure with furosemide as necessary (dose should be increased cautiously to avoid overly aggressive preload reduction and consequent hypotension). Some patients will benefit from digoxin administration.

3. Phlebotomy (by reducing blood viscosity and improving cardiac output) will benefit the patient whose hematocrit exceeds 50%.

4. Vasodilators should be used only for selected patients in a controlled setting. Risks with vasodilator therapy include worsened hypoxia, hypotension, and death. Some patients, however, have been shown to benefit from high doses of calcium channel–blocking agents.

5. Surgical thromboendarterectomy is the procedure of choice in patients with accessible thromboemboli who are surgical candidates, whose mean Pao_2 is greater than 30 mm Hg, and who have clinical evidence that the arterial obstruction has been present for at least 6 months.

6. Chronic anticoagulation with warfarin is appropriate for patients with pulmonary hypertension due to thromboembolism if there are no contraindications.

7. LUNG TRANSPLANTATION: Patients with end-stage pulmonary vascular disease and an anticipated survival of 12–18 months are candidates for lung transplantation. The 2-year postsurgical survival rate in appropriate candidates has been reported to be between 62 and 72%. In the patient with pulmonary vascular disease accompanied by right ventricular failure a combined heart-lung transplant may be the procedure of choice in the appropriate candidate.

Laor T, DeLuca SA: Pulmonary hypertension. Am Fam Physician, November 1989, pp 195–198.
Rich S, Levitsky S, Brundage BH: Pulmonary hypertension from chronic pulmonary thomboembolism. Ann Intern Med 108:425–434, 1988.
Williams TJ, Patterson GA, Maurer J: Lung transplantation today: What's done, and for whom? J Respir Dis 11:937–948, 1990.

88888888888888

GASTROINTESTINAL DISEASES

KENNETH K. WANG and THOMAS VIGGIANO

I. ESOPHAGEAL DISEASES

A. Reflux Esophagitis

1. RATIONALE FOR THERAPY

Symptoms of gastroesophageal reflux (pyrosis) are common and do not warrant therapy unless they are frequent, cause complications (esophageal strictures or ulcers) or cause histologic changes of inflammation. The basis of therapy for gastroesophageal reflux is correction of the basic mechanisms by increasing the lower esophageal sphincter tone, decreasing episodes of gastric acid reflux, and increasing the clearance of refluxed gastric acid (N Engl J Med 307:1547, 1982).

2. THERAPY

a. General Therapy

1. Avoid foods that decrease lower esophageal sphincter pressure (peppermint, chocolate, fatty foods, caffeine, alcohol, tomato juice, and orange juice);
2. Stop smoking;
3. Discontinue or modify drugs that lower esophageal sphincter pressure (progesterone-containing birth control pills, aminophylline, anticholinergics, beta-adrenergic agonists, alpha-adrenergic antagonists, calcium channel blockers, diazepam).

b. Mechanical Measures to Decrease Reflux or Increase Esophageal Clearance

1. Avoid tight-fitting clothes;
2. Avoid excessive stooping or bending;
3. Elevate head of the bed at least 6 inches;
4. Decrease meal size;
5. Avoid eating 3 hours before sleep;
6. Avoid lying down within 2 hours of eating;
7. Weight loss for obese patients.

c. Pharmacologic Therapy (Table 8–1)

(1). Decreased Acid Production

A. ANTACIDS. Liquid antacids, 30 mL 1 and 3 hours after meals and at bedtime, have traditionally been used to neutralize acid. However, solid tablets, such as calcium carbonate antacids, dissolved in the mouth throughout the day, may provide more symptomatic relief.

B. H$_2$-RECEPTOR ANTAGONISTS. Ranitidine (300 mg qd), cimetidine (800 mg qd), nizatidine (300 mg qd), and famotidine (40 mg qd) are effective in decreasing acid production. For more intensive therapy, dosages of these medications can be increased or divided through the day.

TABLE 8–1. PHARMACOLOGIC THERAPY

INDICATION	DRUG	DOSE	DURATION
Reflux esophagitis	Ranitidine	300 mg po qd	6–8 wk
	Cimetidine	800 mg po qd	6–8 wk
	Nizatidine	300 mg po qd	6–8 wk
	Famotidine	40 mg po qd	6–8 wk
	Omeprazole	20 mg po qd	6–8 wk
	Sucralfate	1 gram po qid	6–8 wk
	Metoclopramide	10 mg po qid	6 wk
	Bethanecol	25 mg po qid	6 wk
Diffuse esophageal spasm	Dicyclomine hydrochloride	10 mg po qid	
	Isosorbide dinitrate	10–30 mg po qid	
	Nifedipine	10–20 mg po qid	
	Verapamil	80 mg po tid	
	Hydralazine	25–50 mg po tid	
Achalasia	Isosorbide dinitrate	10–30 mg po qid	
	Nifedipine	10–20 mg po qid	
Peptic ulcer disease	Ranitidine	300 mg po qd	6 wk
	Cimetidine	800 mg po qd	6 wk
	Nizatidine	300 mg po qd	6 wk
	Roxatidine acetate	150 mg po qd	6 wk
	Famotidine	40 mg po qd	6 wk
	Omeprazole	20–40 mg po qd	6 wk
	Sucralfate	1 gm po qid	6 wk
	Misoprostol	200 μg po qid	
Gastroparesis	Metoclopramide	10–20 mg po 1 hr before meals	
	Bethanecol	25 mg po 1 hr before meals	
Nausea and vomiting	Meclizine hydrochloride	50 mg po bid–qid	
	Diphenhydramine hydrochloride	25–50 mg po qid	
	Prochlorperazine	5–10 mg po tid 25 mg pr bid–qid	
	Butyrophenones	2.5–5.0 mg IM bid	
	Trimethobenzamide hydrochloride	250 mg po bid–qid 200 mg pr bid–qid	
Hiccups	Chlorpromazine	25–50 mg IV	
	Metoclopramide	10 mg IV	
Crohn's disease	Sulfasalazine	1 gm/15 kg po qid	
	Prednisolone	0.25–0.75 mg/kg po qd	
	Metronidazole	10–20 mg/kg po qd	
	Azathioprine	2.5 mg/kg po qd	
Tropical sprue	Folate	10 mg po qd	
	Vitamin B_{12}	100 μg IM qd	
	Tetracycline	250 mg po qid	2 wk
	Sulfamethazine	2 gm/day	2 wk

TABLE 8–1. PHARMACOLOGIC THERAPY *Continued*

INDICATION	DRUG	DOSE	DURATION
Chronic ulcerative colitis	Sulfasalazine	500–1000 mg po qid	
	Osalazine	500 mg po bid	
	Mesalamine (enema)	4 gm pr hs	
	Hydrocortisone (enema)	100 mg pr hs	
	Prednisone	30–60 mg po qd	
	Metronidazole	10–20 mg/kg po qd	
	Azathioprine	2 mg/kg po qd	
Pseudomembranous colitis	Vancomycin	125–500 mg po qid	1–2 wk
	Metronidazole	500 mg po qid	1–2 wk
	Bacitracin	25,000 U po qid	1–2 wk
	Cholestyramine	3 grams po qid	1–2 wk
Infectious proctitis	Tetracycline	500 mg po qid	1 wk
	Ceftriaxone	250 mg IM	
Irritable bowel syndrome	Decyclomine hydrochloride	10–40 mg po qid	
	Amitriptyline	25–50 mg po qd	
Chronic diarrhea	Loperamide	2–4 mg po bid	
	Diphenoxylate and atropine	1–2 tablets po qid	
	Clonidine	0.1–0.4 mg po qd	
	Verapamil	80 mg po tid	

Drug interactions, particularly with cimetidine, have been reported that cause increased blood levels of warfarin, theophylline, phenytoin, diazepam, propranolol, lidocaine, and tricyclic antidepressants.

C. **HYDROGEN-ION PUMP INHIBITOR**. Omeprazole is an effective drug for treating refractory reflux disease. It is more effective than cimetidine in terms of symptom relief and histologic improvement (Gut 31:509, 1990). It can be administered at a dosage of 20 mg qd for 6–8 weeks. Higher doses (40 mg) of omeprazole are more effective in relieving symptoms of reflux esophagitis. Omeprazole has been well tolerated in short-term clinical trials (Scand J Gastroenterol Suppl 166:140, 1989). Omeprazole does affect the P450 system and can interfere with such drugs as warfarin, phenytoin, and diazepam. Because of the profound acid inhibition, drugs that require gastric acid for absorption (e.g., ketoconazole, iron supplements, and ampicillin) may be affected.

(2). Mucosal Protection. Sucralfate can be used to aid in healing of refractory esophagitis as either a tablet or slurry (Scand J Gastroenterol Suppl 156:49, 1989), prepared by placing 1 tablet (1 gm) in water ½ hour before use. The tablet will then dissolve and can be administered po qid for up to 8

weeks. Sucralfate can cause decreased absorption of digoxin, phenytoin, and tetracycline.

(3). *Increasing Lower Esophageal Sphincter Tone.* Antacid therapy has been associated with increased lower esophageal sphincter (LES) tone. Other drugs that increase LES tone as well as esophageal and gastric clearance of acid are cholinergic agents (bethanechol 25 mg qid) and metoclopramide (10 mg qid). Neither of these agents should be thought of as first-line therapy.

3. COMPLICATIONS OF GASTROESPHAGEAL REFLUX DISEASE

a. Barrett's Esophagus. This replacement of squamous epithelium by columnar mucosa is thought to be secondary to chronic reflux esophagitis (Am J Med 74:313, 1983). It is an indication for esophagoscopy and biopsy because of its association with esophageal neoplasms. An esophageal reflux program should be initiated to contain the Barrett's esophagus, but the efficacy of antireflux measures in causing regression of Barrett's esophagus has not been demonstrated (Gastroenterology 92:118, 1987). Omeprazole at a dosage of 40 mg hs has caused some regression of Barrett's esophagus. The cost-effectiveness of surveillance procedures to detect early neoplasm in Barrett's esophagus remains controversial.

b. Esophageal Strictures, Ulcers, and Aspiration Pneumonia. Symptomatic strictures secondary to reflux esophagitis can often be dilated endoscopically. Patients should also be treated for reflux after dilatation. The combination has been successful in managing most strictures. Surgery may be indicated if endoscopic dilatation provides only short-term improvement. Aspiration pneumonia and pulmonary fibrosis may also result from untreated gastroesophageal reflux. If this recurs despite medical therapy, surgery is indicated. Reflux disease can induce esophageal ulcers, most often in association with Barrett's esophagus. Ulcers usually respond to maximal medical management, but surgery is sometimes required. Surgery may also be indicated for gastroesophageal reflux that has persisted despite intensive medical therapy for at least 4–6 months. Before any surgical intervention, 24-hour pH monitoring and esophageal motility studies are essential. Occasionally, bile acid reflux may cause esophagitis as well as gastritis. Bile acid reflux necessitates a surgical drainage procedure different from that for gastric acid reflux. If abnormal esophageal peristalsis is found, surgery should be reconsidered.

B. Strictures of the Esophagus. Strictures discovered on barium swallow may be asymptomatic but should be investigated by endoscopy and biopsy. Schatzki's rings should be dilated if dysphagia can be attributed to their presence. The cervical Plummer-Vinson's web should have periodic rebiopsy because of a 10% incidence of associated malignant disease. Malignant strictures may also be dilated if symptomatic. If dilatation fails in these patients, esophageal stents or percutaneous gastrostomies may be placed to aid in nutrition.

C. Caustic Ingestions. Ingestion of caustic alkali may cause more severe damage to the esophagus than ingestion of acid. However, neither the type of irritant nor symptoms created by ingestion indicate the actual damage. If patients are seen within 1 hour of ingestion, water lavage of the gastric contents should be done. Endoscopy can assess the extent of damage as soon as possible after ingestion unless esophageal perforation is suspected. A soft-rubber nasogastric tube can be placed to stent the lumen of the esophagus and to provide decompression of the stomach. Broad-spectrum antibiotics, not routinely necessary, should be given at the first sign of an infection. Steroids have not been shown to prevent stricture formation and are not recommended (N Engl J Med 323:637, 1990). Dilatation of caustic strictures may be attempted as early as a week after ingestion.

D. Motility Disorders of the Esophagus

1. PHARYNGEAL DYSPHAGIA
Nasal regurgitation of food, coughing, and other evidence of aspiration are signs of pharyngeal dysphagia. This is often secondary to structural lesions such as tumors of the posterior pharynx. However, disorders such as hypothyroidism, amyotrophic lateral sclerosis, polymyositis, and Parkinson's disease must be considered.

Zenker's diverticulum may also cause dysphagia and should be resected if symptoms are severe. Medical management usually involves diet modification to avoid liquids, which commonly are the most difficult to swallow. Endoscopic placement of feeding gastrostomy tubes helps in long-term management of patients with neurologic disorders. Careful assessment should be done to avoid regurgitation and aspiration of enteral feedings.

2. DIFFUSE ESOPHAGEAL SPASM
Diffuse esophageal spasm (DES) often presents as dysphagia or chest pain and is diagnosed by esophageal manometry and provocative agents such as edrophonium (Gastroenterology 81:10, 1981). Gastroesophageal reflux with secondary esophageal spasm should be carefully excluded. Most patients with DES have prolonged high-amplitude contractions in the body of the esophagus, and approximately a third have elevated LES tone pressures. Pharmacologic therapy should be tailored to the individual patient's tolerance. Anticholinergic agents (dicyclomine hydrochloride 10 mg po qid), nitrates (isosorbide dinitrate 10–30 mg po qid), and calcium channel blockers are often good first-line therapy for DES. Nifedipine 10–20 mg po qid is particularly effective for patients with increased lower esophageal sphincter tone, but patient tolerance may limit the use of effective dosages. Verapamil 80 mg po tid or diltiazem 30–60 mg po qid is most effective for symptoms that are related to chest pain. Hydralazine can be considered in a dosage of 25–50 mg po tid. In refractory cases, dilatation may be effective (Gastroenterology 82:1069, 1982). Some patients with hypertensive LES pressures and dysphagia may respond to pneumatic dilatations. Occasionally medical therapy fails, and patients may be referred for a Lowell myotomy.

3. ACHALASIA
This progressive denervation of the smooth muscle of the lower ⅔ of the esophagus often leads to dysphagia. Patients who have characteristic manometric findings of achalasia should still have esophagoscopy to eliminate the possibility of esophageal tumors that mimic this entity. If symptoms are not severe and changes noted on barium x-ray are slight, pharmacologic therapy with nifedipine 10–20 mg po qid or isosorbide dinitrate 10–30 mg po qid may aid in decreasing LES pressure and improve esophageal clearance (Gastroenterology 80:39, 1981). Unfortunately, although some symptoms may be relieved with medications, the majority persist (Am J Gastroenterol 84:1259, 1990). Usually, pneumatic dilatation is required for relief of dysphagia. Surgical myotomy should be considered if pneumatic dilatation is unsuccessful on 2 consecutive attempts. However, myotomy is associated with a high incidence of gastroesophageal reflux.

E. Infectious Esophagitis. Immune suppression caused most commonly by chemotherapy predisposes patients to infection by *Candida albicans* and viruses of the herpes family. Although these often cause oral manifestations and odynophagia, patients may be totally asymptomatic and discovered only at endoscopy to have characteristic discrete punched-out ulcerations or vesicles in herpes virus or yellowish-white plaques in *Candida* infection. Mild localized *Candida* esophagitis may be treated with nystatin, usually in dosages of 500,000 U po qid. If this is not successful in relieving symptoms within 48 hours, the dose may be increased to 200,000 U every 2 hours. Clotrimazole may also be used for mild candidiasis as a 10-mg troche dissolved in the mouth qid. Ketoconazole can be used as a single tablet 200 mg/day po as an alternative to nystatin therapy. Therapy should be continued for 1–2 weeks if symptoms disappear and associated problems (e.g., neutropenia) resolve. If there is evidence of systemic candidemia or neutropenia in a patient with severe esophagitis, amphotericin B should be used.

Varicella zoster, cytomegalovirus, and herpes simplex may cause viral esophagitis. For varicella zoster, acyclovir is the treatment of choice (10 mg/kg IV or 800 mg/day po over a 5-day treatment course). The drug is usually given in a dilute solution to avoid possible crystallization in the kidneys. Coadministration of other nephrotoxic drugs should be avoided. Acyclovir infusion has been associated with femoral phlebitis, reversible CNS side effects, and reduced renal clearance. Gancyclovir is recommended for systemic cytomegalovirus infections at a dosage of 5 mg/kg bid.

F. Esophageal Cancer. Medical management of esophageal carcinoma consists primarily of screening for premalignant lesions (Table 8–2). Although screening standards have not yet been established, many gastroenterologists recommend periodic screening of patients with lesions that have a greater disposition to development of carcinoma. Such lesions include strictures from caustic ingestions, Plummer-Vinson's webs, Barrett's esophagus, achalasia, and tylosis palmaris et plantaris. Although peptic esophagitis may be associated with a small increase in incidence of esophageal carcinoma, screening is probably not indicated.

TABLE 8–2. SCREENING FOR GASTROINTESTINAL CARCINOMA

CONDITION	CANCER TYPE	PROCEDURE	INTERVAL (YR)
Barrett's esophagus	Esophageal	EGD*	1–2
Achalasia	Esophageal	EGD	1–3
Gastric adenomas	Gastric	EGD	1–3
Gastric dysplasia	Gastric	EGD	1–3
Polyposis coli	Gastric	EGD	1–3
	Small intestine		
	Colon	Colonoscopy	1
Colonic dysplasia	Colon	Colonoscopy	1–3
Colonic adenomas	Colon	Colonoscopy	1–3
Ulcerative colitis	Colon	Colonoscopy	1–3
Gynecologic cancer	Colon	Barium enema	1–3
Breast cancer	Colon	Barium enema	1–3

*EGD = Esophagogastroduodenoscopy.

Palliative therapy for esophageal carcinoma is nutritional support via percutaneous gastrostomies, laser photoablation of the tumor, dilatation of esophageal strictures, or placement of a stent. Stents have also been used to treat tracheoesophageal fistulas.

Dehn TC, Shepherd HA, Colin-Jones D, et al: Double blind comparison of omeprazole (40 mg od) versus cimetidine (400 mg qd) in the treatment of symptomatic erosive reflux oesophagitis, assessed endoscopically, histologically and by 24 h pH monitoring. Gut 31:509, 1990.

Walan A: The clinical utility and safety of omeprazole. Scand J Gastroenterol (suppl) 166:140, 1989.

Sontag SJ, Hirshowitz B, Holt S, et al: Two doses of omeprazole versus placebo in symptomatic reflux esophagitis: the U.S. multicenter study. Gastroenterology 102:109, 1992.

Ros E, Pujol A, Bordas JM, Grande L: Efficacy of sucralfate in refractory reflux esophagitis. Results of a pilot study. Scand J Gastroenterol (suppl) 156:49, 1989.

Anderson KD, Rouse TM, Randolf JG: A controlled trial of corticosteroids in children with corrosive injury of the esophagus. N Engl J Med 323:637, 1990.

Winters C, Spurling TJ, Cattau WJ, et al: Barrett's esophagus: A prevalent, occult complication of gastroesophageal reflux disease. Gastroenterology 92:118, 1987.

London RL, Ouyand A, Snape WJ, et al: Provocation of esophageal pain by ergonovine or edrophonium. Gastroenterology 81:10, 1981.

Goldin MR, Burns TW, Herrington JP: Treatment of nonspecific esophageal motor disorders: Beneficial effects of bougienage. Gastroenterology 82:1069, 1982.

Traube M, Dubovik S, Lange RC, McCallum RW: The role of nifedipine therapy in achalasia: Results of a randomized, double-blind, placebo-controlled study. Am J Gastroenterol 84:1259, 1989.

II. STOMACH DISORDERS

A. **Peptic Ulcer Disease.** Peptic ulcer disease results from breakdown in the balance between acid pepsin secretion and relevant mucosal defense mechanisms. Duodenal ulcers are frequently associated with increased basal and maximal acid secretion. Almost all duodenal ulcers are benign; however, approximately 5% are malignant. Gastric ulcers usually occur in patients with normal or even reduced rates of acid secretion. Reflux of bile and pancreatic juice from the duodenum through an incompetent pyloric sphincter appears to play a role in the breakdown of mucosal protection seen in gastric ulcer disease. This condition is associated with cigarette smoking, presumably because of diminished bicarbonate secretion by the pancreas. Gastric ulcer is associated with the use of alcohol, aspirin, and NSAIDS as well as the presence of *Helicobacter pylori*. Goals of treatment in peptic ulcer disease include symptom relief, ulcer healing, and prevention of recurrence and complications.

1. *HELICOBACTER PYLORI*

A gram-negative spiral organism, *Helicobacter pylori*, originally named *Campylobacter pylori,* has been demonstrated in patients with a number of peptic conditions, including gastric and duodenal ulcers, gastritis, and duodenitis. Several observations have been made about its role in ulcer disease. Almost all patients with duodenal ulcers harbor the organism, and its eradication decreases the ulcer relapse rate (Rev Infect Dis 12 (suppl 1):S87–93, 1990). However, ulcer healing occurs even if the organism is not eradicated, and maintenance of antiulcer therapy prevents recurrence despite the presence of the organism. Currently therapy has not been widely accepted, although it seems that colloidal bismuth subcitrate in combination with 2 antibiotics such as amoxicillin, tetracycline, or ciprofloxacin and metronidazole is needed to eradicate the organism (J Clin Gastroenterol 11 (suppl 1):S49–53, 1990).

2. DRUG THERAPY

a. **H$_2$ Receptor Antagonists.** H$_2$ receptor antagonists inhibit basal and stimulated gastric acid secretion. Cimetidine 800 mg qd, ranitidine 300 mg qd, nizatidine 300 mg qd, roxatidine acetate 150 mg qd, and famotidine (Pepcid) 40 mg qd are all effective and safe in reducing the secretion of hydrochloric acid. Cimetidine may occasionally cause confusion in older patients, especially in the presence of renal insufficiency, and it has an antiandrogenic effect that can cause gynecomastia and impotence. Also, cimetidine is metabolized by the microsomal oxidase enzyme system; thus there may be drug interactions with other drugs (theophylline, phenytoin, and warfarin) metabolized in the liver. Ranitidine and famotidine are thought to cause less mental confusion, are not antiandrogenic, and do not inhibit the metabolism of other drugs markedly, although interactions with theophylline have been reported. Famotidine, nizatidine, and roxatidine acetate have not been reported to have significant side effects, but they have not been used as long as previous agents.

b. **Drugs That Neutralize Acid and Antacids.** The concentration of acid can be reduced by neutralizing the intraluminal acid. The antacids most frequently used contain magnesium and/or aluminum hydroxide. The goal of antacid treatment is to buffer gastric acid. An antacid taken in the fasting state will buffer acid for only 30 minutes. However, if antacids are taken 1 hour after eating, they will buffer stomach acid an additional 2 hours. In fasting, antacids should be given hourly to keep the gastric pH at an acceptable range. In patients who are eating, 100 mEq of an antacid 1 hour and 3 hours after meals and at bedtime is the recommended dose. Antacids provide prompt pain relief and should be given as needed. Liquid antacids are more effective than antacid tablets. An antacid should be chosen by its buffering capacity, sodium content, and patient tolerance. Aluminum hydroxide binds phosphate and may cause hypophosphatemia. Magnesium-induced diarrhea and aluminum-induced constipation are usually offset by the use of magnesium hydroxide and aluminum hydroxide combinations.

c. **Proton Pump Inhibitor.** Acid secretion is accomplished in the parietal cell by an H^+/K^+-ATPase pump. This is the site of action of a new class of drugs. Omeprazole, an irreversible pump inhibitor, has been released for treatment of reflux disease and has been used in Europe to treat peptic ulcers. Dosages have ranged between 20 mg/day and 40 mg/day with the higher dosage being more effective than H_2 receptor antagonists. The primary concern with this drug is profound hypochlorhydria and resultant hypergastrinemia and bacterial colonization of the stomach. Omeprazole inhibits the P450 enzymes.

d. **Sucralfate.** Sucralfate is an aluminum hydroxide salt of sucrose that has been modified by maximal sulfation and is not absorbed following its usual dose of 1 gm 4 times daily. The mechanism of action of sucralfate is unclear. Recent studies suggest that sucralfate may also stimulate mucus production and prostaglandin release. It is probably the drug of choice in pregnant women. The primary side effect is constipation.

e. **Prostaglandins.** Prostaglandins are synthesized in the gastroduodenal mucosa and have been found to stimulate mucus production, increase bicarbonate secretion, enhance mucosal blood flow, and increase cellular tranport processes. In addition to their cytoprotective effects, higher doses of some prostaglandins inhibit hydrochloric acid secretion. Misoprostol, a prostaglandin E_1 analogue, at 200 μg qid is used for ulcer prevention during therapy with NSAIDs. Diarrhea is the major side effect, occurring in 13% of patients; it usually is self-limited. Misoprostol also produces increased uterine contractions and is contraindicated in women of childbearing age.

f. **Bismuth Compounds.** Bismuth compounds are thought to act by forming a protective coating over the ulcer. De-nol (tripotassium dicitrato bismuthate) has been used extensively in Europe but is not yet available in the United States. The unique property of this agent is its effect on *H. pylori,* which it may eradicate (Rev Infect Dis 12 (suppl 1):S115–119, 1990). Bismuth subsalicylate (Pepto-Bismol) is available in the U.S. and has been shown to inhibit the urease activity of *H. pylori,* but clinical efficacy has not been established.

3. **DIET**
All meals stimulate acid production; thus, no specific diet is indicated in peptic ulcer treatment. Patients should avoid foods that cause irritating symptoms. Eating before bedtime should be avoided because

it stimulates gastric acid secretion at a time when the acid is not well buffered.

4. **TREATMENT STRATEGIES**

a. **Duodenal Ulcer.** Therapy should be begun with H_2 receptor antagonists because of their convenience and lower costs. Alternative therapy should be antacids and sucralfate. Therapy should be continued for 6 weeks with anticipated symptomatic improvement in about 5 days. If relapse occurs after therapy is discontinued, the patient should receive maintenance therapy, and gastrinomas should be excluded. Maintenance therapy usually consists of a single bedtime dose of an H_2 receptor antagonist for a period of at least a year. Patients with renal failure should not be treated with antacids or sucralfate to avoid the accumulation of magnesium. Combined therapy with H_2 receptor antagonists and a mucosal protective agent or treatment with omeprazole should be considered for resistant ulcers. In patients with *H. pylori* and recurrent or refractory ulcers, triple therapy with bismuth, 1 tablet qid, tetracycline 500 mg qid, and metronidazole 400 mg tid can be given for 2 weeks. This therapy is associated with eradication of *H. pylori* in 80% of cases, but relapse occurs in 11% and side effects develop in 30% of treated patients.

b. **Gastric Ulcers.** Therapy is similar to that for duodenal ulcers except that if healing is not documented within 8 weeks of adequate medical therapy, surgical resection should be considered because of the possibility of malignancy.

c. **Complications.** Bleeding from peptic ulcer disease can be treated medically. However, patients with continued or recurrent bleeding from duodenal ulcers should have surgery, as should those with bleeding gastric ulcers. Ulcers that cause obstruction or perforation or fail to respond to 6–8 weeks of intensive medical therapy are candidates for surgical intervention.

B. Gastritis

1. **ACUTE GASTRITIS**
Acute gastritis results from mucosal injury that allows back diffusion of acid. Certain drugs—especially aspirin, alcohol, and NSAIDs—disrupt the mucosal barrier. Stress ulcers, commonly seen in trauma or surgery, are thought to result from ischemia. Gastritis can sometimes be attributed to events such as irradiation, ingestion of alkali, or, rarely, bacterial infection (phlegmonous gastritis).

a. **Prevention of Erosive Gastritis.** Erosive gastritis can be prevented by increasing gastric pH to greater than 4.0 with a proton pump inhibitor, H_2 blocker, or a combination of these with antacids. Patients at highest risk of ulceration (with severe burns, trauma, septicemia, CNS damage, respiratory failure, or renal failure) should receive prophylaxis.

b. **Therapy of Acute Erosive Gastritis.** After initial lavage with tap water, endoscopy should be performed. If diffuse bleeding is seen from superficial erosions, infusion of a solution made from 12 mg of norepinephrine ditartrate in 200 mL normal saline into the stomach for 15 minutes may be helpful. If bleeding is from discrete ulcerations, endoscopic cautery can be performed. If bleeding continues, angiography can be done with the selective infusion of vasopressin. Bleeding does not respond to medical therapy in approximately 20% of patients and may require surgical intervention.

c. **Therapy of Alkaline Reflux Gastritis.** Although diagnosis is difficult, once it is established this entity can generally be managed by antacids, 30 mL 2–3 hours after meals and 60 mL at bedtime. Antacids appear to have significant ability to absorb bile salts. Cholestyramine can also be used at a dosage of 1 package 2–3 hours after meals and at bedtime. Surgery is seldom successful in relieving pain in these patients and should be attempted only if additional symptoms are present.

2. CHRONIC GASTRITIS

Chronic gastritis can be classified by histologic appearance (superficial versus atrophic) and by the anatomic location of the inflammation (type A, fundus and body; type B, antrum). In type A atrophic gastritis, circulating antibodies against parietal cells and pernicious anemia are often present. In type B atrophic gastritis, antibodies against gastrin-producing cells have been reported. Currently, based upon epidemiologic evidence, it is thought that *H. pylori* is the etiologic agent for chronic gastritis. The organism is thought to initially cause a type B form of gastritis involving the antrum and causing hypochlorhydria. In chronic infection, type A pattern may appear. The role of *H. pylori* in benign gastric ulcer and gastric cancer associated with chronic gastritis is unclear. No specific treatment is currently indicated for idiopathic chronic gastritis.

3. ZOLLINGER-ELLISON SYNDROME

This consists of peptic ulceration, acid hypersecretion, the presence of a non–islet cell tumor, and increased serum gastrin. Its treatment should be surgical excision if a tumor mass can be defined. If tumors cannot be localized, medical therapy should be instituted. Omeprazole is the treatment of choice for this condition. Octreotide, a somatostatin analogue, has been effective in decreasing symptoms and may decrease tumor growth.

C. Motility Disorders

1. GASTROPARESIS

This diagnosis is made by the exclusion of obstructing lesions in the stomach and duodenum and demonstration of delayed emptying of either solid or liquid material by radionuclide scintigraphy. Therapy is concentrated on the underlying disorder, including electrolyte abnormalities, diabetes mellitus, and medications (anticholinergics, antidopaminergics, beta-adrenergic agonists, calcium channel blockers). Dietary manipulation is often necessary, with the use of liquid supplements if tolerated. Bypassing the stomach with nasal–jejunal feeding tubes may be effective if the small bowel is not involved.

Bethanechol is often used as a prokinetic agent, but it is not well tolerated. Metoclopramide may be used in dosages of 10–20 mg a ½ hour before meals and at bedtime. Side effects include akathisias, increased prolactin secretion, agitation, and sedation.

2. **NAUSEA AND VOMITING**
After identification of the cause of vomiting, therapy can be initiated. With peripheral vestibular dysfunction, 25 mg of meclizine hydrochloride may be used 2 or 4 times a day or 50 mg po before activity. Diphenhydramine hydrochloride can also be used in a dosage of 25–50 mg 4 times a day. Both are antihistamines that can cause sedation. Scopolamine transdermal patches applied 4 hours before a provocative event and every 3 days afterward can be effective. Nausea postoperatively or due to gastroenteritis responds well to prochlorperazine, 5–10 mg orally 3 times a day or 25 mg as a rectal suppository 2–4 times a day. Butyrophenones are also useful in dosages of 2.5–5.0 mg IM 2 times a day but may cause extrapyramidal side effects. Trimethobenzamide hydrochloride is used in dosages of 250 mg orally 2 or 4 times a day or 200 mg rectally as suppositories 2 to 4 times a day. High-dose metoclopramide 1–2 mg/kg IV has been particularly effective in decreasing nausea due to chemotherapeutic agents.

3. **HICCUPS**
This nonspecific symptom should be evaluated for possible causes such as diaphragmatic irritation and medication effects. Symptomatic therapy with chlorpromazine 25–50 mg IV or metoclopramide 10 mg IV can be helpful.

Driks MR, Craven DE, Celli BR, et al: Nosocomial pneumonia in intubated patients given sucralfate as compared with antacids or histamine type 2 blockers: The role of gastric colonization. N Engl J Med 317:1376, 1987.
Peterson WL: Helicobacter pylori and peptic ulcer disease. N Engl J Med 324:1043, 1991.
Marshall BJ: Campylobacter pylori: its link to gastritis and peptic ulcer disease. Rev Infect Dis 12(suppl 1):S87–93, 1990.
Eberhardt R, Kasper G: Effect of oral bismuth subsalicylate on Campylobacter pylori and on healing and relapse rate of peptic ulcer. Rev Infect Dis 12(suppl 1):S115–119, 1990.
Tytgat GN, Rauws EA, de Koster EH: Campylobacter pylori. Diagnosis and treatment. J Clin Gastroenterol 11(suppl 1):S49–53, 1989.
Wolfe MM, Jensen RT: Zollinger-Ellison syndrome. N Engl J Med 317:1200–1209, 1987.

III. SMALL-BOWEL DISEASE

A. **Crohn's Disease.** This is an idiopathic inflammatory bowel disease that discontinuously involves the entire GI tract. It is characterized by a cobblestone appearance to the mucosa and the formation of deep linear ulcers. Transmural bowel wall involvement distinguishes it from idiopathic ulcerative colitis and predisposes patients to fistula formation and rectal fissures.

1. **DRUGS**

   a. **Sulfasalazine.** This drug consists of sulfapyridine linked to 5-aminosalicylic acid, which is thought to be the active ingredient. Most of the drug reaches the colon unchanged until the 5-ASA is released by action of bacterial azoreductase. The principal side effects are secondary to the sulfapyridine moiety, which is readily absorbed in the colon. These include nausea, anorexia, dyspepsia, reticulocytosis, rash, oligospermia, bronchospasm, neutropenia, and aplastic anemias. This drug is believed to exert its primary effect on arachidonic acid metabolism. Sulfasalazine has been used at a dosage of 1 gm/15 kg to treat mild to moderate Crohn's colitis and ileocolitis. However, evidence concerning its efficacy in ileitis alone is conflicting. It has not been demonstrated to be effective in preventing relapse of Crohn's disease.

b. **Aminosalicylic Acid.** Since up to ⅓ of patients with inflammatory bowel disease are unable to tolerate sulfasalazine because of reactions to the sulfa component, several new drugs have been developed that are constructed solely of 5-aminosalicylic acid (5-ASA). Differences in these drugs are mainly in their coatings, which determine where the drug is released. Currently, osalazine (Dipentum) has been released at a dosage of 500 mg bid for ulcerative colitis in patients intolerant of sulfasalazine. Taken orally, it is released primarily in the colon and would not be useful in ileitis. Mesalamine (Rowasa) is available as a rectal suppository (4 gm/60 mL) to be used at bedtime and retained for 8 hours in patients with proctosigmoiditis.

c. **Corticosteroids.** Corticosteroids have long been recognized as effective in severe Crohn's disease. At doses of 0.25 mg/kg to 0.75 mg/kg, depending on severity, **prednisolone** has been effective in treating ileal disease (Gastroenterology 77:847, 1979). Therapy with corticosteroids does not prevent relapse.

d. **Metronidazole.** Metronidazole has been shown in European studies to be as effective as sulfasalazine in the treatment of colonic Crohn's disease and more effective in ileal and perianal disease. In dosages used (10–20 mg/kg/day), however, it often induces nausea, a metallic taste, alcohol intolerance, and a peripheral neuropathy that requires discontinuation of therapy. Almost half the patients treated with this drug complain of numbness and tingling in their fingers and toes. Nonetheless, this drug may be substituted for sulfasalazine in appropriate cases.

e. **Immunosuppressive Agents.** Immunosuppressive agents such as azathioprine or its active metabolite 6-mercaptopurine have been used successfully in the treatment of Crohn's disease, although azathioprine is generally reserved for those who suffer from refractory steroid-dependent disease with severe steroid side effects, postsurgical patients with rapid recurrence of disease, diffuse jejunoileitis with severe symptoms, and intractable perianal disease or fistulas not amenable to surgery. Azathioprine is slowly effective in treating active Crohn's disease, and it must be given for 3 months to achieve results. Azathioprine therapy is usually begun at a dose of 50 mg/day and gradually increased to 2.5 mg/kg. Blood counts should be followed weekly during initiation of therapy and, if they remain stable, may be followed monthly.

2. TREATMENT STRATEGY

Medical therapy should be dictated by the disease severity. New-onset Crohn's disease with symptoms solely of diarrhea and abdominal cramping without weight loss or evidence of abdominal masses should be treated with sulfasalazine, 500 mg twice a day increased gradually over a week to 500–1000 mg 4 times daily. If mild symptoms persist, a trial of antispasmodic agents for relief of cramping such as dicyclomine hydrochloride 20 mg 4 times a day or antidiarrheal agents such as diphenoxylate and atropine 2.5–5 mg every 6 hours may be added. Tapering to a maintenance dose of sulfasalazine of 2 gm/day should not be attempted unless symptoms are relieved and the original dose has been given at least 3 months. Patients with more active inflammation involving significant weight loss, fever, severe diarrhea, or abdominal pain should be treated initially with steroids, beginning with 40–60 mg of prednisone a day in a single dose. Sulfasalazine can be started simultaneously at a dosage of 500 mg twice a day if colonic involvement is found. After symptom abatement the steroid dosage may be tapered by 5 mg/week until the patient is receiving no more than 20 mg/day. Then the tapering should be done more slowly, at a rate of 5 mg/month until prednisone can be discontinued. During this time, sulfasalazine should be continued at a maintenance dose of 2 gm/day.

Patients with active Crohn's disease involving an inflammatory mass, abscesses, or evidence of malnutrition should be hospitalized and parenteral nutrition and antibiotic therapy started. Parenteral steroids may be started in these patients at a dosage of 40–60 mg/day once an infectious process can be excluded. Patients with recurrent Crohn's disease should be assessed for severity of recurrence, appearance of *Clostridium difficile,* and development of malabsorption as a result of short-bowel syndrome, bacterial overgrowth, or bile salt–induced diarrhea. If recurrent disease is a cause of the patient's symptoms, treatment may be instituted as for new disease. The clinician must always be alert for extraintestinal complications of Crohn's disease, such as iritis, uveitis, peripheral arthritis, erythema nodosum, pyoderma gangrenosum, sclerosing cholangitis, cholelithiasis, and cholecystitis.

a. Nutritional Therapy. Nutritional support is essential in patients with Crohn's disease. Assessment of nutritional deficiencies should be made and replacements given as needed. Elemental diets have even been found to lead to remissions as often as steroid usage has in selected patients. Total parenteral nutrition should be considered in presurgical candidates, children with growth failure, and in patients with malnutrition unable to tolerate oral feedings. Fistula outputs will decrease with total parenteral nutrition, but complete closure is unlikely.

b. Surgical Treatment of Crohn's Disease. Approximately 78% of Crohn's disease patients have a surgical resection within 20 years of onset of symptoms. However, surgery should be a last resort, and the minimal amount of bowel should be resected to relieve symptoms. The most common indications for surgery are bowel obstruction, fistula unresponsive to medical therapy, and abscesses. Abscesses usually will not respond to simple drainage and will require surgery. Toxic megacolon occurs less frequently in Crohn's disease than in chronic ulcerative colitis and usually responds better to conservative measures.

B. Malabsorption. Fat malabsorption is best defined as greater than 7 gm of fat in a 24-hour stool collection while the patient is receiving a 100-gm/day fat diet. Fat malabsorption may occur with factors that impair lipolysis (rapid intestinal transit, decreased bile circulation from bowel resection or liver disease), pancreatic insufficiency, or decreased absorptive area (Crohn's disease). Protein digestion depends on pancreatic enzymes as well as mucosal peptidases. Only in rare disorders such as Hartnup's disease or cystinuria is there preferential malabsorption of amino acids. Carbohydrate malabsorption may occur because of decreased pancreatic amylase, decreased mucosal disaccharidases, or general dysfunction of the brush border. Although certain nutritional deficiencies may predominate, most common malabsorptive syndromes affect absorption of a variety of minerals and vitamins. Excess fat in the stool contributes to increased diarrhea secondary to stimulation of colonic secretion by fatty acids. Fatty acids also form a complex with calcium, leaving oxalate to be absorbed, thus causing renal stone formation. Deficiencies of fat-soluble vitamins may lead to secondary hyperparathyroidism and osteoporosis with vitamin D deficiency and increased bleeding with vitamin K deficiency secondary to deficits of factors II, VII, IX, and X; demyelination of the CNS with vitamin E deficiency has been reported. Disaccharidase deficiencies more commonly cause watery acidic diarrhea and increased flatulence.

1. CELIAC SPRUE
This disorder is caused by increased sensitivity of the small-bowel mucosa to gliadin proteins found in grains such as barley, oats, wheat, and rye. It has been reported that beer should also be excluded because of the hordein contained in malt (Clin Chim Acta 189:123–130, 1990). Although celiac sprue may present as a selective deficiency in iron (anemia), vitamin K (coagulopathy), or vitamin D (osteoporosis), it most commonly presents as a cause of moderate steatorrhea and weight loss. Diagnosis can be established only by histologic demonstration of blunted small-bowel villi with recovery of the villi after gluten withdrawal (Clin Chim Acta 163:1, 1987). Although patients usually recover within 2 months of therapy, some require up to a year.

Complications of celiac sprue include small-bowel lymphoma in up to 13% of patients. There has also been an increased incidence of malignant GI disease, small-bowel ulcerations, and a syndrome similar to subacute combined degeneration of the spinal column. Vitamin supplementation should be considered in very ill patients. In patients with unresponsive celiac sprue, after exclusion of tropical sprue, lymphoma, bacterial overgrowth syndromes, and Zollinger-Ellison syndrome, the use of steroids may be indicated. Prednisone should be given, 40 mg/day, and then decreased to a maintenance dosage of

10 mg/day to sustain near-normal serum protein levels. A report has suggested that cyclosporine may be effective in a refractory pediatric case (Gastroenterology 95:199–204, 1988).

2. INFECTIOUS CAUSES OF MALABSORPTION

   a. **Tropical sprue** occurs in patients who have recently visited tropical areas such as the Far East, the Caribbean, or the Middle East (Gastroenterology 80:590, 1981). The histologic appearance of the small bowel is identical to that in celiac sprue; however, these patients should be treated with vitamin supplementation (folate, 10 mg/day and B_{12}, 100 μg/day IM) as well as tetracycline, 250 mg 4 times/day. In patients unable to tolerate tetracycline, either sulfamethazine 2 gm/day or chloramphenicol 500 mg 4 times a day may be used until nutritional parameters and small-intestinal villi improve (approximately 3–4 weeks).

   b. **Bacterial overgrowth** may cause malabsorption by deconjugation of bile salts or direct utilization of vitamins. This spectrum of diseases may be caused by motility disturbances such as scleroderma or pseudo-obstruction or by disturbances of the anatomy of the small intestine, as occurs in Crohn's disease, small-bowel diverticula, fistula formation, or creation of afferent loops. Careful culturing of at least 10^6 aerobic organisms/mL or 10^4 anerobes from the small intestine is diagnostic. Broad-spectrum antibiotics can be used to suppress bacterial overgrowth. Tetracycline 250 mg 4 times/day for a course of 1–2 weeks should be used. Patients may require repeated courses of therapy, alternating antibiotics such as metronidazole, ampicillin, trimethoprim-sulfamethoxazole, or neomycin. Some gastroenterologists have advocated C14–glycocholate breath tests to monitor treatment success.

   c. **Whipple's disease** is a systemic bacterial infection that causes hyperpigmentation, fever, arthralgias, diarrhea, and confusion (Mayo Clin Proc 63:539–551, 1988). Although the organism has never been cultured, it can be observed in the intestinal mucosa, peripheral lymph nodes, cardiovascular system, pulmonary system, and CNS. Recommended therapy is trimethoprim-sulfamethoxazole 1 double-strength tablet twice daily for at least 1 year. If CNS involvement is evident at initiation of therapy, use of penicillin and streptomycin IM for the first 2 weeks of therapy has been associated with fewer relapses. Nutritional supplementation is given as folic acid 2 mg/day. Alternatives to trimethoprim-sulfamethoxazole are chloramphenicol 250 mg 4 times/day for 6–12 months, oral penicillin 250 mg 4 times/day, or oral tetracycline 250 mg 4 times/day. Long-term therapy for at least 2 years with tetracycline has been suggested to reduce the number of relapses.

   d. **Giardia lamblia** is one of the most common parasitic infections causing malabsorption and may be seen in either stool or duodenal aspirates. Therapy should begin with either metronidazole 250 mg 3 times/day for 1 week or quinacrine hydrochloride 100 mg 3 times/day for 5 days. A second course may be necessary in up to 10% of patients. Other protozoan causes of malabsorption include the *Cryptosporidium* species and *Isospora belli,* which are currently being found as a cause of malabsorption in immunosuppressed patients. No current therapy has yet been demonstrated to be successful in the eradication of *Cryptosporidium.* Trimethoprim-sulfamethoxazole one double-strength tablet po qid for 1 week and then bid for 3 weeks is currently recommended for the treatment of *I. belli.*

3. DISACCHARIDASE DEFICIENCIES

Lactose intolerance due to the brush border deficiency of lactase is a common cause of bloating and diarrhea. It may be diagnosed by oral administration of lactose or by hydrogen breath tests. Deficiency of lactase activity may also be secondary to diseases that injure the brush border mucosal cells such as infectious diarrheas, Crohn's disease, and celiac disease. Treatment is either avoidance of lactose-containing foods or use of lactase packets added to milk products to predigest the lactose.

4. SHORT-BOWEL SYNDROME

The loss of more than 100 cm of terminal ileum is associated with malabsorbtion of fat. However, a small bowel that is 100 cm or longer will still allow oral nutrition with supplementation. Patients with resection of the terminal ileum should receive supplementary B_{12} 100 μg IM each month. Cholestyramine can be titrated to control diarrhea if less than 100 cm of terminal ileum has been removed. The use of pancreatic extracts such as Viokase or Pancrease 3 or 4 capsules with each meal may aid in fatty digestion. H_2 receptor antagonists may be useful in the first month after lengthy small-bowel resections because of the hyperacidity that occurs in this period. Antidiarrheal agents such as loperamide or diphenoxylate and atropine may help decrease "dumping" and increase mucosal contact time with nutrients. Use of medium-chain triglycerides (6–10 carbon fatty acids) bypasses the need for micellar formation and supplies vital calories. Fat-soluble (A, D, K, E) and water-soluble (B, C, folate) vitamins and minerals (calcium, magnesium, iron, zinc) should also be supplemented as needed. Somatostatin analogues (100 μg sc bid) have been shown to decrease the volume of diarrhea and the amount of fluid needed for maintenance in these patients (Digestion 45(suppl 1):77–83, 1990).

C. **Intestinal Ischemia and Obstruction.** For management purposes, small-bowel obstruction should be divided into mechanical obstruction and ileus. Ileus may be treated with fluid resuscitation and stomach decompression using suction. If symptoms are chronic, intestinal pseudo-obstruction should be considered after drug effect is excluded. Mechanical small-bowel obstructions must be divided further into partial small-bowel obstruction (which is treated like an ileus) and complete mechanical small-bowel obstruction (which should be managed surgically because of the high incidence of small-bowel ischemia). With mechanical small-bowel obstruction, a tube should be placed beyond the ligament of Treitz for intermittent suction and decompression. Small-bowel ischemia may be caused by embolism or thrombosis and should be treated either by surgery or angiography with angioplasty. Nonocclusive mesenteric insufficiency may be treated with arteriographic infusion of papavarine. Despite these measures, the mortality in mesenteric ischemia approaches 50%.

Brandt LJ, Berstein LH, Boley SJ, et al: Metronidazole therapy for perineal Crohn's disease: A follow-up study. Gastroenterology 83:383, 1982.

Summers RW, Switz DM, Sessions JT, et al: National Cooperative Crohn's Disease Study: Results of drug treatment. Gastroenterology 77:847, 1987.

Goldstein F: Immunosuppressant therapy of inflammatory bowel disease. Clin Gastroenterol 91:982, 1987.

Davidson AG, Bridges MA: Coeliac disease: A critical review of aetiology and pathogenesis. Clin Chim Acta 163:1, 1987.

Ellis HJ, Freedman AR, Ciclitira PJ: Detection and estimation of the barley prolamin content of beer and malt to assess their suitability for patients with coeliac disease. Clin Chim Acta 189:123–130, 1990.

Bernstein EF, Whitington PF: Successful treatment of atypical sprue in an infant with cyclosporine. Gastroenterology 95:199–204, 1988.

Clinical Conference. Tropical sprue in travelers and expatriates living abroad. Gastroenterology 80:590, 1981.

Fleming JL, Wiesner RH, Shorter RG: Whipple's disease: Clinical, biochemical, and histopathologic features and assessment of treatment in 29 patients. Mayo Clin Proc 63:539–551, 1988.

Nightingale JM, Walker ER, Burnham WR, et al: Short bowel syndrome. Digestion 45(suppl 1):77–83, 1990.

IV. COLONIC DISEASES

A. Chronic Ulcerative Colitis. This is an idiopathic inflammatory disease of the colonic mucosa and submucosa that causes symptoms of tenesmus, pain, and repeated episodes of bloody diarrhea. Its peak incidence is in the 20- to 40-year-old age group. It has been associated with an increased risk of colon cancer and development of primary sclerosing cholangitis. Treatment depends on its extent and severity.

1. THERAPY

   a. **Disease Assessment.** Extent is best established with colonoscopy during a period of relative quiescence. Involvement may be purely distal as in ulcerative proctitis (disease limited to the distal 12 cm of the colon), proctosigmoiditis, or any proximal extension of disease including the entire colon. Primarily left-sided disease (proctitis or proctosigmoiditis) may respond to topical agents. Severity is generally established by clinical parameters:

   (1). Mild disease usually implies fewer than 4 bowel movements a day with minimal systemic symptoms (fever, weight loss) and very little hematochezia.

   (2). Moderate disease involves approximately 4–10 bowel movements a day, with low-grade fever (not exceeding 101°F), mild abdominal pain, and no evidence of nutritional deficiencies.

   (3). Severe disease usually involves high fever, severe abdominal pain, evidence of nutritional compromise, severe GI bleeding requiring transfusions, or evidence of toxic megacolon. Generally, moderate to severe disease should be treated in the hospital with parenteral anti-inflammatory agents.

b. **Sulfasalazine.** Sulfasalzine is a first-line agent in treatment of chronic ulcerative colitis, in disease of any severity with involvement of more than the rectum. Sulfasalazine, as in Crohn's disease, is usually given in a dosage of 3–4 gm/day in 2–4 divided doses. Administration should be gradually increased to therapeutic dosages over a 1-week period, starting from 500 mg 2 times a day. Dosages higher than 4 gm/day rarely prove beneficial. There is usually a response to sulfasalazine within a 2-week period. If no response occurs, sulfasalazine should still be continued with the addition of other agents. If there is response to sulfasalazine, therapy should be continued until clinical and endoscopic evidence of remission is seen. Then the drug may be decreased to 2 gm/day for maintenance. Patients with limited proctitis or proctosigmoiditis on initial treatment may not need maintenance therapy. If maintenance therapy is begun, it should be continued for at least 3 years. Sulfasalazine may cause exacerbation of ulcerative colitis. If side effects occur, desensitization schemes are available that involve stopping the drug for about 2 weeks and then restarting it at 250–500 mg/day, with increases of 250 mg/week. If severe allergic reactions occur, the drug should be discontinued.

c. **5-Aminosalicylic Acid.** 5-ASA is thought to be the active moiety in sulfasalazine. Osalazine (Dipentum) is available (500 mg bid) for ulcerative colitis in patients intolerant of sulfasalazine. Mesalamine (Rowasa) is available as a rectal suppository (4 gm/60 mL) to be used at bedtime and retained for 8 hours in patients with proctosigmoiditis. The role of oral 5-ASA would be as a second-line agent after failure of or intolerance to sulfasalazine. The enema form should be used as a substitute for cortisone enemas or as treatment in those cases unresponsive to corticosteroid enemas.

d. **Corticosteroids.** Cortisone enemas can be given as first-line therapy for left-sided disease. Ulcerative proctosigmoiditis or proctitis can be treated with a once-a-night steroid enema (100 mg hydrocortisone hs), which should be retained for 8 hours. This is usually initiated for a 2-week trial period that may be increased to a twice-daily regimen. It should not be continued longer than a month without response. Oral steroids can be used in mild to moderate colitis that does not respond to sulfasalazine. Prednisone is usually started at 30–60 mg/day and continued for about a 2-week period. If a response is noted, the dosage can be withdrawn at a rate of approximately 5 mg/week. Limited distal colitis that is unresponsive to local therapy and sulfasalazine usually is unresponsive to systemic steroids as well. Therefore, therapeutic trials of oral prednisone in these patients should be kept brief. Severe ulcerative colitis should be treated with systemic steroids, usually given as a continuous infusion of prednisolone 60–80 mg/day or methylprednisolone 40–60 mg/day. Corticotropin has been advocated by some authorities as more efficacious in patients who have not had steroids in the past. The dosage is 120 U/day. Patients should be gradually weaned from corticosteroids if possible and a maintenance dosage of sulfasalazine (500 mg qid) continued to prevent relapse.

e. **Immunosuppressive Agents.** Azathioprine and its metabolite, 6-mercaptopurine, have been used in therapy of refractory ulcerative colitis. Most often, azathioprine is administered in a dosage of 2.0 mg/kg/day and will permit a decrease in steroid use. Mean time of onset of symptomatic relief is 3 months after initiation of therapy. Monthly monitoring of blood counts is necessary because of possible bone marrow suppression. Drug therapy should be halted if leukocyte counts fall below 4000. Side effects of medication include rash, fever, joint pain, hepatitis, pancreatitis, and immune suppression. Because of the unknown potential for malignancy, most authorities would recommend discontinuing azathioprine within a year.

f. **Antidiarrheal Agents.** These may be used in patients with minimally active disease to control symptoms of diarrhea. Loperamide, tincture of opium, belladonna, and diphenoxylate with atropine have all been used to decrease the number of bowel movements. These agents may be used for patients who have episodes of nocturnal diarrhea that cannot be controlled with other methods, but should not be used in any patient with acute moderate to severe symptoms because of the risk of precipitating toxic megacolon.

g. **Nutrition.** Although no specific diet has been found to be helpful in ulcerative colitis, it is important for patients to avoid foods that seem to create increased diarrhea, bloating, and flatulence. Calcium supplementation should be considered in patients receiving steroids. Iron and folate replacement is sometimes necessary in patients with chronic disease. For the seriously ill, TPN should be used to improve overall status if oral intake is going to be restricted for longer than 2 weeks.

2. COMPLICATIONS

a. **Toxic Megacolon.** Toxic megacolon occurs in severe colitis with fever, tachycardia, abdominal pain, abdominal distention, and radiologic evidence of dilatation of the transverse colon greater than 6 cm in diameter. It is usually found in recurrent ulcerative colitis as opposed to the initial presentation. Other causes of fulminant colitis such as *Clostridium difficile, Salmonella, Shigella,* and *Campylobacter* should be excluded. Supportive care is extremely important, with careful management of fluid and electrolyte balances, blood transfusions, broad-spectrum antibiotics, and large doses of prednisolone (100–200 mg IV). Any anticholinergics or opiates should be discontinued.

Patients should be kept NPO, with nasogastric tube placement and suction to help decompress the GI tract. Abdominal flat plates should be taken every day for the first 3 days to determine whether the colon is decreasing in diameter. If the colon continues to distend or does not shrink after 3 days, colectomy is generally recommended because of the high incidence of perforation. If the patient responds to these measures, steroids should be continued at high dosage for another 2 weeks. Some believe that Crohn's disease has a decreased incidence of perforation in toxic megacolon than with chronic ulcerative colitis and that it should be treated medically for a longer period. Patients responding to medical therapy are more prone to redevelop toxic megacolon in later flares of colitis and require colectomy (Am J Surg 147:106, 1984).

   b. Colon Cancer Risks. Colon cancer rates in ulcerative colitis are highest in those who were less than 20 years of age at disease onset, in pancolitis, and in disease of more than 8 years' duration. The incidence of colon cancer has been estimated at 1.4% after 14 years. Colonic cancer associated with ulcerative colitis appears endoscopically to be flatter than cancers in the general population, thereby making diagnosis more difficult. *Surveillance colonoscopy is usually recommended after disease has been present longer than 8 years* (Med Clin North Am 74:189, 1990). If no dysplasia is found, barium enema study can be alternated with colonoscopy and multiple biopsies on a yearly basis for continued surveillance. If moderate to severe dysplasia is found, colonoscopy with multiple biopsies should be done within 3 months. The area of dysplasia should be carefully identified and colectomy performed because of the high association of occult malignancy with dysplasia.

   c. Indications for Surgery. Colectomy generally should be recommended in patients with refractory toxic megacolon, suspected colon perforation, uncontrollable colonic hemorrhage, and severe ulcerative colitis that does not improve despite 2 weeks of intensive therapy. Other indications are dictated by the functional abilities of the patient, toxicities of medical therapy, and the long-term risk of malignant disease. Patients with longstanding disease would be considered for colectomy despite mild symptoms because of the increasing malignancy risk. It is useful to note that the operative mortality is approximately 3% in elective colectomy.

B. Pseudomembranous Colitis. Pseudomembranous colitis is most commonly found as a sequela of prior antibiotic therapy (ampicillin, clindamycin, cephalosporins, penicillin), usually occurring a week after administration (Rev Infect Dis 12(suppl 2):S243, 1990). In the absence of antibiotic exposure, the disease is usually more difficult to eradicate and has a higher relapse incidence. Symptoms generally are fever, bloody diarrhea, and abdominal pain. Although the disease is produced by proliferation of *Clostridium difficile,* it can be diagnosed by detection of the toxin in the stool as well as by culture. Endoscopic evaluation may reveal small yellowish-white plaque-like pseudomembranes.

   Vancomycin is highly effective in the therapy of pseudomembranous colitis when given orally 125–500 mg 4 times a day. Although it is poorly absorbed, it should be carefully monitored when given in the presence of renal failure (Med Clin North Am 66:655, 1982). Metronidazole, 500 mg 4 times/day has been found to be equally effective and much less expensive. Bacitracin is also used as treatment (25,000 U 4 times/day). Generally these regimens should be continued for 1–2 weeks. Ion exchange resins such as cholestyramine have been used to bind the toxin of *Clostridium difficile* and decrease diarrhea. Cholestyramine may be given in dosages of 3 gm 4 times/day. Unfortunately, relapses may occur in as many as 20% of the patients within 3 weeks of discontinuing therapy. Several methods have been advocated to deal with such relapses, including reinstituting a course of metronidazole and adding cholestyramine during the last days of therapy and continuing it for another week after discontinuing antibiotic therapy.

C. **Diverticular Disease.** This is diagnosed by the presence of multiple herniations of the colonic mucosa through the muscular colonic wall. Diverticuli are associated with increasing age and long exposure to a "Western" diet. It is generally believed that diverticuli occur secondary to high intraluminal pressure caused by colonic hypermobility and decreased intraluminal mass resulting from lack of dietary fiber. Patients are usually asymptomatic; however, spasmodic left lower quadrant pain may be present. Therapy involves increasing stool bulk with such agents as psyllium, methylcellulose, and bran. In patients with abdominal pain, antispasmodics such as probanthine bromide, 15 mg 3 times/day, have been found effective.

Diverticulitis occurs in approximately ⅕ of patients with diverticulosis. Most commonly, pain and fever are the presenting symptoms. This may be associated with upper GI upset as well as changes in bowel habits. The diagnosis is most often made clinically with the prior diagnosis of diverticulosis. However, careful flexible sigmoidoscopy can be valuable in diagnosing acute diverticulitis. If the pain is localized and there are no peritoneal symptoms, broad-spectrum antibiotics such as ampicillin or a cephalosporin can be utilized. However, if there is high fever, leukocytosis, or evidence of peritoneal irritation, the patient should be admitted to the hospital, nasogastric suction instituted, and broad-spectrum parenteral antibiotics given with anaerobic coverage. Antibiotics should be given for approximately 1 week–10 days unless there is perforation of the colon. Complications from diverticulitis include the formation of enteroperitoneal abscesses and bowel obstruction secondary to stricture. Fistulas may form between the colon and any adjacent organ, including the bladder, vagina, or small bowel. Fistulas to the bladder are the most common and are difficult to identify. However, computed tomography of the bladder appears to be very sensitive in demonstrating air in the bladder, confirming the presence of a fistula. Surgical resection is necessary when abscesses, fistulas, or strictures appear.

D. **Irritable Bowel Syndrome.** Irritable bowel syndrome (IBS) is the most common GI disorder faced by the practitioner. Its cardinal manifestations are abdominal pain and either constipation or diarrhea. IBS generally occurs in the 20- to 30-year-old age group and should be diagnosed only when other conditions are excluded. Its cause is unknown; however, several studies have indicated that patients have an increased response to colonic distention in terms of pain perception. There may also be a relationship between increased cluster contractions in the small bowel and the pain. Patients need to be educated about the excellent prognosis of this disorder but should also be reminded of its chronic nature. High-fiber diets should be initiated in most patients, while recognizing that most will have some exacerbation within the first month of therapy. Bulking agents also should be added, with increased liquid intake to prevent stools from becoming too dehydrated from the stool softener's hydrophilic properties. Antispasmodic anticholinergic agents such as decyclomine hydrochloride may be used, starting at 10 mg 4 times/day, with gradual increases to as high as 40 mg 4 times/day. Newer antimuscarinic agents such as cimetropium bromide (50 mg po tid) are under study. Patients primarily with diarrhea may respond to the addition of either diphenoxylate and atropine 2.5–5 mg 4 times/day or loperamide 2–4 mg 3 times/day. Analgesics such as pentazocine 50–100 mg 4 times/day may be prescribed for short periods. Antiflatulents may also provide some relief in patients who complain of bloating. Simethicone 2–4 tablets 4 times/day or activated charcoal 4 tablets 4 times/day supplies some gas relief. Depression may be present in these patients and can be treated with a single bedtime dosage of amitriptyline 25–50 mg. There is no convincing evidence that any therapy is uniformly effective in IBS (Gastroenterology 95:232, 1988).

E. Constipation. Constipation is a common symptom reported by 21% of American women (Dig Dis Sci 34:1153, 1989). It is difficult to define and is usually related to the individual's expectations. However, 2 or fewer stools per week is generally considered evidence of constipation. Constipated stools are hard and contain less than 50% water. Constipation may be caused by any mechanism that decreases stool transit time, increases colonic absorption of fluid, or disturbs the bacterial content of the colon. Lesions such as anal fissures or hemorrhoids may cause pain and decreased evacuation of the colon. Hirschsprung's disease is usually detected in childhood but may be diagnosed in adults by anal manometry and a rectal biopsy showing aganglionosis. When the cause is idiopathic, several modifications may be made. Increasing dietary bulk corrects constipation in about ⅔ of patients (Clin Ther 11:572, 1989). Some patients feel less urge to defecate and require modification of their daily schedule in an attempt to defecate at least once a day. Glycerin suppositories may help them by lubricating the stool, thus assisting in emptying the rectum. Inability to relax the rectosigmoid angle during defecation may require the use of biofeedback techniques to re-train rectal reflexes. Some patients, predominately female, have markedly increased colonic transit times, symptoms of abdominal bloating, pain, and a history of laxative abuse. Their symptoms may be aggravated by increased dietary fiber.

F. Chronic Diarrhea. This is defined as diarrhea of longer than 6 weeks' duration. It may be divided into 2 subgroups: osmotic and secretory, based on stool osmolality and persistence of diarrhea with fasting. The osmolar gap found in chronic osmotic diarrheas is most often secondary to either factitial causes with unabsorbed cations such as magnesium or disaccharidase deficiencies such as lactose intolerance. Chronic secretory diarrhea persists with fasting and most commonly is due to bile salt and fatty acid malabsorption. Factitial diarrhea from laxative abuse is common when there are no other detectable causes. Endocrine tumors such as VIPoma (VIP = vasoactive intestinal peptide) and carcinoid syndrome also produce secretory diarrhea.

Therapy consists primarily of careful fluid management, especially with stool outputs greater than 1 L/day. Various oral rehydration solutions are available that primarily supply glucose in combination with sodium, taking advantage of their co-transport mechanism in the small intestine. Opiates, diphenoxylate and atropine 1–2 tablets 4 times/day, loperamide 2–4 mg two times/day, and codeine 30–60 mg 4 times/day can be used to decrease the symptoms of chronic diarrheas. Most of these have side effects such as drowsiness, nausea and vomiting, and respiratory depression. However, loperamide can be used in dosages up to 35 mg/day without significant toxicity. Alpha-adrenergics such as clonidine may be used for chronic diabetic diarrheas in particular. It should be started at 0.1 mg/day and gradually increased to 0.3–0.4 mg/day as tolerated. Patients often develop postural hypotension and drowsiness at high dosages. Calcium channel blockers such as verapamil 80 mg 3 times/day may be used with loperamide to control diarrhea. Prostaglandin inhibitors such as indomethacin 50 mg 3 times/day, may be helpful in selected patients with increased mucosal prostaglandin production.

In patients with VIPomas, medications such as lithium 300 mg/day and prednisone 60 mg/day are helpful in controlling diarrhea. Lithium has well-known hematologic, CNS, and cardiovascular side effects. Prednisone should be started at 60 mg/day but should be decreased as soon as possible to decrease side effects. Somatostatin, given as 100 µg subcutaneous injections twice daily, has been found to decrease diarrhea secondary to endocrine tumors, but produces steatorrhea and decreased glucose tolerance as its side effects. Methylsergide and cyproheptadine are selective serotonin antagonists used in carcinoid diarrhea. Often a combination of these drugs with Imodium may be necessary to control the diarrhea associated with the syndrome.

G. **Colonic Polyps.** Incidental small colonic polyps less than 1 cm discovered on colon x-ray should generally be followed by colonoscopy for biopsy and surveillance for further polyps. A 50% chance of discovering synchronous adenomatous polyps exists. If histologically the polyp is a tubular, tubulovillous, or villous adenoma, the patient should undergo another colonoscopy in a year to be sure the colon is free of polyps. If it is, surveillance of the colon should be instituted with colonoscopy alternating with barium enema study every 2–3 years. Recent reports suggest that hyperplastic polyps may be a marker for adenomatous polyps, but further surveillance with the sole finding of hyperplastic polyps is not recommended. Polyps larger than 1 cm have at least a 1% chance of malignancy, and they should be removed and examined histologically. The need for polyp removal is increased based on size and the patient's history. If adenomatous polyps are found, surveillance should be instituted as with small adenomatous polyps. Patients with a family history of hereditary colon cancer require early colonoscopy starting by age 18. In familial polyposis syndromes, screening should begin at age 10 and be continued until at least age 40 to be certain that polyps do not develop.

V. ANORECTAL DISORDERS

A. **Hemorrhoids.** Hemorrhoids are a submucosal venous plexus found in the upper anal canal. External hemorrhoids are those dilated veins that are found below the dentate line. External hemorrhoids usually cause pain only when thrombosed. Frequently this pain persists only for the first 48 hours. If the patient is seen within that time, excision of the clot is the treatment of choice. If the pain has already begun to subside, sitz baths are usually sufficient.

Internal hemorrhoids are the dilated venous plexus found above the dentate line. These are usually responsible for the rectal outlet bleeding the patient experiences and are treated by decreasing abdominal straining and by fixing the prolapsing hemorrhoidal tissue. Decreased abdominal straining can be accomplished by giving bulk-forming agents and thereby decreasing strain in defecation. If substantial prolapse of internal hemorrhoids exists, the tissue may be fixed by rubber band ligation, injection, or hemorrhoidectomy. Infrared coagulation can be used but may be associated with a greater risk of recurrent hemorrhoids (Surg Clin North Am 68:1401, 1989). Treatment of hemorrhoids in HIV + patients should be as conservative as possible as there have been recent reports of abscess formation after rubber band ligation.

B. **Anal Fissure.** An anal fissure is a tear of the squamous cell–lined portion of the anal canal. It is generally less than 1 cm in size and produces severe burning pain during bowel movements. It may also be a cause of rectal outlet bleeding. Most anal fissures are secondary to passage of very firm and large stools. Acute anal fissures should be treated with sitz baths, topical anesthetics, and stool bulking agents. Patients should be able to pass stools without discomfort if this therapy is to succeed. If the fissure becomes chronic, surgical intervention, usually in the form of a lateral sphincterotomy, is indicated.

C. **Rectal Abscesses and Fistulas.** Rectal abscesses are generally characterized by severe rectal pain, tenderness, and high fever. Suspected abscesses should be surgically evaluated and drained. Fistulas are most often secondary to prior incompletely healed rectal abscesses. They usually begin in the anal canal crypt and extend into the perianal skin region. Fistulas rarely heal by themselves, requiring surgical intervention.

D. **Infectious Proctitis.** Most cases of infectious proctitis are sexually transmitted. *Chlamydia trachomatis,* probably the most common cause of sexually transmitted disease, can now be easily cultured. Therapy is usually tetracycline 500 mg 4 times/day for 1 week. Gonococcal proctitis may occur in homosexual males or in females, spreading from gonococcal cervical disease. Penicillin therapy is recommended unless a resistant strain of organism is present. Then treatment with ceftriaxone 250 mg IM can eradicate the organism. In homosexuals, empiric therapy with penicillin (4.8 million U procaine penicillin IM and probenecid 1 gm po) followed by tetracycline 100 mg po bid may be beneficial for early relief of symptoms pending cultures (JAMA 260:348, 1988). Herpetic rectal infections cause severe pain and may lead to constipation. The presence of characteristic erythematous grouped vesicles usually confirms the diagnosis. Topical acyclovir ointment may decrease the duration of viral replication. Oral acyclovir 400 mg 5 times/day also decreases viral replication, formation of new lesions, and leads to earlier resolution of symptoms (JAMA 259:2879, 1988).

E. **Pruritus Ani.** Pruritus ani is common but may be a symptom of many systemic illnesses such as diabetes mellitus, jaundice, or lymphomas. *Candida* may involve this region and can be treated by topical 1% clotrimazole cream. A program of anal hygiene by careful cleansing of the region with a moist towel can decrease symptoms. Contact dermatitis may also be the cause of pruritus ani, from scented toilet paper, bath soaps, or laundry detergents. Removal of the agent and application of 1% topical hydrocortisone can speed relief.

Klotz U, Maier K, Fischer C, et al: Therapeutic efficacy of sulfasalazine and its metabolites in patients with ulcerative colitis and Crohn's disease. N Engl J Med 303:1499, 1980.
Schroeder KW, Tremaine WJ, Ilstrup DM: Coated oral 5-aminosalicyclic acid therapy for mildly to moderately active ulcerative colitis: A randomized study. N Engl J Med 317:1625, 1987.
Grant CS, Dozois RR: Toxic megacolon: Ultimate fate of patients after successful medical management. Am J Surg 147:106–110, 1984.
Binder V: Incidence of colonic cancer in inflammatory bowel disease. Scand J Gastroenterol (suppl) 170:78 (discussion pp 81–82), 1989.
Korelitz BI: Considerations of surveillance, dysplasia, and carcinoma of the colon in the management of ulcerative colitis and Crohn's disease. Med Clin North Am 74:189–199, 1990.
Bartlett JG: Clostridium difficile: Clinical considerations. Rev Infect Dis 12(suppl 2):S243–251, 1990.
Tedesco FJ: Pseudomembranous colitis: Pathogenesis and therapy. Med Clin N Am 66:655, 1982.
Klein KB: Controlled treatment trials in the irritable bowel syndrome: A critique. Gastroenterology 95:232–241, 1988.
Snape WJ Jr: The effect of methylcellulose on symptoms of constipation. Clin Ther 11:572–579, 1989.
Everhart JE, Go VL, Johannes RS, et al: A longitudinal survey of self-reported bowel habits in the United States. Dig Dis Sci 34:1153–1162, 1989.
Shouler P, Keighley MRB: Changes in colorectal function in severe idiopathic constipation. Gastroenterology 90:414, 1986.
Dennison AR, Wherry DC, Morris DL: Hemorrhoids. Nonoperative management. Surg Clin North Am 68:1401–1409, 1988.
Rompalo AM, Mertz GJ, Davis LG, et al: Oral acyclovir for treatment of first-episode herpes simplex virus proctitis. JAMA 259:2879–2881, 1988.
Rompalo AM, Roberts P, Johnson K, Stamm WE: Empirical therapy for the management of acute proctitis in homosexual men. JAMA 260:348–353, 1988.

VI. PANCREATIC DISEASES

A. **Sphincter of Oddi Dysfunction.** The sphincter of Oddi is thought to cause biliary colic by either stenosis of the lumen or hypertonicity of the sphincter (dyskinesia). The diagnosis can be established by endoscopic retrograde cholangiopancreatography (ERCP) and biliary manometry. Dysfunction is suggested by the elevation of serum alkaline phosphatase on at least 2 occasions. Both stenosis and dyskinesia of the sphincter can be treated with sphincterotomy (N Engl J Med 320:82, 1989).

B. Acute Pancreatitis. This is known to occur in association with alcohol ingestion, gallstones, trauma to the pancreas, viral infections (mumps, herpes viruses, coxsackie, hepatitis), ischemia, hypertriglyceridemia, hypercalcemia, drugs (steroids, diuretics, sulfas, alpha methyldopa, and azathioprine), collagen vascular diseases, malignant disease, penetrating ulcers, and ERCP. The process is perpetuated by inappropriate activation of pancreatic enzymes and decreased inactivation by trypsin inhibitors. Therapy for acute alcoholic pancreatitis is determined by the severity of the disease. This can be established by using the Ranson criteria (Am J Gastroenterol 77:633, 1982), which consist of:

1. Criteria on entry: Age greater than 55; WBC greater than 16,000/mm^3; blood sugar greater than 200 mg/dL; LDH greater than 350 IU/dL; SGOT greater than 250 IU/dL;
2. Criteria present during the first 48 hours: 10% or more decrease in hematocrit; 5 mg/dL rise in BUN; calcium below 8 mg/dL; more than 6 L of fluid retention; arterial Pao$_2$ less than 60 mm Hg; and a base deficit of more than 4 mEq/L.

If fewer than 3 criteria are present, pancreatitis may be classified as mild; if more than 4 are present, severe pancreatitis with a poor prognosis is suggested. The degree of pancreatic necrosis may be correlated to the number of Ranson criteria present.

The Glasgow scoring system is accepted in Europe; it has simplified criteria and is based totally on admission findings (Br J Surg 75:460, 1988).

CRITERIA	LEVEL OF SIGNIFICANCE
Age	>55 years
Serum transaminase	>100 (U/L)
WBC	>16 (thousand/mm^3)
Blood glucose	>10 (mmol/L)
Serum urea	>16 (mmol/L)
Arterial oxygen	<60 (mm Hg)
Serum calcium	<2 (mmol/L)
Serum albumin	<3.2 (gm/dL)
Serum LDH	>600 (U/L)

If 2 or fewer criteria are present, the pancreatitis can be classified as mild; more than 2 suggest severe pancreatitis. It has been proposed that either transaminase or age can be deleted from the criteria to increase the sensitivity of the system, which appears to be valid for gallstone-related as well as alcoholic pancreatitis.

1. TREATMENT OF MILD PANCREATITIS

1. Rehydration should be given immediately, with careful attention to fluid and electrolyte balance.
2. Nasogastric suction should be used only if ileus or nausea and vomiting is present.
3. Analgesia should be supplied with meperidine, 50–75 mg IM every 4 hours as needed.

4. Food should be reinitiated after pain subsides and the patient's appetite returns. This should occur within the first week of hospitalization with serum amylases approaching normal levels. Liquids should be given initially as 6 small meals/day to reduce acid secretion, which in turn decreases pancreatic secretion. During this time, acid should be suppressed by giving antacids 1 hour postprandially or by an H_2 receptor blocker.

2. THERAPY FOR SEVERE PANCREATITIS

1. Severe pancreatitis warrants ICU admission and careful fluid management with either wedged pulmonary artery pressures or a central venous pressure monitor. If fluid loss exceeds 5 L, colloid replacement should be initiated.

2. Nasogastric tube placement should be instituted with antacids given every hour as needed to keep the gastric pH greater than 4.

3. Meperidine may be given for pain in dosages of 50–100 mg IM every 4 hours.

4. Cardiac, renal, and pulmonary function should be monitored for evidence of congestive heart failure, arrhythmias, acute tubular necrosis, atelectasis, pneumonia, pleural effusions, and ARDS.

5. Metabolic complications, for example, **hyperglycemia,** may necessitate institution of insulin therapy early in the disease. **Hypocalcemia** may occur secondary to loss of serum albumin. If loss is severe, calcium can be replaced with 10 mL (1 gm) of 10% calcium gluconate, which provides only 93 mg of elemental calcium. IV calcium should be administered over 10–15 minutes with careful monitoring for cardiac arrythmias. Calcium should not be administered until hypokalemia is corrected. **Magnesium may be depleted concomitantly** with hypocalcemia and can be replaced by providing 8–40 mEq/L of fluid given over 4–6 hours.

6. Parenteral nutrition should be instituted within 2 days of admission if nutritional intake is expected to be curtailed for a prolonged period. Standard parenteral nutrition formulas may be used. No deleterious effects have been ascribed to IV lipids.

7. Prophylactic antibiotics are generally not indicated in acute pancreatitis unless it is thought to be due to biliary obstruction. Then ciprofloxacin has been proposed to be the best agent because of its ability to cross the blood-pancreas barrier (Am J Surg 158:472, 1989).

8. ERCP should be performed in cases of biliary pancreatitis to remove the common bile duct stone as soon as possible. Sphincterotomy appears to decrease complications and decrease mortality.

3. COMPLICATIONS

Disseminated intravascular coagulation may occur and should be treated by replacement of blood factors with fresh frozen plasma. Bleeding may appear secondary to stress ulceration, esophageal varices, and bowel infarctions due to vascular thrombosis from pancreatic inflammation. Acidosis may be secondary to ketoacidosis from hyperglycemic or alcoholic causes, lactic acidosis resulting from decreased perfusion, or ingestion of salicylate- or ethylene glycol–containing drugs. Jaundice may be intrahepatic, secondary to the disease process, or extrahepatic, due to retained common bile duct stones or edema of the head of the pancreas. Pancreatic abscess is a dreaded complication with almost 100% mortality if not surgically debrided. Diagnosis should be established by CT scan to look for gas in either pseudocysts or a pancreatic phlegmon. If infection is suspected, some authors suggest that aspiration of pancreatic fluid via CT and culturing for bacteria may be beneficial. Use of peritoneal lavage in patients with severe pancreatitis is controversial. Some believe that in patients with profound pancreatitis with pancreatic ascites and evidence of shock, peritoneal lavage may be instituted with a peritoneal dialysis catheter and infusion of standard dialysis fluids into the abdomen (N Engl J Med 312:399, 1985). This fluid can be gravity drained continuously to "wash out" toxic pancreatic substances. Recent studies have advocated the combination of surgical debridement with local lavage (World J Surg 12:255, 1988). Somatostatin analogue, at a dosage of 100 µg/hour after a loading dose of 250 µg, has been used for the first 48 hours of acute pancreatitis. Results in a very small number of patients suggest that this therapy may decrease complications, although mortality rates have not been altered.

C. Chronic Pancreatitis. This diagnosis implies end-stage organ failure with endocrine insufficiency (diabetes mellitus) or exocrine insufficiency with steatorrhea. Chronic pain is also present in approximately 85% of patients. The diagnosis is most reliably made by duodenal intubation and collection of stimulated pancreatic secretions that are analyzed for bicarbonate and pancreatic enzyme content (Gastroenterology 88:1973, 1985).

1. THERAPY FOR PAIN
Treatable causes of chronic pancreatitis such as hypercalcemia, hypertriglyceridemia, and hemochromatosis should be ruled out. Use of alcohol should be discontinued. Anatomic lesions such as localized strictures of the pancreatic duct or pancreatic pseudocysts should be sought. Pseudocysts larger than 4 cm in diameter that have been present for more than 6 weeks and are causing symptoms should be considered for surgical drainage procedures. CT or ultrasound-guided needle aspiration of pseudocysts may lead to their resolution. Some authorities believe pancreas divisum to be a cause of chronic pancreatitis (Gastroenterology 89:1431, 1985). Sphincterotomy should be considered with caution in these patients. Narcotic analgesics should be used sparingly because of the high potential of addiction. Celiac ganglion blocks have been reported to have some success in pain treatment. Surgical options include total pancreatectomy and ligation of the pancreatic duct. Some authorities have advocated enzyme replacement with dosages similar to those used for pancreatic exocrine

insufficiency to inhibit pancreatic secretion and decrease pain (Gastroenterology 87:44, 1984).

2. **THERAPY FOR EXOCRINE INSUFFICIENCY**
Dietary modifications should be begun early in pancreatic insufficiency. These include increasing protein intake and decreasing fat to less than 20% of daily calories. Medium-chain triglycerides that do not require pancreatic digestion for absorption should be the major source of fat calories. Enzymes can be replaced with supplements such as Viokase 8 tablets with each meal, Cotazym 6 capsules with each meal, or Pancrease (microencapsulated) 3 capsules with each meal. Enzyme supplements should be divided to give ⅓ of the dose before eating, ⅓ during the meal, and ⅓ after the meal. If supplementation fails to correct the steatorrhea, other causes of malabsorption should be sought. If none are found, the addition of bicarbonate (650 mg with meals) or H_2 receptor antagonists may be necessary.

3. **THERAPY FOR ENDOCRINE INSUFFICIENCY**
Insulin therapy in chronic pancreatitis must be carefully monitored because of the lability of glucose absorption secondary to exocrine insufficiency and the absence of counterregulatory peptides such as glucagon during periods of hypoglycemia. Systems of insulin administration that increase flexibility and monitoring are advised.

D. Cystic Fibrosis. Sweat sodium and chloride secretion more than 60 mEq/L with appropriate clinical findings is diagnostic of this autosomal recessive illness. The genetic abnormality has been identified, and gene therapy may someday correct the disease. Nutritional supplementation is the primary GI management problem with this disease that causes pancreatic insufficiency. Intestinal obstruction may occur secondary to viscous intestinal secretions mixed with partially digested food. This may result from noncompliance or overcompliance with pancreatic enzyme supplementation. 1 tablespoonful of mineral oil given with each meal usually relieves this problem. If it persists, a Gastrografin enema diluted with water to ⅓ strength is usually successful. Rectal prolapse occurs in 20% of patients but is usually amenable to increased pancreatic enzyme supplementation. Abnormal gallbladder function leading to a microgallbladder or cholelithiasis is found in upwards of 40% of patients. Surgery is generally not indicated unless the patient has symptoms. Fatty liver is also commonly found in up to 30%. Liver disease may lead to cirrhosis and portal hypertension in as many as 5% of patients. Bleeding esophageal varices should be treated initially with sclerotherapy. Shunt procedures should be considered if the patient has sufficient pulmonary reserve.

Geenen JE, Hogan WJ, Dodds WJ, et al: The efficacy of endoscopic sphincterotomy after cholecystectomy in patients with spincter-of-Oddi dysfunction. N Engl J Med 320:82–87, 1989.
Ranson JHC: Etiological and prognostic factors in human acute pancreatitis. Am J Gastroenterol 77:633, 1982.
Leese T, Shaw D: Comparison of three Glasgow multifactor prognostic scoring systems in acute pancreatitis. Br J Surg 75:460–462, 1988.

Ihse I, Evander A, Holmberg JT, et al: Influence of peritoneal lavage on objective signs in acute pancreatitis. N Engl J Med 312:399, 1985.
Niederan C, Grendell JH: Diagnosis of chronic pancreatitis. Gastroenterology 88:1973, 1985.
Steinberg WM, et al: Diagnostic assays in acute pancreatitis. Ann Intern Med 102:576, 1985.
Bradley EL III: Antibiotics in acute pancreatitis. Am J Surg 158:472–478, 1989.
Cotton PB: Pancreas divisum—Curiosity or culprit. Gastroenterology 89:1431, 1985.
Slaff J, Jacobson J, Tillman R, et al: Protease specific suppression of pancreatic exocrine secretion. Gastroenterology 87:44, 1984.
Berger HR, Buchler M, Bittner R, et al: Necrosectomy and post-operative local lavage in patients with necrotizing pancreatitis: Results of a prospective clinical trial. World J Surg 12:255–262, 1988.

VII. MISCELLANEOUS

A. Chronic Idiopathic Abdominal Pain. By definition, chronic idiopathic abdominal pain consists of pain of more than 6 months' duration, absence of physical or laboratory abnormalities, lack of response to symptomatic therapy, and deterioration of functional status. Treatment should be based on the understanding that chronic pain primarily comes from the evaluative brain centers rather than the peripheral nerves. Therapy should be based on:

1. Confirmation of the reality of the pain to the patient;
2. Careful explanation of the chronic nature of the pain and the likelihood that the pain will persist;
3. Behavior modification techniques to increase physical activity and the patient's coping skills with the assistance of psychiatric consultation;
4. Avoidance of medications such as aspirin, narcotics, and benzodiazepines, as these are primarily effective only with acute pain;
5. Use of tricyclic antidepressants in patients with depressive symptoms.

Treatment of chronic pain depends on the combined efforts of primary care physicians, physical therapists, and psychiatrists to bring patients to a functional level.

B. Gastrointestinal Bleeding

1. UPPER GASTROINTESTINAL BLEEDING

Upper GI bleeding remains a diagnostic and therapeutic challenge because its 10% mortality rate has not decreased in the past 30 years. Any degree of upper GI bleeding must be considered major until proven otherwise. The patient's hemodynamic status must be assessed. Orthostatic changes in blood pressure (a decrease in diastolic blood pressure of more than 15 mm of mercury or an increase in pulse rate of 20 beats/minute) indicate a 15% loss of blood volume. Hypotension at rest indicates a blood volume loss of at least 25%. Large-bore IV lines should be established and crystalloid given immediately. Laboratory tests should investigate the presence of chronic anemia, hemolysis, coagulation abnormalities, liver dysfunction, or renal dysfunction. Packed red blood cells may be used for blood replacement, 1 unit of fresh frozen plasma being given for every 5 units of packed red blood cells given. Gastric lavage should be instituted with a large-bore tube and infusion of about 200–300 mL of tap water with a 50-mL syringe. There is no evidence that lavage with vasoconstrictive agents is routinely effective. Because 85–90% of upper GI bleeding stops on its own in the first 24 hours, endoscopy of all patients is not necessary. If gastric lavage reveals no evidence of active bleeding, patients may be carefully monitored and treated with either antacids or H_2 receptor blockers. There is currently no evidence to suggest that medical therapy for active GI bleeding is effective. However, common practice is to start acid suppression in hopes of preventing future rebleeding. Patients who are actively bleeding or who are not actively bleeding but are older than 60, hemodynamically unstable, require more than 3 U of blood, have a coagulopathy, or have bleeding while hospitalized should have endoscopy at the earliest opportunity. Depending on the results of this procedure, therapy can be instituted as follows:

a. **Gastric or Duodenal Ulcer** (40% of hemorrhages). Antacids, H_2 receptor blockers, or sucralfate may be used if there are no active signs of bleeding. If bleeding is present or a vessel is visible at the base of the ulcer (associated with more than 5 units of blood loss within 24 hours and a 50% chance of emergency surgery), the use of electrocoagulation, heater probe, or laser therapy is indicated (Gastroenterology 90:217, 1986). If bleeding continues, surgical intervention is warranted. If no active bleeding is seen, medical therapy may be sufficient unless bleeding recurs.

b. **Gastritis and Duodenitis** (25% of hemorrhages). These usually respond to removal of the irritating drug and administration of antacids, IV H_2 receptor blockers, omeprazole, or sucralfate. In stress-related gastritis (severe trauma, CNS injury, or hepatic coma), IV H_2 receptor blocker therapy and antacids should be utilized to keep the pH greater than 4. Although there has been recent evidence that decreased gastric acidity may lead to increasing morbidity and mortality from bacterial colonization, the severity of the hemorrhage should determine the agents of choice (N Engl J Med 317:1376, 1987).

c. **Variceal Bleeding.** If active variceal bleeding is present, IV administration of vasopressin at a rate of 0.2–0.9 U/minute and balloon tamponade with a Sengstaken-Blakemore tube or Minnesota tube should be initiated. Evidence exists that the addition of nitroglycerin, either sublingual or IV, may potentiate the effects of vasopressin and decrease its side effects. Balloon tamponade should generally be withdrawn within 24 hours to prevent pressure necrosis of the esophagus. Sclerotherapy should be initiated at the earliest opportunity. Somatostatin (4.2 μg/minute) has been used to treat variceal hemorrhage and has been successful in initially stopping bleeding, but its use is still controversial (Am J Gastroenterol 85:804, 1990). Surgical intervention is reserved for those patients who have either bled repeatedly despite sclerotherapy or are continuously hemorrhaging. The role of propranolol in preventing rebleeding after initial variceal bleeding has not been established.

d. Esophagitis. Antacids and omeprazole 20 mg qhs for 4–6 weeks should be used to treat esophagitis or esophageal ulcers. If bleeding recurs, a sucralfate suspension made from dissolving 1 gm of sucralfate in about 30 mL of water or sorbitol may be useful. Continued bleeding may necessitate the addition of IV vasopressin, and if this is unsuccessful, surgical resection of the involved area may be required.

e. Mallory-Weiss Tear. This usually occurs at the gastroesophageal junction and may be treated initially with antacids, H_2 receptor blockers, or omeprazole. If the patient is vomiting, antiemetics can be given. In 90%, bleeding stops spontaneously; however, continued bleeding may necessitate the use of endoscopic therapy. Rarely, surgical intervention is necessary.

f. Aortoenteric Fistula. If this is identified on endoscopy, surgery should be undertaken immediately. If massive hemorrhage is continuing despite normal results of upper GI endoscopy and an aortic graft is present, surgery is indicated. If no GI bleeding is noted, CT with IV contrast medium is sensitive for detecting aortic enteric fistulas.

g. Bleeding Neoplasms. If hemorrhage continues, electrocoagulation, heater probe, or laser therapy is indicated. Resection of the tumor should be undertaken if this is thought to be possible.

2. LOWER GASTROINTESTINAL BLEEDING
Initial evaluation of lower GI bleeding should begin by excluding the presence of upper GI bleeding. Resuscitation and laboratory tests are similar to those in upper GI bleeding. Evaluation of major active bleeding should consist of a careful anal examination. This will usually detect rectal varices, rectal ulcers, and inflammatory bowel disease. If rapid bleeding persists, arteriography is the procedure of choice. This can localize the source of bleeding and also provide a method of therapy with intra-arterial vasopressin administration or injection of thrombotic material. Bleeding scans have been controversial because of their low yield but may be valuable before arteriography to establish the presence of profuse bleeding. If major bleeding has ceased, colonoscopy can be performed with a rapid Golytely preparation. If the GI bleeding is chronic and minimal, full evaluation should again begin with careful anal examination, proctoscopy followed by colonoscopy, and then upper GI endoscopy. If all of these fail to reveal a bleeding source, small-bowel x-rays may be obtained. Enteroclysis has been found by some investigators to be of greater sensitivity in detecting bleeding lesions. Radionuclide scans are usually not useful in chronic bleeding because of the variability of active bleeding. Angiography may be of value in detecting arteriovenous

malformations when results of all other studies have been negative. Recently, small-bowel endoscopy has been used with some success in this situation. However, at present this remains an investigative approach.

a. **Diverticular Bleeding.** Diverticular bleeding most commonly occurs from diverticula in the right colon (60%). It is usually secondary to arterial bleeding and is most often self-limited. It recurs in less than half the patients. If bleeding is major or recurrent, angiography is the best means to document the site. Emergency colonoscopy can often be deceived by the presence of clots in nonbleeding diverticula. If the site of bleeding is found, intra-arterial vasopressin can be given. Definitive therapy is usually surgical resection of the involved diverticula.

b. **Arteriovenous Malformations.** These are becoming increasingly recognized as a cause of chronic GI bleeding. Usually they appear as a discrete erythematous mucosal lesion on the right side of the colon. Endoscopy is the initial diagnostic procedure of choice and may be useful in treatment of limited lesions with BICAP, heater probe, or laser photocoagulation. Careful and repeated endoscopic evaluation is usually necessary to discover these lesions. Angiography may be useful for continued occult bleeding. Estrogen-progesterone therapy (0.05 mg ethinylestradiol and 1 mg norethisterone qd po) has been found to be effective in severe bleeding from vascular malformations (Lancet 335:953, 1990).

c. **Colonic Ulcers.** Solitary ulcers with arterial bleeding are very uncommon but may be associated with massive hemorrhage. Treatment is by endoscopic coagulation or surgical oversewing of the ulcer if endoscopy is not possible.

d. **Colonic Varices.** These form in portal hypertension and may be managed with injection sclerotherapy. If this is unsuccessful, portal systemic shunt operations are used.

e. **Meckel's Diverticulum.** This should be a consideration in lower GI hemorrhage in any young person. Technetium 99m pertechnetate or Meckel's scans are useful in demonstrating this diverticulum. Surgical resection is indicated.

f. **Postpolypectomy Bleeding.** Commonly, immediately after polypectomy the bleeding stalk can be resnared, tamponaded, and cauterized. If delayed hemorrhage occurs, usually an ulcer site is present, and either injection sclerotherapy or coagulation with a heater probe is necessary.

g. **Radiation Colitis.** This usually causes minor GI bleeding but may bring continuous discomfort to a patient. It can respond to cortisone enemas, but if bleeding points can be seen, endoscopic therapy with heater probe or electrocoagulation may be tried. Laser coagulation may be more useful if involvement is diffuse and surgery is not contemplated.

h. **Hemorrhoids.** If hemorrhoids are a cause of continuous bleeding, injection sclerotherapy or rubber band ligation is usually effective.

Fleischer D: Endoscopic therapy of upper gastrointestinal bleeding in humans. Gastroenterology 90:217–234, 1986.

Saari A, Klvilaakso E, Inberg M, et al: Comparison of somatostatin and vasopressin in bleeding esophageal varices. Am J Gastroenterol 85:804–807, 1990.

Driks MR, Craven DE, Celli BR, et al: Nosocomial pneumonia in intubated patients given sucralfate as compared with antacids or histamine type 2 blockers: The role of gastric colonization. N Engl J Med 317:1376, 1987.

van Cutsem E, Rutgeerts P, Vantrappen G: Treatment of bleeding gastrointestinal vascular malformations with oestrogen-progesterone. Lancet 335:953–955, 1990.

999999999999999

LIVER DISEASES

ROBERT L. CARITHERS, JR.

I. ACUTE LIVER DISEASE

The major causes of acute hepatocellular injury include **viral hepatitis, drug-induced hepatitis,** and **ingestion of toxins.** Patients with mild to moderate acute hepatitis rarely require hospitalization. The emphasis in these disorders is on preventing spread of infectious agents and avoiding further liver damage when the underlying cause is drug-induced or toxic hepatitis. Patients with fulminant hepatitis require special management because of the rapid progression of their disease and the potential need for urgent transplantation.

A. Viral Hepatitis. 5 hepatitis viruses have been identified: hepatitis A, B, C, D, and E. **Hepatitis A and E** are contracted through water or food contaminated with the viruses or through close contact with infected patients. Travelers are at high risk for infection with these viruses when visiting underdeveloped countries. Hepatitis A also is endemic in the United States. Individuals at high risk include children in day care centers, homosexuals, and family members of patients with acute hepatitis A. **Transmission of hepatitis A can be prevented by prophylaxis with immune serum globulin. Family members and sexual contacts of patients with acute hepatitis A should receive 0.02 mL/kg** as soon as possible after identification of the index case. Hepatitis B, C, and D virus infections are blood borne. Infection can follow transfusion of contaminated blood products, IV drug abuse, exposure of health care workers to blood and blood products of infected individuals, sexual contact, and maternal-fetal transfer from a chronically infected mother to her newborn. The current recommendations for hepatitis B virus prophylaxis are outlined in Table 9–1. Since hepatitis D occurs only in patients infected with hepatitis B, this prophylaxis also is effective in preventing transmission of hepatitis D. The use of **immune serum globulin** for prevention of hepatitis C virus infection remains controversial, but **0.06 mL/kg is recommended following needle-stick accidents** (MMWR 39:1–25, 1990).

B. Drug-Induced Hepatitis. A variety of drugs can cause hepatocellular injury. Evidence of liver injury is most commonly seen 4–6 weeks after

TABLE 9–1. PROPHYLAXIS FOR HEPATITIS B VIRUS INFECTION

	HBIG*	VACCINE
Newborn of HBsAG carrier	0.5 mL at birth	1 wk, 1 mo, 6 mo
Sexual contact	0.06 mL/kg within 14 days	Immediately, 1 mo, 6 mo
Health care worker	0.06 mL/kg within 7 days	Immediately, 1 mo, 6 mo

*Hepatitis B immune globulin.

TABLE 9–2. DRUGS ASSOCIATED WITH ACUTE HEPATITIS

Allopurinol	Doxapram
Phenylbutazone	Disulfiram
Indomethacin, ibuprofen,	Dantrolene
naproxen	Halothane
Chlorzoxazone	Valproic acid
Phenytoin	Sulfonamides
Oxacillin, carbenicillin, cloxacillin	Mithramyin, L-asparaginase,
Isoniazid, rifampin	streptozocin
Aprinidine	Propylthiouracil
Cimetidine	

initiation of treatment with the offending agent. If injury is identified early and the drug is discontinued, complete recovery is the rule. Once hepatocellular injury is recognized, a patient should never receive the offending medication again. Table 9–2 lists commonly used agents that can result in severe hepatocellular injury.

1. **Isoniazid**
10–15% of patients receiving isoniazid develop mild transaminase increase 3–4 weeks after initiation of therapy, which resolves despite continuation of the drug. However, elevated transaminase levels noted after 6 months of treatment should be followed carefully, and the drug should be discontinued if there is a persistent rise in transaminase values or evidence of synthetic dysfunction, because of the significant risk of fatal hepatitis among patients with isoniazid hepatotoxicity (Am Rev Respir Dis 40:700–705, 1989). Combined use of isoniazid and rifampin appears to enhance the risk of hepatotoxicity.

2. **Phenytoin** hepatotoxicity is seen most frequently after 4–6 weeks of treatment and is associated with fever, diffuse lymphadenopathy, maculopapular rash, splenomegaly, leukocytosis, and atypical lymphocytosis, suggesting infectious mononucleosis or lymphoma. Continuation of therapy despite these symptoms can result in fulminant hepatitis.

3. **Allopurinol** therapy occasionally results in systemic vasculitis manifested by fever, rash, eosinophilia, hepatitis, and renal failure.

4. **Acetaminophen**
Suicidal overdose with acetaminophen is a common cause of severe liver injury. Ingestion of 10–15 gm of the drug is usually required for significant hepatotoxicity. However, **chronic alcoholics** and patients receiving **isoniazid** can develop severe liver injury after exposure to much lower doses of acetaminophen (Ann Intern Med 104:399–404, 1986; 113:799–800, 1990). Plasma acetaminophen levels greater than 200 mg/L 4 hours after ingestion or 50 mg/L 12 hours after ingestion suggest a high likelihood of severe liver damage. **N-acetylcysteine (Mucomyst)** is effective in preventing or limiting the degree of liver

damage if given within 12 hours of acetaminophen ingestion. The recommended **initial dose is 140 mg/kg po followed by 70 mg/kg po every 4 hours for a total of 72 hours.** Charcoal infusion should be avoided because it can interfere with absorption of N-acetylcysteine. Signs most predictive of a poor prognosis and the need for urgent liver transplantation following acetaminophen overdose are hypoglycemia, metabolic acidosis, and the development of hepatic encephalopathy.

C. Toxins. Liver injury can result from ingestion of hepatotoxins such as carbon tetrachloride, *Amanita* mushrooms, and large doses of acetaminophen. The presence of toxic liver injury is suggested by massively elevated transaminase values and a high frequency of fulminant hepatitis.

D. Management of Fulminant Hepatitis

1. CLASSIFICATION
Fulminant hepatitis is defined as the development of hepatic encephalopathy within 8 weeks of the onset of acute liver disease. The early features of this devastating illness are indistinguishable from those of uncomplicated hepatitis; however, patients with fulminant hepatitis develop hepatic encephalopathy and marked prolongation of prothrombin time values frequently in excess of 30–60 seconds. Classification of various stages of encephalopathy is helpful in understanding the clinical features in these patients (Table 9–3).

2. TREATMENT
A variety of medical treatments have been touted to improve survival in patients with fulminant hepatitis. These include total body plasma exchange, charcoal hemoperfusion, corticosteroids, hepatitis B immune globulin for patients with fulminant hepatitis B, and prostaglandins. However, none has been proved in randomized controlled trials to improve survival. The most impressive recent results have been reported in patients who have undergone liver transplantation. Thus the emphasis in managing patients with fulminant hepatitis currently is oriented toward keeping them in the best possible condition for urgent transplantation. Most patients with fulminant hepatitis are young and have few other medical problems. Nevertheless, within hours a number of devastating complications can occur. Successful prevention and management of these complications are the cornerstones of modern management of fulminant hepatitis. This can best be accomplished in an ICU with experienced physicians and

TABLE 9–3. STAGES OF HEPATIC ENCEPHALOPATHY

STAGE	MENTAL CHANGES	REFLEXES
I	Disorientation	Mild increase; no asterixis
II	Confusion	Increased; asterixis
III	Stupor	Clonus; asterixis
IVa	Comatose	Decreased; flaccid
IVb	Unresponsive	Decerebrate

nurses in a center with liver transplantation readily available. The most common potential complications in fulminant hepatitis include respiratory depression, hypoglycemia, GI bleeding, renal failure, acute respiratory distress syndrome, and cerebral edema.

Patients with fulminant hepatitis have a complex coagulopathy that includes diminished synthesis of coagulation factors, impaired fibrinolysis, and diminished number and function of platelets. The usual cause of **bleeding** is **stress ulceration.** This can be prevented by **aggressive management of gastric pH with H_2 blockers.** Maintenance of electrolyte balance, normotension, and reasonable nutritional input also helps to prevent this often devastating complication. Many patients have volume depletion with borderline hypotension and oliguria on admission to the ICU. Placement of a Swan-Ganz catheter to monitor wedge pressure, pulmonary artery pressure, and cardiac output is essential to maintain optimal hemodynamic parameters and to prevent acute tubular necrosis. When renal insufficiency persists despite maximization of intravascular hemodynamics, the cause is usually **hepatorenal syndrome,** the underlying pathogenesis of which is marked selective vasoconstriction of the renal vasculature. The overall prognosis in patients with the hepatorenal syndrome is dismal, with survival rates less than 10%; however, the syndrome is reversed by successful liver transplantation.

Another rapidly evolving and devastating complication that can occur in patients with fulminant hepatitis is the **adult respiratory distress syndrome** (**ARDS**). The usual underlying causes are sepsis, blood products, and the multisystem failure associated with fulminant hepatitis. When ARDS develops, profound hypoxia can obviate any hope of a successful transplant. Fortunately, some patients recover spontaneously. Aggressive respiratory support with 100% oxygen and positive end-expiratory pressures are necessary to maintain the arterial Po_2 at an acceptable level. The final and most devastating complication of fulminant hepatitis is **cerebral edema,** which is a frequent cause of death in patients awaiting transplantation; furthermore, a significant number of patients who have successful transplants suffer perioperative brain death due to cerebral edema. Most patients with fulminant hepatitis have increased intracranial pressure. For this reason, a number of transplant units directly monitor intracranial pressure in all patients with stage III or IV encephalopathy, despite the hazards of infection and bleeding. The safest device is the Ladd extradural monitor. With such monitoring, sudden changes in intracranial pressure can be detected early and can be effectively controlled by hyperventilation, bolus infusion of mannitol, or hypothermia. Patients in whom transplantion is performed earlier have much better results than those in whom transplantation is performed with stage IV encephalopathy (Ann Intern Med 107:337–341, 1987).

Centers for Disease Control: Protection against viral hepatitis: Recommendations of the Immunization Practices Advisory Committee. MMWR 39:1–25, 1990.

Moulding TS, Redeker AG, Kanel GC: Twenty isoniazid-associated deaths in one state. Am Rev Resp Dis 140:700–705, 1989.

Seeff LB, Cuccherine BA, Zimmerman HJ, et al: Acetaminophen hepatotoxicity in alcoholics: A therapeutic misadventure. Ann Intern Med 104:399–404, 1986.

Murphy R, Swartz R, Watkins PB: Severe acetaminophen toxicity in a patient receiving isoniazid. Ann Intern Med 113:799–800, 1990.

Bismuth H, Samuel D, Gugenheim J, et al: Emergency liver transplantation for fulminant hepatitis. Ann Intern Med 107:337–341, 1987.

II. CHRONIC LIVER DISEASE

A number of liver diseases can result in progressive hepatocellular injury and cirrhosis. Appropriate treatment can arrest the progression of disease and result in normal or near-normal life expectancy for patients with many of these diseases. Patients with diseases for which no medical therapy is available may require transplantation.

A. Alcoholic Liver Disease

1. CLINICAL FEATURES

Symptomatic patients with alcoholic hepatitis and cirrhosis describe a variety of complaints, including vague abdominal pain, anorexia, nausea and vomiting, weakness, diarrhea, weight loss, and fever. The most common physical finding is hepatomegaly. Other findings include hepatic tenderness, an audible bruit over the liver, jaundice, spider angiomas, splenomegaly, ascites, edema, and, in more severe cases, the presence of varying degrees of hepatic encephalopathy. A temperature as high as 104–105°F is seen in many patients, and prolonged fever lasting for weeks is not unusual. Other common findings include testicular atrophy, peripheral neuropathy, and Dupytren's contracture. Only modest elevations of transaminase values are seen, even when the disease is severe. AST levels are usually less than 300–500 IU and are associated with trivial elevation of ALT levels, resulting in the increased AST/ALT ratio characteristic of alcoholic liver disease.

2. PROGNOSIS

Because patients with alcoholic hepatitis can experience a wide spectrum of liver injury, the **prognosis** can vary dramatically. Patients with severe disease have high short-term mortality, approaching that of patients with fulminant hepatitis. In contrast, patients with mild disease are primarily at risk for developing alcoholic cirrhosis. The clinical features indicating severe disease include the presence of hepatic encephalopathy, marked prolongation of prothrombin time, elevation of serum bilirubin above 25 mg/dL, depressed serum albumin, elevated serum creatinine, and older age. The prognosis in patients with alcoholic cirrhosis depends on the degree and number of complications experienced and whether they can abstain from alcohol. Individuals with alcoholic cirrhosis who abstain can often return to full function. Those who have experienced no major complications have a 5-year survival rate of almost 90%, whereas patients who have previously experienced jaundice, ascites, or hematemesis have a 60% chance of surviving 5 years (Am J Med 44:406–420, 1968).

3. **Management**

Clinical and biochemical signs of protein-calorie **malnutrition** are seen in 75% of patients hospitalized with moderate to severe alcoholic hepatitis or cirrhosis. Particular attention should be paid to vitamin and mineral deficiencies, including vitamins A and D, vitamin B_{12}, folic acid, thiamine, pyridoxine, zinc, magnesium, and phosphorus. A conscientious dietitian often can find foods that are palatable. Positive nitrogen balance can be achieved and encephalopathy avoided in patients with cirrhosis by use of oral branched-chain amino acids, but these supplements are very expensive. The role of hyperalimentation for patients with alcoholic hepatitis and cirrhosis remains controversial. Branched-chain amino acids and other special hyperalimentation preparations have not been shown to increase survival or to speed recovery. Therapy with propylthiouracil, anabolic steroids, and colchicine has not been shown to improve survival in patients with alcoholic hepatitis or cirrhosis; however, patients with severe alcoholic hepatitis manifested by hepatic encephalopathy or marked prolongation of prothrombin time and high serum bilirubin values may benefit from treatment with prednisone 40 mg daily for 1 month followed by 20 mg for 1 week and 10 mg for 1 week (Ann Intern Med 10:685–690, 1989). No benefit has been shown in patients with milder disease.

B. **Chronic Hepatitis.** Chronic hepatitis is defined as continued elevation of transaminase values for 6 months or longer. A variety of clinical conditions can produce the clinical syndrome of chronic hepatitis, including autoimmune hepatitis, chronic viral hepatitis, and drug-induced liver disease, as well as a number of metabolic diseases. Differentiating these causes is important because the treatment of each is quite different.

1. **Autoimmune Hepatitis**

This is most commonly seen in young girls and postmenopausal women. Most patients have positive antinuclear and anti–smooth muscle antibodies and hyperglobulinemia. Patients with progressive liver disease manifested by histologic features of bridging fibrosis, submassive necrosis, or active cirrhosis have a poor prognosis. In these patients **corticosteroid therapy** usually results in marked improvement in survival (Semin Liver Dis 101:613–616, 1984). **The usual starting dose is 60 mg/day for 1 week followed by 40 mg/day for 2 weeks, 30 mg/day for 2 weeks, and then 20 mg/day.** Most patients respond dramatically, with resolution of symptoms, normalization of transaminase values, and improvement in synthetic function within 2–3 months. There is a high complication rate with long-term corticosteroid therapy, especially in patients who receive more than 20 mg/day for extended periods; therefore, only patients with severe progressive life-threatening disease should be treated. Liver biopsy is essential in selecting appropriate patients for therapy. In patients who require extended therapy, an attempt should be made to reduce the corticosteroid dose to 5–10 mg/day. Addition of azathioprine 1.5 mg/kg/day is helpful in minimizing the dose of corticosteroids in some patients.

2. CHRONIC VIRAL HEPATITIS

5–10% of patients infected with the hepatitis B (HBV) virus develop chronic infection and are at risk for progression to cirrhosis and hepatocellular carcinoma. 30% of patients with chronic HBV infection have a good response to interferon-alpha therapy with disappearance of HBeAg and significant reduction in viral replication within 6 months (N Engl J Med 323:295–301, 1990). With longer follow-up many of these patients also lose HBsAg and appear to be cured of HBV infection. Interferon should not be given to patients with evidence of decompensated liver disease. The recommended dosage of interferon is 10 million U administered sq 3 times/week for 4–6 months. Side effects include malaise, flu-like symptoms, depression, and occasionally hypothyroidism or hyperthyroidism. Blood counts should be monitored during therapy for evidence of significant leukopenia and thrombocytopenia. Patients infected with chronic hepatitis C virus have a 40% chance of developing chronic liver disease. There is often insidious progression to cirrhosis, and patients are at risk for the development of hepatocellular carcinoma. Interferon-alpha 3 million U 3 times/week for 6 months is effective in normalizing transaminase values in the majority of these patients; however, the relapse rate is high following cessation of treatment (N Engl J Med 321:1501–1505, 1989).

3. DRUG-INDUCED CHRONIC HEPATITIS

Liver injury from continued use of hepatotoxic drugs can produce a picture indistinguishable from autoimmune chronic hepatitis. Patients may or may not have positive antinuclear or anti–smooth muscle antibodies. The most common offending agents include alpha-methyldopa, dantrolene sodium, isoniazid, nitrofurantoin, and nonsteroidal anti-inflammatory drugs. If the cause of chronic hepatitis can be identified before the development of cirrhosis, complete resolution usually occurs with cessation of administration of the offending drug.

4. METABOLIC DISEASE

The most common metabolic diseases causing chronic hepatitis are Wilson's disease, alpha$_1$-antitrypsin deficiency, and hemochromatosis.

a. Wilson's Disease. This is an autosomal recessive disorder manifested by deficient biliary copper elimination. Patients gradually accumulate copper in the liver during the first 2–3 decades of life. At some point, usually between the ages of 15 and 25 years, patients develop hepatitis, which often is associated with hemolysis and renal tubular abnormalities. Occasional patients have acute or fulminant hepatitis; however, a more common manifestation is chronic hepatitis. There may be mild neurologic dysfunction with loss of concentration or emotional outbursts, which may lead to psychiatric intervention. Diagnosis during the hepatic phase is essential because both the hepatic and neurologic sequelae can be prevented by administration of 1–2 gm of **penicillamine** daily (Gastroenterology 100:762–767, 1991). Common side effects include fever, pruritus, and a rash. Less common are leukopenia and thrombocytopenia. Patients who develop severe toxic reactions to penicillamine can be treated effectively with **trientine,** in a dosage of 1–2 gm/day.

b. **Alpha₁-Antitrypsin Deficiency.** The most common clinical presentations of alpha₁-antitrypsin deficiency include (1) chronic obstructive pulmonary disease affecting primarily the lower lobes; (2) cholestatic jaundice in infants often progressing to cirrhosis before the age of 10; and (3) chronic hepatitis in adults. Depressed serum alpha₁-antitrypsin levels and demonstration of sequestered alpha₁-antitrypsin granules within hepatocytes on liver biopsy establish the diagnosis. Liver transplantation is the only effective therapy.

c. **Hemochromatosis.** Hemochromatosis is the most common genetic disorder causing liver failure. This autosomal recessive defect in iron absorption results in slowly progressive accumulation of iron in the liver, pancreas, heart, and brain. Patients are commonly in their 50s and 60s with hepatomegaly and chronic hepatitis. If the disease is not recognized, progression to diabetes, cardiomyopathy, and pituitary failure often occurs. Hemochromatosis should be suspected in patients with transferrin saturation greater than 50% who have marked elevation of serum ferritin levels. Marked elevation of the hepatic iron concentration confirms the diagnosis. If the disorder is detected prior to the development of cirrhosis, all manifestations of hemochromatosis can be prevented by regular phlebotomy.

Powell WJ, Klatskin G: Duration and survival in patients with Laennec's cirrhosis. Am J Med 44:406–420, 1968.

Carithers RL Jr, Herlong HF, Diehl AM, et al: Methylpredisolone therapy in patients with severe alcoholic hepatitis. Ann Intern Med 110:685–690, 1989.

Czaja AJ: Natural history, clinical features, and treatment of autoimmune hepatitis. Semin Liver Dis 101:613–616, 1984.

Perrillo RP, Schiff ER, Davis GL, et al: A randomized, controlled trial of interferon alfa-2b alone and after prednisone withdrawal for the treatment of chronic hepatitis B. N Engl J Med 323:295–301, 1990.

Davis GL, Balart LA, Schiff ER, et al: Treatment of hepatitis C with recombinant interferon alpha. A multicenter, randomized, controlled trial. N Engl J Med 321:1501–1505, 1989.

Schilshy ML, Scheinberg IH, Sternlieb I: Prognosis of wilsonian chronic active hepatitis. Gastroenterology 100:762–767, 1991.

III. CHOLESTATIC LIVER DISEASES

Cholestatic hepatobiliary disorders are characterized by marked elevation in alkaline phosphatase values with or without jaundice. Major causes include extrahepatic biliary obstruction, cholestatic drug reactions, primary biliary cirrhosis, and sclerosing cholangitis.

A. **Extrahepatic Biliary Obstruction.** Mechanical extrahepatic obstruction most commonly results from malignant disease or gallstones. Malignant biliary obstruction usually occurs in older patients. Characteristic clinical features include painless jaundice and weight loss. Ultrasound reveals dilated intrahepatic ducts. Except when the tumor is resectable, treatment is palliative, achieved by endoscopic placement of a biliary stent or by bypassing the obstruction through percutaneous insertion of a drainage catheter. The former is preferred because patients do not need a percutaneous catheter; however, endoscopically placed stents have to be replaced periodically because of obstruction. Biliary obstruction due to gallstones usually is accompanied by right upper quadrant pain, fever, and jaundice. The diagnosis is suspected by finding dilated intrahepatic biliary radicals on ultrasound and may be confirmed by percutaneous or endoscopic cholangiography. Most patients respond clinically to treatment with nasogastric suction, intravenous fluids, and antibiotics. Surgical exploration of the common duct and cholecystectomy make up the standard approach in younger patients. In patients who are poor surgical candidates, extrahepatic biliary stones can be removed endoscopically. This can be combined with laparoscopic cholecystectomy. The latter approach may soon replace surgical cholecystectomy and common duct exploration for most patients.

B. Cholestatic Drug Reactions. The agents most commonly associated with cholestatic reactions include chlorpromazine and other phenothiazines, gold, chlorpropamide, oral contraceptives, and erythromycin estolate. Although resolution may be slow, complete recovery usually occurs after discontinuation of the offending agent.

C. Primary Biliary Cirrhosis. Primary biliary cirrhosis (PBC) is an uncommon disorder that occurs most often in middle-aged women. Patients frequently complain of pruritus. There is marked elevation of alkaline phosphatase levels. Associated biochemical features include elevated IgM levels and positive antimitochondrial antibodies. Many patients have associated autoimmune features, particularly Sjögren's syndrome, autoimmune thyroiditis, and renal tubular acidosis. Liver biopsy typically shows inflammation around small bile ducts and nonsuppurative cholangitis. With advancing disease there is increasing fibrosis and progression to cirrhosis. Severe pruritus can be a significant clinical problem, and these patients are at risk for malabsorption of fat-soluble vitamins and zinc. Vitamins A, E, and K levels should be measured and deficiencies replaced. However, the most significant clinical problem for PBC patients is bone disease characterized by impaired osteoblastic activity and accelerated osteoclastic activity. Calcium and vitamin D should be carefully monitored and appropriate replacement instituted. In addition, vigorous physical activity should be encouraged.

There currently is no specific treatment for PBC other than liver transplantation. Penicillamine, colchicine, chlorambucil, corticosteroids, and azathioprine have been studied in controlled clinical trials. None of these agents has been shown to prevent progression of the disease or to prolong survival (Hepatology 8:668–676, 1988). Cyclosporine has resulted in some improvement but is too toxic for general use. Methotrexate and ursodeoxycholic acid are currently being tested in large randomized controlled clinical trials (N Engl J Med 324:1548–1554, 1991).

D. Primary Sclerosing Cholangitis. Sclerosing cholangitis is characterized by inflammation and fibrosis of the biliary tree typically associated with ulcerative colitis. Involvement can include the extrahepatic bile ducts, the intrahepatic ducts, or both. Most patients are young men. Symptoms include fatigue, pruritus, jaundice, abdominal pain, and recurrent fever due to repeated episodes of bacterial cholangitis. Biochemical findings are marked elevations in alkaline phosphatase, intermittent elevations in bilirubin, and minimal increases in transaminase values. The diagnosis is confirmed by endoscopic cholangiography, which reveals multifocal areas of stricture and dilatation giving a beaded appearance to the involved portions of the extrahepatic and intrahepatic biliary tree. Liver transplantation is the only definitive form of therapy. Other surgical treatments are contraindicated. The clinical course is quite variable. Although many patients remain asymptomatic for long periods, most ultimately become symptomatic and develop liver failure, leading to death or the need for liver transplantation. Age, bilirubin and hemoglobin concentrations, the presence of ulcerative colitis, and the histologic stage on liver biopsy are independent predictors of prognosis.

Wiesner RH, Grambsch PM: Clinical and statistical analyses of new and evolving therapies for primary biliary cirrhosis. Hepatology 8:668–676, 1988.
Poupon RE, Balkau B, Eschwege E, et al: A multicenter, controlled trial of ursodiol for the treatment of primary biliary cirrhosis. N Engl J Med 324:1548–1554, 1991.

IV. MAJOR COMPLICATIONS OF CHRONIC LIVER DISEASES

Patients with chronic liver disease are prone to a number of potentially life-threatening complications. Included among these are variceal hemorrhage, ascites, spontaneous bacterial peritonitis, and hepatic encephalopathy. The opportunity for the patient to undergo successful transplantation often rests on effective management of these complications.

A. Variceal Hemorrhage. Bleeding from esophageal varices is particularly common in patients with decompensated cirrhosis who have large varices and red wales observed on endoscopic examination. **Beta blockers** are effective in reducing the risk of variceal hemorrhage (N Engl J Med 317:856–861, 1987). Treatment should be started with 40 mg bid of propranolol with a goal of reducing the pulse rate by 25%. When a patient with cirrhosis has upper GI hemorrhage, a large-bore IV line should be placed and replacement with packed red cells immediately instituted. **Early endoscopy** is essential, for over 50% of upper GI hemorrhages originate from sites other than esophageal varices, including Mallory-Weiss tears, diffuse gastritis, portal gastropathy, and duodenal ulcers.

If bleeding from esophageal varices is confirmed, **IV Pitressin** (20 U 200 ml of saline at 0.25–0.5 U/m) should be initiated. Complications include tachyarrhythmias, myocardial ischemia, diffuse abdominal pain, and ischemia to peripheral extremities. These side effects of vasopressin can be ameliorated by simultaneous IV infusion of nitroglycerin (Hepatology 6:410–413, 1986). **Sclerotherapy** is effective in controlling bleeding in 75% of cases (JAMA 255:497–500, 1986). If bleeding continues or if sclerotherapy is contraindicated, hemorrhage can be controlled by placement of a Sengstaken-Blakemore or Minnesota tube; however, these patients should be intubated and treated in specialized ICUs where the nursing personnel are well trained in the use of these tubes and potential complications. Some patients have recurrent episodes of variceal bleeding. **Repeated sclerotherapy** can eradicate varices and prevent recurrent hemorrhage (Hepatology 5:827–830, 1985). Patients in whom sclerotherapy fails should be considered for surgery. The choice of operations depends on the stage of the patient's liver disease and local surgical expertise. Child's classification and its various modifications (Table 9–4) provide the best means for preoperative assessment of surgical risk (Hepatology 1:673–676, 1981). Patients with well-compensated disease (scores of 5–8) are good candidates for a distal splenorenal shunt. This technically difficult operation does not increase the risk associated with subsequent liver transplantation (Ann Surg 203:454–462, 1986). The operation of choice for patients with uncontrolled variceal hemorrhage who are imminent liver transplant candidates is a mesocaval shunt. Portacaval shunts should not be created in patients who are potential liver transplant candidates, since these operations do not prolong survival and significantly increase the risk of subsequent transplantation.

B. Ascites

1. GENERAL MANAGEMENT

Although the pathogenesis is controversial, avid renal sodium retention is an essential feature of ascites formation. Dietary sodium restriction is a basic ingredient of any effective treatment program. A **2-gm sodium diet** is the minimum tolerable for outpatients. Diuretic therapy can be quite effective in treating **mild to moderate ascites. Spironolactone** (200–400 mg/day) is the most commonly used diuretic. Because spironolactone results in potassium retention, *salt substitutes should be avoided.* Furosemide and other loop diuretics are useful in patients who fail to respond adequately to spironolactone therapy. When used to treat patients with **severe ascites,** diuretics result in a high incidence of hyponatremia, volume depletion, precipitation of hepatic encephalopathy, and renal insufficiency. Vigorous **paracentesis** is safer and more cost-effective in patients with refractory ascites (Ann Intern Med 112:889–891, 1990). 3–5 L of fluid can be removed

TABLE 9–4. PUGH'S MODIFICATION OF CHILD'S CLASSIFICATION

	POINT SCORE FOR INCREASING ABNORMALITY		
	1	2	3
Encephalopathy (grade)	none	1 or 2	3 or 4
Ascites	absent	slight	moderate
Bilirubin	1.0–2.0	2.0–3.0	>3.0
Albumin (gm/dL)	>3.5	2.8–3.5	<2.8
Protime (sec > control)	1–4	4–6	>6

Adapted from Pugh RNH, Murray-Lyon IM, Dawson JL: Transection of the oesophagus for oesophageal varices. Br J Surg 60:646–649, 1973.

daily without deleterious hemodynamic changes. LeVeen and Denver shunts have fallen into disfavor because of the high incidence of occlusion and recurrent infection. However, in selected patients they can be beneficial as a short-term bridge while hepatic function recovers. These shunts are particularly effective in alcoholic hepatitis and massive ascites with a good prognosis (N Engl J Med 321:1632–1638, 1989).

2. **BACTERIAL PERITONITIS**
One of the major life-threatening complications of ascites is **spontaneous bacterial peritonitis** (SBP). Common symptoms include diffuse abdominal pain, fever, and the unexplained onset of hepatic encephalopathy. Any patient hospitalized with ascites should have diagnostic paracentesis to rule out SBP. Gram stains of ascitic fluid are rarely positive. The presence of more than 500 white cells, particularly when polymorphonuclear leukocytes are greater than 75%, should raise the possibility of SBP, and antibiotic therapy should be initiated until ascitic fluid culture results return. The most common organisms causing spontaneous peritonitis are *Escherichia coli, Klebsiella,* and nonenterococcal streptococci. In presumptive cases of SBP, antibiotic therapy should include coverage against gram-negative and -positive organisms; however, aminoglycosides should be avoided because of the high risk of nephrotoxicity in liver disease patients. Unfortunately, 75% of patients successfully treated for SBP have recurrence within a year. Prophylactic therapy with norfloxacin (400 mg/day) reduces the incidence of recurrent infection; nevertheless, transplant candidates who develop SBP should have surgery as soon as possible.

C. **Hepatic Encephalopathy.** Hepatic encephalopathy is a neuropsychiatric syndrome that can occur in patients with acute or chronic liver disease. Accumulation of ammonia, interaction between ammonia, mercaptans, and fatty acids, and false neurotransmitter-induced neural inhibition have all been implicated as causes. The **stage of encephalopathy** (Table 9–3) is a sensitive measure of hepatocellular injury in patients with acute liver failure. In patients with chronic liver disease, encephalopathy generally occurs more gradually, is more commonly associated with extrahepatic precipitating factors, and is more easily reversed. The most common **precipitating factors** are the use of sedative drugs, GI bleeding or excessive protein ingestion, hypokalemia, volume depletion, and infection, particularly spontaneous bacterial peritonitis. These precipitating causes should be searched for whenever a patient develops encephalopathy.

Once the precipitating factors have been addressed, effective management of encephalopathy consists of cleansing the gut with **sorbitol** or another purgative, restricting protein intake, and of therapy with lactulose. The usual starting dosage of **lactulose** is **30 mL 4 times daily.** The objective of therapy is to eliminate the encephalopathy and for the patient to have 1 or 2 soft formed stools daily while avoiding diarrhea. The best measure of the effectiveness of therapy is the number connection test, in which a patient is asked to connect 25 numbered circles as quickly as possible. The test can be repeated periodically and diet and lactulose therapy modified accordingly.

Pascal J-P, Cales P, Multicenter Study Group: Propranolol in the prevention of first upper gastrointestinal tract hemorrhage in patients with cirrhosis of the liver and esophageal varices. New Engl J Med 317:856–861, 1987.
Gimson AES, Westaby D, Hegarty J, et al: A randomized trial of vasopressin and vasopressin plus nitroglycerin in the control of acute variceal hemorrhage. Hepatology 6:410–413, 1986.
Larson AW, Cohen H, Zweiban B, et al: Acute esophageal variceal sclerotherapy. Results of a prospective randomized controlled trial. JAMA 255:497–500, 1986.
Westaby D, Macdougall BR, Williams R: Improved survival following injection sclerotherapy for esophageal varices: Final analysis of a controlled trial. Hepatology 5:827–830, 1985.
Conn HO: A peak at the Child-Turcotte classification. Hepatology 1:673–676, 1981.
Warren WD, Henderson JM, Millikan WJ, et al: Distal splenorenal shunt versus endoscopic sclerotherapy for long-term management of variceal bleeding. Preliminary report of a prospective, randomized trial. Ann Surg 203:454–462, 1986.
Kellerman PS, Linas SL: Large-volume paracentesis in treatment of ascites. Ann Intern Med 112:889–891, 1990.
Stanley MM, Ochi S, Lee KK, et al: Peritoneovenous shunting as compared with medical treatment in patients with alcoholic cirrhosis and massive ascites. N Engl J Med 321:1632–1638, 1989.

V. LIVER TRANSPLANTATION

Liver transplantation is the treatment of choice for patients with end-stage liver disease from a variety of causes (Table 9–5); however, patients must be in suitable physiologic condition to undergo major surgery and must be able to comply with the complex medical regimen required after surgery. The operation's timing influences survival and postoperative complications after liver transplantation. Moribund patients who are referred to a transplant center have little possibility of survival. In contrast, patients who are referred in good physiologic condition have an excellent chance at achieving long-term good quality of life.

A. **Indications.** Liver transplantation is the only effective treatment for patients with cirrhosis due to hepatitis C virus infection, alpha$_1$-antitrypsin deficiency, primary biliary cirrhosis, and sclerosing cholangitis. Patients with autoimmune chronic hepatitis in whom there is decompensation with ascites, jaundice, or variceal bleeding also are excellent

TABLE 9–5. INDICATIONS FOR LIVER TRANSPLANTATION

Fulminant hepatitis
Chronic hepatitis with cirrhosis
  Autoimmune hepatitis
  Chronic hepatitis C
Alcoholic cirrhosis
Cryptogenic cirrhosis
Metabolic disorders causing cirrhosis
  Alpha$_1$-antitrypsin deficiency
  Hemochromatosis
  Wilson's disease
Biliary cirrhosis
  Primary biliary cirrhosis
  Sclerosing cholangitis
Controversial indications
  Chronic hepatitis B
  Hepatobiliary cancer

candidates. Patients with alcoholic cirrhosis being considered for transplantation should have abstained from alcohol for 6–12 months to maximize the potential for spontaneous recovery. These patients should have effectively dealt with their alcoholism through a successful treatment program before being considered for transplantation. Many patients who undergo transplantation have cirrhosis for which no cause can be found (N Engl J Med 321:1014–1022, 1989). Patients with cirrhosis secondary to hepatitis B virus infection are not good candidates because of a high incidence of severe recurrent disease after the operation. Those with unresectable hepatocellular carcinoma and cholangiocarcinoma are also not good candidates because of possible recurrent and metastatic tumor.

B. Timing. In many instances the most difficult decision is the **best time for transplantation.** Any patient with chronic liver disease who develops hepatic encephalopathy or ascites should be considered for transplantation. Unfortunately there are no clearly defined means for selecting the best time. Child's classification (Table 9–4) offers helpful information. For example, patients with scores of 5–8 have excellent survival for 5–10 years without transplantation; in contrast, those with scores over 12 have less than a 50% chance of surviving 6 months unless transplantation is performed (Hepatology 7:122–128, 1987; Gut 26:1359–1363, 1985).

C. Postoperative Management. After successful liver transplantation liver function returns quickly. Early indications of graft function include prompt bile flow, spontaneous correction of coagulation factors within 48–72 hours, and steady improvement in aminotransferase and bilirubin values. In the first 48 hours after liver transplantation the most common serious complications are **primary graft failure** and **intra-abdominal hemorrhage** requiring reoperation. Primary graft failure is shown by persistent jaundice and coagulopathy associated with poor bile flow, metabolic acidosis, and renal insufficiency. Urgent retransplantation is the only option for these patients. Surgery is required for intra-abdominal hemorrhage when there is a persistent need for large-volume transfusions and difficulty in maintaining hemodynamic stability. Fortunately these patients do well if they can be returned to the operating room in good physiologic condition.

1. EARLY MANAGEMENT
In the first 2 weeks after liver transplantation the major concerns are **infection, hepatic artery thrombosis,** and **allograft rejection** (N Engl J Med 321:1092–1099, 1989). Early infectious complications are usually due to nosocomial infections associated with indwelling lines and catheters. The most common organism is *Staphylococcus epidermidis.* Treatment consists of removal of potentially infected lines and antibiotic treatment with vancomycin. Hepatic artery thrombosis can present either as massive hepatic necrosis or as a silent occlusion. The diagnosis is suspected from Doppler sonography showing absence of hepatic artery flow and is confirmed by angiography. If the diagnosis can be made early, revascularization can be successfully performed. Otherwise, retransplantation usually is required. Rejection, which occurs in 60–70% of patients, typically results in modest

nonspecific increases in serum bilirubin and aminotransferase values. The diagnosis is made by liver biopsy, which reveals lymphocytic invasion of biliary endothelium and vascular epithelium. Most rejection episodes respond to bolus corticosteroid treatment of 1 gm of methylprednisolone daily for 3–5 days or monoclonal OKT3 antibody therapy 5 mg daily for 10–14 days.

2. LATE COMPLICATIONS

Later complications include **infection, rejection, biliary tract complications, portal vein thrombosis,** and complications of immunosuppressive therapy. Infection is the leading cause of death after liver transplantation. Late infections, including cytomegalovirus (CMV) and fungal infections, are primarily due to opportunistic organisms. CMV infection occurs in more than half of patients after transplantation. Hepatitis due to CMV can be confused with rejection because of nonspecific changes in bilirubin and aminotransferase values. However, liver biopsy shows focal inflammation of hepatocytes with CMV inclusion bodies. Most patients respond well to reduction in immunosuppressive therapy plus IV **ganciclovir therapy** (5 mg/kg/day) for 10–14 days. Fungal infections, particularly *Candida* and *Aspergillus,* are major causes of death after liver transplantation. If the diagnosis can be established early, treatment with amphotericin or fluconazole can be lifesaving. The most common surgical complications after liver transplantation involve the biliary tract. Diagnosis is usually established by cholangiography. Although surgical intervention may be required, many biliary complications can be effectively treated with radiographic or endoscopic placement of biliary stents.

After hospital discharge of liver transplant recipients, most complications result from **side effects of immunosuppressive therapy.** Hypertension, excessive hair growth, gingival hyperplasia, and renal insufficiency are common side effects of cyclosporine therapy. Complications can be minimized by careful monitoring of cyclosporine levels and appropriate dosage adjustment, particularly in patients with early signs of hypertension and azotemia. Cyclosporine-induced hypertension can be effectively treated with calcium channel blockers such as nifedipine (30–60 mg qid) and beta blockers such as metoprolol (50–100 mg qd). Side effects of prolonged corticosteroid therapy include truncal obesity, bone loss with pathologic fractures, diabetes, cataracts, and aseptic necrosis of the femoral heads. Minimization of dosage levels over time is the best preventive treatment, but oral calcium replacement and avoidance of diuretics also are helpful in reducing osteoporosis. Azathioprine is associated with leukopenia and thrombocytopenia; thus any patient treated with this agent requires careful monitoring of blood counts. Late complications of immunosuppressive therapy include malignant disease, particularly lymphomas and skin cancer.

Starzl TE, Demetris AJ, Van Thiel D: Liver transplantation. N Engl J Med 321:1014–1022, 1989.
Gines P, Quintero E, Arroyo V, et al: Compensated cirrhosis: Natural history and prognostic factors. Hepatology 7:122–128, 1987.
Keating JJ, Johnson RD, Johnson PJ, Williams R: Clinical course of cirrhosis in young adults and therapeutic potential for liver transplantation. Gut 26:1359–1363, 1985.
Starzl TE, Demetris AJ, Van Thiel D: Liver transplantation. N Engl J Med 321:1092–1099, 1989.

10 10 10 10 10 10 10 10 10

HEMATOLOGY AND TRANSFUSION MEDICINE

THOMAS H. PRICE
LAWRENCE R. SOLOMON

I. RED CELL DISORDERS

A. Anemia

1. **DEFINITION.** Hemoglobin is under 14 gm/dL for men and under 12 gm/dL for women, *but* **"low" levels may be appropriate** if tissue oxygen requirements are decreased (e.g., hypothyroidism) or if tissue oxygen delivery is enhanced by a decrease in hemoglobin oxygen affinity. **"Normal" levels may be inadequate** if tissue oxygen delivery is impaired by pulmonary insufficiency, cardiac disorders, or an increase in hemoglobin oxygen affinity.

2. **CLASSIFICATION** (Table 10–1)

   a. **Decreased red cell production or increased red cell destruction** is distinguished by the **reticulocyte index** (a measure of the number of "young" red cells released by the marrow relative to normal each day) calculated as follows:

   $$\text{Reticulocyte count } (\%) \times \text{hematocrit}/45 \times 1/\text{"shift factor"}$$

   The ratio of the patient's hematocrit to the normal value of 45 corrects for anemia severity while the "shift factor" (2.0 for anemia of moderate severity) adjusts for the increased life span of the reticulocyte in the blood due to increased erythropoietin levels (indicated by polychromatophilic red cells on the peripheral smear). In the steady state, values over 3.0 indicate increased destruction or blood loss, while values under 2.0 indicate decreased production. **The ratio of erythroid to myeloid precursors in the marrow (E/G ratio)** separates production defects into **hypoproliferative** disorders (E/G ratio normal or low) and disorders characterized by **ineffective erythropoiesis** due to intramedullary destruction of marrow erythroid precursors (E/G ratio high).

   b. **Normocytic, macrocytic, or microcytic** is distinguished by the **mean corpuscular volume (MCV)**. Most anemias are normocytic; microcytosis suggests a cytoplasmic maturation disorder, and macrocytosis suggests a nuclear maturation disorder. A high MCV also occurs with reticulocytosis, thyroid disorders, alcohol abuse, marrow damage, multiple myeloma, and hyperosmolar states. Regardless of the MCV, the **peripheral blood smear** should be examined for mixtures of red cells of different sizes, abnormal red cell shapes, red cell inclusions, and abnormal white cells and platelets.

3. **THE DIAGNOSTIC APPROACH** involves reticulocyte count, MCV and examination of the peripheral smear initially followed, if appropriate, by measures of nutrients in blood or serum and by a therapeutic trial. A bone marrow aspirate defines the E/G ratio, the type of maturation,

TABLE 10–1. KINETIC CLASSIFICATION OF ANEMIA

DECREASED RED CELL PRODUCTION (reticulocyte index <2.0%)
Hypoproliferative (E/G < 1/2) (MCV *usually* normal)
   Marrow damage (aplasia; hypoplasia): Drugs, tumor, immune, toxins, fibrosis, idiopathic, radiation, infection, congenital
   Decreased marrow stimulation
     Decreased oxygen requirement: hypothyroidism, hypopituitarism
     Increased oxygen release to tissues: low-affinity hemoglobins, hyperphosphatemia
     Decreased erythropoietin production: chronic renal failure, anemia of chronic disease
   Decreased iron supply: iron deficiency, anemia of chronic disease

Ineffective (E/G > 1/1)
   Nuclear maturation defects (MCV *usually* high): B_{12} deficiency, myelodysplastic disorders, folate deficiency, cytotoxic drugs
   Cytoplasmic maturation defects (MCV *usually* low): iron deficiency, thalassemias, sideroblastic anemias, hemoglobin E

INCREASED RED CELL DESTRUCTION (reticulocyte index > 3.0)
   (MCV normal or high)
   Membrane abnormalities (e.g., hereditary spherocytosis; PNH)
   Enzyme defects (e.g., G6PD deficiency)
   Hemoglobin abnormalities (e.g., sickle cell disease)
   Intracellular parasites (e.g., malaria, babesiosis, bartonella)
   Hypersplenism
   Immune (e.g., idiopathic, drugs, infections, lymphoproliferative or rheumatologic disorders)
   Microangiopathic (e.g., vasculitis, intravascular prostheses, TTP, DIC)
   Physical and chemical agents (e.g., bacterial toxins, snake and insect venoms, fresh water drowning, marching or jogging)

the presence of iron stores, and the presence of abnormal cells. A bone marrow biopsy provides complementary information on marrow cellularity and on the presence of fibrosis, granulomas, vasculitis, or tumor. Since anemia is often a secondary process, studies to define an underlying disorder are usually also required.

4. **HYPOPROLIFERATIVE ANEMIAS**

   a. Aplastic anemia is characterized by persistent pancytopenia with decreased marrow hematopoietic cells; it may be congenital, idiopathic, or secondary to drugs, toxins, radiation, viral infections, or immune dysfunction.

     (1). Diagnosis is by bone marrow biopsy.

     (2). Therapy begins with stopping of all suspect drug or chemical exposures. Supportive care includes **red cell transfusion** for symptomatic anemia (p. 369), platelet transfusion for active bleeding (p. 360), and antibiotics for infections. Transfusions should be given sparingly to improve prospects for marrow transplantation and to limit transfusion reactions, iron overload, and platelet sensitization. Good dental and body hygiene decreases infection risk. Bone marrow transplantation cures 50–80% of patients over 40 with severe aplasia (i.e., reticulocyte index <1.0%; granulocytes <500/μ^3; platelets <20,000/μ^3, and marrow cellularity <25%) and an HLA-identical sibling. Results are better if performed before transfusion and/or significant infection. Patients and their families should be HLA-typed at diagnosis, and conditioning should begin within 72 hours of initial administration of blood products; transfusions from family members should be avoided. Risks include death within 3 months after transplant (10–25%) and chronic graft versus host disease (35%). Antithymocyte globulin (ATG) benefits 40–80% of patients, but the potency of different preparations is variable, and optimal regimens are not well defined. Toxicity includes phlebitis, fever, skin rash, anaphylaxis, serum sickness, neutropenia, and thrombocytopenia. Corticosteroids are usually given with ATG and for 7 days thereafter to minimize local and systemic reactions. Although response often occurs within 6 weeks, maximum benefit may not occur for 3–6 months. Immunosuppression (e.g., cyclosporine, cyclophosphamide, azathioprine, steroids) is rarely effective; it may worsen cytopenias and increase infection risk.

Androgens can benefit patients with less severe aplasia. Therapy for 4–6 months is often required and relapse may follow drug withdrawal. Oral agents (e.g., fluoxymesterone 1 mg/kg/day; oxymetholone 2–5 mg/kg/day) are used in patients with severe thrombocytopenia; IM agents (e.g., testosterone propionate or nandrolone decanoate, 2–4 mg/kg/week) are more effective and less hepatotoxic. Patients refractory to one androgen may respond to another.

b. **Iron deficiency anemia** is initially normochromic/normocytic but hypochromia/microcytosis develops with increasing severity and duration. In adult males or postmenopausal females it is most often due to GI bleeding, and the GI tract **should be studied even when tests for occult blood are negative**. Other causes include malabsorption, pulmonary hemosiderosis, chronic intravascular hemolysis (urinary iron loss), or relatively inadequate intake (pregnancy, infancy).

(1). Diagnostic Tests. Low serum iron and increased serum iron binding capacity and red cell protoporphyrin. A low serum ferritin value confirms the diagnosis, but the value may be normal if inflammation, malignant disease, uremia, or liver disease is present. Since inflammation and malignant disease also lower serum iron and raise red cell protoporphyrin values, histologic assessment of marrow iron stores may be required.

(2). Therapy. **Ferrous sulfate** po (300 mg tid) increases hemoglobin at least 2 gm/dL in 4 weeks and should be continued for 6 months after hemoglobin is normal to replenish stores. Absorption is better if ferrous sulfate taken when fasting.

Side effects (nausea, epigastric discomfort, constipation, diarrhea) may abate if the dose is decreased or given with meals. Parenteral iron dextran (50 mg/mL of iron) is given if oral iron is malabsorbed, poorly tolerated, or insufficient to keep up with continuing iron losses. The dose is calculated as follows:

$$\text{mg iron} = \frac{(\text{hematocrit deficit})(\text{total blood volume})}{(\text{RBC iron content})}$$

$$= \frac{(0.45 - \text{patient hematocrit})(70 \text{ mL/kg} \times \text{kg body wt})}{(0.7 \text{ mg/mL RBC})}$$

An additional 500 mg of iron is needed to replace stores. Doses of 100–200 mg are given by deep zigzag intramuscular injection into the upper outer quadrant of the buttock, but this requires repeated injections, leads to skin staining, and rarely causes tumors at the injection site. Alternatively, the total dose can be diluted into 500 mL of 0.9 N saline and given as a single IV infusion over 4–6 hours. Since anaphylaxis can occur with either route, a 0.5-mL test dose is given 30 minutes before the treatment dose. Other side effects include headache, malaise, fever, arthralgias, and lymphadenopathy.

c. Anemia of Chronic Disease. This accompanies overt malignant disease and inflammatory disorders but may be the presenting feature of an otherwise occult process. The MCV is usually normal but may be low. The anemia is shown by low serum iron and iron binding capacity and increased serum ferritin and red cell protoporphyrin. Histologic evaluation of marrow iron stores may be required to exclude iron deficiency. Iron therapy should be avoided and the underlying disorder treated.

d. Anemia of Chronic Renal Disease. This condition is due to decreased erythropoietin production; MCV is normal. Acidosis and hyperphosphatemia lower hemoglobin-oxygen affinity and improve tissue oxygen delivery. Thus, symptoms rather than the hemoglobin level should be used as an indication for red cell transfusion.

(1). Diagnostic tests. Exclude concomitant folate or iron deficiency that may accompany hemodialysis.

(2). Therapy. Recombinant erythropoietin (30–150 U/kg 3 times/week IV or SQ) is effective in almost all patients. Side effects include hypertension, hyperkalemia, seizures, and clotting of dialysis fistulas. Androgens may potentiate erythropoietin, permitting use of lower doses (10–25 U/kg). Parenteral androgens (nandrolone decanoate 100 mg/week or testosterone propionate 200 mg/week IM) are given for 3–6 months. Oral androgens are less effective and more hepatotoxic.

(3). Aluminum toxicity occurs mainly in hemodialysis patients. MCV may be normal or low. Diagnosis involves assessing aluminum in bone biopsy specimens; serum aluminum before and after deferoxamine infusion is less reliable. Aluminum-containing drugs are discontinued; aluminum-free water used for dialysis; deferoxamine administered (p. 358).

5. **NUCLEAR MATURATION DISORDERS (MEGALOBLASTIC ANEMIAS)**

   a. **General Considerations in Vitamin B_{12} and Folic Acid Deficiencies.** Macrocytosis and hypersegmented granulocytes are common, but the MCV may be normal, particularly if iron deficiency or thalassemia coexists. Folate doses over 0.5 mg/day are effective in B_{12} deficiency, but improvement of anemia is incomplete, and neurologic symptoms may develop and progress. B_{12} doses over 100 μg/day also are effective in folate deficiency. Thus, these disorders must be distinguished before vitamin therapy is begun. Therapy produces brisk reticulocytosis in 4–7 days followed by a rapid increase in hemoglobin, but the MCV can remain high for 2–3 months. Further evaluation is needed if hemoglobin levels fail to become normal. Red cell transfusions are needed only for severe symptomatic anemia, and small volumes should be infused slowly to avoid volume overload.

   b. **Vitamin B_{12} deficiency** most often results from malabsorption due to gastric disorders (e.g., pernicious anemia), pancreatic insufficiency, disorders of the terminal ileum, certain infections (e.g., *Diphyllobothrium latum*; bacterial overgrowth) and some drugs (e.g., cholestyramine; colchicine, high-dose vitamin C, cimetidine, possibly ethanol). Neurologic symptoms (dementia, personality change, impaired vibratory sense and proprioception, and spastic paraparesis) can dominate the clinical picture and may occur without either anemia or a high MCV. Diagnosis is by low serum vitamin B_{12} levels (also seen in primary folate deficiency, myeloma, other gammopathies), high urine methylmalonic acid excretion and serum homocysteine levels, and reticulocyte response to low-dose B_{12} (1–2 μg/day). Cyanocobalamin or hydroxocobalamin 1.0 mg is given IM or SQ 3 times/week for 4–6 weeks then 1.0 mg/month for life. Oral doses of 1 mg/day may also be effective in pernicious anemia. Patients with pernicious anemia and atrophic gastritis should be screened regularly for gastric cancer.

   c. **Folic acid deficiency** usually results from poor dietary intake and/or alcohol abuse; less common causes include malabsorption due to inflammatory small-bowel disease, altered metabolism due to certain drugs (e.g., oral contraceptives, diphenylhydantoin, methotrexate, trimethoprim, pentamidine), and increased requirements due to pregnancy, hemolytic anemia, hyperthyroidism, and some malignant diseases. Diagnosis is made by low serum folate level (indicates limited delivery to marrow at the time of evaluation; most sensitive to early depletion; corrects rapidly with food or vitamin intake); low red cell folate value (indicates limited delivery to marrow in the preceding 2–3 months; may be normal in early deficiency and in transfused patients; also low in primary B_{12} deficiency); and reticulocyte response to low-dose folate (0.1–0.2 mg/day). To treat this deficiency, 1 mg/day of folic acid po (or parenterally in patients with malabsorption) is given.

d. **Refractory Anemia and Idiopathic Sideroblastic Anemia.** Clonal myelodysplastic disorders, particularly in the elderly or after exposure to drugs or toxins (e.g., alkylating agents; organic solvents). Sideroblastic anemia may also be hereditary or secondary to drugs (e.g., ethanol, isoniazid, chloramphenicol, lead), chronic inflammation, malignant or other hematologic disorders. Thrombocytopenia and granulocytopenia are common, and the MCV may be high, normal, or low. Leukemia may develop, but morbidity more often results from infection, bleeding, and iron overload. Diagnostic tests exclude B_{12} and folate deficiencies and identify associated disorders and drug exposures. Suspect drugs should be stopped and underlying disorders treated. No treatment or only occasional red cell transfusions for symptomatic anemia may be needed. Folic acid (1–2 mg/day po) prevents deficiency, but improvement in anemia is unlikely. Iron stores should be quantitated and deferoxamine therapy may be needed to prevent or treat symptomatic iron overload. Efforts to improve cytopenias are seldom effective and include androgens; differentiation therapy with low-dose cytosine arabinoside (10 mg/m^2 SQ every 12 hours or 20 mg/m^2/day by continuous IV infusion for 7–21 days) or *cis*-retinoic acid; immunosuppression with corticosteroids, cyclophosphamide, or azathioprine; splenectomy (may cause postoperative thrombocytosis and thrombosis); and bone marrow transplantation for young patients with severe de novo myelodysplasia. **Pyridoxine** (100 mg po 3 times/day for 3–4 months), pyridoxal 5′-phosphate, L-tryptophan, and vitamin C benefit occasional patients with hereditary or idiopathic sideroblastic anemias. Chemotherapy is appropriate for overt leukemia, but success is limited by patient age and refractoriness of leukemias induced by chemical carcinogens.

6. **CYTOPLASMIC MATURATION DISORDERS**

a. **The Thalassemias.** Hereditary defects in synthesis of α or β chains of hemoglobin primarily in Mediterranean, African, and Asian populations. Microcytosis and hypochromia are prominent, even when anemia is mild and splenomegaly is common, but severity of anemia depends on the number of globin chain genes affected. A thalassemia phenotype may also result from structurally abnormal hemoglobins such as hemoglobin E in Southeast Asian subjects. Anemia may increase during pregnancy, infection, or use of oxidant drugs (hemoglobin H disease; hemoglobin E).

(1). *Diagnostic Tests.* Elevated hemoglobin A_2 and/or F levels on hemoglobin electrophoresis (β-thalassemia trait; β-thalassemia [thalassemia major]); hemoglobin H (tetramers of excess β chains) on hemoglobin electrophoresis or Heinz body preparations (α-thalassemia, hemoglobin H disease); in vitro studies of reticulocyte and marrow globin chain synthesis; family studies; tests to exclude iron deficiency, which can suppress hemoglobin A_2 synthesis. If anemia is severe, the presence of unrelated complicating disorders should be considered.

(2). Therapy. Genetic counseling is provided, as is monitoring for iron overload and avoiding iron therapy, folate supplements are given. Oxidant drugs (hemoglobin H disease; hemoglobin E) must be avoided. Splenectomy benefits selected patients with hemoglobin H disease or thalassemia major but should be preceded by polyvalent pneumococcal vaccine. Deferoxamine infusions are given prophylactically in thalassemia major and therapeutically when iron overload develops in other forms of thalassemia. The purpose of chronic red cell hypertransfusion is to maintain hemoglobin levels of 10–12 gm/dL in children with thalassemia major (suppresses erythropoiesis, limits marrow expansion, and prevents bone deformities).

7. HEMOLYTIC ANEMIAS

a. Hemolytic anemia is defined as a rapid fall in hematocrit (acute) or a stable hematocrit with sustained reticulocytosis (chronic) in the absence of bleeding. Reticulocytosis begins 3–7 days after onset of hemolysis. Low serum haptoglobin and elevated serum LDH and bilirubin levels occur with both intravascular and extravascular destruction but are insensitive and nonspecific. Intravascular hemolysis causes hemoglobinemia and hemoglobinuria (often transient) while hemosiderinuria develops 4–14 days later. All patients with chronic hemolysis require folate therapy and monitoring for cholelithiasis, iron overload (if extravascular), and iron depletion (if intravascular). Hemolysis may increase with infections (e.g., sickle cell disease) or the use of oxidant drugs (e.g., G6PD deficiency). Aplastic crises may result from parvovirus infections and require intensive transfusion support.

b. Sickle cell disorders are due to inheritance of a structurally abnormal β chain that forms insoluble polymers under hypoxic conditions. **Heterozygotes** are not anemic, and symptoms are rare, but hematuria and impaired renal concentrating ability may occur, and genetic counseling is needed. **Homozygotes** have chronic intravascular hemolysis and recurrent vaso-occlusive events leading to infarctive crises characterized by bone, chest, and abdominal pain; fever; and neurologic and visual changes that are difficult to distinguish from complicating disorders such as osteomyelitis, cholecystitis, hepatitis, appendicitis, pneumonia, marrow emboli, and meningitis. Hemoglobin electrophoresis is used for diagnosis. Treatment involves avoidance of dehydration and cold exposure; analgesics; correction of hypoxemia and acidosis; and treatment of infections. Exchange transfusions to reduce hemoglobin S levels below 40% may be used therapeutically (for neurologic, cardiac, or retinal symptoms; hypoxemia; priapism; severe prolonged or infarctive crises; acute splenic sequestration [infants]; and chronic leg ulcers) or prophylactically (during pregnancy or before general anesthesia). Long-term exchange/transfusion may be useful in selected patients with severe neurologic, retinal, or cardiac symptoms. Attempts to modify sickling with urea, cyanate, and induced hyponatremia have had little success.

c. **Hereditary Deficiencies of Red Cell Enzymes of Glycolysis, the Hexose Monophosphate Shunt, or Nucleotide Metabolism.** Extravascular hemolysis is diagnosed by specific enzyme assays. In X-linked G6PD deficiency, self-limited hemolysis occurs with infection or the use of oxidant drugs (Table 10–2) if enzyme deficiency is limited to older red cells, while chronic hemolysis occurs if both young and old red cells are affected. Diagnosis may require measuring G6PD activity 3–4 months after recovery. Splenectomy can benefit patients with severe hemolysis due to pyruvate kinase, hexokinase, glucose phosphate isomerase, or G6PD deficiency.

d. **Hereditary spherocytosis.** Extravascular hemolysis is due to hereditary defects of red cell membrane proteins. Hyperchromic microspherocytes on the peripheral smear may be infrequent and also occur with autoimmune hemolytic anemia. The diagnosis is indicated by increased sensitivity to hypotonic lysis on the incubated osmotic fragility test. In treatment, splenectomy is done in cases of severe hemolysis or chronic leg ulcers.

e. **Paroxysmal Nocturnal Hemoglobinuria (PNH)** is an acquired clonal myeloproliferative disorder with intermittent intravascular hemolysis due to complement–mediated membrane damage, a thrombotic diathesis, thrombocytopenia, and neutropenia. PNH may arise from or present as aplastic anemia. Hemolysis increases during correction of iron deficiency or the administration of blood products, while thrombosis increases during surgery or pregnancy. Increased sensitivity of red cells to lysis on incubation with sucrose or acidified serum (Ham test) and low leukocyte alkaline phos-

TABLE 10–2. SOME HEMOLYTIC OXIDANT DRUGS AND CHEMICALS IN G6PD-DEFICIENT PATIENTS

ANTIBIOTICS	ANTIPYRETICS	MISCELLANEOUS
Primaquine	Phenacetin	Acetanilid
Quinacrine		Naphthalene
Nalidixic acid		Phenylhydrazine
Nitrofurantoin		Toluidine blue
Sulfonamides (sulfanilamide,		Methylene blue
sulfacetamide, sulfapyridine,		Trinitrotoluene
salicylazosulfapyridine,		
sulfamethoxazole)		
Diaminodiphyenylsulfone		
Niridazole		

phatase level indicate the diagnosis. Therapy of anemia involves androgens, steroids (prednisone 60 mg/night tapered to 10–40 mg on alternate days), hypertransfusion (hemoglobin >10 gm/dL), particularly perioperatively and during pregnancy or iron replacement. Therapy or prevention of thrombosis is done with prednisone, heparin, and Coumadin. The roles of antiplatelet and fibrinolytic agents have not been established. Bone marrow transplant is an option for young patients with severe disease.

f. **Immune Hemolytic Anemia (IHA).** This is due to binding of immunoglobulin or complement to red cells and is characterized by microspherocytes on the peripheral smear. The condition may be idiopathic or secondary to drugs (Table 10–3), infection, malignant disease, lymphoproliferative diseases, or rheumatologic disorders. Reticulocytopenia occurs if antibody binds to reticulocytes or red cell precursors. Warm-reactive antibodies (often IgG) are most active at 37°C and cause extravascular hemolysis; cold-reactive antibodies (often IgM) are most active below 37°C, bind transiently, fix complement, and cause intravascular hemolysis. Cold agglutinins may react with red cell I or i antigens and cause hemolysis when present in high titers. Drugs or drug metabolites may bind to red cells to form new antigens (haptenic mechanism) or they may modify red cell membranes permitting autoantibody formation (autoimmune mechanism). Drugs may also cause non-specific binding of immunoglobulin and/or complement leading to a positive Coombs' test without hemolysis (e.g., cephalosporins). The direct antiglobulin (Coombs') test is used for diagnosis; it is negative in 5–10% of cases. The first step in therapy is to identify associated disorders and stop suspect drugs. Therapy of warm IHA is **prednisone** (40–60 mg/m²/day—up to 21 days to respond); splenectomy (response **not** predicted by splenic red cell uptake studies); immunosuppressive agents (cyclophosphamide or azathioprine 1–2 mg/kg/day for 3–4 months, but marrow suppression may worsen anemia); and danazol (200 mg 3–4 times/day only

TABLE 10–3. SOME DRUGS ASSOCIATED WITH IMMUNE HEMOLYTIC ANEMIA

HAPTEN MECHANISM (Strong Drug–RBC Binding)

Penicillins	Tetracycline	
Cephalosporins	Streptomycin	

HAPTEN MECHANISM (Weak Drug–RBC Binding)

Quinine	Sulfonamides	Isoniazid
Quinidine	Sulfonylureas	p-aminosalicyclic acid
Phenacetin	Thiazides	Chlorpromazine
Rifampicin		

AUTOIMMUNE MECHANISM

Aldomet	Mefenamic acid	Procainamide
Levodopa	Ibuprofen	

occasionally effective.) Plasma exchange and high-dose immune globulin therapy are rarely helpful. Therapy of cold IHA begins with keeping the patient warm. Immunosuppressive agents and plasma exchange may be of benefit; steroids and splenectomy are rarely effective. Identifying compatible blood may be difficult but transfusions are indicated when anemia is life threatening.

B. Erythrocytosis

1. **DEFINITION.** Hemoglobin > 17.5 gm/dL in men; > 16 gm/dL in women.

2. **CLASSIFICATION** (Table 10–4). A high red cell mass (> 36 mL/kg for men; > 32 mL/kg for women) distinguishes **absolute** from **relative** (low plasma volume) erythrocytosis. Low serum erythropoietin levels distinguish primary marrow proliferative disorders from disorders secondary to systemic hypoxia, renal hypoxia, or autonomous erythropoietin production (high values).

3. **RELATIVE ERYTHROCYTOSIS.** Only associated disorders (e.g., hypertension) are treated.

4. **ERYTHROCYTOSIS DUE TO SYSTEMIC HYPOXIA** (Table 10–4). High red cell mass compensates for increased oxygen needs.

TABLE 10–4. CLASSIFICATION OF ERYTHROCYTOSIS

RELATIVE ERYTHROCYTOSIS (normal red cell mass; low plasma volume)
ABSOLUTE ERYTHROCYTOSIS (high red cell mass)
  Erythropoietin independent (autonomous)
    Polycythemia vera
  Erythropoietin dependent (secondary)
  Systemic Hypoxia
  Hypoxemic disorders (Low *measured* hemoglobin-oxygen saturation)
    High altitude
    Pulmonary insufficiency
    Intrapulmonary shunts (cirrhosis, hereditary telangiectasia)
    Alveolar hypoventilation (obesity)
    Cardiac disorders (right-to-left shunts)
  Non-hypoxemic disorders (Normal hemoglobin-oxygen saturations)
    Increased hemoglobin-oxygen affinity (low P_{50})
      Abnormal hemoglobins: hereditary (autosomal dominant), acquired
        (carboxyhemoglobin; methemoglobin)
      Decreased 2,3-DPG
  Renal hypoxia
  Cysts
  Tumors
  Hydronephrosis
  Renal artery stenosis
  Chronic pyelonephritis
  Renal transplant rejection
  Non-hypoxic (autonomous erythropoietin production)
  Idiopathic
  Familial (autosomal recessive)
  Ectopic erythropoietin production: hypernephroma, hepatoma, uterine
    leiomyoma, cerebellar hemangioblastoma

a. **Diagnostic Tests. Arterial blood gases** (P_{O_2} <60 mm Hg; measured hemoglobin-oxygen saturations <92%, but may fall only during sleep or when patient is supine); P_{50} (<20 mm Hg with high–oxygen affinity hemoglobin); carboxyhemoglobin (>4% in smokers); hemoglobin electrophoresis (rarely useful).

b. **Therapy** is composed of continuous or nocturnal oxygen for hypoxemia; surgery for intracardiac shunts; weight loss; cessation of smoking. Phlebotomy can improve mental alertness, work performance, and headache by increasing blood flow, but blood oxygen-carrying capacity decreases. Thus the optimum hematocrit must be empirically derived for each patient.

5. **ERTHROCYTOSIS DUE TO RENAL DISEASES OR NONHYPOXIC DISORDERS.** Red cell mass exceeds tissue oxygen demands. Treatment of underlying disorder and phlebotomy can improve symptoms.

6. **POLYCYTHEMIA VERA** is acquired clonal myeloproliferative disorder characterized by erythrocytosis, granulocytosis, thrombocytosis, splenomegaly, and thrombosis. Iron deficiency, basophilia, pruritus, and hyperuricemia are also common, and acute leukemia or myeloid metaplasia may develop later.

a. **Diagnostic indications** include high leukocyte alkaline phosphatase, increased serum B_{12} binding proteins, abnormal marrow cytogenetics, and autonomous in vitro erythroid colony growth; causes of secondary erythrocytosis should be excluded.

b. **Therapy**

(1). Phlebotomy. Hematocrit should be reduced to 42–45% by removing 0.5–1 unit of blood daily or every other day with less frequent removal of smaller volumes in the elderly and in patients with cardiac disorders. Blood counts should be checked monthly and hematocrit maintained below 45%. As iron deficiency develops, the need for phlebotomy decreases, and iron supplements are given only if symptoms develop (e.g., cheilosis, glossitis, weakness). Phlebotomy can **increase the risk of thrombosis** and does not affect splenomegaly, thrombocytosis, or signs and symptoms due to increased marrow turnover (hyperuricemia, pruritus, weight loss, fatigue).

(2). Myelosuppressive Therapy. Indicated with advanced age (>70), continued need for frequent phlebotomy, prior thromboses, symptoms due to splenomegaly, hypermetabolic state, and perhaps for platelet counts $>1 \times 10^6$ (an association between thrombocytosis and thrombosis is not established). Phlebotomies are also needed for several weeks until a response occurs. [32]P is convenient for elderly patients whose limited life expectancy offsets the risk of treatment-related leukemia. A single dose (2.3 mCi/m^2 intravenously; total dose <5 mCi/m^2) decreases the red cell mass in 2–3 months; a second dose may be required at 12 weeks, and unmaintained remissions last 6–18 months. Hydroxyurea (15–20 mg/kg/day po continuously) or busulfan (4–6 mg/day po until remission and then intermittently as needed) may be less leukemogenic

than chlorambucil. Blood counts should be checked weekly or bimonthly and dosages adjusted for thrombocytopenia or leukopenia, which may be protracted after busulfan. Rarely, prolonged use of busulfan can cause pulmonary fibrosis, hyperpigmentation, or a wasting syndrome.

(3). Allopurinol (300 mg/day) for hyperuricemia; *Cyproheptadine* (4 mg 3–4 times/day) or *Cimetidine* (300 mg 4 times/day) for pruritus.

(4). Antiplatelet agents (aspirin, dipyridamole) may *not* prevent thrombosis and may increase the risk of gastrointestinal hemorrhage.

C. Iron Overload

1. **CLASSIFICATION.** Iron overload results from red cell transfusions and/or increased absorption of dietary iron due to idiopathic hemochromatosis, thalassemia, chronic hemolytic anemias, myelodysplastic syndromes, and congenital dyserythropoietic anemias. Iron may be deposited in reticuloendothelial cells with little associated toxicity or in parenchymal cells with tissue damage resulting in cirrhosis, cardiomyopathy, diabetes mellitus, hypogonadism, and arthritis.

2. **DIAGNOSTIC TESTS.** Serum iron >160 μg/dL with transferrin saturations >60% (also occur with ineffective erythropoiesis, chronic hemolysis, and marrow hypoplasia without iron overload); serum ferritin >400 mg/dL (also increased by inflammation, cancer, and liver disease); urinary iron loss >2.2 mg/day after deferoxamine (10 mg/kg intramuscularly); but this test may be insensitive to early parenchymal iron overload. Liver biopsy with histologic and quantitative analyses of iron content is the best index of total body iron stores, iron distribution (parenchymal vs reticuloendothelial), and tissue damage (cirrhosis). Another diagnostic marker is a family history of anemia or signs and symptoms of iron overload.

3. **THERAPY.** Tea with meals decreases absorption; transfusions should be limited. Removal of iron by phlebotomy (1–2 U/week until iron deficiency develops and then 3–4 U/year) in idiopathic hemosiderosis or by subcutaneous infusion of deferoxamine (1–4 gm over 12/24 hours with dose adjusted to achieve maximum urinary iron loss) in primary hematologic disorders prolongs survival and improves, stabilizes, or prevents cardiac dysfunction, cirrhosis, hyperpigmentation, and hypogonadism. Although vitamin C (100–200 mg/day po) increases the effectiveness of deferoxamine, its use should be discouraged since it may cause cardiac decompensation as iron is released from reticuloendothelial sites. Initially, serum ferritin, serum iron, and MCV are measured monthly and then 2–3 times/year after iron stores are depleted. HLA typing of patients with idiopathic hemochromatosis and their families permits identification of obligate homozygotes and carriers and appropriate genetic counseling.

Hillman RS, Finch CE: The red cell manual. 5th ed. Philadelphia, FA Davis Co, 1985.
Storb R, Thomas ED, Buckner CD, et al: Marrow transplantation for aplastic anemia. Semin Hematol 22:27–36, 1984.
Gordeuk VR, Bacon BR, Brittenham GM: Iron overload: Causes and consequences. Ann Rev Nutr 7:485–508, 1987.

Chanarin J: Investigation and management of megaloblastic anaemia. Clin Haematol 5:747–763, 1976.
Berk PF, Goldberg JD, Donovan PB, et al: Therapeutic recommendations in polycythemia vera based on polycythemia vera study group protocols. Semin Hematol 23:132–143, 1986.

II. LEUKOCYTE DISORDERS

Malignant leukocyte disorders including acute and chronic leukemias, lymphomas, and plasma cell dyscrasias are discussed in Chapter 11.

A. Neutrophilia (>10,000 cells/μL) occurs most commonly as a normal marrow response to inflammation or infection but may also occur in response to epinephrine or corticosteroids, or as part of a myeloproliferative disorder. Neutrophilia per se produces no adverse effects, and therapy is directed toward the underlying disorder.

B. Neutropenia (<1800 cells/μL) may occur as an isolated finding or in association with anemia and/or thrombocytopenia. It may be due to decreased marrow production (drug toxicity, intrinsic marrow disease, marrow infiltration, B_{12} or folate deficiency), increased neutrophil destruction (drug effect, overwhelming bacterial infection, immune neutropenia), or increased margination (inflammation, splenomegaly). **Unexplained isolated neutropenia** is most often drug induced and all unnecessary drugs should be discontinued. Recombinant cytokines (G-CSF, GM-CSF) shorten the period of chemotherapy-associated neutropenia and may prove to be effective in other neutropenic states. Antibiotic management of infections in patients with neutropenia is discussed in Chapter 3. Severely neutropenic patients with documented bacterial infection are candidates for neutrophil transfusion therapy if they do not respond to appropriate antibiotic therapy within 24–48 hours.

III. DISORDERS OF HEMOSTASIS

A. Bleeding Disorders. Pertinent diagnostic information includes the type of bleeding, the nature of inciting events (spontaneous vs surgery or trauma), prior drug or transfusion therapy, the presence of any significant medical disorders, and family history. However, definitive diagnosis of a bleeding disorder depends upon adequate laboratory data. Initial workup should include a full coagulation screen:

1. Platelet count. The relationship between the platelet count and bleeding due to thrombocytopenia is discussed on page 360.
2. Bleeding time (BT), normally 4–8 minutes, is a measure of in vivo platelet plug formation. With normal platelet function, BT = 30 − platelet count/4000. If BT exceeds the predicted value, platelet dysfunction is present. Abnormalities in platelet plug formation are usually clinically significant only if the BT is greater than 12–15 minutes.
3. Fibrinogen. Clinically significant bleeding due to hypofibrinogenemia is not likely to occur unless the fibrinogen level is less than 80–100 mg/dL. Values below 80 mg/dL will result in prolongation of the other clotting tests.
4. Thrombin time will be prolonged in the presence of dysfibrinoge-

nemia/hypofibrinogenemia or fibrin degradation products. The test is most valuable as a sensitive indicator for the presence of heparin.

5. Prothrombin time (PT) measures extrinsic pathway clotting and reflects levels of factor VII as well as the common pathway factors (X, V, II, fibrinogen). Clinically important factor deficiency usually prolongs the PT at least 4–6 seconds.

6. Partial thromboplastin time (PTT) measures intrinsic pathway clotting and reflects levels of factors XII, XI, IX, VIII as well as the common pathway factors (X, V, II, fibrinogen). Clinically important factor deficiencies usually prolong the PTT at least 8–12 seconds.

7. Fibrin degradation products will generally be increased with significant fibrinolysis.

Depending on the results of the screening tests, specific coagulation factor assays and other special tests may be performed to further define the problem.

1. PLATELET DISORDERS

 a. **Thrombocytopenia** may be due to decreased production, increased destruction, or splenic sequestration. The peripheral blood smear should be examined to confirm the degree of thrombocytopenia, assess platelet morphology (large platelets suggest a high platelet turnover), and detect abnormalities in other cell lines. Examination of bone marrow megakaryocyte numbers provides an estimate of platelet production.

   In addition to treating any underlying disorders, general management includes **minimizing the chance of bleeding** by avoiding intramuscular injections, drugs that inhibit platelet function (e.g., aspirin), and activities that carry significant risk of trauma. Menses can be suppressed by hormonal therapy. In the absence of platelet dysfunction, spontaneous bleeding will not occur in most patients until the platelet count drops below 5000/μL. Bleeding may occur at higher levels (20,000–40,000/μL) in patients with platelet dysfunction (e.g., uremia, sepsis, exposure to drugs that impair platelet function). With trauma or surgery, counts as high as 50,000–100,000/μL may be needed for effective hemostasis. In the absence of significant bleeding, **platelet transfusions** should be reserved for patients with platelet counts under 5000–10,000/μL or for patients with counts below 50,000–100,000/μL who are about to undergo an invasive procedure.

 b. **Drug-induced thrombocytopenia** is common after cytotoxic drug therapy. It may also occur as an unanticipated reaction to other drugs on either a marrow suppressive or antibody-mediated basis. Unnecessary drugs should be discontinued. **Platelet transfusions** may be necessary, but often are not effective in immune-mediated cases. Therapy with **corticosteroids** has not proved useful. **Plasma exchange** has been reported to be rapidly effective in some cases of quinine/quinidine-induced thrombocytopenia.

 c. **Autoimmune thrombocytopenia purpura (AITP)** is an antibody-mediated disorder with decreased platelet survival and normal or increased numbers of megakaryocytes in the marrow. There may be large platelet forms and BT shorter than predicted by the platelet count. Increased amounts of IgG can usually be demonstrated on the platelet surface. The disorder may be primary or may be seen in association with systemic lupus erythematosus, non-Hodgkin's lymphoma, chronic lymphocytic leukemia, or HIV infection. Diagnosis depends on exclusion of other causes of thrombocytopenia. Prednisone 1–2 mg/kg should be given as initial therapy. 80% of patients will respond; the initial response usually occurs within 2–3 days, but may take as long as 1–2 weeks. Once a maximum or normal platelet count is achieved, the drug dose should be tapered to ascertain the dose required to maintain an acceptable count. Of responding patients, 10–15% will be cured. Splenectomy is indicated for patients in whom steroid therapy has failed or for those in whom the maintenance dose is unacceptably high. Approximately 80% of patients will respond to splenectomy and ⅔ of these will be cured. Splenectomy can usually be performed without excessive bleeding or the need for platelet transfusions, even in patients with severe thrombocytopenia. Approximately 75% of patients will respond to IV gamma globulin (0.4 gm/kg/day for 5 days). The effect is short-lived, with severe thrombocytopenia usually recurring within 1–3 weeks. However, the transient improvement may be useful in getting the patient through an acute episode of bleeding or a surgical procedure. For patients in whom the above therapy has failed, favorable results have been reported with danazol (an attenuated androgen) and with immunosuppressive agents (e.g., vincristine, vinblastine, azathioprine, cyclophosphamide). Plasma exchange has not proved generally efficacious.

Platelet transfusions are normally reserved for patients with life-threatening hemorrhage, since the life span of the transfused cells is usually very short. However, platelet survival does vary, and administration of a trial platelet transfusion is reasonable for patients with significant bleeding or with severe thrombocytopenia if the diagnosis is uncertain.

d. **Thrombotic thrombocytopenic purpura (TTP)** is characterized pathologically by widespread deposition of platelet aggregates in the microvasculature and clinically by microangiopathic hemolytic anemia, thrombocytopenia, neurologic abnormalities, renal dysfunction, and fever. The syndrome is closely related to the hemolytic uremic syndrome and is often associated with infection by toxigenic strains of *Escherichia coli*. Untreated, TTP is often fatal. The principal therapeutic approach involves plasma exchange or plasma infusion. In severely affected patients, daily plasma exchange (1–1.5 plasma volumes) should be started immediately with the replacement fluid being 50–100% plasma. Alternatively, if the cardiovascular status permits, 4–8 U of plasma may be infused initially followed by 3–4 U/day. The intensity of this therapy may be adjusted, depending on the patient's response but should be continued at least 7–10 days before it is concluded that no effect is likely to occur. Less severely affected patients may be treated less aggressively, and some will respond to much less plasma. Prednisone (1–2 mg/kg/day) probably improves the response rate, and the dose can be tapered rapidly after maximal response is attained. Antiplatelet agents (aspirin 325–1300 mg/day with or without dipyridamole 400 mg/day) have been shown to be important in therapy in some cases and should probably be given and continued for 3–6 months if there is not significant bleeding. About 75% of cases will respond to this approach with improvement in neurologic status and platelet count apparent after a few days. Therapy with vincristine, IV gamma globulin, or splenectomy may be effective in refractory cases. Platelet transfusions are usually not necessary in patients with TTP, and some reports have suggested that they may be detrimental.

e. **Post-transfusion purpura** is a rare disorder characterized by thrombocytopenia occurring about 1 week after transfusion in a patient who either has previously been pregnant or undergone transfusion. Platelet counts are usually less than 10,000/μL. Megakaryocytes are plentiful in the marrow, and high-titer platelet antibodies are demonstrable. Most commonly in patients negative for the platelet–specific antigen PIA1, a previously made anti-PIA1 antibody has been recalled resulting in the destruction of both autologous and transfused platelets. Untreated, thrombocytopenia may persist for weeks. High-dose prednisone (2–4 mg/kg/day), IV gamma globulin (0.4 gm/kg/day for 2–5 days), or plasma exchange may improve the platelet count within a few days. Platelet transfusion is ineffective.

f. **Dilutional Thrombocytopenia** may occur in massive transfusion. Platelet counts should be monitored in patients transfused with more than 1 blood volume and platelet transfusion considered for clinically significant thrombocytopenia.

g. **Qualitative Platelet Abnormalities.** Acquired platelet function abnormalities occur with uremia, myeloproliferative disorders, paraproteinemias, disseminated intravascular coagulation, sepsis, and the use of drugs known to impair platelet function. Congenital platelet function abnormalities include von Willebrand disease and other more rare disorders. **The hallmark of platelet dysfunction is prolonged bleeding time** not explainable by the platelet count. Management of acquired platelet dysfunction involves treatment of the underlying disorder. The platelet defect in uremia is usually improved by dialysis. In both congenital and acquired disorders, platelet function may be transiently improved by cryoprecipitate (10–15 bags), deamino-D-arginine vasopressin (DDAVP [0.3 μg/kg]), or platelet transfusion. The patient should avoid drugs that impair platelet function.

h. **Thrombocytosis.** Extremely high platelet counts may be associated with abnormal bleeding or, less frequently, with venous or arterial thrombosis. These clinical manifestations are almost always limited to patients with myeloproliferative disorders and severe thrombocytosis (platelets $\geq 10^6/\mu L$). They do not occur in patients with secondary thrombocytosis. Therapy with myelosuppressive and antiplatelet agents is discussed in the section on essential thrombocythemia and polycythemia vera. If symptoms are life threatening, plateletpheresis will decrease the platelet count rapidly, but the effect is transient and the count will rebound within a few days.

2. **COAGULATION FACTOR ABNORMALITIES.** The distinction between congenital and acquired coagulation factor abnormalities is usually apparent from the history, although the condition in some patients with mild congenital factor deficiencies may not become apparent until adulthood, often after a hemostatic challenge. In congenital disorders, the defect is usually the deficiency of a single coagulation factor; with acquired disorders there are usually multiple factor deficiencies.

   a. Hemophilia. Congenital deficiencies of factor VIII (hemophilia A) or factor IX (hemophilia B) are X-linked disorders. Patients with factor levels less than 1% of normal usually suffer frequent spontaneous hemorrhage. Spontaneous hemorrhage is unusual in patients with levels of 1–5%. With levels greater than 5%, bleeding may occur if patients are subjected to hemostatic challenge. Management involves factor replacement at the time of hemorrhage, patient and family education, genetic counseling, psychological support, and inclusion of dentists and orthopedic surgeons on the health care team. Active but sensible exercise is encouraged to increase muscle tone and minimize the chance of bleeding. Patients should avoid aspirin-containing drugs as well as IM injections.

   The basic principle of therapy for bleeding episodes is that they be treated early; thus the widespread use of home treatment. There must be a high level of suspicion that any unexplained symptom is an episode of bleeding. Pain usually occurs before any other evidence of bleeding, and treatment should not be withheld simply because there are no physical signs. Superficial cuts and bruises can usually be handled by local measures. If sutures are required, factor replacement should be provided. Initial factor levels of 30–40% should be attained with uncomplicated hemarthrosis, hematuria, and minor hematomas, with daily repetition of this dose until resolution. Surgery or major muscle hematomas require initial factor levels of 60–100% with minimum levels of 30–50% maintained over the next 10–14 days. Factor levels should be monitored to ensure that the expected levels are being attained. Patients with head injury, even if only a hard blow, should be given factor replacement to initial levels of 50–60% even if there are no neurologic signs or symptoms. CT should be performed on any patient with neurologic abnormalities; if positive, a full surgical regimen of factor replacement is initiated. For oral surgical procedures or dental extractions, a single infusion of factors to bring the level to 50–100% is followed by administration of epsilon-aminocaproic acid (EACA) to inhibit clot lysis (see below).

   The component and dose required to achieve the above factor levels depend upon the particular factor involved and the patient's baseline level. For factor VIII, replacement is with either cryoprecipitate or factor VIII concentrate. The administration of 1 U/kg will result in an increase in plasma levels of 2%. Since the half-life of factor VIII is about 10 hours, the dose may have to be repeated every 12 hours. Factor IX replacement can be achieved with fresh frozen plasma or factor IX concentrate. Fresh frozen plasma is preferred if the necessary volume can be given without compromising the patient's cardiovascular status. Because of the extravascular distribution of factor IX, the dose is twice that of factor VIII. The half-life of factor IX is approximately 24 hours; thus the repeated dose, if required, need be administered only every 24 hours. Although factor replacement is normally not indicated in the absence of bleeding, prophylactic replacement may be appropriate for frequent repeated hemorrhage.

EACA, a fibrinolytic inhibitor, is effective in achieving clot stabilization following dental or oral surgical procedures. The usual dose is 50 mg/kg every 6 hours for 7–10 days. Antifibrinolytic therapy is contraindicated in urinary bleeding or if commercial factor IX concentrates have been used.

DDAVP (0.3 μg/kg IV) mobilizes extravascular factor VIII and increases plasma levels by 2–3 fold. Its use in patients with mild hemophilia A who have acute bleeding or before scheduled minor surgery may eliminate the need for blood products. The effect is rapid, factor VIII levels being maximal within an hour and declining with the usual 10-hour to 12-hour half-life. Patients may be refractory to a second dose for 48 hours. Factor VIII levels should be monitored. DDAVP is not effective in hemophilia B.

Joint bleeding is a common manifestation of severe hemophilia. Treatment consists of early factor replacement and **joint immobilization** during the period of pain. Routine joint aspiration is not indicated, but may be considered, if factor levels are adequate, for relief of severe pain and as a diagnostic procedure if infection is suspected. Chronic synovitis is best handled by prophylactic factor replacement and isometric exercises. Joint replacement can be accomplished with adequate factor replacement.

Approximately 10–15% of patients with severe hemophilia A develop antibodies to factor VIII. In most cases the inhibitor titer will increase dramatically if factor VIII is given, making subsequent treatment difficult. Thus management of mild bleeding episodes is limited to immobilization and analgesia. With more severe bleeding episodes, commercial factor IX concentrates are often effective, presumably because of the presence of activated factors that "bypass" factor VIII in the coagulation sequence. Treatment with recombinant factor VII$_a$ or porcine factor VIII may be effective. If the inhibitor concentration is low, large doses of factor VIII concentrate may be effective, but one may have only a few days before the titer increases to the point that further therapy is not possible. In desperate situations, inhibitor concentrations can be lowered with plasma exchange. Corticosteroids or cytotoxic agents have not proved useful. A state of "immune tolerance" may be induced in ½–⅔ of cases by daily infusion of factor VIII. After several months, the inhibitor titers fall and may disappear. Factor IX inhibitors develop in only 1% of patients with hemophilia B;

management is similar to that of patients with factor VIII inhibitors.

b. Von Willebrand Disease. Von Willebrand disease (VWD) results from an inherited abnormality of von Willebrand factor (VWF). The most common form, type I, is an autosomal dominant disorder characterized by a deficiency of all multimeric forms of the protein (15–60% of normal levels). Type II is characterized by selective deficiency of the larger VWF multimers; type III, by severe deficiency of all multimeric forms. VWF is necessary for the maintenance of factor VIII levels, which will be reduced in proportion to the level of total VWF protein. All forms of VWD are characterized by long BTs. Therapy is aimed at restoring the circulating level of VWF–factor VIII. For minor bleeding or for scheduled minor surgery, DDAVP (0.3 μg/kg) is effective in achieving adequate factor levels. This therapy is not effective in type II VWD and may be detrimental in the type IIb subtype, in which it may cause thrombocytopenia. For replacement of VWF–factor VIII, cryoprecipitate is preferred to factor VIII concentrate because the latter may lack the high molecular weight VWF multimers necessary for correction of the platelet function defect. Factor VIII levels necessary for hemostasis are those outlined above for hemophilia A. After infusion of cryoprecipitate the BT correction lasts 4–6 hours, whereas correction of the factor VIII level is prolonged (24–48 hours). For surgery, component administration is needed at most once a day. As with hemophilia A, EACA is useful in patients undergoing oral surgery.

c. Other Factor Deficiencies. Deficiencies of other coagulation factors are inherited as autosomal recessive disorders and may also be associated with clinical bleeding. As with hemophilia, treatment of bleeding episodes is based on replacement of the factors to hemostatic levels (Table 10–5). With the exception of hypofibrinogenemia, which is treated with cryoprecipitate, replacement is with fresh frozen plasma.

d. Vitamin K Deficiency/Antagonism. Vitamin K deficiency may occur with malabsorption syndromes, biliary obstruction, poor diet in combination with broad-spectrum antibiotic therapy, therapy with certain third-generation cephalosporins, and high-dose aspirin therapy. Warfarin, a vitamin K antagonist, induces functional vitamin K deficiency. Screening test values include a normal fibrinogen level but prolonged PT and PTT, which correct to normal after mixture with normal plasma. Management depends on the urgency with which the hemostatic abnormality needs to be corrected. In patients with little or no bleeding, therapy with vitamin K_1 10–15mg IV is sufficient and will correct the hemostatic abnormality within 24–72 hours if liver function is normal. Vitamin K deficiency can be reversed immediately with fresh frozen plasma, but this should be reserved for patients with significant bleeding or those about to undergo an invasive procedure. Factor IX concentrates should not be used to reverse vitamin K deficiency because of the risk of hepatitis and of thrombosis due to the presence of activated clotting factors. In warfarin-treated patients,

TABLE 10–5. PLASMA COAGULATION FACTORS

FACTOR	MINIMUM LEVEL NECESSARY FOR SURGERY (%)	NORMAL IN VIVO HALF-LIFE (HOURS)
II	15	100
V	15–20	25
VII	10–15	5
VIII	25	10
IX	20–25	20
X	15–20	65
XI	10–25	65
XIII	5	150

restoration to proper control may be achieved within a few days by adjusting the dose of either the anticoagulant or interacting drugs.

e. **Liver Disease.** Coagulation factor abnormalities in liver disease may be due to decreased factor synthesis, biliary obstruction with vitamin K deficiency, decreased clearance of fibrin degradation products, or dysfibrinogenemia. The PT and PTT are typically prolonged. For clinically significant abnormal laboratory values alone, therapy with vitamin K_1 (10 mg IV) is appropriate, but factor replacement is not required. If the patient is bleeding or is about to undergo an invasive procedure, coagulation factors should be provided, using fresh frozen plasma, or, if the patient also needs red cells, whole blood. Because of the increased risk of thrombotic and viral complications, factor IX concentrates should not be given to patients with liver disease. Factor replacement may be compromised in patients with ascites, since the volume of distribution of the administered factors is greatly increased.

f. **Defibrination Syndromes.** Disseminated intravascular coagulation (DIC) is often associated with malignant disease, sepsis, tissue necrosis, shock, abruptio placentae, brain injury, and complement-mediated intravascular hemolysis. Diagnostically the most important laboratory findings are thrombocytopenia and hypofibrinogenemia. The PT and PTT are typically mildly to moderately prolonged. The thrombin time and BT may be prolonged because of the presence of fibrin degradation products. Clinical manifestations are most commonly bleeding and less commonly end-organ ischemia. Management of DIC is directed primarily toward correction of the underlying abnormality. Component replacement is usually appropriate only in patients who are bleeding or who require an invasive procedure. Most patients can be satisfactorily treated with a combination of **platelet transfusions** to keep the platelet count above 30,000–50,000/μL and **cryoprecipitate transfusion** to keep the fibrinogen above 80–100 mg/dL. Treatment with heparin is contraindicated unless the clinical manifestations are primarily tissue ischemia. Primary fibrinolysis occurs rarely except as a result of administration of fibrinolytic agents. It is manifested principally by hypofibrinogenemia. If treatment is necessary, hypofibrinogenemia may be reversed with cryoprecipitate.

g. **Massive Transfusion.** Patients who require large volumes of packed red blood cells may experience significant dilution of clotting factors. The extent of transfusion needed to produce a clinically important hemostatic abnormality depends on the baseline levels of the coagulation factors, but factor levels would be expected to be at 15–20% of the starting levels after the exchange of 2 blood volumes. Patients with laboratory evidence of clinically significant coagulation abnormalities may be treated with whole blood or with fresh frozen plasma. Dilutional thrombocytopenia will also occur under these circumstances and is nearly always of more clinical importance than dilution of the coagulation factors.

h. **Circulating Anticoagulants.** Spontaneous inhibitors may develop to specific coagulation factors; the most common is directed toward factor VIII and may occur in association with rheumatologic, lymphoproliferative, and other disorders. Factor VIII inhibitors occurring in patients with hemophilia are discussed on page 364. The PTT is prolonged and does not correct on mixing with normal plasma; the diagnosis is confirmed by specific factor inhibitor assay. Management is similar to that in hemophiliacs with inhibitors, with three important differences: (1) spontaneous inhibitor titers usually do not rise in response to factor administration, so one can be more liberal in attempts to overwhelm the inhibitor with factor VIII infusion, (2) treatment with corticosteroids (prednisone 1 mg/kg/day) and/or cytotoxic agents is often effective, and (3) most spontaneous inhibitors do not cross-react with porcine factor VIII. Lupus inhibitors are immunoglobulins that interfere with clot generation in vitro. They occur in patients with disorders such as systemic lupus erythematosus, rheumatoid arthritis, drug reactions, and neoplasms, as well as in otherwise healthy individuals. These inhibitors are only rarely associated with a bleeding tendency; rather, they have been associated with an increased incidence of venous or arterial thrombosis and of spontaneous abortions. No specific therapy is indicated for the laboratory finding per se; if they are associated with thrombosis or frequent abortion, management includes anticoagulation therapy and immunosuppression with corticosteroids or cytotoxic agents.

3. **VASCULAR DISORDERS.** Purpura in the absence of identifiable hemostatic abnormalities can be seen in patients with vasculitis, scurvy, connective tissue disorders, Cushing's syndrome, Kaposi's sarcoma, cryoglobulinemia, and hyperglobulinemic purpura, as well as in patients with no obvious underlying disorder. Therapy is directed toward the underlying disorder.

B. **Thrombotic Disorders.** Thrombotic states of clinical importance include deep venous thrombosis, pulmonary embolus, and coronary or cerebral artery thrombosis or thromboembolism. These disorders are discussed in Chapters 4 and 7.

Karpatkin S: Autoimmune thrombocytopenic purpura. Semin Hematol 22:260–288, 1985.

Kasper CK, Dietrich SL: Comprehensive management of haemophilia. Clin Haematol 14:489–512, 1985.

Thompson AR: Acquired complex coagulation factor disorders. *In* Rossi E, Simon T, Moss G (eds): Principles of Transfusion Medicine. Baltimore, Williams & Wilkins, 1991.

IV. MYELOPROLIFERATIVE DISORDERS

A. Classification. Clonal stem cell disorders, which include **polycythemia vera, chronic myelogenous leukemia, paroxysmal nocturnal hemoglobinuria, agnogenic myeloid metaplasia with myelofibrosis**, and **essential thrombocythemia**.

B. Agnogenic Myeloid Metaplasia with Myelofibrosis. Characterized by marrow fibrosis and extramedullary hematopoiesis leading to splenomegaly and anemia (often macrocytic) with granulocytosis, thrombocytosis and teardrop-shaped red cells, nucleated red cells, large platelets and immature granulocytes on the peripheral smear. Basophilia, eosinophilia, platelet dysfunction, hyperuricemia, and high serum lactic dehydrogenase levels are common. Leukocyte alkaline phosphatase may be high, normal, or low.

1. **DIAGNOSTIC TESTS.** Increased reticulin and collagen on bone marrow biopsy (but may be hypercellular or hypoplastic, and additional sampling may be needed); exclusion of folate and B$_{12}$ deficiencies and disorders that cause secondary marrow fibrosis, such as other hematopoietic neoplasms (e.g., lymphomas, mastocytosis), solid tumors (e.g., prostate cancer), infections (e.g., tuberculosis), disorders with abnormal bone metabolism (e.g., renal osteodystrophy), rheumatologic diseases, and miscellaneous disorders (e.g., sarcoidosis, radiation therapy).

2. **THERAPY** includes transfusions (for symptomatic anemia); folate; allopurinol (for hyperuricemia). Androgens (p. 349) or pyridoxine (200–300 mg/day po) may improve anemia. **Splenectomy** relieves local symptoms and improves cytopenias (but operative mortality is high and preoperative platelet transfusions may be needed for thrombocytopenia or platelet dysfunction); splenic radiation relieves pain of splenic infarction and decreases spleen size in poor surgical candidates (but cytopenias may worsen from radiation of marrow included in the port). **Myelosuppressive agents** (e.g., busulfan 2–4 mg/day, 6-thioguanine 20–40 mg/day; ^{32}P) are given for splenomegaly or hypermetabolic symptoms (fever, fatigue, weight loss), but cytopenias may worsen. **1,25-Dihydroxyvitamin D$_3$** may improve anemia and thrombocytopenia, but hypercalcemia may occur. **Bone marrow transplantation** may be useful in young patients with severe disease.

C. Essential Thrombocythemia. Characterized by thrombocytosis (>600,000 platelets/mm^3 with giant forms on smear and atypical megakaryocytes in the marrow), bleeding, venous or arterial thromboses (less common), anemia, granulocytosis, and splenomegaly. Spurious elevations in serum potassium and acid phosphatase levels may occur. Diagnosis is shown by bone marrow biopsy; platelet function tests, and BT (less consistently prolonged); exclude reactive thrombocytosis due to iron deficiency, acute hemorrhage, hemolysis, inflammation or cancer (platelet function and morphology normal and pathologic bleeding or thrombosis does not occur); exclude other myeloproliferative disorders (e.g., polycythemia vera with complicating iron deficiency). **No treatment may be required** in patients less than 30 years old. **Myelosuppressive agents** in older patients (hydroxyurea 15–20 mg/kg/day po; busulfan 4–6 mg/day po) decrease platelet counts in 4–6 weeks. α-**Interferon** may decrease the platelet count within 1–2 weeks. **Plateletpheresis, nitrogen mustard** (0.4 mg/kg IV) or hydroxyurea (30 mg/kg/day po) is used for rapid reduction of platelet count in patients with acute bleeding or thrombosis. **Antiplatelet agents** (aspirin, dipyridamole, sulfinpyrazone) may help patients with digital ischemia or transient ischemic attacks, but risk of bleeding may be increased.

Gilbert HS: The spectrum of myeloproliferative disorders. Med Clin North Am 57:355–393, 1973.
Murphy S, Hand H, Rosenthal D, Laslo J: Essential thrombocythemia: an interim report from the polycythemia vera study group. Semin Hematol 23:177–183, 1986.

V. TRANSFUSION THERAPY

Modern transfusion therapy is based on the administration of specific components that are either collected directly from donors by apheresis techniques or separated from donated whole blood. Components can be divided into those containing red cells and those used to effect hemostasis.

A. Blood Components

1. COMPONENTS CONTAINING RED CELLS

a. Indications for Transfusion. A hematocrit value below which transfusions are universally required cannot be defined. The patient's age, underlying condition, symptoms, and the rate of change of the degree of anemia must be considered. Symptoms that may indicate a need for additional red cells include extreme fatigue, headache, dyspnea, angina, and palpitations. Patients rarely need transfusion if the hematocrit is over 30%. Patients who are otherwise healthy can often tolerate hematocrits of 15–20% without adverse effect. Patients with cardiorespiratory disease may develop symptoms when the hematocrit falls below 30%, but most patients do not do so until it falls below 25%. Each red cell unit can be expected to raise the hematocrit 3–4% in an adult recipient.

In patients with acute hemorrhage, the immediate goal of maintaining intravascular volume can be achieved mostly, if not entirely, by administration of salt solutions or colloid preparations. Most patients without serious underlying disease can tolerate hemodilution to a hematocrit in the low 20s; thus it is probably reasonable to begin blood transfusion after loss of 30–40% of the blood volume, assuming the baseline hematocrit was normal.

b. Available products include whole blood/modified whole blood, packed red blood cells, and other specialized red cell products. Whole blood/modified whole blood units contain approximately 200 mL red cells. If cryoprecipitate has been prepared from the unit, the suspending plasma will contain one half of the initial fibrinogen and 15–20% of the initial factor VIII, but other factors will be normal. With storage, factor VIII levels will fall to 30% of baseline in 2–3 days; factor V, to 20% of baseline in 3 weeks; other coagulation factors remain at baseline levels. There are no functional platelets or neutrophils. Packed red cells contain approximately 200 ml red cells suspended in a small amount of plasma or crystalloid solution (hct 70–80%). There is no significant amount of coagulation factors and no functional platelets or neutrophils. Leukocyte-poor blood may be prepared by centrifugation or filtration, techniques that remove more than 90% of the white blood cells. Leukocyte-poor blood is indicated for transfusion in patients with repeated febrile transfusion reactions. Saline washed cells are indicated for patients with severe adverse reactions to plasma constituents and perhaps for patients with complement-mediated immune hemolytic anemia. Previously frozen deglycerolized red cells are suspended in a crystalloid solution and contain very few white cells and no coagulation factors.

Whole blood is appropriate for patients who require both intravascular volume and increased oxygen-carrying capacity (i.e., patients who are bleeding significantly). Hypovolemic patients may also be supported with packed red cells and colloid/crystalloid solutions, but if large volumes are required, supplementation with coagulation factors may be necessary. Patients who are not hypovolemic should be given packed red cells. Administration of whole blood to such patients may result in circulatory overload and also represents a waste of plasma components.

c. **Compatibility Testing.** Patients should not be transfused with (1) red cells to which they have circulating antibodies, (2) red cells to which they are likely to form antibodies (Rh system), or (3) large amounts of plasma containing antibodies to the patient's red cells (small amounts of such plasma, as would be present in a unit of packed red cells, are usually not harmful). Although patients usually receive ABO group–specific components, appropriate substitutions are permissible (Table 10–6). A full crossmatch includes typing, testing the patient's serum for unexpected antibodies, and compatibility testing between the patient's serum and the donor's cells. If there is not time to complete compatibility testing, type-specific (ABO and Rh) blood or uncrossmatched O Rh-negative cells may be given.

d. **Administration of Blood.** Circulatory overload may occur if blood is given too quickly. Otherwise healthy patients with chronic

TABLE 10–6. BLOOD TYPE SUBSTITUTIONS

BLOOD TYPE	PERMISSIBLE BLOOD TYPE SUBSTITUTIONS Red Cells	Plasma
O	None	A, B, AB
A	O	AB
B	O	AB
AB	A, B, O	None

anemia can be given packed red cells safely at a rate of 3–4 mL/kg/hour. Patients with severe anemia and/or hypervolemia should not be given blood any more rapidly than 1 mL/kg/hour. All blood products should be administered through a filter. Blood should not be mixed with any fluid except isotonic saline.

2. COMPONENTS FOR HEMOSTASIS

   a. **Platelets.** The indications for platelet transfusions are discussed on page 360. Platelet concentrates are prepared from units of whole blood or by apheresis techniques. A unit is defined as the number of platelets obtained from 1 unit of blood (approximately 0.7×10^{11} cells). Platelets obtained by apheresis usually contain the equivalent of about 6 units. Platelets are suspended in the donor's plasma and may be stored at room temperature for up to 5 days. Platelets should not be refrigerated. Transfusion of 1 unit of platelets will elevate the adult recipient's platelet count approximately 8000–10,000/μL. The usual adult dose is 4–8 units. Ideally platelets should be ABO identical, but substitutions may be made. Rh-positive platelets should not be given to Rh-negative women of childbearing potential. A platelet count should be obtained before and 1 hour after completion of the transfusion. In patients with sepsis, splenomegaly, autoimmune platelet disorders, or platelet alloimmunization, the life span of transfused platelets may be so short that the post-transfusion platelet count is no different from the baseline. Management of alloimmunization depends on providing platelets from more closely HLA-matched donors. Other measures such as IV IgG or plasma exchange have not generally proved useful.

   b. **Cryoprecipitate.** Cryoprecipitate is prepared from single units of plasma by freeze/thaw techniques. Each bag contains approximately 100 factor VIII/VWF units, 250 mg fibrinogen, and 25% of the factor XIII in the original unit of blood. Cryoprecipitate is suspended in 10–20 mL (per bag) of either plasma or saline. Cryoprecipitate is indicated for documented deficiencies of factor VIII, VWF, or fibrinogen. The adult dose is generally 10–20 bags.

   c. **Factor VIII Concentrates.** Commercial factor VIII concentrates are prepared from large volumes of plasma and are supplied as a lyophilized powder. Modern manufacturing techniques have essentially eliminated the risk of HIV transmission by these products. The dose is calculated on the basis of the patient's estimated blood volume, the increase in factor VIII level desired, and the assumption that 100% of the transfused factor will circulate. Transfusion of factor VIII concentrate is indicated for the treatment of patients with factor VIII deficiency. Cryoprecipitate is preferred to factor VIII concentrate for the treatment of von Willebrand disease, since high–molecular weight VWF multimers are not present in many of the factor VIII concentrates.

   d. **Factor IX Concentrates.** These are commercially prepared concentrates of factors II, IX, and X, with or without factor VII. Use of these preparations is generally limited to the treatment of patients with hemophilia B and of patients with factor VIII inhibitors. Doses for patients with hemophilia B are based on the level of factor IX desired and the assumption that 50% of the transfused dose will be retained in the plasma. Factor IX concentrates should be used with caution in patients with liver disease, since decreased clearance of activated factors may result in disseminated intravascular coagulation or thrombosis.

e. **Fresh Frozen Plasma.** A unit of fresh frozen plasma varies in volume from 200–350 mL and contains all of the coagulation factors in normal amounts. Transfusion of fresh frozen plasma is indicated for the treatment of documented factor deficiencies that cannot be treated more efficiently with other component preparations. Common indications include congenital factor deficiencies, liver disease, reversal of oral anticoagulation, and dilutional coagulopathy. Transfusion is usually indicated only in patients who are actually bleeding or are about to undergo an invasive procedure. In a 70-kg adult, factor levels will increase 2–3% per unit of plasma infused; thus reversal of oral anticoagulation will require approximately 4 units.

B. Transfusion Reactions

1. HEMOLYTIC. Intravascular hemolytic reactions are usually due to ABO incompatibility and are preventable; most commonly they result from clerical errors, mislabeled tubes, and improper identification of the recipient. Symptoms include chills, fever, chest pain, back pain, and nausea. If a hemolytic reaction is suspected, the transfusion should be stopped, the blood pressure carefully monitored, and the clerical work checked. 2–10 mL of the patient's blood should be centrifuged and the plasma examined immediately. If a significant hemolytic reaction has occurred, the plasma will be red. If a reaction is confirmed by examination of the plasma, attempts should be made to maintain urine flow at > 100 mL/hour with diuretics (furosemide 20–80 mg IV) and sufficient IV fluids. Renal function and coagulation status should be monitored closely. A post-transfusion blood sample should be sent to the blood bank to determine the cause of the reaction. Delayed hemolytic transfusion reactions occur in patients who have been previously sensitized to a red cell antigen; the antibody, however, is undetectable at the time of transfusion. The transfusion itself is uneventful. An anamnestic response is triggered, and transfused red cells bearing the relevant antigen are destroyed. The patient's hematocrit suddenly drops 3–10 days after the transfusion. In addition, there may be fever, hemoglobinuria, and hyperbilirubinemia. The direct antiglobulin test may be positive if there are any remaining antigen–positive red cells. The indirect antiglobulin test will reveal a red cell alloantibody not present at the time of the transfusion. Since all sensitized red cells may be rapidly destroyed, severe anemia may result, and additional transfusions using antigen-negative blood may be required.

2. FEBRILE TRANSFUSION REACTIONS are usually due to antibodies to white blood cells and are most often manifested by chills and/or fever beginning ½–2 hours after the start of the transfusion. Since chills

and fever can also be the only symptoms of a hemolytic transfusion reaction, it is important to rule out this possibility. Therapy with aspirin or acetaminophen is usually effective; corticosteroids and meperidine may be required for more severe reactions. The transfusion need not be discontinued if the reaction is mild, but slowing the infusion rate may be helpful. Patients with two consecutive febrile reactions should be provided with leukocyte-poor blood for subsequent transfusions.

3. **ALLERGIC TRANSFUSION REACTIONS** are due to antibodies to plasma proteins. Urticaria is most common, although hypotension and bronchospasm can also occur. Serious reactions may result from antibodies to IgA, particularly in IgA-deficient patients. For mild cases, diphenhydramine 50 mg (either po or IV) usually suffices. The transfusion may be slowed but should not be discontinued if urticaria is the only problem. For more severe reactions, the transfusion should be discontinued and therapy with corticosteroids or epinephrine considered.

C. Other Adverse Effects of Transfusion

1. **TRANSMISSION OF INFECTION.** The incidence of post-transfusion hepatitis C is probably less than 0.1%. Transmission of HIV by transfusion has been exceedingly rare since the institution of anti-HIV screening of blood donors. Cytomegalovirus (CMV) transmission to immunocompetent recipients may result in a mononucleosis-like syndrome. CMV transmission to profoundly immunosuppressed recipients, such as bone marrow transplant recipients, may result in serious infection. For such immunosuppressed patients not previously infected with CMV (i.e., negative for antibody to CMV), transmission of CMV by transfusion can be prevented by supplying blood products only from donors who are also seronegative.

2. **ALLOIMMUNIZATION.** Approximately 2–3% of transfusion recipients will develop red cell alloantibodies. Platelet alloimmunization occurs in 20–50% of patients receiving frequent transfusions.

3. **GRAFT-VERSUS-HOST DISEASE.** Graft-versus-host disease may occur if immunocompetent lymphoid cells are transfused into severely immunosuppressed recipients. Gamma irradiation (1500–5000 rads) eliminates the possibility. All blood products provided for intrauterine transfusions, for neonatal exchange transfusions, and for transfusion in patients who have Hodgkin's disease or who have undergone bone marrow transplantation should be irradiated.

4. **CITRATE TOXICITY.** Blood for transfusion is collected in a citrate-based anticoagulant that prevents clotting by chelation of calcium. With extremely rapid transfusion of whole blood or plasma (500–1000 mL/10 min over a prolonged period) symptoms or signs of hypocalcemia may occur, and supplemental calcium (do not mix the calcium with the blood) should be considered.

Slichter SJ: Controversies in platelet transfusion therapy. Ann Rev Med 31:509–540, 1980.
Greenwalt TJ: Pathogenesis and management of hemolytic transfusion reactions. Semin Hematol 18:84–94, 1981.
Barton JC: Nonhemolytic, noninfectious transfusion reactions. Semin Hematol 18:95–121, 1981.

11 11 11 11 11 11 11 11 11

ONCOLOGIC THERAPEUTICS

OLIVER W. PRESS, CAROLYN COLLINS,
JOANNE MORTIMER, and ROBERT LIVINGSTON

I. PRINCIPLES OF CANCER THERAPY

Cancer currently afflicts an estimated 1,040,000 new patients annually and causes 510,000 deaths per year (Table 11–1), making it the second leading cause of death in the United States. Since epidemiologic studies have suggested that environmental risk factors are operative in the multifactorial pathogenesis of 80–90% of cancer cases, avoidance of carcinogenic factors (such as cigarette smoke, alcohol, and asbestos) is the most desirable method of reducing cancer morbidity and mortality. Unfortunately, intervention trials aimed at primary prevention of cancer have been limited in scope and efficacy, making therapy of established cancer an important medical priority. Three major types of treatment are used to treat neoplasms: surgery, radiation therapy, and systemic chemotherapy. Surgery and radiation therapy are generally used in attempting to cure localized malignancies, whereas chemotherapy is used for disseminated neoplasms. Recently, the advantages of combined therapy have become evident, and an increasing number of tumors are now managed with combinations of these three therapeutic approaches (e.g., Ewing's sarcoma, ovarian carcinoma, osteosarcoma). The rationale for such combination therapy comes from observations that surgery is most likely to fail locally at the edges of tumor resection ("positive surgical margins"), radiation therapy is most likely to fail in the center of tumors, and chemotherapy is most likely to fail in the presence of bulk disease.

Laboratory studies have validated clinical observations that small tumors are more likely to respond to chemotherapy than are large tumors. Small tumors generally have high "growth fractions" (i.e., most of the cells are actively proceeding through the cell cycle), whereas larger tumors have higher percentages of dormant cells resistant to cell cycle–active agents. Furthermore, smaller tumors are statistically less likely to contain cells that have acquired drug resistance by somatic mutation (estimated to occur every 10^6 cell divisions). Studies have shown that combination chemotherapy regimens with agents having different modes of action and exhibiting different forms of toxicity are more likely to be curative than single-agent therapy, since the chance of double resistance to 2 drugs is much less (10^{-12}) than the risk of single-drug resistance (10^{-6}). Maximally tolerated drug doses should be used because the fraction of cells killed is proportional to the dose employed. Single drugs, low doses, and long intervals between chemotherapy cycles encourage the development of resistant tumor cell clones.

Based on preliminary promising results, future treatments for selected tumors may include hormonal therapy, biologic response modifiers, hyperthermia, and monoclonal antibodies. The maximally tolerated doses of standard chemotherapeutic agents may be extended by the co-administration of growth factors such as granulocyte-macrophage colony stim-

TABLE 11–1. ESTIMATED RELATIVE CANCER INCIDENCES AND DEATHS BY SITE AND SEX (1990)*

SITE	RELATIVE INCIDENCES		CANCER DEATHS	
	Male (%)	Female (%)	Male (%)	Female (%)
Lung	20	11	34	21
Colorectal	15	15	11	13
Breast	<1	29	<1	18
Prostate	20	—	11	—
Leukemia/lymphoma	7	6	8	7
Pancreas	3	3	5	5
Ovary	—	4	—	5
Uterus	—	9	—	4
Urinary	10	4	5	3
Oral	4	2	2	1
Melanoma	3	3	2	1
Other	18	14	20	20

*Data from Silverberg E, Boring C, and Squires T: Cancer statistics, 1990. Ca: A Cancer Journal for Clinicians 40:9–26, 1990. Nonmelanoma skin cancer and carcinoma in situ have been excluded.

ulating factor (GM-CSF) and interleukin-3 (IL-3). GM-CSF and IL-3 may mitigate the severity and abbreviate the duration of drug-induced myelosuppression, which currently is the dose-limiting toxicity of most chemotherapy regimens.

II. CHEMOTHERAPY

This brief introduction to the major chemotherapeutic agents currently in use presents standard doses for each drug given as a single agent. When given in combination, these doses may need to be modified. Expected side effects are summarized in Table 11–2. Before prescribing such agents, a physician should have a thorough pharmacologic understanding of these drugs, beyond that which can be provided here.

A. **Alkylating Agents.** Alkylating agents are widely used cytotoxic chemotherapeutic agents having mutagenic and carcinogenic effects. Most alkylating agents form positively charged carbonium ions, which then attack the nucleophilic (electron-rich) sites on nucleic acids and proteins, resulting in formation of a covalent bond and subsequent cross-linking of DNA. Single-strand breaks occur primarily in the process of DNA repair and generally do not produce lethal damage. Most alkylating agents are cell cycle–phase nonspecific. Although the alkylating agents share a common mechanism of action, they do not display cross-resistance in experimental systems and are not uniformly effective against the same malignancies.

1. CYCLOPHOSPHAMIDE (**Cytoxan**) requires activation by hepatic microsomal enzymes to the active moiety, phosphoramide mustard. A toxic metabolite, acrolein, may cause hemorrhagic cystitis. Cytoxan is well

absorbed orally and commonly administered in a daily, continuous oral dose of 50–150 mg/m². The IV dose is 500–1000 mg/m² every 3–4 weeks. Hemorrhagic myopericarditis is the dose-limiting toxicity of cyclophosphamide when given at maximal doses (120 mg/kg) in preparative regimens for bone marrow transplantation. This drug is active in the treatment of breast carcinoma, non-Hodgkin's lymphoma, small cell lung cancer, and ovarian carcinoma.

2. IFOSFAMIDE (Ifex) differs from Cytoxan only in the placement of one of its alkylating side chains. Hemorrhagic cystitis occurs commonly with this drug unless it is given with the uroprotectant mesna, which binds to acrolein in the urine. The standard dosage is 1.8–2.4 gm/m² IV daily for 4–5 days every 3–4 weeks. Mesna is given IV at a dose 20% of the ifosfamide dose before, 4 hours, and 8 hours after ifosfamide. Ifosfamide is active in the treatment of soft tissue sarcomas and testicular carcinomas as well as some lymphomas.

3. NITROGEN MUSTARD (Mechlorethamine) is an analogue of mustard gas and was the first chemotherapeutic drug to be tested clinically. The usual dosage is 8 mg/m² IV day 1 and day 8 every 4 weeks. This drug has largely been replaced by cyclophosphamide, though it is still used in some regimens for Hodgkin's disease and non-Hodgkin's lymphomas.

4. CHLORAMBUCIL (Leukeran) is well absorbed orally and is generally given in a daily dose of 3–6 mg/m². Intermittent administration reduces the risks of irreversible bone marrow damage and secondary acute myelogenous leukemia that may occur with prolonged use. Chlorambucil is used in chronic lymphocytic leukemia, non-Hodgkin's lymphoma, and multiple myeloma.

5. BUSULFAN (Myleran) is well absorbed orally and given in a dose of 2–4 mg/m² daily on an intermittent schedule. As with chlorambucil, myelosuppression may be prolonged and irreversible if excessive doses are used. This drug is used almost exclusively in the treatment of chronic myelogenous leukemia.

6. MELPHLAN (Alkeran, L-PAM, phenylalanine mustard) is given orally in spite of its variable absorption because no IV formulation is available. The usual dosage is 8–10 mg/m² orally for 4–6 days every 4–6 weeks, adjusted to bone marrow tolerance. Secondary leukemia may occur with prolonged oral use. It is administered most frequently to patients with multiple myeloma.

7. NITROSOUREAS. Carmustine (BCNU) and Lomustine (CCNU) are highly lipid-soluble and cross the blood-brain barrier, producing CSF drugs levels that are 30–50% of plasma levels. BCNU is given in a dose of 200–225 mg/m² IV and CCNU 100–150 mg/m² orally. Because these drugs produce delayed neutropenia and thrombocytopenia, they are administered every 6–8 weeks. BCNU is active in Hodgkin's disease, multiple myeloma, non-Hodgkin's lymphoma, brain tumors, and melanoma. CCNU is principally used in the treatment of brain tumors.

TABLE 11–2. TOXICITIES OF CHEMOTHERAPEUTIC AGENTS

DRUG/ROUTE*	WBC†	PLATE-LETS‡	NAUSEA	OTHER GI	PUL-MONARY	RENAL	NEUROLOGIC	INFERTILITY	ALO-PECIA	VESI-CANT§	OTHER
Alkylating Agents											
Cyclophosphamide (PO, IV)	3+	1+	2+	—	Fibrosis	Hemorrhagic cystitis	—	+	+	—	SIADH
Ifosfamide (IV)	2+	2+	1–2+	—	—	Hemorrhagic cystitis	+	—	+	—	—
Nitrogen mustard (IV, topical)	3+	3+	3+	—	—	—	—	+	+	+	—
Chlorambucil (PO)	2+	2+	1+	—	—	—	—	+	—	—	Leukemogenic
Busulfan (PO)	3+	3+	1+	—	Fibrosis	—	—	+	—	—	Skin toxicity
Melphalan (PO)	2+	2+	1+	—	—	—	—	+	—	—	Leukemogenic
Nitrosoureas (PO, IV)	3+	3+	2+	—	Fibrosis	1–2+ nephrotoxicity	—	+/−	—	—	Leukemogenic
Cisplatin (IV, IA, IP)	1+	1+	3+	—	—	3+ nephrotoxicity	2+	—	—	—	Ototoxic
Carboplatin (IV)	3+	3+	1+	—	—	—	—	—	—	—	—
Anti-tumor Antibiotics											
Doxorubicin (IV)	3+	2+	2+	Mucositis	—	—	—	+/−	+	+	Cardiotoxic
Bleomycin (IV, IM, SC)	—	—	1+	—	Fibrosis	—	—	—	—	—	Skin, allergic reactions
Dactinomycin (IV)	3+	3+	2+	Mucositis, diarrhea	—	—	—	—	+	+	Radiation recall
Mitomycin C (IV)	3+	3+	2+	Mucositis	Fibrosis	Hemolytic-uremic syndrome	—	—	+/−	+	Cardiotoxic

Plant Alkaloids									
Vincristine (IV)	1+	1+	—	—	3+	—	—	+	SIADH
Vinblastine (IV)	3+	3+	—	—	—	+/-	+	—	Myalgias
Etoposide (PO, IV)	2+	1-2+	Mucositis	—	—	+/-	+	—	Hypotension, Allergic rxn
Anti-metabolites									
Thioguanine (PO, IV)	2-3+	1+	Stomatitis	—	—	—	—	—	Hepatotoxic
Mercaptopurine (PO)	2-3+	1+	—	—	—	—	—	—	Hepatotoxic
Cytarabine (IV, SC, IT)	3+	2+	Mucositis, pancreatitis	—	Ataxia	+/-	+	—	Hepatotoxic, conjunctivitis
Fluorouracil (IV)	1-2+	1+	Stomatitis, diarrhea	—	Ataxia	—	—	—	Conjunctivitis, angina,
Methotrexate (IV, IT, PO, IM)	2-3+	1+	Stomatitis	Fibrosis 2+ nephrotoxicity	+	—	+	—	Hepatotoxic
Miscellaneous									
DTIC (IV)	1+	3+	—	—	—	—	—	+	Flu-like syndrome

Toxicity Severity: 1+, mild; 2+, moderate; 3+ marked. SIADH = syndrome of inappropriate anti-diuretic hormone.
*Routes of administration: IV, intravenous; IM, intramuscular; IT, intrathecal; IP, intraperitoneal; IA, intra-arterial; SC, subcutaneous; PO, oral.
†Likelihood of producing leukopenia.
‡Likelihood of producing thrombocytopenia.
§Vesicants cause extravasation ulcers.

379

8. **CIS-DIAMMINEDICHLOROPLATINUM (Cisplatin, Platinol)** is extensively protein bound with a tissue half-life of 5 days. 20–75% is
excreted in the urine within 24 hours of administration. The incidence
of renal toxicity can be significantly reduced by vigorous saline
hydration (e.g., 250 cc/hr) for 4 hours before and 8–12 hours after
cisplatin administration. The standard dose is 100–120 mg/m^2 IV
every 3–4 weeks or 20 mg/m^2 daily for 5 days every 3 weeks. There
is evidence that administering this drug in split doses (weekly or
daily) may decrease the toxicity and increase its cytotoxic activity (J
Clin Oncol 4:1707, 1986). At high doses, the dose-limiting toxicities
are peripheral sensory neuropathy and cumulative myelosuppression.
Cisplatin is active against testicular cancer, ovarian carcinoma, non-
Hodgkin's lymphoma, non-small cell lung cancer, small cell lung
cancer, and squamous cell carcinomas of the head and neck.

9. **CARBOPLATIN (Paraplatin, CBDCA)** is a non-nephrotoxic but myelosuppressive analogue of cisplatin. Its administration does not require
hydration. For patients with normal renal function, the standard
dosage is 300–360 mg/m^2 IV every 4 weeks. Doses must be adjusted
for renal dysfunction to prevent severe myelosuppression, particularly
thrombocytopenia (J Clin Oncol 7:1748, 1989).

B. Antitumor Antibiotics

1. **ANTHRACYCLINES. Doxorubicin (Adriamycin)** and **Daunorubicin
(Daunomycin)** are produced by species of *Streptomyces* and exert
their cytotoxic effects by several different mechanisms. These compounds intercalate between the base pairs of DNA, forming a high
affinity complex that results in both single- and double-strand breaks.
Both of these antibiotics undergo extensive hepatic metabolism and
biliary excretion. The usual dose of Adriamycin is 60–90 mg/m^2 via a
short IV infusion or as a prolonged infusion over 96 hours. It is also
given as 15–20 mg/m^2 IV weekly. Daunomycin is given in a dose of
30–60 mg/m^2 IV daily for 3 days. A 50% dose reduction is required
in the presence of hepatic dysfunction (bilirubin > 2 mg/dL). These
drugs should probably be withheld if the bilirubin is more than 3
mg/dL. Three forms of cardiac toxicity are produced by anthracylines,
the most important of which is a chronic dilated congestive cardiomyopathy; this is dose and schedule dependent. The risk is < 10%
with a total dose of Adriamycin < 450 mg/m^2. The incidence of
congestive heart failure is significantly less if Adriamycin is administered either by continuous infusion or on a weekly schedule (Ann
Intern Med 99:745, 1983). At high total cumulative doses, cardiac
function should be followed with serial left ventricular ejection
fractions. Adriamycin is active against a variety of malignancies,
including non-Hodgkin's lymphoma, Hodgkin's disease, breast carcinoma, sarcomas, small cell lung cancer, ovarian cancer, and thyroid
cancer. Daunorubicin is used primarily in the treatment of acute
myelogenous and lymphocytic leukemias.

2. **BLEOMYCIN** is a mixture of small molecular weight glycoproteins
produced by a species of *Streptomyces*. It induces single- and double-

stranded breaks in DNA through formation of superoxide and hydroxyl radicals. As almost all of the drug is excreted unchanged in the urine, doses should be reduced 50–75% for a creatinine clearance less than 40 cc/min. The usual dosage is 10–20 mg/m^2 IV weekly or 15 mg/m^2 by continuous infusion daily for 4 days. The most important toxicity is interstitial pneumonitis, most likely to occur in elderly patients with underlying pulmonary disease, previous pulmonary irradiation, and with cumulative doses of more than 400 mg. Subsequent oxygen exposure may precipitate respiratory failure, and if patients who have received bleomycin require surgery, the FIO$_2$ should be kept as low as possible. Bleomycin is active against squamous cell carcinomas, non-Hodgkin's lymphoma, Hodgkin's disease, and testicular carcinomas.

3. **DACTINOMYCIN (Actinomycin D)** is a high molecular weight antibiotic isolated from a species of *Streptomyces* that intercalates between DNA strands blocking the DNA's ability to act as a template both for DNA and RNA synthesis. Actinomycin D is administered in doses of 2.5 mg/m^2 IV every 3–4 weeks in treatment of gestational choriocarcinoma, Wilms' tumor, rhabdomyosarcoma, Ewing's sarcoma, and testicular cancer.

4. **MITOMYCIN C (Mutamycin)** is a purple antibiotic isolated from a species of *Streptomyces*. The drug requires metabolic activation and produces damage to DNA either by alkylation or through generation of free radicals. The recommended dose is 10–20 mg/m^2 IV. Mitomycin produces prolonged, cumulative bone marrow suppression and should be administered every 6–8 weeks. This drug is used for gastrointestinal carcinomas, non-small cell lung cancer, and bladder carcinomas.

C. Plant Alkaloids

1. **VINCA ALKALOIDS.** The vinca alkaloids are derived from the ornamental shrub *Vinca rosea*. They bind to tubulin, inhibiting the assembly of microtubules and disrupting the mitotic apparatus. Spindle formation is the most sensitive to the action of these drugs, but they are not absolutely phase specific. Minute concentrations of these alkaloids kill sensitive cells. As vincristine and vinblastine undergo extensive hepatic metabolism, a dose reduction is advised in patients with bilirubin over 2 mg/dL.

   a. **VINCRISTINE (Oncovin)** is given in doses of 1.0–1.4 mg/m^2 IV weekly. Most oncologists do not administer over 2 mg in a single dose. The dose should be reduced 50% if the bilirubin is over 2 mg/dL. The most important side effect is a sensory peripheral neuropathy that usually resolves with time but may progress to muscle weakness. Loss of deep tendon reflexes is an indication to discontinue the drug. Oncovin is active in acute lymphocytic leukemia, non-Hodgkin's lymphoma, and Hodgkin's disease.

   b. **VINBLASTINE (Velban)** is given in doses 4–8 mg/m^2 IV weekly. In contrast to vincristine, the dose-limiting toxicity of vinblastine is myelosuppression. Velban is used in the treatment of testicular cancer, Hodgkin's disease, breast carcinoma, and non-small cell lung cancer.

2. **VP-16 (Etoposide)** is a podophyllotoxin derived from the mandrake plant. It has no effect on microtubule assembly but does arrest cells in the G_2 portion of the cell cycle. VP-16 is a schedule-dependent drug; the usual dose is 50–150 mg/m^2 daily for 3–5 days (total dose 300 mg/m^2). Because the drug is excreted in the urine, the dose should be reduced in the presence of renal dysfunction. It is active against testicular carcinoma, small cell lung cancer, non-Hodgkin's lymphoma, Hodgkin's disease, Kaposi's sarcoma, and acute myelogenous leukemia.

D. **Antimetabolites.** Antimetabolites act as fraudulent substrates for biochemical reactions, either inhibiting essential synthetic steps or becoming incorporated into molecules and interfering with cellular function or replication. They exert their major effect during the S phase of the cell cycle and therefore are most effective against actively replicating cells.

1. **PURINE ANTAGONISTS.** Thioguanine and mercaptopurine are analogues of the natural purines guanine and hypoxanthine, respectively. After activation, both drugs are capable of inhibiting multiple steps in purine synthesis and of incorporation into DNA.

   a. **Thioguanine (6-thioguanine, 6-TG)** should be taken between meals to facilitate oral absorption. With a standard dose of 2 mg/kg daily, 6-TG is active in acute myelogenous and lymphocytic leukemias.

   b. **Mercaptopurine (6-mercaptopurine, 6-MP)** is administered in the maintenance phase of acute lymphocytic leukemia treatment at a dose of 2.5 mg/kg daily (adjusted to bone marrow tolerance). Allopurinol creates a metabolic block of 6-MP metabolism, and the dose of 6-MP needs to be reduced if allopurinol is given concurrently.

2. **PYRIMIDINE ANTAGONISTS**

   a. **Cytarabine (Cytosine Arabinoside, Ara-C)** is an analogue of deoxycytidine that is converted to its active form, ara-cytidine triphosphate, by enzymes of the salvage pathway. It inhibits DNA polymerase and is an S phase–specific agent. It is rapidly inactivated and principally excreted in the urine as the inactive metabolite Ara-U. It is distributed readily into total body water and crosses the blood-brain barrier. Ara-C is administered as a continuous infusion in a dosage of 100–200 mg/m^2 IV every 24 hours for 5–7 days. It is also given in higher doses as 3 gm/m^2 IV every 12 hours for 6–12 doses. Low-dose Ara-C (20 mg/m^2 IV or SQ daily for 14–21 days) is used in treatment of myelodysplastic syndromes. The usual intrathecal dose is 50 mg/m^2. The duration of myelosuppression depends on the dose administered. Unique toxicities of high-dose Ara-C include cerebellar ataxia and pancreatitis. This drug is effective only against tumors with high growth fractions such as acute myelogenous and lymphocytic leukemia, and non-Hodgkin's lymphoma.

b. **Fluorouracil (5-fluorouracil; 5-FU)** is an analogue of thymine that has two distinct mechanisms of action after conversion to the nucleotide fluorouridine monophosphate (FUMP). The major mechanism of action of 5-FU when it is administered by continuous infusion is incorporation of its ribose-triphosphate (5-FUTP) into RNA, thereby modulating protein synthesis. When 5-FU is administered in intravenous boluses, a second derivative, 5-FdUMP, inhibits thymidylate synthetase preventing DNA synthesis. The dosage and scheduling of 5-FU significantly alters its toxicity profile. The dose-limiting toxicity of IV boluses of 5-FU (12 mg/kg daily for 4 days, maximum of 800 mg daily) is hematologic. Continuous infusions of 5-FU (1000 mg/kg daily for 4 days or 200–300 mg/m² daily for 4 to 6 weeks) produce significantly more GI side effects, particularly diarrhea and stomatitis. Patients with coronary atherosclerosis may experience chest pain, ischemic ECG changes, and myocardial infarction when given 5-FU, due to vasospasm of the coronary arteries. 5-FU or FUdR have also been infused via the hepatic artery to treat liver metastases, usually from colon cancer. Because there is extensive first-pass hepatic metabolism, only limited amounts of the drug administered in this manner reach the systemic circulation. 5-FU is used in treatment of breast cancer, colorectal carcinoma, gastric carcinoma, and pancreatic cancer.

3. **FOLATE ANTAGONISTS**

a. **Methotrexate (MTX),** a 4-NH methylfolate derivative, inhibits dihydrofolate reductase, the enzyme that replenishes the intracellular pool of reduced folates. At lower concentrations (10^{-8}) of MTX, the deficiency of tetrahydrofolate blocks the synthesis of thymidylate, a precursor of DNA. At higher concentration (10^{-7}) it blocks purine nucleotide synthesis. To overcome potential resistance from either an altered dihydrofolate reductase or increased dihydrofolate reductase levels resulting from gene amplification, MTX has been given in very high doses (1500 mg/m² or more) followed by leucovorin (N_5-formyltetrahydrofolate) rescue. The dose of leucovorin required depends on the dose of MTX administered and the measured plasma levels of MTX and may be as high as 100–200 mg/m² every 6 hours for 48 hours or longer. These doses of MTX should be administered only by experienced physicians. The usual regimen of MTX IV or IM as a single agent is 30–60 mg/m² every 7–14 days. It is also administered intrathecally (12 mg). Because 90% of the drug is excreted by the kidneys, administration in the presence of renal dysfunction is potentially toxic. The risk of renal failure in patients receiving high doses can be lessened by vigorous hydration and alkalinization of the urine to increase the solubility of MTX. MTX accumulates in third-space fluids that act as a depot, slowly releasing the drug into the systemic circulation producing unexpected toxicity. Hepatitis is most frequent in patients who are receiving low continuous oral doses but may also occur after single high doses. Liver biopsy is the only reliable method of determining the extent of liver damage. Intrathecal MTX can produce potentially permanent neurotoxicity consisting of motor weakness, cranial nerve palsies, coma or seizures, as well as an acute arachnoiditis within 48 hours. MTX is active in acute lymphocytic leukemia, trophoblastic tumors, squamous cell carcinomas of the head and neck, breast cancer, non-small cell lung cancer, and osteosarcoma.

E. Miscellaneous

1. DACARBAZINE (DTIC, Imidazole carboxamide-dimethyl triazeno) is activated by hepatic microsomes producing an active methyl cation and exerts its cytotoxic action through alkylation of DNA. The usual dosage is 250 mg/m² IV daily for 4 days every 4–6 weeks. It is used in treatment of melanoma, soft tissue sarcomas, and Hodgkin's disease.

Chabner B, Collins JM: Cancer Chemotherapy: Principles and Practice. Philadelphia, JB Lippincott Co., 1990.
Dorr RT, Fritz WL: Cancer Chemotherapy Handbook. New York, Elsevier, 1983.

III. ONCOLOGIC EMERGENCIES

A. The Superior Vena Cava Syndrome. The superior vena cava syndrome (SVCS) occurs in 3–8% of patients with lung cancer or lymphoma because of extrinsic compression, thrombosis, or occlusion of the thin-walled SVC, resulting in impaired venous drainage of the head, thorax, and upper extremities. Malignancies are responsible for approximately 90% of cases of SVCS, with bronchogenic carcinoma (especially small-cell carcinoma) and lymphoma (especially diffuse large-cell lymphoma) accounting for the majority of cases. Most authorities now believe that optimal management of SVCS requires knowledge of the underlying pathology, and disagree with previous recommendations for immediate empiric radiation therapy, since this may obscure the interpretation of subsequent biopsies (Ca 35:238–251, 1985). Although SVCS has traditionally been called an "oncologic emergency," recent studies have shown that this may be an overstatement. Delaying therapy for more than 1 week generally does not have a significant deleterious impact on the patient's survival (Cancer 57:847–851, 1986.)

1. THERAPY. Traditional management of SVCS involves external beam radiation therapy with 400 cGy fractions for 3–4 days to the mediastinal mass, followed by continuation with 200 cGy fractions to a total dose of 2000–4000 cGy for lymphomas and 4000–6000 cGy for lung cancer. Approximately 83% of patients will respond to such management with symptomatic relief within 2 weeks of initiation of therapy. The degree of symptomatic relief correlates poorly with the magnitude of objective tumor response; dramatic resolution of symptoms commonly occurs without substantial reduction in tumor size. Supplemental oxygen, diuretics, and corticosteroids are often administered concurrently with radiation therapy. Anticoagulant or thrombolytic therapy is generally considered to be of insufficient benefit to warrant

the increased risk of hemorrhage in these patients who have elevated venous pressures. Chemotherapy is as effective as radiotherapy in alleviating SVCS caused by small cell carcinoma of the lung or lymphoma. Chemotherapy is usually the treatment of choice since these cancers generally require early institution of systemic therapy. When chemotherapy is to be the primary treatment, venous access should be obtained via lower extremity veins until SVC obstruction is relieved.

2. **PROGNOSIS.** Although more than 80% of patients will obtain relief with the measures suggested above, the median survival of patients with SVCS is only 5.5 months, with an overall 24% 1-year survival and a 9% 5-year survival. Survival depends highly on the histology of the underlying malignancy, with lymphoma patients enjoying a 41% 5-year survival compared with 5% for small cell lung cancer and 1% for non-small cell lung cancer patients. Recurrence of SVCS occurs in 10–20% of patients and is generally treated with symptomatic measures, chemotherapy, stenting, or surgery, since maximally tolerated radiation is usually administered at initial presentation.

Helms SR, Carlson MD: Cardiovascular Emergencies. Semin Oncol 16:463–470, 1989.
Armstrong BA, Perez CA, Simpson JR, et al: Role of irradiation in the management of superior vena cava syndrome. Int J Radiat Oncol Biol Phys 13:531–539, 1987.
Sculier JP, Evans WK, Feld R, et al: Superior vena caval obstruction syndrome in small cell lung cancer. Cancer 57:847–851, 1986.
Stanford W, Doty DB: The role of venography and surgery in the management of patients with superior vena cava obstruction. Ann Thorac Surg 41:158–163, 1986.

B. **Pericardial Tamponade.** Neoplastic involvement of the heart is found in 3.4% of general autopsies and 11.6% of autopsies performed on patients dying of cancer. Two-thirds of these patients have pericardial metastases; of these, 29% become symptomatic and 16% develop life-threatening cardiac tamponade. Lung cancer (37%), breast cancer (22%), hematologic malignancies (17%), sarcomas (4%), and melanoma (3%) are the most common causes of pericardial metastatic disease.

1. **EMERGENCY MANAGEMENT.** Acute pericardial tamponade is a medical emergency that mandates prompt withdrawal of pericardial fluid. Pericardiocentesis is effective in 87% of cases but is associated with a 7% major complication rate (fatal dysrhythmias, right ventricular lacerations). Most of these untoward events can be avoided if pericardiocentesis is preceded by echocardiographic confirmation of pericardial fluid and performed in a catheterization laboratory under fluoroscopy with ECG guidance of the exploring needle. Pericardiocentesis should be avoided in patients with thrombocytopenia (platelets <50,000/cu mm), small effusions (<200 mL), or loculated effusions. In some institutions with a high complication rate from pericardiocentesis, subxiphoid pericardiostomy can be substituted as a safe, rapid, and effective procedure (see below). In situations in which immediate pericardiocentesis or subxiphoid pericardiostomy cannot be performed, IV infusion of fluids may be used temporarily to support cardiac output.

2. **LONG-TERM MANAGEMENT.** Although simple pericardiocentesis is generally effective in relieving acute symptoms and hemodynamic compromise, rapid reaccumulation of fluid generally leads to relapse within a few days unless more definitive measures are instituted.

a. **Intrapericardial Instillation of Tetracycline.** This is the most popular approach for solid tumors (e.g., lung cancer and breast cancer) (Table 11–3). An 18-gauge catheter is inserted into the pericardial space from a subxiphoid approach; the space is then aspirated dry, anesthetized with a small amount (10 mL) of 1% xylocaine, and sclerosed with 500–1000 mg of tetracycline hydrochloride (dissolved in 20 mL of saline). Daily thereafter, the pericardial cavity is aspirated via the catheter, and if significant fluid is present (> 25 mL), tetracycline is reinstilled. This technique is successful in resolving 81–91% of malignant effusions after an average of 2.8 instillations of tetracycline (J Clin Oncol 2:631–636, 1984). Major complications are uncommon with this approach, though moderate pain (11%), fever (36%), and asymptomatic dysrhythmias (18%) may occur. Other agents that have been used for intrapericardial instillation include talc, nitrogen mustard, 5-FU, thiotepa, bleomycin, and a variety of radioisotopes, but none have been used as extensively or as effectively as tetracycline.

b. **Surgery.** Operative relief of pericardial tamponade has historically involved the creation of a pleuropericardial window by an anterior thoracotomy approach. This technique is usually effective at achieving lasting relief of tamponade (94% of survivors) but is associated with significant morbidity and 8% operative mortality. Unfortunately, debilitated, hemodynamically unstable patients with advanced cancer and tamponade are often poor candidates for general anesthesia and major intrathoracic surgery. In recent years, subxiphoid pericardiostomy has become a more popular means of providing pericardial decompression than the traditional pleuropericardial window. This procedure can be done under local anesthesia in 30 minutes, with negligible morbidity, no mortality, and virtually 100% efficacy. Radical pericardiectomy should be reserved for cases of constrictive pericarditis.

TABLE 11–3. THERAPY OF NEOPLASTIC PERICARDIAL TAMPONADE

THERAPY	RESPONSE RATE (%)	RELAPSE RATE (%)	CONSTRICTIVE PERICARDITIS (%)	MAJOR COMPLICATIONS
Tetracycline sclerosis	85	0–6	0–2	1–2
Radiation therapy (external beam)	61	NA*	NA	NA
Subxiphoid pericardiostomy	90–100	0–3	0–6	0–5
Pleuropericardial window	100	0–6	0	12

*NA = not available.

c. **Radiation Therapy.** External beam radiation therapy (2500–3000 cGy in 150–200-cGy fractions over 3 to 4 weeks) has waned in popularity for management of malignant tamponade, since its efficacy rate (61% overall) is inferior to that of the aforementioned methods. It is most effective for hematologic malignancies (90–100% success rate) and breast cancer (69%).

d. **Systemic Chemotherapy.** Chemotherapy often achieves rapid remission of hematologic malignancies and may successfully cure pericardial disease without adjunctive local therapy in patients with leukemia or lymphoma.

3. **PROGNOSIS.** The survival of patients presenting with malignant pericardial tamponade is generally dictated by the progression of extrapericardial cancer. The methods mentioned can control pericardial involvement in 80–100% of cases with under 5% recurrence. Survival in a typical series varies from over a month to several years, with a median survival of less than a year

Davis S, Rambotti P, Grignani F: Intrapericardial tetracycline sclerosis in the treatment of malignant pericardial effusion: An analysis of 33 cases. J Clin Oncol 2:631–636, 1984. *The best article on intrapericardial instillation therapy.*

Press OW, Livingston R: Management of malignant pericardial effusion and tamponade. JAMA 257:1088–1092, 1987. *A comprehensive review of the literature.*

Thurber DL, Edwards JE, Achor RW: Secondary malignant tumors of the pericardium. Circulation 26:228–241, 1962. *An old but excellent autopsy series.*

C. Pleural Effusion. Pleural effusion results from either obstruction of mediastinal lymphatics by centrally located tumor (cytology negative) or pleural involvement with tumor by direct extension or seeding (cytology usually positive). Lung cancer is the most common cause of a malignant effusion in men and is second only to breast cancer as a cause in women. A pleural effusion may be asymptomatic when small but is usually associated with chest pain, cough, or dyspnea as it progresses. The best management of pleural effusions in patients with chemotherapy-responsive tumors (leukemia, lymphoma, small cell lung cancer) is systemic chemotherapy. For other tumors, sclerodesis (usually with tetracycline or bleomycin) is generally required. Unfortunately, sclerodesis itself, regardless of the sclerosing agent employed, is often ineffective and may be associated with chronic pain as well as loculation of the pleural fluid. When an effusion is loculated, localization under ultrasonographic guidance is essential for safe therapeutic thoracentesis.

Ruckdeschel JC: Management of malignant pleural effusion: An overview. Semin Oncol (suppl 3):24–28, 1988.

D. Hypercalcemia of Malignancy. Neoplastic hypercalcemia occurs with an incidence of 150 cases per million people per year and is responsible for 20–25% of the cases of hypercalcemia diagnosed in the United States. The tumors most commonly associated with this condition include squamous cell carcinoma of the lung, head and neck cancers, breast cancer, prostate carcinoma, renal cell carcinoma, and multiple myeloma.

1. MANAGEMENT

   a. **Tumor Cytoreduction.** The most successful long-term approach to the hypercalcemia of malignancy is eradication of systemic tumor by surgery, radiation therapy, or chemotherapy. These definitive modalities should be used with the following palliative, temporizing measures.

   b. **Hydration and Furosemide.** Initial management of all patients with malignant hypercalcemia should include vigorous hydration (e.g., 300 mL/hr of saline) to correct volume depletion and to promote calciuresis. Furosemide (20–40 mg IV) should be utilized to prevent volume overload and to augment renal calcium wasting. Standard hydration therapy generally leads to a 2–3 mg/dL fall in the serum calcium level over 48 hours, but complete, sustained control is unusual.

   c. **Diet.** Low-calcium diets have not generally been effective, since most patients with malignancy-associated hypercalcemia have reduced serum levels of 1,25-dihydroxycholecalciferol and reduced intestinal calcium absorption.

   d. **Mobilization.** Patients should be encouraged to remain ambulatory and physically active, since immobilization stimulates osteoclastic bone resorption.

   e. **Calcitonin.** Calcitonin is a potent inhibitor of osteoclastic bone resorption and also has a direct calciuretic effect at the level of the proximal tubule in the kidney. Commercial salmon calcitonin (4–12 IU/kg SQ q 8–12 hr) causes rapid reduction of elevated serum calcium levels in more than 80% of cases, but in 2–3 days osteoclasts "escape" from the effects of the hormone and calcium levels begin to rise again. Interrupting therapy when "escape" occurs restores responsiveness to the drug after a few days. Concomitant use of corticosteroids (prednisone, 10 mg qid) delays the development of the calcitonin escape phenomenon for 4–9 days (Lancet 21:907–910, 1985).

   f. **Corticosteroids.** Glucocorticoids (40–60 mg prednisone daily) improve hypercalcemia in 50% of cases, particularly those due to multiple myeloma, other hematologic malignancies, and breast cancer. Disadvantages of corticosteroid therapy for this condition include prolonged latency before clinical response occurs (5–10 days), immunosuppressive and catabolic side effects of steroids, and induction of skeletal demineralization by glucocorticoids.

   g. **Phosphate Therapy.** Oral phosphate therapy (250 mg po qid of elemental phosphate) is safe and moderately effective in patients with hypophosphatemia. Careful dosage escalation (up to 2–3 gm/day in divided doses) should be tried if no clinical response is observed after several days, though doses above 2 gm/day often cause intolerable diarrhea. Serum phosphate and creatinine levels should be monitored and phosphate therapy discontinued if hyperphosphatemia or renal insufficiency develop.

   h. **Plicamycin (Mithramycin).** This antineoplastic antibiotic inhibits osteoclast activity, reduces renal tubular calcium reabsorption, and lowers serum calcium levels. It is nearly always effective at a dosage of 25 μg/kg IV (over 4–6 hours) and usually has an onset of action in the first 24 hours and an effect that lasts 5–7 days. If no improvement in hypercalcemia is evident within 48 hours, a second dose of plicamycin should be given. Toxicity reported with plicamycin therapy includes hemorrhage due to thrombocytopenia, elevation of the prothrombin time and transaminases, and renal failure. The platelet count, prothrombin time, liver transaminase values, and creatinine level should be monitored during therapy.

i. **Diphosphonates (Bisphosphonates).** The most promising agents for treating hypercalcemia are the diphosphonates: ethane hydroxydiphosphonate (EHDP, etidronate disodium), aminohydroxypropylidine diphosphonate (APD), and dichloromethylene diphosphonate (Cl_2MDP). These pyrophosphate analogues are incorporated into the hydroxyapatite of bone in areas of high bone turnover (e.g., metastatic lesions). All three compounds inhibit osteoclastic bone resorption. In a double-blind, controlled trial of EHDP (7.5 mg/kg IV qd over 2–3 hours for 3–5 days) versus placebo in patients receiving hydration and furosemide, normocalcemia was attained in 92% of patients receiving EHDP plus hydration as opposed to 33% of control patients. Oral maintenance EHDP is given at a dose of 20 mg/kg/day. Toxicity associated with diphosphonate administration has consisted of mild fever (APD), phlebitis at the infusion site (APD), and mild gastrointestinal toxicity. Osteomalacia can occur with prolonged use of EHDP.

j. **Gallium Nitrate.** A randomized trial demonstrated the superiority of gallium nitrate (200 mg/m^2 IV for 5 days by continuous infusion) compared with calcitonin (8 IU/kg IM every 6 hours for 5 days) in achieving normocalcemia (75 versus 31%) and in duration of normocalcemia (> 11 days versus 2 days). Nephrotoxicity was the major adverse effect.

2. **PROGNOSIS.** The survival of patients with hypercalcemia associated with malignancy is poor, with a median survival of 39 days despite achievement of normocalcemia. Death nearly always results from progressive disseminated disease. The only patients who survive longer than 6 months are those in whom systemic remissions can be achieved with radiation therapy, chemotherapy, or hormonal therapy.

Ritch PS: Treatment of cancer-related hypercalcemia. Semin Oncol 17 (suppl 5):26–33, 1990.

Ralston SH, Gallacher SJ, Patel U, et al: Cancer-associated hypercalcemia: morbidity and mortality. Ann Intern Med 112:499–504, 1990.

Fetchick DA, Mundy GR: Hypercalcemia of malignancy: diagnosis and therapy. Compr Ther 12:27–32, 1986.

Singer FR, Fernandez M: Therapy of hypercalcemia of malignancy. Am J Med 82 (suppl 2A):34–40, 1987.

E. **The Tumor Lysis Syndrome.** Acute tumor lysis syndrome results from the rapid release of large quantities of intracellular potassium, phosphate, and nucleic acids from dying tumor cells, with resultant hyperkalemia, hyperphosphatemia, hypocalcemia, and hyperuricemia. The metabolic consequences include weakness, lethargy, paresthesias, muscular twitching, seizures, vomiting, ventricular dysrhythmias, and oliguric renal failure. Patients at risk for tumor lysis syndrome are those with bulky tumors that have high cell turnover rates and are sensitive to chemotherapeutic agents (especially Burkitt's and lymphoblastic lymphomas and acute leukemias). Most cases occur within 2–3 days of the initiation of chemotherapy.

1. **MANAGEMENT.** Prevention of tumor lysis syndrome is preferable to therapy. Patients at risk should be well hydrated (e.g., 3000 mL/m^2/d) for 24 hours before chemotherapy, and a brisk diuresis should be maintained with diuretics if necessary. Alkalinization of the urine (e.g., 50 mEq of sodium bicarbonate per liter of fluid) may inhibit deposition of uric acid crystals in the kidney (urine pH > 7). Allopurinol (200–500 mg/m^2 po or IV) is administered for 24 hours before therapy and for a week after therapy to inhibit the generation of uric acid from nucleic acids. Electrolytes, uric acid, and creatinine levels should be measured before chemotherapy and daily thereafter for several days in patients at high risk. If the syndrome evolves despite prophylactic measures, dialysis may be necessary to normalize metabolic parameters until renal function recovers.

F. Spinal Cord Compression. Spinal epidural metastases (especially from lung, breast, prostate, unknown primary tumors, and lymphomas) cause spinal cord compression in 5% of patients with disseminated malignancies. Typical manifestations include back pain exacerbated by recumbency, paraparesis, spinal sensory deficits, and sphincter dysfunction.

1. **MANAGEMENT.** Immediate intervention is mandatory in neoplastic spinal cord compression, since progression can be rapid and lost neurologic functions are usually not regained. Emergency myelography or MRI should be performed in patients suspected of having cord compression and dexamethasone therapy initiated (16–100 mg/day in divided doses q 6 hr). Radiation therapy is promptly begun in patients with slow progression (weeks to months), incomplete block on myelography, radiosensitive tumors (e.g., lymphomas), or contraindications to major surgery (e.g., terminal disease). Patients with a complete block confirmed on myelography, rapid progression, cervical compression, and an unknown primary tumor should receive prompt decompressive laminectomy. Accessible tumor should be excised, and consideration should be given to removal of associated diseased vertebral bodies with subsequent stabilization using methylmetacrylate prostheses. Adjunctive postoperative radiation therapy (3000–4000 cGy over 2–4 weeks) has been shown to improve the final outcome compared with surgery alone (44 versus 26% ambulatory [Arch Surg 87:137–142, 1963]). Treatment outcome according to tumor types and preoperative motor status is presented in Table 11–4.

2. **PROGNOSIS.** Patients with neoplastic spinal cord compression generally have advanced cancer and short survival (16–20% 1-year survival). Favorable treatment outcomes are most likely to occur in patients with an insidious onset of symptoms, minimal neurologic

TABLE 11–4. TREATMENT OUTCOME FOLLOWING NEOPLASTIC SPINAL CORD COMPRESSION

PARAMETER	AMBULATORY POST THERAPY (%)
Primary tumor type	
Lymphoma	52
Multiple myeloma	50
Breast	33
Prostate	31
Lung	14
Kidney	10
Preoperative motor status	
Ambulatory	60
Paraparetic	35
Paraplegic	7

Modified from Bruckman JE, Bloomer WD: Semin Oncol 5:135–140, 1978.

impairment at diagnosis, hematologic malignancies, and lesions in the lower thoracic spine (T5–T12) as opposed to the upper spine (T1–T4).

Bruckman JE, Bloomer WD: Management of spinal cord compression. Semin Oncol 5:135–140, 1978.

Lozes G, Fawaz A, Devos P, et al: Operative treatment of thoraco-lumbar metastases, using methylmetacrylate and Kempf's rods for vertebral replacement and stabilization. Acta Neurochir 84:118–123, 1987.

Pedersen AG, Bach F, Melgaard B: Frequency, diagnosis, and prognosis of spinal cord compression in small cell bronchogenic carcinoma. Cancer 55:1818–1822, 1985.

Zevallos M, Chan PYM, Munoz L, et al: Epidural spinal cord compression from metastatic tumor. Int J Radiat Oncol Biol Phys 13:875–878, 1987.

G. The Serum Hyperviscosity Syndrome. Marked overproduction of monoclonal serum paraproteins resulting in elevation of the serum viscosity is seen in Waldenström's macroglobulinemia, multiple myeloma (especially with immunoglobulin A[IgA]), and lymphomas. In patients with plasma viscosities > 4.0 centipoise, the serum hyperviscosity syndrome may supervene and cause bleeding, visual disturbances, and neurologic derangements.

1. MANAGEMENT. Patients should receive plasmapheresis to avoid stroke, seizures, congestive heart failure, blindness, and hemorrhage. Dehydration should be corrected and rapid blood transfusion avoided, since these conditions will increase plasma viscosity and cause clinical deterioration. The efficacy of plasmapheresis depends on the biodistribution of the causative paraprotein. IgM dysproteinemias are most effectively managed because 80% of IgM is confined to the vascular space, and removal of a liter of plasma can reduce IgM levels by 15–20% and reduce relative viscosity by 50–100%. Reduction of IgG levels is much less satisfactory because of the large extravascular pool available for redistribution following plasmapheresis. Concomitant antineoplastic therapy (generally with chlorambucil, melphalan, or cyclophosphamide and prednisone) must be administered to prevent

recurrence of the syndrome, which generally relapses within 2–3 weeks unless tumor bulk is reduced. Maintenance plasmapheresis at 1–2 week intervals may be necessary.

Patterson WP, Caldwell CW, Doll DC: Hyperviscosity syndromes and coagulopathies. Semin Oncol 17:210–216, 1990.
Crawford J, Cox EB, Cohen HJ: Evaluation of hyperviscosity in monoclonal gammopathies. Am J Med 79:13–22, 1985.

H. Hypercoagulable States Associated with Cancer. Recurrent migratory thrombophlebitis associated with low-grade chronic disseminated intravascular coagulation (Trousseau's syndrome) is most commonly seen with metastatic mucinous adenocarcinomas of the GI tract (pancreas, stomach, colon, and gallbladder), lung, prostate, or ovary. Thromboses are often atypical (superficial, located in upper extremities) and refractory to conventional anticoagulation therapy. Hemorrhagic episodes, nonbacterial thrombotic endocarditis, and arterial emboli often occur.

   1. MANAGEMENT. Acute thrombotic episodes are treated with IV heparin for 5–10 days (adjusted to maintain the APTT 1.5–2 times control). Outpatient therapy with either adjusted-dose subcutaneous heparin or oral warfarin is then given for about 3 months. Warfarin frequently fails to prevent recurrent thromboses, and subcutaneous heparin is favored by many authorities for maintenance therapy. If anticoagulation is contraindicated, vena caval interruption may be advisable. Thrombolytic agents are uncommonly used in cancer patients because of increased hemorrhagic risks (e.g., thrombocytopenia, brain metastases, pericardial metastases). Eradication of the underlying tumor with surgery, radiation, or chemotherapy, which is the best method for preventing recurrent thromboembolism, is seldom feasible.

Levine M, Hirsh J: The diagnosis and treatment of thrombosis in the cancer patient. Semin Oncol 17:160–171, 1990.
Bell WR, Starksen NF, Tong S, et al: Trousseau's syndrome: devastating coagulopathy in the absence of heparin. Am J Med 79:423–430, 1985.
Rickles FR, Edwards RL: Activation of blood coagulation in cancer: Trousseau's syndrome revisited. Blood 62:14–31, 1987.

IV. TREATMENT OF SPECIFIC DISEASE ENTITIES

A. Acute Myeloid Leukemia. Acute myeloid leukemia (AML) is characterized by a marked excess of nonlymphoid blast cells in the bone marrow (> 30% of nucleated cells), in association with circulating blast cells. Seven subtypes have been defined (including myeloblastic [M1] and [M2], promyelocytic [M3], myelomonocytic [M4], monocytic [M5], erythoblastic [M6], and megakaryocytic [M7]), but treatment considerations are similar for all.

   1. CHEMOTHERAPY

      a. **Induction Chemotherapy.** Newly diagnosed AML must be treated aggressively with myelosuppressive agents to achieve complete remission. **Daunorubicin** (30–60 mg/m²/day for 3 days IV) and

cytosine arabinoside (100–200 mg/m²IV by continuous infusion for 7 days) induce complete remissions in 60–85% of patients. Addition of other drugs to this regimen has not convincingly improved the results.

b. **Consolidation Chemotherapy.** Additional cycles of chemotherapy must be given after achievement of complete remission to prevent early relapse. The original induction regimen is repeated as consolidation therapy 3–4 weeks after bone marrow recovery provided patients are ambulatory, afebrile off antibiotics, and have more than 3000 leukocytes per cu mm and more than 100,000 platelets per cu mm. Alternatively, high-dose cytarabine (HDAC; 3 gm/m² IV over 1–2 hours every 12 hours for 6–12 doses), either alone or in combination with daunorubicin or mitoxantrone, may be administered. Patients receiving HDAC should be treated with topical corticosteroids to prevent painful conjunctivitis and must be monitored for early signs of cerebellar toxicity (e.g., nystagmus). Patients over the age of 50–55 should probably receive reduced doses (e.g., 2 gm/m²) or abbreviated cycles (e.g., 6 doses per cycle) of HDAC because of a marked increase in cerebellar toxicity in this age group. The optimal number of cycles of consolidation chemotherapy is currently unknown; most oncologists administer 2–3 postremission cycles.

c. **Maintenance Chemotherapy.** Several trials have investigated the role of prolonged administration of low-dose chemotherapy for 1–2 years after consolidation therapy. Most studies show no benefit to maintenance therapy in AML, provided *aggressive* induction and consolidation therapy is given.

2. **SUPPORTIVE CARE.** Patients usually must be hospitalized for 3–4 weeks with each cycle of chemotherapy. Central venous access, hyperalimentation, hydration, allopurinol, prolonged transfusional support, and empiric antibiotics for neutropenic fevers are usually required. Histocompatibility typing of patients and family members should be done to identify potential platelet and bone marrow donors. Patients with acute promyelocytic leukemia presenting with DIC are often treated with low-dose heparin therapy (10–20 U per kg/hour) during induction, although management with intensive blood product support is equally effective (Blood 69:187–191, 1987).

3. **PROGNOSIS**

a. **Conventional Therapy.** Most AML trials report median remission durations of 12–13 months, median survivals of 20–24 months, and long-term disease-free survival rates of 15–25%. Subtypes M1–M3 have more favorable prognoses than M4–M7. Recent uncontrolled studies of consolidation with HDAC report long-term survival rates of 30–65%, suggesting the possible superiority of this approach.

b. **Salvage Chemotherapy.** Approximately 75% of patients with AML will experience leukemic relapse, and about half of these patients can be reinduced into a second complete remission. Unfortunately, virtually none of these patients will survive long term unless marrow transplantation is undertaken. Drugs commonly used in relapsed patients include HDAC, mitoxantrone plus etoposide (VP-16), idarubicin, 6-thioguanine, m-AMSA, azacytidine, and teniposide (VM-26) (J Clin Oncol 7:1071–1080, 1989).

4. BONE MARROW TRANSPLANTATION FOR AML. Allogeneic bone marrow transplantation has been widely used in patients for whom a suitable HLA-matched marrow donor is available. With histocompatible transplants, long-term disease-free survival may be achieved in 50–60% of patients when performed in first remission, 25–30% in first relapse or second remission, and 10–15% in end-stage refractory leukemia. In patients without suitable matched sibling donors, partially matched transplants, unrelated matched transplants, and autologous transplants are being investigated. Recent studies of autologous transplantation (with and without purging of marrow stored in remission with 4-hydroperoxycyclophosphamide or mafosfamide) suggest that 20–50% of patients who have transplant in second remission may be cured with this approach (Blood 75:1606–1614, 1990).

Champlin R, Gale RP: Acute myelogenous leukemia: recent advances in therapy. Blood 69:1551–1562, 1987.

Wolff SN, Herzig RH, Fay J, et al: High dose cytarabine and daunorubicin as consolidation therapy for acute myeloid leukemia in first remission: long term follow-up and results. J Clin Oncol 7:1260–1267, 1989.

Tallman MS, Kopecky K, Appelbaum FA, et al: Analysis of prognostic factors for the outcome of marrow transplantation or further chemotherapy for patients with acute nonlymphocytic leukemia in first remission. J Clin Oncol 7:326–337, 1989.

B. Acute Lymphoblastic Leukemia. Acute lymphoblastic leukemia (ALL) is the most common childhood malignancy (3.5 cases/100,000 children) and peaks in incidence between 2–7 years of age. ALL is much less common in adults but still constitutes 20% of adult acute leukemias. Patients typically present with fatigue, malaise, epistaxis, fever, bone pain, lymphadenopathy, hepatosplenomegaly, and petechiae. Features that have been associated with an unfavorable outcome include age under 2 years or over 10, immunophenotype (B cell worse than T cell which is worse than common ALL), elevated leukocyte count ($> 25,000$ per cu mm), delayed achievement of remission (> 4 weeks), abnormal karyotype (especially translocations), male sex, hepatosplenomegaly, and the presence of CNS leukemia at diagnosis.

1. MANAGEMENT. Treatment of ALL can be divided into four phases: remission induction, consolidation, low-dose maintenance, and treatment of sanctuary sites (CNS and testicles). Treatment regimens are usually stratified in intensity, depending on the presence or absence of high-risk features (see above).

a. Induction Chemotherapy. The standard remission induction regimen for childhood ALL includes vincristine (1.5 to 2.0 mg/m² IV q week × 4), prednisone (40 mg/m² po qd for 4 weeks), and L-asparaginase (6000 U/m² IM 2–3 times/week) following hydration, urine alkalinization, and allopurinol administration. High-risk childhood ALL and all cases of adult ALL should also be treated with an anthracycline (e.g., daunorubicin, 25–50 mg/m^2 IV on days 1–3) to improve remission rates and durations.

b. **Continuation Chemotherapy.** After complete remission is achieved, chemotherapy must be continued or most patients will have relapse within 1–2 months. Administration of a relatively nontoxic outpatient maintenance regimen of MTX (20 mg/m^2 po every week) and 6-MP (75 mg/m^2 po qd) for 2.5 years prevents relapse and achieves cure in up to 50% of low-risk childhood cases. However, high-risk children and adults do poorly with low-dose maintenance therapy alone and should receive intensive consolidation chemotherapy with additional drugs (e.g., anthracyclines, L-asparaginase, cytarabine, high-dose MTX, cyclophosphamide, and teniposide [VM-26]) for several months after remission is attained and before institution of maintenance. Several regimens have been shown to improve survival (Blood 69:1242–1248, 1987; Semin Hematol 24:12–26, 1987), but no single approach is yet generally accepted. Such patients should be referred to major cancer centers for entry into controlled clinical trials.

c. **Central Nervous System Prophylaxis.** Before the advent of prophylactic measures, CNS leukemia occurred in 50% of childhood ALL cases. Conventional CNS prophylaxis with intrathecal MTX (6 mg in children < 1 yr; 8 mg, 1–2 yr; 10 mg, 2–3 yr; 12 mg, > 3 yr) for 5 doses (given every 3–4 days), in conjunction with cranial irradiation (2400 cGy), reduces the incidence of meningeal leukemia to 5% but is complicated by a substantial decrement in intellectual functioning. Therefore, less aggressive prophylactic measures are currently advocated for standard-risk children. Prolonged intrathecal chemotherapy alone (with MTX alone or combined with intrathecal cytarabine [30 mg/m^2] and intrathecal hydrocortisone [15 mg/m^2]), limitation of cranial irradiation to 1800 cGy, and use of systemic high-dose MTX have all been advocated for low-risk cases of ALL. Patients treated with intrathecal chemotherapy alone must receive intermittent doses over a prolonged period of time (1–2.5 years). Patients who are at high risk for CNS leukemia (infants, leukocyte counts > 100,000 per cu mm, T cell ALL, adults) should receive combined-modality prophylaxis.

Patients with overt CNS leukemia at diagnosis should receive aggressive CNS treatment with cranial irradiation (24 to 28 Gy), weekly intrathecal MTX during induction chemotherapy (for 5–10 doses), and monthly intrathecal MTX for the first year of therapy.

d. **Systemic Relapse**

(1). *Chemotherapy.* Second remissions can be achieved in 70–90% of children and 50% of adults following leukemic relapse using the same chemotherapeutic regimens employed for initial remission induction. The chances of achieving a durable second remission are greatly increased in patients who have relapse after a disease-free interval of at least 18 months, especially if relapse occurs after cessation of maintenance chemotherapy. Second-line drugs that have been found active against disease recurrences refractory to standard regimens include mitoxantrone, rubidazone, HDAC, teniposide, and etoposide.

(2). Bone Marrow Transplantation (BMT). The role of marrow transplantation for ALL is controversial. With improvements in combination chemotherapy, most centers have stopped performing marrow transplantation in first remission (even in high-risk cases) because of the danger of submitting cured patients to potentially fatal treatment. After relapse, however, the chances of achieving cure with conventional chemotherapy are greatly diminished. A recent analysis suggests that children who have relapse within 18 months of first remission while on maintenance chemotherapy have superior long-term survival if they undergo transplantation (44% versus 5% for standard-risk cases; 10% versus 1% for high-risk cases), whereas those with disease-free intervals of over 18 months do as well with conventional chemotherapy as with bone marrow transplantation (20–40% long-term survival versus 30–40%) (Lancet 1:429–432, 1987). Few adults with relapsed ALL can be cured with salvage chemotherapy, and BMT is generally recommended in this setting. Long-term disease-free survival can be achieved in 40–50% of high-risk patients undergoing allogeneic transplantation in first remission and in 20–40% undergoing transplantation in second remission.

2. **PROGNOSIS.** Current regimens are capable of achieving complete remissions in more than 90% of children and 65–80% of adults. Long-term disease-free survival can be expected in 50–75% of children and 30–45% of adults.

Hoelzer D, Gale RP: Acute lymphoblastic leukemia in adults: Recent progress, future directions. Semin Hematol 24:27–39, 1987.

Rivera GK, Mauer AM: Controversies in the management of childhood acute lymphoblastic leukemia: treatment intensification, CNS leukemia, and prognostic factors. Semin Hematol 24:12–26, 1987.

Bleyer WA, Poplack DG: Prophylaxis and treatment of leukemia in the central nervous system and other sanctuaries. Semin Oncol 12:131–148, 1985.

Wingard JR, Piantadosi S, Santos GW, et al: Allogeneic bone marrow transplantation for patients with high risk acute lymphoblastic leukemia. J Clin Oncol 8:820–830, 1990.

C. Chronic Myelogenous Leukemia. Chronic myelogenous leukemia (CML) has an incidence of 1 per 100,000 and is responsible for 20–30% of cases of leukemia in Western countries. The disease typically occurs in middle age and is associated with an unequal reciprocal translocation (the Philadelphia chromosome), which transfers the c-abl oncogene from the 9th to the 22nd chromosome. Three phases of CML occur. An initial **chronic phase**, with a median duration of 42 months, is characterized by minimal symptomatology and responsivity to low-dose chemotherapy. A transitional **accelerated phase** is characterized by progressive leukocytosis, anemia, basophilia, splenomegaly, fever, bone pain, new cytogenetic abnormalities, and increasing blast counts (usually > 10%) despite escalating intensity of chemotherapy. A terminal **blast crisis phase**, with a median duration of 4 months, is associated with more than 30% blasts and promyelocytes in the marrow or blood and is generally refractory to therapy.

1. TREATMENT

   a. **Chronic Phase.** Asymptomatic patients having white cell counts < 50,000/cu mm do not necessarily require treatment, since conventional therapy has not been shown to prolong survival or delay blast crisis. Patients who are symptomatic or who have progressive leukocytosis, anemia, thrombocytosis, or thrombocytopenia should be treated with either hydroxyurea (0.5 to 4.0 gm po qd), α-interferon (e.g., 2–5 million units SC or IM daily), or busulfan (initially 0.1–0.2 mg/kg/d). Hydroxyurea is rapid acting, nearly always effective, and has few side effects. α-interferon initially causes a flu-like syndrome in most patients, achieves hematologic remissions in 80% of cases, and is the only drug capable of inducing cytogenetic remissions (in 10–20% of cases). Busulfan is rarely used now because of its risk of pulmonary toxicity, its long half-life, and the availability of safer drugs. Aggressive combination chemotherapy does not eliminate the leukemic clone and is not recommended for CML in chronic phase. Splenectomy should be employed only in patients with refractory hypersplenism. Leukapheresis is expensive and of evanescent benefit and is recommended only in patients who are pregnant or have leukostasis. All patients over 50 with CML should have HLA typing done on family members for donor purposes in allogeneic bone marrow transplantation. Long-term disease-free survival can be expected in 50–65% of patients undergoing matched allogeneic transplantation. No other therapy results in long-term cure.

   b. **Accelerated Phase.** Escalating doses of hydroxyurea are usually employed in the accelerated phase. Patients with refractory hypersplenism may benefit from splenectomy. Allogeneic bone marrow transplantation from a matched donor, the treatment of choice, results in the cure of 15–30%.

   c. **Blast Crisis.** Myeloid blast crisis occurs in two-thirds of cases of CML and is treated with regimens identical with those used in AML. Unfortunately, only 15–35% of patients will benefit from therapy, and few will be cured. One report suggests that plicamycin (mithramycin) plus hydroxyurea may be effective in returning patients with myeloid blast crisis to a second chronic phase (6 of 6 cases, N Engl J Med 315:1433–1438, 1986), but confirmation is needed. Lymphoid blast crisis occurs in a third of cases of CML and is characterized by lymphoid morphology and terminal deoxynucleotidyltransferase (Tdt) positivity of blast cells. Lymphoid crisis should be treated like ALL, with vincristine and prednisone, with or without L-asparaginase and daunorubicin. With such management, 50–60% of patients can be induced into a remission or second chronic phase, but overall survival is poor, with the reappearance of blast crisis within 2–3 months. Median survival for patients in blast crisis with conventional therapy is 10 weeks (27 weeks if a second CP can be induced). Matched allogeneic marrow transplantation in blast crisis results in approximately 15% long-term disease-free survival and is the treatment of choice.

Talpaz M, Kantarjian H, Kurzrock R, Gutterman J: Update on therapeutic options for chronic myelogenous leukemia. Semin Hematol 27 (suppl 4):31–36, 1990.
Thomas ED, Clift RA, Fefer A, et al: Marrow transplantation for the treatment of chronic myelogenous leukemia. Ann Intern Med 104:155–163, 1986.
Ozer H: Biotherapy of chronic myelogenous leukemia with interferon. Semin Oncol 15 (suppl 5):14–20, 1988.

D. Chronic Lymphocytic Leukemia. Chronic lymphocytic leukemia (CLL) is the commonest type of leukemia in the United States and Europe. It typically is seen in an elderly asymptomatic patient (median age, 60 years) noted to have lymphocytosis on routine blood testing. Monoclonal B lymphocytosis (> 5,000 per cu mm in blood, > 40% in marrow), lymphadenopathy, hepatosplenomegaly, and hypogammaglobulinemia are typical. Most patients survive several years in relatively good health with minimal therapy before developing pancytopenia and succumbing to an infectious complication. Numerous staging systems have been proposed to stratify the risk of death from CLL. One of the most commonly used is that suggested by Rai (Table 11–5). Other prognostic features include the degree of lymphocytosis (> 40,000 per cu mm, unfavorable) and the pattern of marrow infiltration, with a nodular or interstitial pattern being much more favorable than a diffuse pattern.

1. THERAPY. Asymptomatic stage 0–1 patients should not receive therapy because survival is not improved with early drug administration. When patients develop systemic complaints (fever, sweats, fatigue), progressive lymphadenopathy or hepatosplenomegaly, progressive anemia or thrombocytopenia, or recurrent infections, oral chlorambucil (e.g., 0.1 mg/kg/d po) with or without prednisone is usually started. Cyclophosphamide (2–3 mg/kg/d po) may be substituted for chlorambucil in patients with marked thrombocytopenia, since the former has a less profound effect on platelet production. Pulse therapy with chlorambucil (0.7 mg/kg po over 4 days every 3–4 weeks) or cyclophosphamide (20 mg/kg every 2–3 weeks) may be substituted for daily continuous therapy with equivalent efficacy and less hema-

TABLE 11–5. STAGING OF CLL

STAGE	CRITERIA*	MEDIAN SURVIVAL (mo)
0	Lymphocytosis only	>150
1	Lymphadenopathy	101
2	Hepatosplenomegaly	71
3	Anemia (hemoglobin <11 gm/dL)	19
4	Thrombocytopenia (<100,000/mm³)	19

*All stages have lymphocytosis (>15,000/mm³ in blood and >40 per cent in marrow). Cases are assigned stage according to their worst prognostic feature (e.g., lymphocytosis with severe anemia is stage 3 even if lymphadenopathy and hepatosplenomegaly are lacking).

tologic toxicity. Randomized studies from Europe suggest that patients with advanced disease (with significant anemia or thrombocytopenia) may benefit from early institution of combination chemotherapy (e.g., CHOP [cyclophosphamide, doxorubicin, vincristine, prednisone]), though these results remain controversial. Newer agents that show considerable promise in CLL include fludarabine (response rate of 50–75%), 2-deoxycoformycin, 2-chlorodeoxyadenosine, and IV gamma globulin (for patients with recurrent infections [N Engl J Med 319:902–907, 1988]). Severe refractory anemia or thrombocytopenia due to hypersplenism is often ameliorated by splenectomy (Cancer 29:340–345, 1987).

Foon KA, Rai KR, Gale RP: Chronic lymphocytic leukemia: New insights into biology and therapy. Ann Intern Med 113:525–239, 1990.
Cheson BD: Recent advances in the treatment of B cell chronic lymphocytic leukemia. Oncology 4:71–78, 1990.
French Cooperative Group on Chronic Lymphocytic Leukemia: Effects of chlorambucil and therapeutic decision in initial forms of chronic lymphocytic leukemia (Stage A): results of a randomized clinical trial on 612 patients. Blood 75:1414–1421, 1990.

E. Hairy Cell Leukemia (HCL) is a rare chronic leukemia that generally occurs in middle-aged males and is characterized by pancytopenia, splenomegaly, and recurrent infections. The malignant cell is derived from the B lymphocyte lineage and is characterized by numerous cytoplasmic projections (hairy cells) and by acid phosphatase activity that is tartrate resistant (TRAP positive). Conventional management has been splenectomy, which improves the peripheral blood counts in 90% of patients. Unfortunately, at least 50% of patients will have progressive disease following splenectomy. Recent trials of α-interferon (2–3 mU SQ ti week) and 2'-dexycoformycin (4 mg/m^2 IV qo week) demonstrate response rates of over 80% for both agents, though the latter is more rapid acting and induces more complete remissions. The dramatic effectiveness of these new agents has led to their use as first-line therapy in HCL. Recently, 2-chlorodeoxyadenosine (0.1 mg/kg IV qd × 7 days) was reported to have induced durable complete remissions in 11 of 12 patients (N Engl J Med 322:1117–1121, 1990).

Steis RG and Longo DL: Update on the treatment of hairy cell leukemia. Update #6 for Cancer: Principles and Practice of Oncology (DeVita VT, Hellman S, and Rosenberg SA, eds.) Philadelphia, J. B. Lippincott Co., 1988.
Golomb HM, Fefer A, Golde DW, et al: Report of a multi-institutional study of 193 patients with hairy cell leukemia treated with interferon-alfa 2b. Semin Oncol 15 (Suppl. 5):7–9, 1988.

F. Multiple Myeloma. Multiple myeloma is a malignant plasma cell dyscrasia with an incidence of 3–4 cases per 100,000. It is characterized by marrow plasmacytosis (> 10%), monoclonal gammopathy (serum M protein > 3 gm/dL), osteopenia, tissue plasmacytomas, and "punched-out" bone lesions. Patients are typically elderly (median age 62) and present with fatigue, bone pain, anemia, or infection.

1. THERAPY

   a. **Monoclonal Gammopathy of Unknown Significance (Benign Monoclonal Gammopathy)** is characterized by minimal gammopathy (serum M protein < 3 gm/dL in serum and negligible in urine), less than 5% marrow plasma cells, no bone lesions, no anemia, and normal albumin and hematocrit values. In these patients, the disease uncommonly progresses to myeloma and requires no therapy, though regular follow-up with serial serum protein electrophoreses is indicated.

b. **Smoldering or Indolent Myeloma.** Patients with definite but mild myeloma (no anemia, bone lesions, or renal insufficiency) should be monitored with serial serum protein electrophoreses and should not receive treatment until symptoms develop or clear evidence of progression occurs.

c. **Symptomatic or Progressive Myeloma.** Melphalan (0.25 mg/kg po qd for 4 days every 6 weeks) and prednisone (1 mg/kg po qd for 4 days every 6 weeks) have been standard therapy for myeloma for many years. These drugs induce objective regressions (75% decrement in M protein production) in 50–60% of patients (median survival of 2–3 years). A 25% reduction in melphalan dose is prudent for initiation of therapy in patients with modest renal insufficiency. Leukocyte and platelet counts should be checked every 3 weeks to guide dosage titration. A properly adjusted regimen induces modest midcycle cytopenias. At least 3 cycles of therapy should be administered before failure is declared. Therapy should be ended in responding patients when the M protein level reaches a plateau, since melphalan is leukemogenic. Cyclophosphamide (100 mg/m^2 IV every 3–4 weeks) produces response rates and survival durations comparable to those achieved with melphalan. A recent controlled trial has demonstrated prolongation of survival and response duration in patients given α-interferon maintenance therapy after induction chemotherapy (N Engl J Med 322:1430–1434, 1990). The merits of multiagent combination chemotherapy in myeloma remain controversial. Combination therapy may be beneficial to patients with high tumor burdens, but evidence suggesting superior benefit for combination chemotherapy is inconclusive and does not warrant the complexity, cost, and side effects of the newer regimens (Semin Oncol 13:318–325, 1986). Adjunctive radiation therapy for severe bone pain (90% response rate) and IV gamma globulin (300 mg/kg q 3 week) for recurrent infections may be advisable in individual cases.

d. **Refractory Disease.** The salvage regimen of choice is VAD (vincristine, Adriamycin, and dexamethasone), which produces a 65–70% response rate and a 22-month median survival in responders. Patients whose disease is primarily refractory to first-line chemotherapy fare as well with high-dose dexamethasone alone (27% response rate) as with VAD (32% response rate) (Ann Intern Med 105:8–11, 1986). Syngeneic, allogeneic, and autologous bone marrow transplantation also are being investigated for their utility in myeloma therapy (Blood 70:869–872, 1987).

Sporn JR and McIntyre OR: Chemotherapy of previously untreated multiple myeloma patients: An analysis of recent treatment results. Semin Oncol 13:318–325, 1986. *A superb critical review of myeloma chemotherapy regimens.*

Buzaid AC and Durie BGM: Management of refractory myeloma: A review. J Clin Oncol 6:889–905, 1988.

G. Hodgkin's Disease. Hodgkin's disease has an incidence of 3 cases per 100,000 and is responsible for 25% of the lymphomas in the United States. The disease exhibits a bimodal age distribution, with peaks in young adulthood and in late middle age. Patients typically have painless lymphadenopathy, fatigue, night sweats, fever, or weight loss.

1. STAGING. The therapy of Hodgkin's disease depends on accurate staging as outlined by the Ann Arbor Classification:

Stage I: Single lymph node region or focal extralymphatic site
Stage II: Two or more sites on one side of the diaphragm
Stage III: Involved sites on both sides of the diaphragm
Stage IV: Disseminated involvement of an extralymphatic site

Stages are substratified by the absence (A) or presence (B) of fever (>38°C), night sweats, or weight loss (>10% of body weight). A staging laparotomy is performed if its results will affect treatment planning (e.g., if the choice of radiation therapy or chemotherapy would be altered by the discovery of intraabdominal disease [J Clin Oncol 8:257–265, 1990]).

2. MANAGEMENT. Several excellent therapeutic regimens with comparable curative potential are available for Hodgkin's disease. Management varies considerably from institution to institution, but the following recommendations are reasonably standard.

   a. **Initial Therapy**

      (1). *Stages I and II.* Conventional management of stages I and II involves subtotal nodal (mantle, para-aortic, and splenic fields) or total nodal (mantle plus inverted Y fields) irradiation (4000–4400 cGy in 200-cGy fractions), depending on disease location. This approach yields 10-year survivals of 95 and 93% and disease-free survival of 88 and 76% in stages IA and IIA, respectively. Patients with stages IB and IIB fare less well, with 77% overall survival and 69% disease-free survival at 10 years (Cancer 55 [suppl]:2072, 1985). Although several authorities have advised chemotherapy alone or chemotherapy plus radiation therapy for stages IB and IIB, the consensus is that chemotherapy with its toxicities should be reserved for the 30% of patients in whom radiation therapy fails. One subgroup for which the combined-modality approach is generally accepted, however, includes patients with large mediastinal masses (> ⅓ the thoracic diameter) because of unsatisfactory failure rates with radiation therapy alone (J Clin Oncol 7:1059–1065, 1989).

      (2). *Stage IIIA.* Patients with disease limited to the spleen and upper abdominal lymph nodes (stage IIIA$_1$) fare better than those with involved lower abdominal nodes (stage $IIIA_2$), with reported 5-year survival rates of 94 and 65%, respectively, following radiotherapy alone (Ann Intern Med 92:159–165, 1980). The poor outcome in stage $IIIA_2$ has led to the recommendation that combined-modality therapy be used in this subgroup while retaining total nodal irradiation for stage $IIIA_1$. Recent studies demonstrating a 95% complete remission rate and 80–90% disease-free survival 5 years after chemotherapy alone make a strong case for using chemotherapy in all stage IIIA patients (J Clin Oncol 2:892–896, 1984).

(3). Stages IIIB and IV. Combination chemotherapy is essential for the management of patients with stage IIIB or IV disease. Several effective, curative regimens have been devised, including **MOPP** (mechlorethamine, 6 mg/m² on days 1 and 8; vincristine, 1.4 mg/m² IV on days 1 and 8; procarbazine, 100 mg/m² po on days 1–14; and prednisone, 40 mg/m² po on days 1–14), **ABVD** (Adriamycin, 25 mg/m² IV; bleomycin, 10 U/m² IV; vinblastine, 6 mg/m² IV; and dacarbazine, 375 mg/m² IV on days 1 and 15), **alternating MOPP/ABVD, MOPP/ABV hybrid therapy** (half-cycles of MOPP and ABV each month), and **BCVPP** (carmustine [BCNU], cyclophosphamide, vinblastine, procarbazine, and prednisone.). Chemotherapy is given for 6–12 cycles (of 28 days each) or for 2 cycles beyond verification of complete remission (Table 11–6). MOPP has the longest track record, but ABVD appears to be equally efficacious, less leukemogenic, and causes less male sterility. Alternating therapy with MOPP and ABVD may improve cure rates by preventing the emergence of drug-resistant cell clones.

TABLE 11–6. CHEMOTHERAPY OF ADVANCED HODGKIN'S DISEASE

REGIMEN	COMPLETE REMISSION RATE (%)	5-YEAR DISEASE-FREE SURVIVAL (%)	REFERENCE
MOPP*	60–84	40–70	J Clin Oncol 4: 1295, 1986
ABVD*‡	60–80	40–70	Cancer 36: 252–259, 1975
BCVPP	76	64	Ann Intern Med 101: 447, 1984
MOPP/ABVD*	92	77	N Engl J Med 306: 770, 1982
MOPP/ABV†	95	90	Semin Hematol 24 (suppl 1): 35–40, 1987

*Twelve cycles, †eight cycles, ‡six cycles.
Abbreviations: MOPP = mechlorethamine (Mustargen), vincristine (Oncovin), procarbazine, prednisone; ABVD = doxorubicin (Adriamycin), bleomycin, vinblastine, dacarbazine; BCVPP = Carmustine (BCNU), cyclophosphamide, vinblastine, procarbazine, prednisone; ABV = doxorubicin (Adriamycin), vinblastine.

TABLE 11–7. SALVAGE THERAPY OF RELAPSED HODGKIN'S DISEASE

PREVIOUS THERAPY	SALVAGE THERAPY	COMPLETE REMISSION RATE (%)	5-YEAR DISEASE-FREE SURVIVAL (%)	REFERENCE
Radiation therapy	MOPP/ABV	88	79	J Clin Oncol 3:1174, 1985
MOPP	MOPP	59	20–25	Ann Intern Med 90:761, 1979
MOPP	ABVD	59	22	Ann Intern Med 96:139, 1982
MOPP	BCAVe	44	25	Ann Intern Med 101:440, 1984
Variable	Radiation therapy*	88	18–42	J Clin Oncol 5:38, 1987
				J Clin Oncol 5:544, 1987
Variable	BMT	60	20–25	J Clin Oncol 5:1340, 1987
Variable	[131]I antiferritin antibodies	3	NA	J Clin Oncol 3:1296, 1985

*Only for patients whose disease has relapsed at sites not previously irradiated.
BMT = bone marrow transplantation (mixed syngeneic, allogeneic, and autologous); BCAVe = bleomycin, CCNU doxorubicin, vinblastine; NA = not available.

b. **Salvage Therapy for Relapsed Hodgkin's Disease.** Factors predictive of a favorable outcome for salvage therapy of relapsed Hodgkin's disease include a disease-free interval over a year, absence of B symptoms, limited nodal sites of relapse, and treatment in first as opposed to subsequent relapse. Useful salvage regimens and their success rates are summarized in Table 11–7.

c. **Side Effects of Therapy.** Short-term toxicities include nausea, vomiting, alopecia, neuropathy, and radiation pneumonitis (5–20%). Longer-term sequelae include radiation-induced hypothyroidism (3–15%), pulmonary fibrosis, pericarditis, sterility (80–100% of men and > 80% of women over 25 years old after MOPP; 70–100% of men and 40% of women after total nodal irradiation). Most ominous is the occurrence of secondary malignancies. The magnitude of this risk has been estimated to be 17.6% at 15 years, including a 13.2% risk for solid tumors (lung and stomach cancers, melanomas, and sarcomas), 3.3% for AML, and 1.6% for non-Hodgkin's lymphomas. Chemotherapy (especially mechlorethamine and procarbazine) is primarily responsible for the development of secondary leukemias, but both radiation therapy and chemotherapy contribute to secondary solid tumors.

Bonadonna G, Santoro A, Viviani S, Valagussa P: Treatment strategies for Hodgkin's disease. Semin Hematol 25 (suppl 2):51–57, 1988.
Klimo P, Connors JM: An update on the Vancouver experience in the management of advanced Hodgkin's disease treated with the MOPP/ABV hybrid program. Semin Hematol 25 (suppl 2):34–40, 1988.
Tucker MA, Coleman CN, Cox RS, Varghese A, Rosenberg SA: Risk of second cancers after treatment for Hodgkin's disease. N Engl J Med 318:76–81, 1988.
Canellos GP: Can MOPP be replaced in the treatment of advanced Hodgkin's Disease? Semin Oncol 17 (suppl 2):2–6, 1990.

H. Non-Hodgkin's Lymphomas. Non-Hodgkin's lymphomas (NHL) have an incidence of 9 per 100,000 persons. Features adversely affecting outcome include advanced stage, presence of B symptoms, aggressive histology, marrow or liver involvement, advanced age, bulky disease (> 10 cm), elevated lactate dehydrogenase (LDH) levels, male sex, and hemoglobin < 12 gm/dL.

1. MANAGEMENT. Treatment of NHL depends on the histology and stage of disease. For the purpose of this discussion, NHL will be subgrouped as outlined by the International Working Formulation and by Rappaport's classification (Table 11–8).
   a. **Indolent (Low-Grade) Lymphomas.** Stages I–II low-grade lymphomas should be treated with external beam radiation therapy with curative intent ($\geq$ 3500 cGy over 3.5 weeks). Stages III–IV indolent lymphomas are generally considered incurable with conventional management and are treated palliatively. Asymptomatic patients may be followed clinically with no intervention, provided normal organs are not impaired. A Stanford University study of 83 untreated patients revealed a 73% 10-year survival, a 23% spontaneous regression rate, and a necessity for eventual therapeutic intervention in 61% (after a median of 3 years) (J Clin Oncol 3:299–310, 1985). Disseminated symptomatic disease can be treated with single alkylating agents (e.g., chlorambucil, 0.1 mg/kg/d po qd or 0.7 mg/kg po over 4 days every 3–4 weeks) with or without prednisone (1 mg/kg per day initially, followed by a taper over several weeks), with a response rate of about 70%. Relapsing or unresponsive disease can be managed with CVP

TABLE 11–8. CLASSIFICATION OF NON-HODGKIN'S LYMPHOMAS

RAPPAPORT CLASSIFICATION	WORKING FORMULATION
Favorable Prognosis	**Low Grade**
1. Diffuse well-differentiated lymphocytic (DWDL)	1. Small lymphocytic (SLL)
2. Nodular poorly differentiated lymphocytic (NPDL)	2. Follicular small cleaved cell (FSC)
3. Nodular mixed lymphocytic (NML)	3. Follicular mixed small and large cell (FMC)
Intermediate Prognosis	**Intermediate Grade**
1. Nodular histiocytic (NH)	1. Follicular large cell (FLL)
2. Diffuse poorly differentiated lymphocytic (DPDL)	2. Diffuse small cleaved cell (DSC)
3. Diffuse mixed lymphocytic (DML)	3. Diffuse mixed small cleaved and large cell lymphoma (DML)
	4. Diffuse large cell (cleaved/noncleaved) (DLCL)
Unfavorable Prognosis	**High Grade**
1. Diffuse histiocytic (DHL)	1. Diffuse large cell, immunoblastic
2. Diffuse undifferentiated (DUL) (Burkitt's/non-Burkitt's)	2. Small noncleaved cell (SNCC)
3. Lymphoblastic (LB)	3. Lymphoblastic (LB)

TABLE 11–9. COMBINATION CHEMOTHERAPY REGIMENS FOR DIFFUSE, AGGRESSIVE NON-HODGKIN'S LYMPHOMAS*

REGIMEN	COMPLETE REMISSION RATE (%)	5-YEAR DISEASE-FREE SURVIVAL (%)	DURATION OF THERAPY (mo)
CHOP	51	39	4–6
BACOP	48	48	6
COMLA	55	48	9
ProMACE-MOPP	73	60	6–9
M-BACOD	77	57	7.5
MACOP-B	84	75	3

*Data from Ann Intern Med 107:25–30, 1987.
Abbreviations: A and H = Adriamycin (doxorubicin); B = bleomycin; C = cyclophosphamide; D = dexamethasone; E = etoposide; L = leucovorin; M = methotrexate (except in MOPP, in which M = mechlorethamine); O = Oncovin (vincristine); P and Pro = prednisone.

(cyclophosphamide, 400 mg/m^2 IV on days 1–5; vincristine, 1.4 mg/m^2 IV on day 1; prednisone, 100 mg/m^2 po on days 1–5 repeated every 21–28 days) or CHOP (cyclophosphamide, 650 mg/m^2 IV; doxorubicin [Adriamycin], 25 mg/m^2 IV; vincristine, 1.4 mg/m^2, all on day 1; prednisone, 100 mg/m^2 po on days 1–5). α-interferon may also be used with a response rate greater than 50% in patients with follicular lymphomas.

Early intervention with C-MOPP (cyclophosphamide, vincristine, procarbazine, prednisone) or CHOP has been advocated for follicular, mixed small-cleaved and large cell lymphomas on the basis of two studies showing prolonged disease free survival when this histology is treated aggressively (Ann Intern Med 100:651–656, 1984; Proc Am Soc Clin Onc 9:259, 1990). Aggressive therapy of indolent lymphomas with aggressive combination chemotherapy is being compared with conventional therapy in a large trial sponsored by the National Cancer Institute, with early results favoring the intensive therapy group.

b. **Aggressive (Intermediate and High-Grade) Lymphoma.** Stages I–II diffuse aggressive lymphomas (diffuse mixed lymphoma [DML], diffuse large-cell lymphoma [DLCL], etc.) are best treated with combined-modality therapy (e.g., 3 cycles of a doxorubicin-based regimen [CHOP, ACOB] plus 3000 cGy involved-field radiation therapy). This approach yields a 95–99% complete remission rate and 84–96% disease-free survival at 2.5 years (Ann Intern Med 107:25–30, 1987; J Clin Oncol 7:1295–1302, 1989). Bulky stage II and stages III–IV aggressive lymphomas are best managed with one of the high dose–intensity doxorubicin-based chemotherapy regimens shown in Table 11–9. With this approach 50–85% of stages III–IV patients can be expected to achieve complete remission; 40–75% will enjoy long-term disease free survival.

2. MISCELLANEOUS LYMPHOMAS

a. **Cutaneous T Cell Lymphomas (CTCL).** Patients with mycosis fungoides and other CTCLs usually present with chronic skin plaques, tumors, and nodules, which may be associated with circulating cerebriform lymphocytes (Sézary cells), lymphadenopathy, and visceral involvement. Diagnosis is generally elusive for several years while the patient's skin disease is managed with emollients and steroid creams. Aggressive therapy of CTCL with total skin electron beam radiation therapy and chemotherapy can produce major responses in 90% of patients and may cure a minority of patients with early-stage (skin-only) disease. For the majority of patients, however, early institution of aggressive therapy does not appear to improve disease-free survival or overall survival compared with conservative management with topical nitrogen mustard (N Engl J Med 321:1784–90, 1990). Alternative therapies include photochemotherapy with retinoic acid in association with ultraviolet irradiation of lymphocytapheresed cells, topical nitrogen mustard, and psoralen and ultraviolet A (PUVA). Once lymph nodes and visceral organs are involved, CTCL is incurable with conventional therapy. Combination chemotherapy with CVP or CHOP will induce remissions in the majority of patients, but the remission durations are short.

b. **Lymphoblastic Lymphoma.** This is typically a T cell disorder of young men presenting with mediastinal masses. It responds poorly to conventional lymphoma regimens but is curable when treated with ALL-type regimens (Semin Oncol 17:96–103, 1990).

c. **Central Nervous System Disease.** Patients with small noncleaved cell lymphomas, lymphoblastic lymphomas, T cell lymphomas, or large-cell lymphomas with marrow, testicular, or sinus involvement are at high risk for spread to the CNS. Prophylactic therapy involves administration of intrathecal chemotherapy (e.g., intrathecal MTX), cranial irradiation (2400 cGy in 2.5 weeks), or treatment with drug regimens that penetrate the cerebrospinal fluid well (e.g., high-dose methotrexate or cytarabine). Therapy for documented CNS disease is more intensive and usually includes cranial irradiation (3600–4000 cGy) combined with intrathecal methotrexate (12 mg twice a week until the cerebrospinal fluid is clear and then 12 mg intrathecally every 6 weeks for 1.5 years).

3. **BONE MARROW TRANSPLANTATION FOR LYMPHOMAS.** Patients who have relapse following therapy with doxorubicin-based regimens are rarely curable with conventional chemotherapy. Consequently, high-dose chemoradiotherapy in conjunction with syngeneic, allogeneic, or autologous bone marrow transplantation has become increasingly popular as salvage therapy for suitable candidates. Recent series from several institutions indicate that 11–60% of patients with relapsed lymphomas can be cured with marrow transplantation. The prognosis appears to be best for patients transplanted early after relapse with small tumor burdens (preferably after induction of a second remis-

sion). Patients with end-stage, resistant disease and large tumor burdens fare poorly with transplantation.

Portlock CS: Managememt of the low grade non-Hodgkin's lymphomas. Semin Oncol 17:51–59, 1990.

DeVita VT, Hubbard SM, Young RC, Longo DL: The role of chemotherapy in diffuse aggressive lymphomas. Semin Hematol 25 (suppl 2):2–10, 1988.

Hoppe RT: The role of radiation therapy in the management of the non-Hodgkin's lymphomas. Cancer 55 (suppl):2176–2183, 1985.

Petersen FB, Appelbaum FR, Hill R, et al: Autologous marrow transplantation for malignant lymphoma: a report of 101 cases from Seattle. J Clin Oncol 8:638–647, 1990.

Williams SF: The role of bone marrow transplantation in the non-Hodgkin's lymphomas. Semin Oncol 17:88–95, 1990.

I. Breast Cancer

1. **LOCALIZED DISEASE.** Pathologic stage I (primary tumor < 5 cm, negative nodes), stage II (primary tumor < 5 cm, positive nodes) and operable stage III (primary tumor ≥ 5 cm with or without positive nodes, no local contraindication to resection) may be managed by a variety of approaches, from excisional biopsy and irradiation to modified radical mastectomy. These will produce equivalent results if the gross tumor is removed and microscopic tumor that may be present elsewhere in the breast is excised (mastectomy) or sterilized by radiation therapy. *An axillary sampling procedure is essential for pathologic staging*: clinical estimation that an axilla does or does not contain tumor will be wrong in 20–30% of cases.

   a. **Premenopausal Women.** For premenopausal women with positive axillary nodes, adjuvant chemotherapy with an effective combination is indicated for a minimum of 6 monthly cycles. Commonly employed combinations are shown in Table 11–10 (intermittent

TABLE 11–10. COMMON ADJUVANT CHEMOTHERAPY REGIMENS FOR BREAST CANCER

1. Intermittent CMF ("Bonadonna")		
Cyclophosphamide	100 mg/m²/day PO	Day 1–14
Methotrexate	40 mg/m² IV on days 1, 8	Every 4 weeks
5FU	600 mg/m² IV on days 1, 8	
2. Continuous CMF ± VP ("Cooper")		
Cyclophosphamide	60 mg/m²/day PO	Continuously
Methotrexate	15 mg/m²/week IV	
5FU	300 mg/m²/week IV	
(Vincristine)	1–2 mg/week IV to total of 6–10 doses	
(Prednisone)	60 mg/day PO, taper to 10 mg/day then discontinue in 6 weeks	
3. FAC ("M.D. Anderson")		
5FU	400 mg/m² IV days 1, 8	Every 4 weeks
Adriamycin	40 mg/m² IV day 1	to total of 300
Cytoxan	400 mg/m² IV day 1	mg/m² of Adriamycin
5FU	500 mg/m² IV days 1, 8	Every 4 weeks
Methotrexate	30 mg/m² IV days 1, 8	
Cyclophosphamide	500 mg/m² IV day 2	

CMF, continuous CMF, and FAC). Without systemic adjuvant treatment, about 50% of such patients will relapse within 5 years, while about half this percentage will do so on an "effective" chemotherapy program. The greatest benefit is seen in those patients who have 1–3 positive nodes, in whom there is a plateau for disease-free survival with long-term follow-up, suggesting an increased cure rate. Retrospective analysis of the results of many trials indicates that the efficacy of chemotherapy in the adjuvant setting is directly related to drug dosage per unit time ("dose intensity"). Adjuvant chemotherapy exerts beneficial effects in both hormone receptor–positive and –negative disease, and its efficacy does not depend on whether amenorrhea is induced and maintained. These considerations point to a direct cytotoxic effect as the major mechanism of drug action, but there may be an indirect effect as well, mediated via suppression of endogenous estrogen production through the ovaries.

b. **Postmenopausal Women.** In postmenopausal women, adjuvant chemotherapy has not proven as effective, possibly because of underdosing. Recent studies with equal "dose intensity" in this group appear to show significant benefit. For postmenopausal women with positive hormone receptors, the administration of "additive" hormone manipulation in the form of **tamoxifen** alone clearly exerts a beneficial effect on disease-free survival, and the duration of benefit appears to be related to the duration of tamoxifen treatment. Tamoxifen probably acts by a non-cytotoxic growth-arresting effect, preventing the transition of hormone-dependent cells into the "S phase" of DNA synthesis. At the present time, tamoxifen alone may be considered standard treatment for receptor-positive, node-positive postmenopausal patients. Women with negative axillary nodes appear to benefit from adjuvant therapy based on recent controlled clinical trials. However, 70% of such patients are cured by local treatment alone. Tamoxifen also appears to exert positive effects in receptor-positive patients with about the same degree of benefit.

Patients with locally advanced stage III disease or inflammatory breast cancer pose a special problem. A combined modality approach appears to yield the best results, with initial chemotherapy followed by mastectomy and irradiation. Both local control and cure rates are improved, but the majority of these patients still succumb to uncontrolled disease.

2. DISSEMINATED DISEASE
   a. **Hormone Receptor Positive.** For the majority of patients with positive estrogen (ER) or progesterone (PR) receptors, hormone manipulation alone offers a 60% chance of objective remission with minimal morbidity. Although ablative procedures performed at the outset may provide a longer duration of initial disease control, randomized trials did not show survival benefit for women undergoing the major procedures (adrenalectomy, hypophysec-

tomy) initially: today the **first maneuver is oophorectomy in premenopausal women and "additive" therapy in postmenopausal women**. The **concurrent use of chemotherapy and tamoxifen** in postmenopausal women does not appear superior to initial use of tamoxifen alone, possibly because of unfavorable cytokinetic and/or pharmacologic interactions. Although tamoxifen has largely replaced diethylstilbestrol (DES) as "standard" initial management in postmenopausal women because of its lessened toxicity, one controlled trial has reported substantial benefit (50% 5-year survival) in ER-positive patients from the combination of DES and chemotherapy. These results require confirmation. For patients whose disease relapses after hormone therapy, use of "second-line" hormone manipulation provides further useful response in 30–50%; second-line hormones almost never work if there was no initial response. Megestrol acetate has comparable activity to aminoglutethimide but is preferred due to lesser toxicity.

b. **Hormone-Refractory or Receptor Negative.** When a patient has disease progression on hormonal treatment, ER or PR-negative disease, or "grave signs of involvement" (including evidence of hepatic or lymphangitic lung disease), **chemotherapy** should be used. Of the available chemotherapeutic agents, Adriamycin is the most effective as a single drug, and the only one that consistently produces response in 25–30% of patients after multiple other drugs have failed. Partly for this reason, it is often "saved" for second-line management, and non–Adriamycin-containing combinations are used initially. The most common is CMF (cyclophosphamide, methotrexate, and 5-FU). Adriamycin-containing regimens may be of special benefit in hepatic-dominant and ER-negative disease. Most responses to chemotherapy are incomplete, but 50–70% of patients will respond to an effective combination, for a median of 6–9 months. Survival from the start of treatment is 12–18 months on the average and may be improved by programs of high-dose "consolidative" chemotherapy in remission.

Harris JR, Hellman S, Canellos G, Fisher B: *In* DeVita VT, Hellman S, and Rosenberg SA (eds.): Cancer: Principles and Practice of Oncology. 2nd ed. Philadelphia, JB Lippincott Co., 1985, p. 1119.

Kiang DT, Gay J, Goldman A, Kennedy BJ: A randomized trial of chemotherapy and hormonal therapy in advanced breast cancer. N Engl J Med 313:1241, 1985.

Fisher B, Brown A, Wolmark N, et al: Prolonging tamoxifen therapy for primary breast cancer. Ann Intern Med 106:649, 1987.

J. Lung Cancer

1. Treatment of Non–Small Cell Lung Cancer

a. OPERABLE DISEASE. Non–small cell histologies (epidermoid or squamous, adenocarcinoma and large cell) account for 75% of patients with lung cancer. Of these, approximately a third will be candidates for a surgical procedure with curative intent. When possible, the tumor and areas of known nodal involvement in continuity should be removed by a procedure less than pneumonectomy, since the outcome of treatment is not improved by more radical surgery and the patient is left with a worse pulmonary reserve. Operative mortality should be < 3% from lobectomy and < 8% from pneumonectomy. Some patients' tumors that are anatomically resectable will be medically inoperable and should be managed as described for "localized inoperable" disease.

Stage I lung cancer is best treated by surgical resection alone, usually a lobectomy. 5-year disease-free survival is little influenced by cell type and (in properly staged patients) exceeds 60%. In stage II disease with hilar/lobar nodal involvement and in stage III resectable disease, the results of surgery are influenced by histologic type: epidermoid tumors have a better prognosis than large cell or adenocarcinomas due to the greater likelihood of hematogenous dissemination with the latter cell types. The 5-year disease-free survival for resected stages II and III is only 20–35% in the absence of gross mediastinal nodal involvement. When the latter finding is present, most surgeons do not operate, since the mortality of pneumonectomy may be greater than the chance of cure. Whether to operate on patients with *microscopic*, not grossly apparent, involvement of mediastinal nodes, is controversial.

b. LOCALIZED INOPERABLE DISEASE. This includes patients whose tumors are anatomically resectable but medically inoperable, as well as those who have stage III disease without distant metastasis. For these patients, radiation therapy has been the mainstay of treatment. Given 5000–6000 cGy over a period of 5–7 weeks, patients with inoperable disease confined to the lungs have a 2-year survival of about 15% (median 9 months), while those with evidence of extrapulmonary spread have a 2-year survival of 5–8% (median 6 months).

A combination of chemotherapy and irradiation may improve the results of radiation therapy alone in localized inoperable disease. Another approach is to give chemotherapy, with or without irradiation, as initial treatment, followed by an attempt at surgical resection in patients for whom it becomes technically possible. Such combined modality therapy remains investigational and is best conducted in the context of a protocol.

c. EXTENSIVE INOPERABLE DISEASE. There is no standard therapy for these patients, who unfortunately make up 30–40% of the lung cancer population at the time of presentation. They have clinically detectable metastasis beyond the ipsilateral hemithorax and regional nodes. A definitive approach requires systemic chemotherapy. It is important to realize that *palliation* of selected symptoms (e.g., bone pain, hemoptysis, superior vena cava syndrome), may be more reliably achieved with appropriate irradiation, while other symptoms (obstructive atelectasis, hoarseness) rarely are improved by x-ray treatment. Chemotherapy for non–small cell lung cancer is in a state of evolution. Nonprotocol treatment is not indicated for patients who are less than fully ambulatory and is controversial for those who are fully ambulatory. The *best* treatment for the latter group is entry on a protocol study. If this is not possible, a reasonable approach is the administration of a cisplatin-containing chemotherapy program, such as cisplatin plus VP-16 or vinblastine.

2. Treatment of Small Cell Lung Cancer

a. LIMITED (UNRESECTABLE) DISEASE. In these patients (25–40% of the total) clinical staging fails to reveal evidence of spread beyond the ipsilateral hemithorax and regional nodes. It appears that concurrent or rapidly alternating chemotherapy and chest irradiation is superior to chemotherapy alone or use of these modalities in sequence. Cisplatin and VP-16 with irradiation has become a standard form of induction chemotherapy. Whole brain irradiation is used by most centers as prophylaxis against relapse at that site in patients who achieve remission. At the completion of induction treatment, maintenance chemotherapy is no longer administered on a chronic basis. However, administration of pulsed intensive cycles of "reinduction," either with the initially employed program or with one made up of different "non–cross-resistant" drugs, is a subject of promising investigations. With concurrent chemoradiotherapy, 40% of patients with limited disease will survive for 2 years and about 25% for 5 years, a major improvement over supportive care alone (median survival, 12 weeks) or radiation therapy alone (median survival 6 months, and 2-year survival < 5%).

b. EXTENSIVE DISEASE. The majority of patients with small cell lung cancer have clinically evident spread to organs beyond the chest at the time of presentation, reflecting the aggressive growth and early hematogenous dissemination of this cell type. Standard therapy is the use of drugs in combination, with elective whole-brain irradiation to prevent relapse in this "pharmacologic sanctuary" reserved for patients with a complete or near-complete response to chemotherapy. Using a program like CAV (cyclophosphamide, Adriamycin, and vincristine) alternating with cisplatin/VP-16, the median survival is about 8 months, with almost no long-term survivors. About 60% will have tumor regression but only 15% will achieve complete response. Other approaches attempted to date have yielded no reproducible improvement in survival. "Dose-intensive" programs with weekly treatment are promising and currently under investigation.

Minna JD, Higgins GA, Glatstein EJ: Cancer of the lung. *In* DeVita VT, Hellman S, and Rosenberg SA (eds): Cancer: Principles and Practice of Oncology. Philadelphia, JB Lippincott Co., 1985, p. 507.

Dillman RO, Seagren SL, Propert KJ, et al: A randomized trial of induction chemotherapy plus high-dose radiation versus radiation alone in stage III non-small cell lung cancer. N Engl J Med 323:940–945, 1990.

Livingston RB: Lung neoplasms. *In* Cancer Medicine, 3rd ed. Holland JF, Frei E III (eds). Philadelphia, Lea & Febiger (in press).

K. Ovarian Carcinoma. This is the fourth leading cause of cancer deaths in women with 20,000 new cases of ovarian carcinoma and more than 12,000 deaths in 1990. Epithelial neoplasms constitute 80–90% of all ovarian cancers, and 60% of women have advanced stage disease (stages III–IV) at diagnosis.

1. PRIMARY SURGERY. Cytoreductive surgery is critical to adequately stage and optimally treat advanced ovarian carcinoma. Approximately 60–75% of tumors at the time of diagnosis can be satisfactorily debulked (residual nodules < 1–2 cm). This may require resection of large tumor masses and partial bowel resections, in addition to bilateral salpingo-oophorectomy, total abdominal hysterectomy, and omentectomy. Complete staging requires biopsies of the diaphragm and paracolic gutters as well as pelvic and periaortic lymph nodes and cytologic washings of the entire peritoneal cavity. The response rate to chemotherapy, the odds of a pathologic negative second-look operation, and eventual cure are directly related not only to optimal debulking but also to tumor stage and grade.

2. PRIMARY CHEMOTHERAPY. The objective response rates of advanced ovarian carcinoma to single alkylating agents (melphalan, chlorambucil, or cyclophosphamide) range from 15–65%. The vast majority of these responses are partial remissions and the 2-year disease-free survival rate is less than 10%. Cisplatin is the most active chemotherapeutic agent with a response rate of 40%. A recent retrospective review of a number of clinical trials showed that the only predictive factor for an objective response in a number of combination regimens was the dose intensity of cisplatin administered (J Clin Oncol 5:756, 1987). Although high-dose cisplatin (40 mg/m^2 daily for 5 days) has demonstrated impressive activity in refractory ovarian carcinoma, the incidence of disabling neuropathy prevents routine use (J Clin Oncol 3:1246, 1985). Recent studies have demonstrated equivalent therapeutic benefit for carboplatin at a dose of 400 mg/m^2 and cisplatin at 100 mg/m^2.

Randomized trials have now demonstrated significantly improved survival with combination cisplatin-based chemotherapy compared with those attained with single aklylating agents. Combination regimens based on cisplatin or carboplatin and cyclophosphamide given for 6 cycles produce overall objective response rates of 90% with clinical and pathologic complete responses in the range of 40–60% and 25–30%, respectively. However, even with these advances, only 20% of women with advanced ovarian carcinoma are cured of ovarian cancer today. The rise and fall of CA-125, a serum glycoprotein which is elevated in most patients with epithelial ovarian carcinoma, has been correlated with the clinical course of the disease.

3. SECOND-LOOK SURGERY. The value of secondary cytoreductive surgery (a second-look operation) in patients with persistent or recurrent disease after chemotherapy is controversial. Secondary cytoreductive

surgery may assume greater importance if more effective salvage therapy becomes available for those women in whom standard cisplatin-based chemotherapy fails.

4. **PALLIATION.** Intestinal obstruction is the inevitable outcome for most women who have persistent disease. In 85% of obstructed patients undergoing surgical exploration, some type of palliative operation can be performed with a morbidity of 30–40% and a mortality of 12–16%. With the use of parenteral hyperalimentation, these rates can be significantly reduced. The average life expectancy of these patients is 3–4 months.

5. **SALVAGE IV CHEMOTHERAPY.** High-dose cisplatin (40 mg/m^2 daily for 5 days), taxol (a natural product isolated from the western yew tree), ifosfamide, and hexamethylmelamine have all been shown to have activity as single agents in relapsed patients.

6. **SALVAGE INTRAPERITONEAL CHEMOTHERAPY.** Epithelial ovarian carcinoma is a unique disease in that many women do not have evidence of disease involving organs other than the serosal surfaces of the peritoneum. Instillation of drugs such as 5-FU, methotrexate, melphalan, Adriamycin, cytosine arabinoside, cisplatin, and α-interferon (J Clin Oncol 8:1036, 1990) through a Tenckhoff catheter or portacath implanted into the peritoneal cavity achieves local drug concentrations in the peritoneal fluid 10–1000 fold higher than the concentrations achieved with IV therapy. Such intraperitoneal chemotherapy has been promising in pilot clinical trials, particularly in the presence of minimal residual disease at second-look laparotomy. In order to provide adequate exposure of the entire peritoneum, the drugs must be given in large volumes of fluid. Intra-abdominal adhesions may result in poor drug distributions. Complications include bacterial peritonitis, catheter infections, and bowel perforation.

7. **RADIATION THERAPY.** Pelvic irradiation alone is not adequate to control a disease that puts the entire peritoneal surface at risk. Whole abdominal radiation, using either an open-field or moving-strip technique, can be delivered in doses of 3,000–5,500 cGy to the upper abdomen and pelvis, respectively. The role of this type of radiotherapy, however, is limited and is not appropriate for women who have bulky disease. The complications include radiation enteritis and hepatic and renal damage.

Hoskins W: The role of cytoreductive surgery in ovarian cancer. Cancer: Principles and Practice of Oncology. Philadelphia, JB Lippincott Co., 1987, pp. 1, 2.

Redman JR, Petroni GE, Saigo PE, et al: Prognostic factors in advanced ovarian carcinoma. J Clin Oncol 4:515–523, 1986.

Reichman B, Markman M, Hakes T, et al: Intraperitoneal cisplatin and Etoposide in the treatment of refractory/recurrent ovarian carcinoma. J Clin Oncol 7:1327j–1332, 1989.

L. Malignant Melanoma. The incidence of cutaneous melanoma increased 80% from 1973 to 1980. This tumor accounts for 1% of all cancers in the United States; its behavior is unpredictable, ranging from spontaneous regression to rapid progression leading to death. The depth of vertical invasion of a primary melanoma is the most important prognostic factor determining the risk of recurrence or dissemination.

1. **PRIMARY SURGERY.** An excisional, full skin thickness biopsy of any lesion suspected of being a malignant melanoma should be performed with a margin of several millimeters of normal skin. If the lesion is too large for an initial excisional biopsy, an incisional biopsy through the most nodular or elevated portion of the lesion can be done without affecting the overall survival. All skin biopsies, regardless of the physician's clinical diagnosis, should be submitted for pathologic study. After the diagnosis of malignant melanoma is made, the traditional approach has been wide local re-excision with 3–5 cm margins, with skin grafting if necessary. Using this technique, the local recurrence rate is about 7%. Local recurrence following excision of "thin" primary lesions (< 1 mm in depth) is rare; 1-cm margins suffice.

2. **REGIONAL LYMPH NODE DISSECTION.** For patients without lymphadenopathy (clinical stage I), lymph node disssection is controversial. 20% of such patients have occult pathologic nodal micrometastases, but two prospective, randomized trials showed no improvement in survival for patients undergoing lymphadenectomy at the time of diagnosis compared with those undergoing delayed lymphadenectomy when clinically suspicious adenopathy appeared (Cancer 49:2420, 1982; Cancer 41:948, 1978). Careful, expectant follow-up after excision of the primary lesion is probably justified, particularly for thin, minimally invasive lesions and axial lesions, in which the nodal drainage is ambiguous (J Clin Oncol 6:163, 1988). Lymphadenectomy for patients with nodal spread (stage II) represents appropriate, accepted standard practice. The overall survival for this group following surgery is about 20%.

3. **ADJUVANT THERAPY.** No large, prospective randomized trial has demonstrated a survival advantage for adjuvant chemotherapy (DTIC, methyl-CCNU, chemotherapeutic combinations), immunotherapy (BCG, transfer factor, and levamisole), immunochemotherapy (DTIC plus BCG), or vitamin A compared with an untreated control arm. To date, there is no proven benefit for adjuvant chemotherapy or immunotherapy of high-risk stage I or II patients.

4. **METASTATIC DISEASE.** There is no predictable pattern of dissemination of malignant melanoma. Any anatomic site may be involved, including skin, subcutaneous tissue, lungs, lymph nodes, gastrointestinal tract, spleen, liver, CNS, and bone. The disease-free interval before development of metastatic disease may be about 20 years.
   a. **Surgery.** Simple resections of cutaneous melanoma recurrences should be done if the patient can be rendered free of disease without major morbidity. Although surgery in this setting is rarely

curative, palliative resections, particularly of bleeding gastrointestinal lesions, may be helpful. The 5-year survival rate may be as high as 20% after resection of solitary pulmonary metastases.

b. Chemotherapy. DTIC (250 mg/m^2 IV daily for 4 days every 28 days) is the single most active agent in the treatment of disseminated melanoma, with an overall objective response rate of approximately 20%. Patients with subcutaneous, lymph node, or pulmonary metastases have the highest response rates, with a median duration of response approaching 12 months. BCNU (200 mg/m^2 IV q 6–8 weeks) produces objective responses in 15% of patients. Tumors that have responded to DTIC may subsequently respond to nitrosoureas after progression. The combination of DTIC, cisplatin, BCNU, and tamoxifen has the highest reported response rate (50%) (Cancer 63:1292, 1989).

c. Immunotherapy. Several lines of evidence suggest that the immune response of the host alters the growth and dissemination of malignant melanoma. Well-documented cases of spontaneous regression of primary and metastatic lesions have been reported, and intralesional injection of the immunomodulatory agent BCG can induce regression in 65% of skin lesions in immunocompetent patients. Systemic immunotherapy with BCG or *Corynebacterium parvum* alone or in combination with chemotherapy have been beneficial in advanced melanoma in some trials. Recently, DNA recombinant technology has allowed the production of cytokines and monoclonal antibodies, engendering new interest in immunotherapy. The combination of interleukin-2 and lymphocyte-activated killer cells (LAK cells) has produced objective responses in 20–30% of patients with advanced melanoma, including occasional complete responses. Early reports (N Engl J Med 319:1676, 1988) of IL-2 given in association with tumor-infiltrating lymphocytes (TIL) derived from the patient's own melanoma suggest a higher response rate than with LAK cells. About 15% of patients will have objective responses to α-interferon. Autologous tumor vaccines, with or without cyclophosphamide, occasionally produce tumor regression (J Clin Oncol 8:1858, 1990). The combination of cytokines or cytokines given with chemotherapy or monoclonal antibodies may be most active in the setting of microscopic disease after surgical excision.

Balch CM: The role of elective lymph node dissection in melanoma: rationale, results, and controversies. J Clin Oncol 6:163–172, 1988.

Greene MH, Clark WH, Tucker MA, et al: Acquired precursors of cutaneous malignant melanoma. N Engl J Med 312:91–116, 1985.

Koh HK, Sober AJ, Day CL, et al: Prognosis of clinical stage I melanoma patients with positive elective regional node dissection. J Clin Oncol 4:1238–1244, 1986.

M. Soft Tissue Sarcomas. Each year in the United States, there are 4500 new cases of soft tissue sarcomas and 1600 deaths from this malignancy. This rare group of tumors arises primarily from mesodermal structures. The following discussion is primarily applicable to spindle cell sarcomas of the extremities found in adults. The most important predictor of the biological aggressiveness of an individual tumor and its propensity to metastasize is the grade of the tumor. This difficult pathologic assessment is based on the frequency of mitoses and the degree of pre-therapeutic necrosis as well as on the cellularity and nuclear pleomorphism (Semin Oncol 16:273, 1989). Grade I, and to some extent Grade II, tumors are low grade and tend to recur locally rather than systemically. In general, they do not respond as well to chemotherapy as do the high-grade tumors (Grade III), which are malignant, aggressive tumors with a high propensity for systemic dissemination.

1. **PRIMARY SURGERY.** Soft tissue sarcomas commonly present as asymptomatic, slowly enlarging, firm soft tissue masses, which can occur anywhere in the body. An "excisional biopsy" through the tumor's pseudocapsule is not appropriate surgical treatment since residual gross tumor remains after "excisional biopsy" in 50% of cases. The proper biopsy for all lesions > 3 cm is a carefully placed small incisional biopsy, utilizing a longitudinal incision on the extremities. After the diagnosis is established, primary resection of the sarcoma should be performed by wide excision including several centimeters of normal tissue in all directions as well as excision of previous biopsy sites. In general, it is not necessary to perform lymph node dissections. Until recently, the most common surgical procedure for a soft tissue sarcoma of the extremity was amputation, with a subsequent local recurrence rate of 10%. However, with development of multimodality approaches using neoadjuvant chemotherapy and/or preoperative irradiation, the vast majority of these tumors can be handled with limb salvage operations.

2. **NEOADJUVANT CHEMOTHERAPY.** Preoperative or neoadjuvant chemotherapy provides a unique opportunity to pathologically assess the effectiveness of chemotherapy and is under active investigation in soft tissue sarcomas. Necrosis of more than 90% of the cells in the resected specimen has been shown to correlate with improved survival in patients with osteogenic sarcomas, and similar prognostic significance is assumed for soft tissue sarcomas. Preoperative chemotherapy may also facilitate surgery by shrinking tumors, potentially allowing limb salvage surgery rather than amputation.

3. **ADJUVANT CHEMOTHERAPY.** The issue of adjuvant chemotherapy after definitive local therapy is controversial. Adjuvant therapy apparently does not improve disease-free survival or overall survival in patients with low-grade lesions. Only one of five randomized trials using Adriamycin as a single agent for high-grade sarcomas has shown improved disease-free survival for treated patients. There have been four major prospective randomized trials of *combination* adjuvant chemotherapy in sarcomas of the extremities. Of these trials, only two, one employing Adriamycin, cyclophosphamide, and methotrexate (Cancer 58:190, 1986) and one employing vincristine, Adriamycin,

cyclophosphamide and actinomycin D (VACAR) (5th Int Conf Adjuvant Therapy Cancer 14, March 1987) have resulted in improved disease-free or overall survival. Until the issue of adjuvant therapy is resolved, we recommend that patients with high-grade soft tissue sarcomas be entered into controlled trials of adjuvant chemotherapy.

4. RADIATION THERAPY. The local control rate of inoperable soft tissue sarcoma treated with 6000–8000 cGy of conventional photon radiotherapy is only 10–12%. The use of neutrons (which have a higher linear energy transfer and are not dependent on oxygen for cell kill) increases the local control rate to 50% (Am J Clin Oncol 9:397–400, 1986). Standard postoperative photon irradiation in a dose of 5500–6500 cGy in the presence of microscopic residual tumor provides a long-term local control rate of 80–85%. In order to apply a shrinking field technique to the involved compartment and to spare a longitudinal strip of normal skin, precisely shaped fields and immobilization are mandatory.

5. TREATMENT OF RECURRENT OR METASTATIC DISEASE. Isolated pulmonary metastases represent the initial pattern of recurrence in 50% of patients who have relapse. Although the timing of resection of pulmonary metastases and the integration of such surgery with chemotherapy remain controversial, patients treated with this combined approach have a long-term survival rate of 25–40%. Patients who have relapse with an isolated local recurrence should be considered for further operative therapy combined with chemotherapy and radiation. Tumor size is the major predictor of outcome following a local recurrence, though a full re-evaluation should be done to exclude disseminated disease.

Patients who develop widely disseminated sarcoma are treated with chemotherapy. The overall survival is 11 months, with responding patients surviving about 2 years. The most active agent is Adriamycin (50–60 mg/m^2 IV every 3–4 weeks) with an objective response rate of 15–35%. A dose high enough to produce moderate myelosuppression is necessary to achieve an optimal response. Drug combinations that decrease the dosage of Adriamycin have lower response rates than single-agent Adriamycin. DTIC (250 mg/m^2 IV qd × 4 d every 4 weeks) is the next most active drug, with an objective partial response rate of 15–20%. The combination of Adriamycin and DTIC appears to be moderately synergistic with an overall response rate of 45%. Ifosfamide (1.8–2.4 gm/m^2 IV qd × 5d given with mesna) produces a 25–30% response rate in recurrent sarcomas (J Clin Oncol 7:126, 1989).

Antman KH, Eilber FR, Shiu MHJ: Soft tissue sarcomas: Current trends in diagnosis and management. Curr Prob Cancer, Nov/Dec. 1989.
Baker LH, Frank J, Fine G et al: Combination chemotherapy using Adriamycin, DTIC, cyclophosphamide, and actinomycin D for advanced soft tissue sarcomas: a randomized comparative trial. J Clin Oncol 5:851–861, 1987.
Potter DA, Glenn J, Kinsella T, et al: Patterns of recurrence in patients with high-grade soft-tissue sarcomas. J Clin Oncol 3:353–366, 1985.

N. Head and Neck Cancer

Head and neck cancers afflict 42,000 Americans annually and occur 3 times as often in males as females. Each tumor site has a distinct natural history and epidemiology. Alcohol and tobacco abuse have additive carcinogenicity for squamous cell cancers, nickel exposure predisposes to sinus tumors, and Epstein-Barr virus infection, woodworking dust, and residence in southeastern China predispose to nasopharyngeal carcinomas. In general, tumors arising from the anterior head and neck region (lip or anterior tongue) are less aggressive than those arising posteriorly (nasopharynx, hypopharynx, or larynx). Prognosis also depends on tumor stage and differentiation as well as the presence of underlying medical conditions. The frequent occurrence of other medical problems, such as chronic obstructive pulmonary disease, coronary artery disease, and poor nutrition, places these patients at an increased risk for surgery and postoperative complications. As many as 15–30% have a synchronous primary tumor elsewhere in the aerodigestive tract.

1. **LOCALIZED TUMORS.** Either surgery or radiation therapy can be used as the sole treatment modality for small primary tumors (< 2 cm). When tumors are larger or have positive surgical margins or lymph node metastases, pre- or postoperative radiotherapy is commonly added to surgical resection. Although pre- and postoperative radiotherapy have never been compared in a randomized study, they appear equally effective. Adjunctive neck dissection or neck radiotherapy are performed when the risk of lymph node metastases is estimated to be over 15%.

2. **LOCALLY ADVANCED TUMORS.** 60% of patients have tumors too far advanced to allow surgical resection. Radiation therapy alone is curative in under 20% of these patients. In previously untreated epidermoid cancers, cisplatin and 5-fluorouracil (5-FU) regimens produce remissions in 60–90% of patients, but randomized trials have failed to show a survival advantage to adjuvant chemotherapy in this setting compared with radiation therapy alone. Several cooperative groups are currently investigating the possible utility of concurrent radiation and chemotherapy with radiosensitizing agents (e.g., 5-FU or cisplatin) and combined modality therapy with neoadjuvant chemotherapy followed by surgery and postoperative radiotherapy.

3. **METASTATIC DISEASE.** Many chemotherapeutic agents have been shown to have activity against disseminated head and neck cancers. Methotrexate alone produces tumor regression in 30% of patients for a median of 4–6 months. Combination chemotherapy regimens (especially those containing cisplatin and 5-FU), yield higher response rates (35–80%), but randomized trials have failed to demonstrate a survival advantage for the more aggressive chemotherapy regimens compared with methotrexate alone. Large tumor size, prior therapy, and poor performance status all adversely affect the response to chemotherapy.

4. SALIVARY GLAND CANCERS. 90% of parotid tumors and 75% of submandibular tumors are benign and can be treated effectively with surgical resection with or without postoperative irradiation. The most common malignant salivary gland neoplasms are mucoepidermoid and adenoid cystic carcinomas. Prognosis of these tumors depends on the tumor site, grade, stage, and effectiveness of local therapy. Surgical resection of the primary tumor and regional lymph nodes is the primary treatment modality, but adequate tumor margins are often difficult to obtain. Consequently, postoperative radiation therapy is commonly employed, especially for high-grade lesions. This approach is curative in 70–80% of patients. When metastases occur, they are most likely to involve the local region, lung, and bone. 5-FU and doxorubicin appear to be the most active chemotherapeutic agents for these tumors.

Jacobs CD, Goffinet DR, Fee WE: Head and neck squamous cancers. Curr Probl Cancer 14:1–72, 1990.

Snow JB: Surgical management of head and neck cancer. Semin Oncol 15:20–28, 1988.

Clark JR, Frei E: Chemotherapy for head and neck cancer: progress and controversy in the management of patients with MO disease. Semin Oncol 16 (suppl 6):44–57, 1989.

Al-Sarraf M: Head and neck cancer: chemotherapy concepts. Semin Oncol 15:70–85, 1988.

Dimery IW, Legha SS, Shirinian M, Hong WK: Fluorouracil, doxorubicin, cyclophosphamide, and cisplatin combination chemotherapy in advanced or recurrent salivary gland carcinoma. J Clin Oncol 8:1056–1062, 1990.

O. Esophageal Carcinoma. Esophageal carcinoma is responsible for 1.5% of all malignancies and occurs with an incidence of 3.5 cases/100,000 in the US. Tobacco and alcohol abuse are strong risk factors for squamous cell carcinoma of the esophagus, which is responsible for over 90% of esophageal cancers. Historically, surgery has been the primary therapeutic modality for esophageal carcinomas, but 5-year survival following esophagectomy is less than 5%, and operative mortality ranges from 5–20%. Patients with incompletely excised tumors should receive postoperative radiation therapy. The combination of chemotherapy and irradiation has been used to treat locally advanced or regionally inoperable esophageal cancer, and more recently as preoperative neoadjuvant therapy. Cisplatin and 5-FU administered concomitantly with radiation therapy achieves complete remissions in 25–60% of patients, but it is not clear that the overall survival with chemoradiotherapy is superior to that achieved with surgery alone. Palliative chemotherapy for widely metastatic disease utilizes one or more of the following agents: 5-FU, cisplatin, bleomycin, mitomycin C, and MTX. Responses lasting 4–6 months are seen in 20–40% of patients with metastatic disease.

Forastiere AA, Orringer MB, Perez-Tamayo C, et al: Concurrent chemotherapy and radiation therapy followed by transhiatal esophagectomy for local-regional cancer of the esophagus. J Clin Oncol 8:119–127, 1990.

Kelsen, D: Chemotherapy for local-regional and advanced esophageal cancer. Update for Principles and Practice of Oncology (DeVita VT, Hellman S, and Rosenberg SA, eds.) Philadelphia, JB Lippincott Co., 1988.

Coia LR: Esophageal Cancer: Is esophagectomy necessary? Oncology 3:101–110, 1989.

P. Stomach Cancer. Gastric adenocarcinomas occur with an incidence of 10 cases/100,000 people in the US, and typically cause vague abdominal distress, nausea, and dyspepsia. Surgical excision remains the only curative treatment for stomach cancer. Patients with large primary tumors, positive surgical margins, or positive regional lymph nodes may benefit from intraoperative or postoperative radiotherapy with or without concurrent 5-FU. In patients with tumors too advanced for definitive surgery, palliative surgery, radiation therapy, chemotherapy, or a combined-modality approach may be employed. Recently, a combination of 5-FU and methyl-CCNU in conjunction with radiation therapy has been shown to be superior to either modality alone for unresectable disease. 5-FU remains the most active drug for disseminated disease, producing tumor regression in 20–40% of patients for periods of 4–6 months. The addition of other chemotherapeutic agents such as doxorubicin, mitomycin C, and/or BCNU has not been shown to improve survival in randomized trials. The most promising new regimens consist of etoposide in combination with either doxorubicin and methotrexate or 5-FU and leucovorin. These two combinations have been reported to induce objective responses in 50–60% of patients with median survivals of 18 months and 11 months, respectively.

Wilke H, Preussner P, Fink U, et al: New developments in the treatment of gastric carcinoma. Semin Oncol 17 (suppl 2):61–70, 1990.
Douglass HO: Gastric cancer: current status of adjuvant therapy. Oncology 3:61–66, 1989.
Coombes RC, Schein PS, Chilvers CED, et al: A randomized trial comparing adjuvant fluorouracil, doxorubicin, and mitomycin with no treatment in operable gastric cancer. J Clin Oncol 8:1362–1369, 1990.

Q. Pancreatic Cancer. Pancreatic cancer affects 27,000 Americans each year and has an annual mortality rate of 10.4 per 100,000. Because of the paucity of early symptoms, less than 15% of patients with pancreatic cancer present with resectable tumors. Pancreaticoduodenectomy is the treatment of choice for the minority of patients with resectable disease, but it is associated with an operative mortality of 20%. Patients with tumors found to be unresectable at surgery should have a bypass procedure (e.g., gastroenterostomy and cholecystoenterostomy) as well as chemical splanchnicectomy with a neurolytic agent (e.g., 50% alchohol or 6% phenol) for palliation. Intraoperative radiation therapy allows delivery of a large single fraction of radiation locally and may improve local tumor control. Postoperative radiation therapy in conjunction with 5-FU as a radiosensitizer is commonly used adjunctively. Chemotherapy for disseminated disease usually involves 5-FU, with or without mitomycin C, streptozotocin, or doxorubicin. Tumor regression occurs in less than 30% of patients for 4–6 months. A review of 15,000 patients with pancreatic cancer has revealed a 5-year survival of only 0.4% with conventional therapy.

Beazley RM and Cohn I: Update on pancreatic cancer. CA 38:310–319, 1988.
Roldan GE, Gunderson LL, Nagorney DM, et al: External beam versus intraoperative and external beam irradiation for locally advanced pancreatic cancer. Cancer 61:1110–1116, 1988.
Harter KW and Dritschilo A: Cancer of the pancreas: are chemotherapy and radiation appropriate? Oncology 3:27–30, 1989.

Gastrointestinal Tumor Study Group: Further evidence of effective adjuvant combined radiation and chemotherapy following curative resection of pancreatic cancer. Cancer 59:2006–2010, 1987.

R. Colon Carcinoma. Adenocarcinoma of the colon is the second most common malignancy in the US, with 110,000 new cases annually. Potentially curative primary surgical resection (with lymph node sampling) is feasible in 75% of newly diagnosed patients. Approximately 65% of operated patients are cured by surgery, with the remainder developing metastatic disease, most commonly in the liver. Patients with tumor limited to the muscularis of the bowel wall (stage I) have an 80–90% cure rate with surgery alone, and adjuvant therapy is not indicated for this group. Patients with tumor involvement of the regional lymph nodes (stage III) are at high risk for recurrence. Adjuvant chemotherapy with 5-FU and levamisole in such patients has been shown to reduce the risk of relapse substantially and improve the 3-year survival from 55 to 71% (N Engl J Med 322:352–358, 1990). Whether adjuvant therapy will benefit stage II patients (with tumor invasion into the subserosa or invasion of adjacent organs without lymph node metastasis) is currently unknown. Postoperative radiation therapy may be beneficial for selected patients whose primary tumor extends to adjacent viscera, the bladder, the uterus, or the pelvic side wall (Cancer 57:955–963, 1986).

The prognosis with disseminated disease (stage IV) is related to the extent of tumor replacement within the liver as well as to elevations of carcinoembryonic antigen (CEA) and LDH. 5-FU is the most active drug for adenocarcinoma of the colon, producing objective tumor reduction in 20% of patients. Because the morbidity and mortality in colon cancer are due to hepatic metastases and since 95% of metastases derive their blood supply from the hepatic artery, regional therapy with either hepatic artery ligation or hepatic arterial chemotherapy has been tested (Ann Intern Med 107:459–465, 1987). Although these approaches are widely practiced, they have not been shown convincingly to confer a significant survival advantage over that achieved with systemic 5-FU (J Clin Oncol 8:1466–1475, 1990). Although the response rates and survival of patients with metastatic colon cancer have not been altered by the addition of other chemotherapeutic agents (including mitomycin C, BCNU, streptozotocin, and vincristine), recent data suggest the potentiation of 5-FU by folinic acid (leucovorin). Randomized trials comparing 5-FU with the combination of 5-FU with high-dose folinic acid have shown a significantly higher response rate (44 versus 13%) and longer survival (164 versus 120 days) for those patients treated with the combination (J Clin Oncol 8:491–501, 1990).

Minsky BD, Mies C, Rich TA, et al: Potentially curative surgery of colon cancer: patterns of failure and survival. J Clin Oncol 6:106–118, 1988.
Laurie JA, Moertel CG, Fleming TR, et al: Surgical adjuvant therapy of large-bowel carcinoma: an evaluation of levamisole and the combination of levamisole and fluorouracil. J Clin Oncol 7:1447–1456, 1989.
NIH Consensus Conference: Adjuvant therapy for patients with colon and rectal cancer. JAMA 264:1444–1450, 1990.

Poon MA, O'Connell, Moertel CG, et al: Biochemical modulation of fluorouracil: evidence of significant improvement of survival and quality of life in patients with advanced colorectal carcinoma. J Clin Oncol 7:1407–1418, 1989.

O'Connell MJ: Is portal-vein fluorouracil hepatic infusion effective colon cancer surgical adjuvant therapy? J Clin Oncol 8:1454–1456, 1990.

S. Rectal Cancer. Adenocarcinoma of the rectum occurs in 45,000 people per year in the US. The surgical and chemotherapeutic considerations for rectal cancer are similar to those for colon cancer, except that rectal cancer patients have a higher risk of local recurrence after resection (30–50%). Accordingly, *combined* postoperative chemotherapy (5-FU ± methyl-CCNU) and radiation therapy to the pelvis are recommended for patients with rectal tumors extending through the muscularis and deeper (stages II–III) because randomized studies have shown improved local control and survival compared with patients treated with either modality alone or with no adjuvant therapy (N Engl J Med 312:1465–1472, 1985). Although abdominoperineal resection has been the standard operation for rectal carcinomas, conservative sphincter-sparing surgery combined with adjuvant chemoradiotherapy appears adequate for small tumors (J Clin Oncol 7:988–990, 1989).

Willett CG, Tepper JE, Donnelly S, et al: Patterns of failure following local excision and local excision and postoperative radiation therapy for invasive rectal adenocarcinoma. J Clin Oncol 7:1003–1008, 1989.

O'Connell MJ, Gunderson LL, Fleming TR: Surgical adjuvant therapy of rectal cancer. Semin Oncol 15:138–145, 1988.

T. Anal Carcinoma. Epidermoid and cloacogenic carcinomas are responsible for 1–2% of large bowel cancers (approximately 1500 cases/year in the US) and occur with increased frequency in homosexual males, renal transplant patients, and patients with chronic anorectal irritation from anal fistulas, hemorrhoids, and condyloma. Small (< 2 cm) superficial tumors below the dentate line may be locally excised with a cure rate of 45–88%. Traditionally, larger tumors have been treated with anteroposterior (AP) resection and inguinal node dissection with a 55% long-term disease-free survival. Within the past decade, however, it has been possible to cure more than 80% with chemotherapy and irradiation. Chemotherapy includes a 5-day infusion of 5-FU, with or without a bolus of mitomycin C, administered concomitantly with external beam irradiation of the anus and inguinal nodes for 2 weeks. The cycle of chemotherapy and radiation therapy is repeated after a 1-week treatment break, to a total radiation dose of approximately 3000 cGy. Upon completion of chemoradiotherapy, many experts recommend a deep biopsy or local excision to confirm eradication of the tumor. Not only does this therapy spare the sphincter and avoid a permanent colostomy, but long-term survival appears superior to that with AP resection. Patients with disseminated disease may respond to chemotherapy programs containing cisplatin, bleomycin, 5-FU, mitomycin C, or MTX.

Mitchell EP: Carcinoma of the anal region. Semin Oncol 15:146–153, 1988.

Hussain M, Al-Sarraf M: Anal carcinomas: new combined modality treatment approaches. Oncology 2:42–48, 1988.

U. **Cancer of Unknown Primary Site (CUPS).** 5% of patients with cancer have disseminated disease without evidence of a primary tumor on physical examination, blood studies, urinalysis, or chest radiography. The most common presentations are abdominal masses/hepatomegaly (19–84%), lymphadenopathy (11–36%), and bone pain (6–28%). The location of metastases often provides a valuable clue to the primary site. Isolated cervical adenopathy is most commonly caused by occult head and neck cancer. A thorough examination by a head and neck surgeon (including panendoscopy under general anesthesia) should be done before node biopsy. Virchow's nodes (in the left supraclavicular fossa), Sister Mary Joseph's nodules (periumbilical nodes), and Blumer's shelf implants (in the rectovesical or rectouterine pouch) all strongly implicate an underlying GI malignancy. The presence of an abnormal axillary node most likely represents metastatic breast cancer in a woman, though lymphomas and melanomas also present in this manner. Supraclavicular nodes are common metastatic sites for occult lung and breast cancers, whereas inguinal nodes implicate tumors arising in the leg, perineum, prostate, or gonads. Liver metastases generally indicate a GI primary, particularly colon carcinoma.

Exhaustive diagnostic tests are often inappropriate in patients with CUPS. Diagnostic workup should be limited by the premise that the benefits of the established diagnosis should outweigh the expense, time, and risks sustained by the patient. Since only 10–15% of patients with CUPS have tumors responsive to current therapies, most patients will not benefit from an extensive diagnostic workup. The most valuable approach is a careful review of biopsied tumor tissue using histologic, immunocytochemical, electron microscopic, hormone receptor, and gene rearrangement techniques. Measurement of selected serologic tumor markers (e.g., prostate specific antigen, HCG, α-fetoprotein [AFP]) may also yield valuable information. The purpose of these analyses is to identify patients with tumors for which *effective* curative (lymphomas, germ cell tumors, and trophoblastic tumors) or palliative (breast, ovarian, prostatic, endometrial, and head and neck) therapy is available. If a primary tumor is identified, treatment is given accordingly.

If no primary tumor is identified, effective empiric therapy may still be available for certain subgroups. Squamous cell cancers in cervical nodes are curable in 30–50% of patients by wide-field radiation (encompassing primary sites within the head and neck as well as the bilateral neck nodes). Males younger than 50 with poorly differentiated carcinomas presenting in the mediastinum, retroperitoneum, or lymph nodes may have extragonadal germ cell tumors even if HCG and AFP levels are not elevated and should be treated with cisplatin plus etoposide (or vinblastine) with or without bleomycin (Ann Intern Med 104:547–553, 1986). Responses can be obtained in 56% of such patients (including 22% complete responses) and 13% will achieve long-term disease-free survival. Similarly, patients with poorly differentiated tumors with neuroendocrine features on electron microscopy or immunocytochemistry should be treated with cisplatin-based regimens since 72% will experience partial or complete remissions (Ann Intern Med 109:364–371, 1988). Women with peritoneal adenocarcinomas should be treated with cytoreductive surgery and cisplatin chemotherapy; approximately 40% will achieve a complete response with a median survival of 23 months (Ann Intern Med 111:213–217, 1989). Women with axillary adenocarcinomas should be treated for presumptive ipsilateral breast cancer with mastectomy, axillary dissection, irradiation, and adjuvant chemotherapy or hormonal therapy.

Other subgroups of patients have a bleak prognosis, with a median survival of 3–4 months. Empiric chemotherapy is commonly administered with various combinations of doxorubicin, mitomycin C, 5-FU, and cyclophosphamide, but response rates are low (0–30%) and no survival benefit has been demonstrated for this approach. Radiation therapy should be used for palliation of painful metastases and prophylactically for prevention of pathologic fractures from long bone metastases.

Greco AF, Hainsworth JD: The management of patients with adenocarcinoma and poorly differentiated carcinoma of unknown primary site. Semin Oncol 16 (suppl 6):116–122, 1989.

Silverman CL, Marks JE, Lee F, et al: Treatment of epidermoid and undifferentiated carcinomas from occult primaries presenting in cervical lymph nodes. Laryngoscope 93:645–648, 1983.

V. Testicular Cancer. Cancer of the testis affects 5500 males in the US each year and accounts for 1% of malignancies in men. Optimal management depends on the histology and stage (as determined by physical examination, CT scans, lymphangiography, and chest x-rays). Over 90% of testicular carcinomas are germ cell tumors (GCTs) occurring in men between the ages of 15 and 40. Two main types of GCTs are distinguished histologically: seminomas and nonseminomatous GCTs (including choriocarcinoma, embryonal tumors, and endodermal sinus tumors). Approximately 90% of nonseminomatous GCTs have an elevation of at least one tumor marker (α-fetoprotein or HCG) at presentation. Persistent elevations after therapy indicate residual tumor.

1. NONSEMINOMATOUS GERM CELL TUMORS (NSGCTs). Patients with tumors localized to the testis (stage I) have traditionally been treated by inguinal orchiectomy followed by retroperitoneal lymph node dissection (RLND) with surgical cure rates of 80–90%. Recently, the necessity of lymphadenectomy with its risk of infertility has been questioned, and many experts advise orchiectomy alone followed by close observation with monthly serum markers, chest x-rays every 1–2 months, and CT scans of the chest and abdomen every 2–3 months for 2 years (Semin Oncol 15:321–323, 1988; J Clin Oncol 8:4–8, 1990). Cisplatin-based chemotherapy is used to salvage the 25–30% of patients who have relapse during surveillance, and 90–100% of them are cured.

Patients with involvement of retroperitoneal lymph nodes (stage II) are treated with retroperitoneal lymph node dissection if the tumor burden is minimal or moderate (nodes < 5 cm) and with cisplatin-based chemotherapy if bulky nodes larger than 5 cm are present

(Semin Oncol 15:324–334, 1988). If a lymphadenectomy is performed and microscopic disease is identified, two cycles of chemotherapy should be given.

Patients with bulky stage II or Stage III (supradiaphragmatic or extranodal) disease should be treated with cisplatin (20 mg/m² IV qd × 5 days) and etoposide (100 mg/m² qd × 5 days) with or without bleomycin (30 U/week IV) every 3 weeks for 3–4 cycles (J Clin Oncol 7:387–391, 1989). Side effects of chemotherapy include nausea, vomiting, myalgias, alopecia, mucositis, paresthesias, and chronic Raynaud's phenomenon. Durable complete remissions can be obtained in more than 70% of patients with disseminated disease with this regimen. Some patients have persistence of radiographic abnormalities after completion of combination chemotherapy. Resection of these masses reveals necrosis and fibrosis in 40% of cases, adult teratoma in 40%, and residual NSGCT in 20%. Patients having necrosis or teratoma are usually cured with surgery alone, but those with cancer remaining should receive 2 additional cycles of chemotherapy. Patients with refractory disease are treated with regimens containing ifosfamide, vinblastine, double-dose cisplatin, carboplatin, or marrow transplantation (J Clin Oncol 7:932–939, 1989).

Overall, 95–100% of patients with stage I–II and 80% of stage III NSGCTs are cured with modern therapy.

2. **SEMINOMAS.** Pure seminomas account for 30–40% of GCTs and are extremely radiosensitive. Stage I–II seminomas are treated with orchiectomy and retroperitoneal radiation therapy (≥ 3000 cGy) with cure rates of 97% in stage I and more than 80% in stage II. Disseminated seminoma is treated with cisplatin based chemotherapy as described, with cure rates of about 85% (Ann Intern Med 108:513–518, 1988).

Einhorn LH: Complicated problems in testicular cancer. Semin Oncol 15 (suppl 3):9–15, 1988.

Fung CY, Garnick MB: Clinical stage I carcinoma of the testis: a review. J Clin Oncol 6:734–750, 1988.

Williams SD, Loehrer PJ, Nichols CR, et al: Disseminated testicular cancer: current chemotherapy strategies. Semin Oncol 16 (suppl 6):105–109, 1989.

Ozols RF, Ihde DC, Linehan WM, Young RC: Management of high risk patients with advanced testis cancer: National Cancer Institute Approach. Semin Oncol 15:335–338, 1988.

Mason BR and Kearsley JH: Radiotherapy for stage 2 testicular seminoma: the prognostic influence of tumor bulk. J Clin Oncol 6:1856–1862, 1988.

W. Prostate Cancer. Prostate cancer is the second most common malignancy in men with an incidence of 58/100,000 white men and 95/100,000 black men. Presenting complaints include symptoms of urethral obstruction, hematuria, urinary tract infection, and bone pain. 10% of patients have localized tumors discovered incidentally after transurethral prostatectomy (stage A), 15–20% have palpable nodules (stage B), 40% have regional extension to periprostatic tissues (stage C), and 30–35% have metastases to lymph nodes (stage D1) or distant sites (stage D2).

1. **LOCALIZED TUMORS.** Well-differentiated, focal, asymptomatic tumors discovered incidentally after transurethral prostatectomy (stage

A1) may be followed with observation alone since only 2% will progress within 4 years. Patients with more extensive or poorly differentiated adenocarcinoma discovered at transurethral prostatectomy (stage A2) or with palpable prostatic nodules (stage B) may be treated with either radical prostatectomy, interstitial irradiation, or external beam radiation therapy with comparable 10-year survival rates of 55–75%. Prostatectomy has been associated with a high incidence of impotence, but newer nerve-sparing operations now preserve potency in approximately 70% of men. Impotence rates after irradiation are 30–50%, with urinary incontinence rates of 5–10%.

2. **REGIONAL DISEASE.** Patients with extracapsular extension of tumor to the seminal vesicles or regional lymph nodes are best treated with external beam radiation therapy. The combination of surgery and radiation therapy results in an unacceptable incidence of leg, penile, and scrotal edema. The 10-year survival with conventional radiotherapy techniques is 30–40% for stage C and 10–20% for stage D1. Recent studies with fast neutron beam radiotherapy suggest the superiority of neutrons compared with conventional photon therapy (63 versus 18% survival at 8 years) for stages C and D1 (Semin Oncol 15:359–365, 1988).

3. **METASTATIC DISEASE.** 85% of patients with disseminated prostate cancer (stage D2) experience tumor regression following a hormonal manipulation with bilateral orchiectomy, diethylstilbesterol (DES), or luteinizing hormone–releasing hormone (LHRH) analogues. Responses to hormonal manipulation are rapid and effective for a median of 12–18 months. All treatments result in impotence; therefore, choice of therapy is dictated by other side effects. Administration of DES may result in gynecomastia, hypertension, phlebitis, acute myocardial infarction, and cerebrovascular accidents. Because higher doses fail to have an impact on survival owing to cardiovascular complications, a dose of 1 mg tid is recommended. Gynecomastia may be prevented by irradiating the breasts before institution of DES therapy. The LHRH analogue leuprolide has been compared with DES in prospective, randomized trials, with similar response and survival rates (Semin Oncol 15:366–370, 1988). The LHRH analogues are expensive and require daily subcutaneous injection. The addition of antiandrogens such as flutamide to LHRH agonists has been shown in some studies to improve progression-free survival (16.5 versus 13.9 months) and overall survival (35.6 versus 28.3 months) compared with leuprolide alone (N Engl J Med 321:419–424, 1989).

In patients with progressive disease after an initial response to hormones, second-line hormonal therapy is rarely effective. These patients are then candidates for chemotherapy with cyclophosphamide, doxorubicin, MTX, cisplatin, and/or 5-FU. Unfortunately, neither response rates nor duration of response have been convincingly improved with combination chemotherapy. Recently, bone-seeking radioactive samarium chelates have been shown to achieve significant palliation in patients with painful bony metastases unresponsive to other manipulations.

Livingston RB, Bartolucci AA, Becker JA, et al: The management of clinically localized prostate cancer. JAMA 258:2727–2730, 1987.

Walsh PC, Lepor H: The role of radical prostatectomy in the management of prostatic cancer. Cancer 60:526–537, 1987.

Bagshaw MA, Ray GR, Cox RS: Selecting initial therapy of prostate cancer. Radiation Therapy Perspective. Cancer 60:521–525, 1987.

Grayhack JT, Keeler TC, Kozlowski JM: Carcinoma of the prostate. Hormonal therapy. Cancer 60:589–601, 1987.

Raghavan D: Non-hormone chemotherapy for prostate cancer: principles of treatment and application to the testing of new drugs. Semin Oncol 15:371–389, 1988.

12 12 12 12 12 12 12 12 12

ENDOCRINOLOGIC AND RELATED METABOLIC DISORDERS

EDWARD A. BENSON and NORMAN R. ROSENTHAL

I. HYPOTHALAMIC-PITUITARY DISORDERS

A. **General Principles.** The release of the anterior pituitary hormones thyroid-stimulating hormone (TSH), corticotropin (ACTH), luteinizing hormone (LH), follicle-stimulating hormone (FSH), prolactin, and growth hormone is regulated by "releasing" and "inhibiting" hormones produced in the hypothalamus and reaching the pituitary via the hypo-thalamic-pituitary portal venous system. The posterior pituitary stores oxytocin and vasopressin in preparation for release into the general circulation. The hypothalamus and pituitary form an integrated axis that maintains control over much of the endocrine system. Disorders of the hypothalamic-pituitary axis are usually clinically manifested by either syndromes of hormone excess or deficiency or by visual impairment from optic nerve compression. Treatment of pituitary tumors usually includes measures to correct hormone imbalance and reduce tumor mass. Expanding lesions in the pituitary typically cause pituitary hormones to "drop out" in a predictable sequence of growth hormone and gonado-tropins early and ACTH and TSH late. Lesions originating in the pituitary do not cause ADH deficiency (diabetes insipidus) unless the destructive process extends into the hypothalamus.

Deficiencies of ACTH, LH, FSH, and TSH are treated by replacing target organ hormones, i.e., corticosteroids, sex steroids, and thyroid hormone. Glucocorticoid and thyroid hormone replacement are indicated in all patients with hypopituitarism since untreated adrenal insufficiency and hypothyroidism are potentially life-threatening. Replacement of sex steroids improves sexual function and well-being and is indicated in all but the very elderly. Diabetes insipidus, although not life-threatening, causes bothersome polyuria and polydipsia, which can be easily treated. Treatment of growth hormone deficiency is necessary only in children and adolescents.

B. **Treatment of Hypopituitarism**

1. **ACTH Deficiency (Adrenal Insufficiency). Prednisone**, 7.5 mg/day (5 mg in A.M., 2.5 mg in P.M.) or **hydrocortisone**, 30 mg/day (20 mg in A.M., 10 mg in P.M.) provides physiologic replacement of glucocorticoid for most patients. Adequacy of glucocorticoid replacement is indicated by restoration of the patient's sense of well-being, appetite, and weight. Excessive glucocorticoid replacement is indicated by the development of cushingoid features (e.g., rounded face, thin skin, hypertension). Orthostatic hypotension despite glucocorticoid replacement may signify a need for mineralocorticoid. **Fludrocortisone** (Florinef) is usually given as a single daily dose of 0.05–0.3 mg. Hypertension, hypokalemia, edema, or congestive heart failure are indications for a dose reduction.

At the first sign of illness (including minor infections such as gastroenteritis and febrile viral syndromes) patients should double their maintenance dose of glucocorticoid. If vomiting precludes the use of oral medication, arrangements must be made immediately for parenteral administration of corticosteroids. Patients should wear a bracelet or necklace identifying themselves as having hypopituitarism. An injectable form of glucocorticoid (dexamethasone phosphate, 4 mg) for self-injection should be available whenever the patient will be out of reach of medical care for more than a day. Patients with hypopituitarism require coverage with "stress" doses of glucocorticoids during serious illness or surgery.

2. **HYPOTHYROIDISM.** Treatment of hypothyroidism due to TSH deficiency consists of L-thyroxine in appropriate doses. The usual dose is 1.5–1.7 μg/kg body weight. The dose should be adjusted to maintain the patient's free thyroxine index in the midnormal range.

3. **GONADOTROPIN DEFICIENCY–MEN.** In men, gonadotropin deficiency causes testosterone deficiency with accompanying impotence and/or infertility, whereas in boys, delayed puberty or short stature may be the result. Testosterone deficiency can also lead to loss of muscle tone and osteoporosis. This deficiency is treated with a long-acting testosterone preparation such as testosterone enanthate given by IM injection. The frequency of administration must be tailored to the individual, a typical regimen being 200 mg testosterone enanthate IM every 3–4 weeks. The frequency of injections should be adjusted to avoid periods of symptomatic hypogonadism. Since testosterone can stimulate the prostate, careful examination of the prostate is performed to rule out cancer or benign hypertrophy before treatment is initiated.

4. **GONADOTROPIN DEFICIENCY–WOMEN.** In women, gonadotropin deficiency may cause estrogen deficiency symptoms including infertility, amenorrhea, vaginal mucosal atrophy, hot flashes, and breast atrophy. Treatment depends on whether or not fertility is being sought. If fertility is the goal of treatment, gonadotropins can be used in an attempt to induce ovulation. If fertility is not an issue, hypogonadism is treated with estrogens.

C. **Treatment of the Nonfunctioning Pituitary Adenoma.** Clinically silent tumors, i.e., those that produce no neurologic symptoms or endocrine deficiencies, grow slowly, if at all. A reasonable approach to a patient with an incidentally discovered tumor who has normal pituitary function and visual fields is to withhold treatment unless serial measurements of visual fields or tumor size (measured by periodic CT or MRI scanning) indicate tumor enlargement or pituitary hormone deficiency develops. Treatment consists of surgery and/or external irradiation. Surgery is generally recommended for large tumors with suprasellar extension and/or optic nerve compression. External irradiation is given after surgery if removal is incomplete or if the tumor recurs. External irradiation as primary therapy is appropriate for intrasellar tumors that present no immediate threat to surrounding structures. Irradiation usually consists of 4,000 to 5,000 cGy delivered over 4–6 weeks.

D. Treatment of Hormone-Producing Pituitary Tumors

1. **ACROMEGALY.** This is a chronic disease associated with diminished life expectancy. Treatment designed to reduce growth hormone level produces improvement in cardiac function and hypertension. **Transsphenoidal adenomectomy** will initially normalize growth hormone concentration in up to 75% of cases, but in many late relapse occurs. **External pituitary irradiation** is a reasonable choice as primary therapy in patients with mild acromegaly whose tumors are confined to the sella turcica. Mean growth hormone concentration may be expected to fall by about 50% at 5 years after treatment, with 70% of patients attaining a normal growth hormone level by 10 years. For large tumors, external irradiation is often given after surgery. **Bromocriptine** in doses up to 20 mg/day may be of use in the treatment of acromegaly. Although the majority of patients will describe a clinical improvement, only 20–50% will show significant biochemical response.

2. **CUSHING'S DISEASE. Transsphenoidal adenomectomy** or **hypophysectomy** is the treatment of choice for most patients with Cushing's disease. In the hands of an experienced neurosurgeon, pituitary microsurgery is successful in nearly 80% of patients with a microadenoma. The outcome is less favorable for patients with a macroadenoma (tumors > 1 cm in diameter), of whom less than 50% are cured with surgery. Preoperative localization of the pituitary tumor will usually reduce the extent of surgery and thus lessen the likelihood of hypopituitarism from extensive pituitary resection.

   Patients undergoing pituitary surgery require **glucocorticoid coverage** in stress doses, both intra- and postoperatively. Glucocorticoid coverage is usually tapered to physiologic replacement doses over 5–7 days after surgery. After successful adenomectomy, glucocorticoid replacement therapy is often needed for 6–12 months as the remaining pituitary gradually recovers its homeostatic ability to produce ACTH. Pituitary irradiation is most effective in children. The remission rate in children is 70–80%, but there is a lag between treatment and remission of 12–18 months. Remission rates in adults are lower; approximately 50% have a successful response a year after irradiation therapy. Irradiation may be useful as adjunctive therapy for patients not cured by surgery.

3. **PROLACTIN-PRODUCING PITUITARY TUMORS.** The most common functioning pituitary tumor is the **prolactinoma**. Women characteristically have amenorrhea, galactorrhea, and/or infertility. In men, erectile dysfunction and loss of libido can occur. Most prolactinomas are benign microadenomas (<1 cm) and less than 10% of microadenomas will grow over time. Macroadenomas (>1 cm) can cause mass-related symptoms. The decision whether to treat a prolactinoma depends on several factors, including tumor size, the patient's symptoms and age, and the option of fertility. Therapy for microadenomas is directed at restoring gonadal function and reducing galactorrhea. Hyperprolactinemic women over childbearing age might not need

treatment. Suprasellar extension and associated neurologic symptoms are common in macroadenomas, and strategies for therapeutic intervention must consider the growth potential of this tumor.

The treatment choices are surgery, irradiation, or bromocriptine. Successful **transsphenoidal removal** of the microadenoma with preservation of normal pituitary function is achieved in up to 90% of selected patients. External **irradiation therapy** will arrest tumor growth but does not generally normalize prolactin levels or restore menses. The treatment of choice is the dopamine agonist **bromocriptine**. Doses of 2.5–15 mg/day will rapidly suppress prolactin secretion, restoring menses in about 95%. Bromocriptine often produces nausea and lightheadedness and should be initiated gradually with a dose of 1.25 mg (½ tablet) at night with a snack, then 1.25 mg tid, gradually increasing the dose until prolactin level is normalized or menses restored.

Large prolactinomas, even those with suprasellar extension, can be effectively treated with bromocriptine in 70%. Surgical resection or debulking may also be necessary.

When the goal of treatment is to restore fertility, the potential effect of pregnancy on tumor growth must be considered in selecting therapy. Pregnancy is associated with pituitary enlargement due to expansion of pituitary lactotrophs. In a woman with a prolactinoma, expansion of the tumor and/or normal pituitary may compress the optic nerves resulting in visual impairment. The risk appears to be quite small for microadenomas but is of greater concern for macroadenomas. Some authorities recommend surgical extirpation of macroadenomas if pregnancy is the goal of therapy. Although bromocriptine has been used successfully to restore fertility, it has not yet received FDA approval for this indication. If bromocriptine therapy is used to restore fertility, the drug should be discontinued once pregnancy is established.

E. Diabetes Insipidus

1. **GENERAL PRACTICES.** Diabetes insipidus (DI) results from a deficiency of, or resistance to, antidiuretic hormone (ADH). In the absence of ADH, urine volumes may exceed 6 liters a day, making it difficult to maintain water balance by increased fluid intake. Approximately half of patients will have a neoplasm or infiltrative disease of the hypothalamus with the remainder labeled as having "idiopathic" diabetes insipidus.

2. **TREATMENT.** In patients with partial DI, a normal thirst mechanism and free access to water will usually allow maintenance of normal hydration. For those in whom the polyuria, polydipsia, and nocturia are troublesome, several agents are available.

   a. **DDAVP.** Desamino-D-arginine vasopressin (DDAVP), a synthetic analogue of human antidiuretic hormone, is the drug of choice for most patients. It is administered by instillation into the posterior nasal cavity by a nasal spray. The dose is 0.1–0.4 mL at a frequency based on duration of antidiuresis. For some patients, a single administration provides 24-hour antidiuresis, but for most, twice daily dosing is necessary. For patients unable to use the nasal route, DDAVP can be given parenterally in a dose of 2–4 μg SQ or IV.

b. Pitressin. Pitressin tannate in oil given IM provides long-acting (24–72 hour) antidiuresis. Because of vasopressor effects, it may cause headache, increased blood pressure, exacerbation of angina, or uterine cramps. A single dose of 5–10 U will usually provide a 24–72 hour effect. Vigorous shaking of the vial is required to ensure that the active ingredient is adequately suspended.

c. Chlorpropamide. This potentiates the effect of ADH at the renal tubule and, in patients with partial DI, may provide satisfactory relief of symptoms. Chlorpropamide is given once a day in a dose of 100–500 mg. Hypoglycemia may occur, especially at higher doses.

Andreoli TE: The posterior pituitary. *In* Wyngaarden JB, Smith LH (eds): Cecil's Textbook of Medicine. Philadelphia, WB Saunders Co., 1985, pp. 1266–1272.
Besser GM, Wass JAH, Thorner MO: Bromocriptine in the medical management of acromegaly. Adv Biochem 23:191–198, 1980.
Frohman LA: The anterior pituitary. *In* Wyngaarden JB, Smith LH (eds): Cecil's Textbook of Medicine. Philadelphia, WB Saunders Co., 1985, pp. 1251–1265.
Lamberts SWJ, Uitterlinden P, Verschoor MD, et al: Long-term treatment of acromegaly with the somatostatin analogue SMS 201–995. N Engl J Med 313:1576–80, 1985.
March CM, Kletzky OA, Davajan V, et al: Longitudinal evaluation of patients with untreated prolactin-secreting adenomas. Am J Obstet Gynecol 139:835–843, 1981.
Melmed S: Acromegaly. N Engl J Med 322:966–977, 1990.
Schlechte J, Dolan K, Sherman B, et al: The natural history of untreated hyperprolactinemia: A prospective analysis. J Clin Endo Metab 68:412–418, 1989.
Vance ML, Evans WS, Thorner MO: Bromocriptine. Ann Intern Med 100:78–91, 1984.
Wollesen F, Anderson T, Karle A: Size reduction of extrasellar pituitary tumors during bromocriptine treatment. Ann Intern Med 96:281–286, 1982.

II. TREATMENT OF THYROID DISORDERS

A. Hyperthyroidism

1. **GENERAL PRINCIPLES.** Several disorders of the thyroid can cause hyperthyroidism. In Graves' disease, toxic multinodular goiter, and toxic adenoma, overproduction of thyroid hormone occurs. Treatment is aimed at suppressing the overactive gland. The hyperthyroidism of thyroiditis results from uncontrolled release of hormone from the gland. Treatment of thyroiditis is directed toward ameliorating symptoms while waiting for the hyperthyroidism to subside. There are three means of treating an overactive thyroid: **thionamide medication, radioactive iodine, or thyroid surgery**. The thionamides (propylthiouracil and methimazole) are concentrated in the thyroid and interfere with the synthesis of thyroid hormone. Thionamides effectively lower hormone levels but usually do not cure the hyperthyroidism. Radioactive iodine (RAI) or surgery are usually required for definitive treatment. Since RAI accomplishes the same objective as surgery (i.e., ablating an overactive thyroid gland) but without the risks of anesthesia and surgery, it is preferred for most patients. Thyroidec-

tomy is usually reserved for pregnant patients (in whom RAI is contraindicated) who are allergic to antithyroid medication or as definitive therapy for those who refuse RAI.

2. **TREATMENT**

   a. **Thionamides.** The thionamides **propylthiouracil** (PTU) and **methimazole** inhibit thyroxine synthesis by blocking the organification of iodide. In addition, PTU (but not methimazole) partially blocks the peripheral conversion of thyroxine (T_4) to the more metabolically active tri-iodothyronine (T_3). In patients with Graves' disease, thionamides are usually given for 6 to 18 months, then withdrawn to determine whether a remission has occurred. About a third of selected patients will remain euthyroid in long-term remission after a course of thionamides. Patients with mild hyperthyroidism and small goiters are more likely to enter remission.

   The **starting dose of propylthiouracil is 100–200 mg tid or methimazole 5–15 mg tid.** Thyroid function tests should be measured monthly to determine the appropriate maintenance dose. Eventually patients can usually be treated with once or twice daily administration of PTU or methimizole.

   Thionamides have several potential side effects. A maculopapular rash occurs in 2–8% of patients. Rarely, thionamides cause cholestasis and PTU can cause vasculitis. The most serious adverse reaction of thionamides is **agranulocytosis**, a complication seen in approximately 0.5% of patients. Patients should be instructed to report fever, sore throat, or infection. In this situation medication should be witheld until the patient's white blood cell count is known.

   b. **Radioactive Iodine.** RIA is concentrated in the thyroid where radiation causes injury to thyroid cells, rendering some or all incapable of continued hormone production. The result of radiation-induced injury to the thyroid is progressive atrophy and fibrosis, in many cases resulting in hypothyroidism. 20 to 50% of patients treated with RAI become hypothyroid within a year and another 2–3% annually thereafter. At the commonly used doses of RAI (i.e., 5–10 mCi) 80–95% of patients are cured of hyperthyroidism with one dose, usually within 2–4 months. Patients advised to have RAI therapy are often concerned about the potential harmful effects of irradiation. Several studies show no increase in incidence of malignancy or genetic defects in offspring of patients followed for decades after RAI therapy.

   c. **Beta-Adrenergic Blockers.** Several manifestations of hyperthyroidism appear to be due to increased sensitivity to circulating catecholamines. Beta-adrenergic blocking agents are effective in reducing palpitations, tremulousness, nervousness, and tachycardia. **Propranolol**, 40–200 mg/day in divided doses, or **atenolol**, 50–200 mg/day, will ameliorate these symptoms as other steps are taken to treat the underlying thyroid overactivity.

   d. **Oral Cholecystographic Agents.** Certain radiologic contrast agents used for gallbladder imaging inhibit the conversion of T_4 to the more active T_3, and the iodide contained in these agents also blocks all steps of thyroid hormonogenesis. Their rapid onset can be valuable when prompt control of hyperthyroidism is desired. Sodium ipodate (Oragrafin) or iopanoic acid (Telepaque), 1 gm/day or 3 gm every 3 days, produce a dramatic fall in serum T_3 concentration within 48 hours. These agents contain iodide, and their use precludes RAI for a period of several weeks or months. If used in conjunction with a thionamide, these agents are usually given for the first 2 or 3 weeks of therapy, while waiting for the thionamides to take effect.

e. **Overview.** RAI is preferred treatment for most patients with hyperthyroidism. Patients are often treated initially with thionamides since it usually takes 2–4 months to control hyperthyroidism with RAI. If thionamides are used in preparation for treatment with RAI, they should be discontinued for at least a week before RAI is given and, if necessary, resumed a week or more after. For patients with Graves' disease and small goiter, thionamide treatment for 6–12 months is a reasonable alternative to initial treatment with RAI. If hyperthyroidism recurs after thionamide treatment, RAI should be recommended since additional treatment with a thionamide is unlikely to induce a remission. Surgery is usually reserved for large multinodular goiters, pregnant patients who are not able to take thionamides, and patients who decline RAI.

3. **THYROIDITIS.** In subacute or silent thyroiditis there is generalized inflammation of the gland and "leakage" of stored thyroid hormone, usually enough to cause hyperthyroidism. Duration of hyperthyroidism is usually less than 3 months; the symptoms usually mild. Transient hypothyroidism may follow subacute thyroiditis and may be severe enough to require treatment for 3–6 months by which time thyroid function has usually returned to normal.

Treatment is directed toward relieving symptoms rather than suppressing thyroid function. **Beta-blocking agents** are useful for control of tachycardia, palpitations, nervousness, and tremor. **Aspirin**, 2–4 gm per day, is usually effective in treating the pain of subacute thyroiditis. When aspirin fails to provide relief, a short course of prednisone (40 mg/day) is nearly always effective.

4. **SPECIAL CIRCUMSTANCES**

a. **Ophthalmopathy.** The ophthalmopathy of Graves' disease is highly variable in severity and course. Minor symptoms of conjunctival irritation or periorbital edema are treated symptomatically with eye drops and elevating the head of the bed. In the most severe cases, vision may be threatened by ulceration or infection of the cornea or by pressure on the optic nerve. Prednisone (80–120 mg/day) is usually the first measure used in the treatment of severe ophthalmopathy. In patients in whom steroids fail, external orbital irradiation or orbital decompression may be indicated.

b. **Pregnancy.** RAI is contraindicated in pregnant women because of potential harm to the fetal thyroid. PTU is used in preference to methimazole in pregnancy because more of the latter crosses the placenta and is associated with the minor congenital anomaly aplasia cutis. The dose of PTU should be carefully titrated to maintain thyroid hormone levels in the upper normal range. Monthly or more frequent testing of thyroid function is required to ensure that hormone levels are in the upper-normal range, thereby preventing fetal hypothyroidism as a complication of treatment. PTU may be used by breast-feeding mothers. Although present in breast milk, the amount of PTU passed to the infant is insignificant at doses of 300 mg/day or less.

c. **Thyroid Storm.** This is a syndrome of multisystem malfunction and fever resulting from severe hyperthyroidism. In thyroid storm the usual symptoms and signs of hyperthyroidism are grossly exaggerated, the patient seemingly "burning up" with unutilizable energy. The temperature is usually over 38°C; supraventricular tachycardia or atrial fibrillation is usually present and may be associated with high-output cardiac failure. Nausea, vomiting, diarrhea, and jaundice are common GI manifestations. Mental status may be unaffected in the early stages, but agitation, delirium, and coma may occur later. General supportive measures include cooling blankets and acetaminophen for fever (aspirin is contraindicated because it displaces T_4 from thyroid-binding globulin, thereby increasing the proportion of free hormone); digitalis and diuretics for heart failure; sedatives for the management of hyperkinesis and agitation and specific drugs for hyperthyroidism (Table 12–1). These act by several independent mechanisms to lower the concentration, or mitigate the effects, of thyroid hormones and are usually used in combination for **rapid control** of thyroid storm.

B. Hypothyroidism

1. **GENERAL PRINCIPLES.** Defects in the thyroid, pituitary, or hypothalamus can produce hypothyroidism. The most common causes of

TABLE 12–1. DRUGS USED IN TREATMENT OF THYROID STORM

DRUG	DOSAGE
Propylthiouracil (PTU)	200–400 mg q 6 h PO or by NG tube
Iodide	PO: supersaturated potassium iodide (SSKI) 5 drops × 3 times/day
	IV: Sodium iodide, 1 gm IV infusion over 12 hr, q 12 h
Propranolol*	PO: 20–120 mg q 4–8 h
	IV: 1 mg/min to a total dose of 2–10 mg q 3–4 h
Dexamethasone	2 mg PO, IM, or IV q 6 h
Sodium ipodate	1 gm/day PO

*Reserpine, 1–2.5 mg IM q 4–6 h, may be substituted in patients with asthma or congestive heart failure.

hypothyroidism are Hashimoto's thyroiditis and previous surgery or radioiodine for treatment of hyperthyroidism. Hypothyroidism due to TSH deficiency occurs as a relatively late manifestation of destructive lesions of the pituitary.

2. **TREATMENT.** The treatment of hypothyroidism is straightforward and effective. **L-thyroxine (T₄)** (Synthroid, Levothroid) is the agent of choice. Because bioavailability may vary between manufacturers, the use of generic thyroxine is not recommended. The dosage of T_4 is **1.5–1.7 μg/kg body weight/day. Thus for a 75-kg patient, 100–125 μg is a reasonable starting dosage.** A reduction of 25–50 μg might be necessary for elderly and chronically ill patients of comparable weight. Thyroid replacement therapy is best monitored by following the patient's TSH level, which should be maintained in the normal range. Treatment is begun with full replacement doses except for patients with coronary artery disease, who are usually started on lower dosages, 50 μg of L-thyroxine per day, because of the possibility of angina or cardiac arrhythmias. The dose can then be raised by 25–50 μg/day every 2 weeks.

3. **SPECIAL CIRCUMSTANCES**

   a. **Coronary Artery Disease and Hypothyroidism.** The coexistence of coronary artery disease and hypothyroidism is a difficult therapeutic problem since treatment of hypothyroidism increases myocardial oxygen demands. Angina may be exacerbated even with subtherapeutic doses of thyroxine. A trial of propranolol with small increments of thyroxine may allow gradual restoration of euthyroidism without provoking increased angina. In some cases, coronary artery bypass surgery may be required to allow return to a euthyroid state.

   b. **Myxedema Coma.** Untreated, hypothyroidism can progress to myxedema coma, a state of deeply depressed metabolic activity characterized by hypothermia, bradycardia, hypoventilation, coma, and ultimately death. Measures to support circulation, ventilation, and temperature as well as thyroid hormone replacement comprise the essential foundation for treatment.

      (1). Hypotension. Severely myxedematous patients usually have diminished plasma volume requiring volume expansion with isotonic saline guided by central venous pressure monitoring. α-Adrenergic agents should be avoided.

      (2). Ventilation. Although the respiratory failure may be insidious, emergency treatment may be necessary. Enlargement of the tongue, which may be associated with long-standing hypothyroidism, can lead to obstruction of the upper airway. Arterial blood gases indicating hypoventilation (i.e., a P_{CO_2} of more than 45–50 mm Hg) or upper airway obstruction by an enlarged tongue require immediate placement of an endotracheal tube and assisted ventilation.

      (3). Thyroid Hormone Replacement is urgent and takes precedence over concerns of precipitating cardiac arrhythmias or

ischemia. Thyroid hormone should be given IV, *0.3 mg of l-thyroxine* initially, with subsequent daily doses of 0.05–0.2 mg IV until the patient is stable and capable of taking oral medication. Some improvement should be apparent within 6 to 12 hours.

(4). Adrenocorticoid Administration. Glucocorticoids should be administered (100 mg of hydrocortisone IV q 8 h) and tapered gradually over a period of 10 days to 2 weeks.

C. Palpable Abnormalities of the Thyroid

1. **SOLITARY THYROID NODULE.** A palpable thyroid nodule is present in about 1–3% of the population. The low incidence (3–4%) of malignancy and relative benign behavior of the most thyroid cancers argues for a conservative approach to the evaluation of the solitary thyroid nodule. A palpable nodule in a patient with a childhood history of head or neck irradiation should be considered for removal because the risk of malignancy is significantly increased. For other patients, the most cost-effective, accurate, and direct means of differentiating malignant from benign nodules is by fine needle aspiration biopsy. Patients with benign cytology should be examined every 6–12 months for changes in size or shape of the nodule. Any increase in the size of the nodule should reopen the question of malignancy even if the biopsy result was negative. Recent evidence suggests that short-term exogenous thyroxine has no significant effect on the growth of thyroid nodules.

If the biopsy shows malignant cells, surgery is indicated. The usual procedure is a subtotal thyroidectomy, with resection of the involved lobe, isthmus, and most of the opposite lobe, being careful not to damage the parathyroids or recurrent laryngeal nerve. On the day after surgery, l-triiodothyronine (T$_3$, Cytomel) 25 mg tid is started. 6–8 weeks after surgery, Cytomel is stopped. 2 weeks later, the patient is treated with 30–100 mCi of I^{131}, which will ablate remaining thyroid tissue in 80% of patients. A follow-up RAI uptake and scan are done a year later, and patients with persistent RAI uptake are retreated with I^{131}. Lifelong treatment with thyroid hormone replacement is mandatory.

2. **NONTOXIC GOITER.** A small diffuse, nontoxic goiter in a young person may remain small and asymptomatic, may evolve into a multinodular goiter, or may become hypofunctional. Measurement of TSH can help to determine appropriate therapy, since even a slight elevation may contribute to gland growth or indicate mild thyroid insufficiency. In either case, thyroxine therapy may prevent the progression to clinical thyroid disease.

If the TSH is normal, a small (i.e., nonvisible) goiter may be simply followed with serial measurements of gland size. For a large or enlarging goiter, treatment with thyroxine and regular follow-up is recommended.

Blum M: Myxedema Coma. Am J Med Sci 264:432, 1972.
Gharib H, James EM, Charboneau JW, et al: Suppressive therapy with levothyroxine for solitary thyroid nodules: a double-blind controlled clinical study. N Engl J Med 317:70–75, 1987.

Hennemann G, Krenning EP, Sankaranarayanan K: Place of radioactive iodine in treatment of thyrotoxicosis. Lancet 1369–1371, 1986.

Helfand M, Crapo LM: Monitoring therapy in patients taking levothyroxine. Ann Intern Med 113:450–454, 1990.

Ingbar SH: The thyroid gland. *In* Wilson JD, Foster DW (ed): Williams Textbook of Endocrinology. 7th ed. Philadelphia, WB Saunders Co., 1985.

Larsen PR: The Thyroid. *In* Wyngaarden JB, Smith LH (eds): Cecil's Textbook of Medicine. Philadelphia, WB Saunders Co., 1985, pp. 1275–1299.

Sawin CT, Surks MI, London M, et al: Oral thyroxine: variation in biologic action and tablet content. Ann Intern Med 100:641, 1984.

III. TREATMENT OF ADRENAL DISEASE

A. Adrenal Insufficiency

1. **GENERAL PRINCIPLES.** Adrenal insufficiency may result from destruction of the adrenal cortex (Addison's disease), congenital enzyme deficiency (congenital adrenal hyperplasia), or pituitary disease with ACTH deficiency. The most common cause of adrenal insufficiency is suppression of the hypothalamic-pituitary-adrenal (HPA) axis by therapeutic glucocorticoids. Recovery from HPA suppression is slow, and patients remain at risk for adrenal insufficiency during periods of stress for as long as a year after discontinuing glucocorticoid therapy. Chronic adrenal insufficiency usually presents insidiously, the usual symptoms being fatigue, anorexia with weight loss, hypotension, and hypoglycemia. In contrast, adrenal crisis is a dramatic, life-threatening condition characterized by prostration, hypotension, fever, and electrolyte disorders that, if untreated, can progress rapidly to shock and death.

2. **TREATMENT**

   a. **Chronic Adrenal Insufficiency.** Patients with primary adrenal insufficiency **(Addison's disease)** lack all three classes of adrenal corticosteroids: glucocorticoids, mineralocorticoids, and androgens. Prednisone, 7.5 mg/day (5 mg in A.M., 2.5 mg in P.M.) or hydrocortisone, 30 mg/day (20 mg in A.M., 10 mg in P.M.) provides physiologic replacement of glucocorticoid with adjustments for very large or small persons or in patients taking drugs that increase the metabolic clearance of glucocorticoids, such as phenytoin, barbiturates, and rifampin. The adequacy of glucocorticoid replacement is indicated by restoration of the patient's sense of well-being, appetite and weight, and resolution of hyperpigmentation. Hyponatremia suggests inadequate glucocorticoid replacement. Insomnia or cushingoid features may be signs of excess glucocorticoid dose. For mineralocorticoid replacement in patients with adrenal insufficiency (signaled by volume depletion and/or hyperkalemia), the synthetic mineralcorticoid fludrocortisone (Florinef) is usually given as a single daily dose of 0.05–0.3 mg. Hypertension, hypokalemia, edema, or congestive heart failure call for a reduction in dosage. Changes in fludrocortisone dosage are usually made in increments of 0.05 mg/day.

   The primary goal in patients with adrenal insufficiency is the prevention of adrenal crisis. At the first sign of illness (including minor infections such as gastroenteritis and febrile viral syndromes) patients should double their maintenance dose of steroid. If vomiting precludes the use of oral steroids, arrangements must be made immediately for parenteral administration of corticosteroids. Patients should wear a bracelet or necklace identifying them as having adrenal insufficiency. An injectable form of glucocorticoid such as dexamethasone phosphate (4 mg) should be taken along whenever the patient is out of reach of medical attention.

b. Acute Adrenal Insufficiency (Adrenal Crisis). Glucocorticoid requirements increase dramatically during stress. During events such as surgery, infection, or trauma, persons with adrenal or pituitary insufficiency are at risk of developing adrenal crisis. The diagnosis of adrenal crisis must be made on clinical grounds since treatment cannot wait for laboratory confirmation of the diagnosis. After a blood sample is taken (to measure serum cortisol and possibly ACTH levels later), treatment is started immediately.

Hydrocortisone, the steroid preparation of choice for acute adrenal insufficiency, is given 100 mg IV, followed by a continuous infusion of 100 mg q 8 h. IV is continued for 48 hours, after which oral hydrocortisone can usually be substituted in a dose of 50 mg q 8 h for the next 2 days. Initial fluid replacement is 5% dextrose and isotonic saline (D_5NS), given at a rate of 500–1000 mL/hr for the first several hours, until the extracellular volume deficit is corrected. Patients with adrenal insufficiency may have a $\geq 10\%$ deficit in extracellular volume and require 4 to 6 L of fluid in the first 24 hours. Serum sodium and potassium levels need to be monitored frequently during the early stages of treatment. If the serum potassium is greater than 6.9 mEq/L (or over 6.5 mEq/L in a patient with cardiac arrhythmia), 2 ampules (89 mEq total) of sodium bicarbonate should be added to each liter of IV $D_5\frac{1}{2}NS$) until the potassium drops to a safer level.

c. Perioperative Management. Patients with known or suspected adrenal insufficiency (including those receiving exogenous steroids) require high doses of glucocorticoid to withstand the stress of anesthesia and surgery. Hydrocortisone 100 mg IV should be given in the morning of surgery, followed by hydrocortisone 100 mg IV q 8 h given over the day of surgery. In uncomplicated cases the dosage may be reduced by 50% each day thereafter until maintenance dosage is achieved.

d. Steroid Treatment and Withdrawal. When glucocorticoids are used as pharmacologic agents, in doses exceeding physiologic replacement, suppression of the hypothalamic-pituitary-adrenal (HPA) axis occurs. The degree is a function of the dose and duration of therapy. The correlation between the dose and duration of steroid therapy potential HPA axis suppression is shown in Table 12–2. The patient may remain at risk for adrenal insufficiency during periods of stress for months after steroids have been discontinued. In a patient who has previously received steroids, adrenal responsiveness to stress can be assessed by measuring cortisol before and after an infusion of synthetic ACTH (cosyntropin). A normal

TABLE 12–2. RELATIONSHIP BETWEEN DOSE AND DURATION OF PREDNISONE THERAPY AND ADRENAL SUPPRESSION

DOSE	DURATION			
	1 week	1 month	6 months	1 year
Replacement (<7.5 mg/day)	−	−	−	−
Alternate day (any dose)	−	−	−	−
10 mg/day*	−	−	+/−	+
15 mg/day*	−	+/−	+	+ +
>30 mg/day*	+	+ +	+ + +	+ + +

From Thygeson M: Glucocorticoid withdrawal. *In* Metz R and Larson E (eds): Bluebook of Endocrinology. Philadelphia, W.B. Saunders Co., 1985.
*Single daily dose in the morning. Pluses and minuses indicated likelihood of adrenal suppression: − rare; +/− some patients; + many patients; + + most patients; + + + all patients.

response (stimulated plasma cortisol > 20 ng/dL, 30 min following 250 µg cosyntropin IV) implies steroid coverage during surgery is not necessary. An alternative and perhaps more practical approach is to simply provide steroid coverage for any patient who has received pharmacologic doses of steroids in the previous year.

When glucocorticoids are no longer required for the treatment of an illness, they should be discontinued. The major concern during and after steroid withdrawal is the development of acute adrenal insufficiency. The stress of an acute illness or injury may precipitate adrenal crisis in patients with adrenal suppression. If therapeutic steroids are to be discontinued, the main issue is whether to reduce the dose gradually. Tapering the dose of steroids does not protect patients from adrenal crisis or steroid withdrawal symptoms but does delay eventual recovery of the HPA axis. The rate at which steroids are withdrawn should be based on the dose of steroid necessary to maintain remission. Gradual reductions in dose are more useful in situations when the goal is to find the lowest dose required for optimal control of disease. Steroids should be reinstituted if the patient develops an intercurrent illness or signs of adrenal insufficiency such as hypotension, fever, nausea, and vomiting.

B. Hyporeninemic Hypoaldosteronism

1. **GENERAL PRINCIPLES.** Isolated aldosterone deficiency is most often due to a deficiency in renin, i.e., hyporeninemic hypoaldosteronism. The typical patient with this condition is elderly, diabetic, and has mild renal insufficiency with hyperkalemia, hyperchloremic acidosis, mild elevation of serum creatinine, and the absence of alternative explanations for hyperkalemia. Blood pressure may be high, normal, or low.

2. Treatment. When hyperkalemia is severe enough to need therapy, treatment depends on the patient's blood pressure. If the patient is hypertensive, a loop diuretic such as furosemide lowers blood pressure and tends to reverse the hyperkalemia. With normal or low blood pressure, fludrocortisone (Florinef) provides mineralocorticoid replacement, reversing the hyperkalemia and acidosis. The dose of fludrocortisone may need to be higher than for adrenal insufficiency, i.e., over 0.2 mg/day.

Beta blockers, prostaglandin synthetase inhibitors, angiotensin-converting enzyme inhibitors, potassium-sparing diuretics, and potassium supplements may exacerbate hyperkalemia and should be avoided.

C. Adrenocortical Excess (Cushing's Syndrome)

1. General Principles. Cushing's syndrome can result from pituitary overproduction of ACTH (Cushing's disease), a benign or malignant cortisol-producing adrenal tumor, or ectopic production of ACTH. Thus the first step in Cushing's syndrome therapy is to identify its cause. Restoring normal adrenal function in patients with Cushing's syndrome is not always possible, and in some cases treatment may leave the patient with temporary or permanent cortisol deficiency.

2. Treatment

   a. Pituitary Cushing's Syndrome (Cushing's Disease). See "Treatment of Cushing's disease" under Pituitary disorders.

   b. Adrenal Neoplasm. Surgical removal of a functional benign adrenal cortical tumor will cure Cushing's syndrome. Postoperatively, patients have temporary adrenal insufficiency due to atrophy of the contralateral adrenal gland, which should be treated for adrenal insufficiency when the overactive adrenal is removed. Glucocorticoid therapy can be tapered and withdrawn over a period of several months. Adrenal carcinomas are usually unresectable at the time of diagnosis. In these patients the adrenolytic agent o,p',DDD can retard tumor growth as well as lower cortisol production, although toxicity may limit its usefulness. The starting dosage is 250 mg qid, increased gradually to tolerance or 24 gm daily, as required to induce and maintain remission. Hypoadrenalism may accompany use of o,p',DDD in which case corticosteroids are given concomitantly. Ketoconazole, metyrapone, and aminoglutethimide, drugs that block cortisol production, can also be used to lower cortisol level in patients with adrenal carcinoma.

   c. Ectopic ACTH. Ectopic ACTH production with Cushing's syndrome may occur in a number of tumors, most commonly oat cell carcinoma of the lung, bronchial carcinoid, and pancreatic islet cell tumors. The ideal treatment of Cushing's syndrome due to ectopic ACTH production is removal of the underlying malignancy. If the tumor is unresectable, drugs that block cortisol production can benefit the symptoms of the Cushing's syndrome. Ketoconazole, the antifungal agent, also inhibits adrenal steroid synthesis, and in doses up to 1200 mg per day may normalize serum cortisol levels. The drug is given orally in 4 divided doses, beginning at 600 mg/day. Elevated serum transaminase levels can occur and rarely an idiosyncratic hepatitis may develop. A second agent can be added if cortisol levels are not controlled on 1200 mg/day. Metyrapone, an inhibitor of 11β-hydroxylase, in doses of 250–500 mg tid will normalize cortisol level in many patients. Aminoglutethimide blocks the conversion of cholesterol to Δ-5-pregnenolone and in doses of 250–500 mg qid can be used to suppress excess cortisol production. Both agents can produce adrenal insufficiency, and serial measurements of serum or urine cortisol levels should be used to determine dosage.

D. Pheochromocytoma. This is a tumor of the adrenal medulla or the extra-adrenal chromaffin system, present in approximately 0.1% of patients with persistent diastolic hypertension. About 10% are bilateral or multiple and nearly 10% are malignant. The medical treatment of pheochromocytoma involves preparing the patient for surgery. Careful preoperative medical management of blood pressure and volume status is essential to prevent complications. These patients are often hypertensive, vasoconstricted, and volume depleted; removal of the tumor without proper premedication can result in hypotension and shock. Use of adrenergic blocking agents before surgery reverses the effects of excessive catecholamines. α-Adrenergic blocking agents lower blood pressure and reexpand blood volume. **Oral phenoxybenzamine,** a long-acting alpha blocker, is preferred. The starting dose is 10 mg twice daily, increased by 10–20 mg/day to a maximum of 200 mg/day or until the blood pressure is stabilized. Even patients with normal blood pressure should be so treated before surgery to avoid sudden volume reexpansion when the tumor is removed. Extra saline may be needed to maintain normal upright blood pressure as the intravascular space expands. A 1–2 week period of adrenergic blockade is usually recommended before surgery. Propranolol, 10–40 mg q 6 h, may be added if tachycardia or atrial arrhythmias occur.

For unresectable tumors, metyrosine (α-methyl-*para*-tyrosine), an inhibitor of tyrosine hydroxylase, can reduce catecholamine production by 50–80%. Metyrosine is administered orally in an initial dose of 250 mg qid, with daily increments of 250–500 mg. The maximal recommended dosage is 4 gm daily.

Aron DC, Findling JW, Fitzgerald PA, et al: Cushing's syndrome: problems in management. Endocrin Rev 3:229–244, 1982.
Bayliss RIS: Adrenal cortex. Clin Endocrinol Metab 9:477–486, 1980.
Baxter JD: Adrenocortical hypofunction. *In* Wyngaarden JB, Smith LH (eds): Cecil's Textbook of Medicine. Philadelphia, WB Saunders Co., 1985, pp. 1425–1430.
Boggan JE, Tyrrell JB, Wilson CB: Transsphenoidal microsurgical management: report of 100 cases of Cushing's disease. J Neurosurg 59:195–200, 1983.
Bondy PK: Disorders of the adrenal cortex. *In* Wilson JD, Foster DW (ed): Williams Textbook of Endocrinology. 7th ed. Philadelphia, WB Saunders Co., 1985.
Bravo EL, Gifford RW: Pheochromocytoma: diagnosis, localization and management. N Engl J Med 311:1298–1303, 1984.
Schteingart DE: Cushing's syndrome. Endocrinol Metab Clin North Am 18:311–330, 1989.
Schambelan M, Sebastian A: Hyporeninemic hypoaldosteronism. Adv Intern Med 24:385–405, 1979.

IV. HIRSUTISM

A. General Principles. The definition of hirsutism, excessive androgen-dependent hair in women, is to some extent subjective and depends on both cultural standards of beauty and the patient's self-image. Mild to moderate hirsutism of gradual onset is rarely a sign of serious illness and usually is a cosmetic rather than a medical problem. If in addition to hirsutism there is evidence of masculinization or virilization, a serious disorder is present. Signs of virilization include temporal balding, thinning of scalp hair, deepening of the voice, male body habitus, and clitoromegaly. Treatment depends on the cause. Congenital adrenal hyperplasia is treated with physiologic doses of glucocorticoids. Ovarian or adrenal neoplasms are treated surgically.

B. Treatment. In most cases this should be limited to simple cosmetic measures, such as bleaching. Shaving, although unappealing to most women, is effective and does not increase the rate of hair growth. Depilatory waxes and creams can be effective but may cause skin sensitization. Electrolysis results in permanent removal of individual hair follicles but is expensive, uncomfortable, and requires many treatments to produce a noticeable effect. When hirsutism is severe, widespread, or psychologically distressing, medical therapy may be helpful.

1. **SPIRONOLACTONE.** This interferes with testosterone synthesis and also competes with testosterone for cytosol and nuclear receptors in androgen-sensitive tissues, including hair follicles. Most patients with simple hirsutism have improvement, usually within 6 months, when treated with spironolactone in doses of 100–200 mg daily in divided doses. Side effects include menstrual irregularity and breast tenderness.

2. **ORAL CONTRACEPTIVE AGENTS (OCAs).** Ovarian androgen production is stimulated by LH and estrogen and progesterone suppress it, thus producing a fall in ovarian androgen output. Oral contraceptive therapy is effective in only about 30% of patients. When contraception is desirable, OCAs are suitable agents for treatment of hirsutism, either alone or in combination with spironolactone. Of the progestins contained in the OCA, ethynodiol diacetate has less androgenic potential than norethindrone acetate.

3. **DEXAMETHASONE.** Dexamethasone is the drug of choice for hirsutism of congenital adrenal hyperplasia (CAH). In addition to the typical case of CAH, which involves precocious puberty and virilization at an early age, a milder variant, late-onset 21 hydroxylase deficiency, may produce hirsutism that appears after puberty. In this condition, dexamethasone in a daily dose of 0.5 mg at bedtime has been uniformly successful. Dexamethasone at this dose does not generally depress the ACTH-adrenal response to stress. The effect of glucocorticoid suppression in simple hirsutism has generally been disappointing.

Biffignandi P, Massucchetti C, Molinatti GM: Female hirsutism: pathophysiological considerations and therapeutic implications. Endocrinol Rev 5:498–509, 1984.
Ehrmann DA, Rosenfield RL: An endocrinologic approach to the patient with hirsutism. J Clin Endocrinol Metab 71:1–4, 1990.

V. MENOPAUSE

A. General Principles. The decline in estrogen levels that occurs at menopause can be associated with a number of effects including hot flashes, emotional lability, atrophy of the urogenital tissues, and, most seriously, osteoporosis and its consequences, vertebral compression fractures and hip fractures. Estrogen replacement therapy can be used to relieve specific symptoms as well as to help preserve bone mass and urogenital tissue. If estrogens are given for treatment of hot flashes, therapy should be discontinued every 12–18 months to see if continued treatment is necessary. Atrophic vaginitis may require treatment for several years. To be maximally effective in treatment and prophylaxis of osteoporosis, estrogens should be started early after menopause and continued indefinitely. Whatever the indications for estrogens, the goals of treatment should be discussed with the patient and her preferences incorporated in the treatment plan. Past history of uterine or breast cancer and history of venous thromboembolic disease or gallbladder disease are contraindications to estrogen use. The unopposed use of estrogens is associated with a 3–8 fold increase in incidence of uterine malignancy. Progestational agents antagonize the proliferative effect of estrogen on the endometrium and, when given in conjunction with estrogen, reduce the risk of endometrial carcinoma.

B. Treatment. Women who have had a hysterectomy should take estrogens daily, starting with a dose of 0.625 mg conjugated estrogen (Premarin). If hot flashes persist, the dose should be increased to 1.25 mg per day. For women with an intact uterus, a progestational drug such as medroxy-progesterone (Provera) should be given in association with estrogen. One schedule of administration is to give estrogen cyclically 25 days per month with progesterone (Provera 10 mg) given on days 15–25. Both hormones are withheld for the last 5 days of the month. On this regimen, most women will have withdrawal bleeding during the 5 days off hormones; bleeding at other times during the cycle is abnormal and if recurrent should be evaluated with an endometrial biopsy. An alternative to cyclic administration is to give estrogen and progesterone daily in combination (Premarin 0.625–1.25 mg and Provera 2.5–5.0 mg/day). This combination is preferred by most women since it does not result in withdrawal bleeding and is easier to remember. Breakthrough bleeding can occur with the initiation of continuous therapy and is easily controlled by increasing the progestin dosage. The bone-sparing effect of estrogens occurs with doses of 0.625 mg conjugated estrogen (Premarin) or 25 µg ethinyl estradiol or more. Although estrogen by injection is effective, it offers no advantages over oral administration and is less cost-effective. Symptoms of urogenital atrophy can be effectively treated with estrogen vaginal cream 1 gm 2–3 times/week. Transdermal estrogen (Estraderm) requires only twice-a-week administration.

Gambrell RD Jr: The menopause: benefits and risks of estrogen-progesterone replacement therapy. Fertil Steril 37:457–474, 1982.
Hammond CB, Maxson WS: Current status of estrogen therapy for the menopause. Fertil Steril 37:5–25, 1982.
Prough SG, Aksel S, Wiebe RH, Sheperd J: Continuous estrogen/progestin therapy in menopause. Am J Obstet Gynecol 157:1449–1453, 1987.

VI. TREATMENT OF CALCIUM DISORDERS

A. Hypercalcemia

1. GENERAL PRINCIPLES. Conditions that cause hypercalcemia vary in pathogenesis and treatment. Hypercalcemia, even when asymptomatic and found incidentally on routine blood testing, can be associated with long-term sequelae such as kidney stones and osteoporosis. More severe hypercalcemia can cause lethargy, anorexia, constipation, and eventually death from obtundation or cardiac arrhythmia. The two most common causes of hypercalcemia are hyperparathyroidism and malignancy. Ideally, treatment of hypercalcemia is directed toward curing its underlying cause. Surgical removal of a parathyroid adenoma cures the hypercalcemia of hyperparathyroidism. A serum calcium concentration of greater than 14 mg/dL requires immediate therapy.

2. TREATMENT. Several agents are generally used in combination for rapid lowering of serum calcium. (Table 12–3).
   a. Forced Saline Diuresis. Since many patients are volume-depleted initially, normal saline should be infused until intravascular volume is normal. This is followed by a forced saline diuresis using furosemide and normal saline to accelerate calcium excretion. Careful monitoring of electrolytes is mandatory, as potassium and magnesium depletion are likely to occur. In some patients central venous pressure monitoring may be needed.
   b. Mithramycin. The cytotoxic antibiotic mithramycin is effective in treatment of hypercalcemia of any cause. A single dose will normalize serum calcium in 75% of hypercalcemic patients within 48 hours; this can persist for about a week. Subsequent doses of mithramycin should be withheld until and unless calcium begins to rise again, since the duration of calcium-lowering activity varies and depends partially upon other steps taken to lower calcium. The toxic effects of mithramycin (thrombocytopenia, hepatic, and renal toxicity) are rarely seen when only 1 or 2 doses are given.
   c. Etidronate Disodium. The diphosphonate etidronate disodium (Didronel) reduces normal and abnormal bone resorption. Etidronate disodium restores serum calcium to normal in approximately 60% of patients with hypercalcemia of malignancy. Etidronate is given IV daily for 3 days, and its effect in normalizing the calcium level may persist for several weeks.
   d. Glucocorticoids. Glucocorticoids in pharmacologic doses increase urinary calcium excretion and decrease calcium absorption from the intestine. They are effective in treating hypercalcemia associated with myeloma, sarcoidosis, and occasionally breast cancer but have little effect on serum calcium in patients with primary hyperparathyroidism. Because their maximum calcium-lowering effect may not occur for several days, glucocorticoids should be used in conjunction with other modes of therapy for acute hypercalcemia.

TABLE 12–3. EMERGENCY TREATMENT OF HYPERCALCEMIA

Saline diuresis	Up to 6 L isotonic saline IV over 24 hr with furosemide, 40–100 mg IV q 2–4 h as needed, to maintain a urine output of 200–300 ml/hr (electrolytes and volume status must be monitored closely)
Mithramycin	25 µg/kg body weight by IV bolus or infusion; repeat q 24–72 h only as needed
Etidronate disodium	7.5 mg/kg IV daily for 3 successive days
Glucocorticoids	Prednisone, 40–100 mg po in divided doses, or hydrocortisone, 200–400 mg/day IV infusion
Calcitonin	25–50 units q 6–8 h SC, IM, IV (concomitant use of glucocorticoids may prolong the effect of calcitonin)
Phosphate	Fleet's Phospha-soda (3.3 gm sodium phosphate per 5 ml), 5 ml po or rectally 3–4 times/day to keep serum phosphate in normal range (use only if serum phosphate is low)
Dialysis	Hemodialysis or peritoneal dialysis with calcium-free dialysis fluid; 1st choice in hypercalcemia complicated by severe renal failure

e. Calcitonin. This inhibits release of calcium from bone and increases renal calcium excretion. By itself, calcitonin is only mildly effective, and escape from its calcium-lowering effect is usually seen within the first hours or days of use. However, the concomitant use of glucocorticoids appears to block this escape phenomenon. The potential advantages of calcitonin are the rapid (although mild) therapeutic effect and lack of toxicity.

f. Phosphates. Oral phosphate will lower serum calcium and may be useful in the treatment of hypercalcemia associated with a low or normal serum phosphate. The deliberate induction of hyperphosphatemia by IV or high-dose oral phosphate has been advocated, but this protocol is not recommended because of the risks of hypocalcemia and metastatic calcification.

g. Gallium Nitrate. Preliminary studies indicate that the antiresorptive actions of gallium can treat cancer-related hypercalcemia safely and effectively when given IV. This drug has been approved recently for clinical use.

B. Hypocalcemia

1. **GENERAL PRINCIPLES.** Hypocalcemia may present with either acute or chronic symptoms, depending upon the level and rate of fall of serum calcium. Chronic mild hypocalcemia may lead to cataracts, calcification of the basal ganglia, and metastatic calcification of soft tissues. Tetany, seizures, and laryngospasm requiring immediate diagnosis and treatment may be the first manifestations of hypocalcemia. Acute hypocalcemia is most often seen in hospitalized patients after removal of or damage to the parathyroid glands during neck surgery. Hypocalcemia due to other causes is usually mild and typically involves chronic symptoms such as fatigue, myalgias, muscle cramps, or cataracts.

2. **TREATMENT**

   a. Chronic Hypocalcemia. Treatment usually requires a combination of supplemental calcium and vitamin D. The treatment regimen must be individualized and followed carefully. To correct the hypocalcemia of hypoparathyroidism usually requires vitamin D in doses of 50,000 to 150,000 units/day along with 0.5 to 2 gm elemental calcium/day. Calcium and vitamin D in these doses frequently induce hypercalciuria and, with it, a risk of calcium stone formation. Drug dosage should be adjusted to maintain the serum calcium in the low-normal range while at the same time avoiding excessive urinary calcium excretion (24-hour urine calcium > 4 mg/kg/day). A thiazide diuretic and restricted sodium diet can help to reduce urinary calcium losses. In renal insufficiency, $1,25(OH)_2$ vitamin D (calcitriol, Rocaltrol) 0.5 to 2 μg/day is preferred to vitamin D for the treatment of hypocalcemia. Serum calcium levels must be monitored frequently, especially at the onset of treatment because of the danger of hypercalcemia.

TABLE 12–4. ORAL CALCIUM PREPARATIONS

PREPARATION	ELEMENTAL CALCIUM
Calcium lactate (650 mg tablets)	85 mg
Calcium gluconate (1 gm tablets)	90 mg
Calcium carbonate (Tums)	200 mg
(Tums E-X)	300 mg
Oyster shell calcium (Os-cal 250)	250 mg
(Os-cal 500)	500 mg

b. Acute Hypocalcemia. Tetany, laryngospasm, or seizures require immediate treatment with IV calcium (**10% calcium gluconate**). Initially, 10–30 mL are infused over 10–15 minutes. If the patient can swallow, oral calcium should be given in a dose of 200 mg q 2 h, increasing to 500 mg q 2 h if necessary. The calcium content of various calcium preparations is listed in Table 12–4. If the patient is unable to swallow, or if tetany returns within 6 hours, administration of calcium by continuous IV infusion is indicated. 1 gm of calcium (approximately 100 mL of 10% calcium gluconate) is added to 1 liter of a 5% dextrose solution and infused at a rate sufficient to prevent tetany—usually between 30 and 100 mL/hour. Serum magnesium should be measured because hypomagnesemia may inhibit both the release and action of parathyroid hormone. If the magnesium level is low (less than 0.8 mg/L), magnesium sulfate is given IV (1–2 gm $MgSO_4$ as a 10% solution over 15 min) or by intramuscular injection (1 gm of 50% solution every 4 hours) until the magnesium level has returned to normal. Once stabilized, the patient may, depending upon the cause of hypocalcemia, need to be started on vitamin D in addition to calcium.

Arnaud CD: The parathyroid glands, hypercalcemia and hypocalcemia. In Wyngaarden JB, Smith LH (eds): Cecil's Textbook of Medicine. Philadelphia, WB Saunders Co., 1985, pp. 1425–1430.

Ryzen E, Martodarm RR, Traxel M, et al: Intravenous etidronate in the management of malignant hypercalcemia. Arch Intern Med 145:449–452, 1985.

Schneider AB, Sherwood LM: Pathogenesis and management of hypoparathyroidism. Metabolism 24:871, 1975.

Scholz DA, Purnell DC: Asymptomatic primary hyperparathyroidism: 10-year prospective study. Mayo Clin Proc 56:473–478, 1981.

Singer FR, Fernandez M: Therapy of hypercalcemia and malignancy. Am J Med 82:34–41, 1987.

Suki WN, Yium JJ, Von Minden M, et al: Acute treatment of hypercalcemia with furosemide. N Engl J Med 283:836, 1970.

VII. TREATMENT OF METABOLIC BONE DISEASE

A. General Principles. Pathologic loss of bone mineral density is most often due to osteoporosis or osteomalacia. These two disorders differ both in their pathogenesis and treatment. Osteoporosis, an age-related thinning of bone, is primarily a disease of postmenopausal women, 25% of whom will experience wrist, vertebral, or hip fracture after age 65. Osteomalacia, a defect in calcification of bone osteoid, is associated with low levels of circulating vitamin D. Conditions that interfere with intestinal absorption of vitamin D or hydroxylation of vitamin D in the liver or kidney may be associated with reduced levels of activated vitamin D and osteomalacia. Certain drugs may contribute to osteopenia. Glucocorticoids interfere with GI absorption of calcium and inhibit bone formation and their extended use can be associated with the development of osteopenia. Phenytoin and the barbiturates interfere with the 25-hydroxylation of vitamin D in the liver, leading to osteomalacia in some patients.

B. Treatment of Osteoporosis

1. NONPHARMACOLOGIC THERAPY. Risk factors for osteoporosis include sedentary lifestyle, excess alcohol consumption, and smoking. Eliminating these factors is the first step in treating postmenopausal osteoporosis. A regular exercise program is particularly helpful in maintaining bone mineral density. Elderly people should be encouraged to walk or swim regularly. Early restoration of mobility after a period of enforced bed rest should also be encouraged.

2. CALCIUM. Ensuring an adequate calcium intake is a basic requirement of any therapeutic regimen. The premenopausal female requires 1000 mg/day of calcium to maintain calcium balance and the estrogen-deficient woman needs 1500 mg/day to meet this goal (Table 12–5).

3. ESTROGENS. Estrogens slow postmenopausal bone loss, and the bone-protecting effect of estrogen occurs with doses of 0.625 mg of conjugated estrogen (Premarin) or 25 μg of ethinyl estradiol or greater. Estrogens are contraindicated in women with a history of breast or endometrial cancer, venous thromboembolic episodes, or

TABLE 12–5. SOURCES OF CALCIUM SUPPLEMENTATION

SOURCE	ELEMENTAL CALCIUM (mg)	DAILY DOSAGE*
Calcium lactate (650 mg tablet)	85	18 tablets
Calcium gluconate (1 gm tablet)	90	17 tablets
Calcium carbonate (Tums tablets)	200	7 tablets
Oyster shell calcium (Tums E-X tablets)	300	5 tablets
Os-cal 250 tablet	250	6 tablets
Os-cal 500 tablet	500	3 tablets
Milk (1 cup)	300	1 ¼ quarts

*No. of tablets needed to provide 1500 mg elemental calcium per day.

gallbladder disease. Blood pressure should be monitored in women taking estrogens.

4. **ETIDRONATE.** Etidronate (Didronel) is a diphosphonate compound that reduces bone resorption by inhibiting osteoclastic activity. When given cyclically, etidronate can increase bone mineral density and reduce risk of fracture in postmenopausal women with osteoporosis. Etidronate is given as a single daily dose of 400 mg. It is poorly absorbed and should be given between meals. Etidronate is taken cyclically for 2 weeks every 3 months. To provide the substrate for new bone formation, the patient should take calcium 500 mg daily, but not within 2 hours of etidronate. Long-term effects (> 2–3 years) are not known.

5. **OTHER AGENTS.** Vitamin D, though effective in treating osteomalacia, is of uncertain benefit in the treatment of osteoporosis. Addition of pharmacologic doses of vitamin D does not reduce fracture rate and may lead to hypercalcemia and hypercalciuria. Fluoride will increase bone density but recent studies have shown no reduction in risk of fracture in patients treated with fluoride. Androgens, calcitonin, IV calcium, and synthetic parathyroid hormone have been used to treat osteoporosis, but their effectiveness in preventing fractures has not been proved.

6. **RECOMMENDATIONS.** Calcium supplements are virtually free of side effects and should be recommended to women of all ages as a means of reducing the risk of osteoporosis. In the absence of contraindications, estrogens should be prescribed for postmenopausal women with osteoporosis and those at increased risk because of race, body habitus, diet, or lifestyle. Etidronate is effective in increasing bone density in postmenopausal women with osteoporosis. Although there are virtually no contraindications to its use, current enthusiasm must be tempered by the lack of long-term data.

C. **Treatment of Osteomalacia.** Osteomalacia responds dramatically to treatment with vitamin D. For patients with nutritional osteomalacia, oral vitamin D, 50,000 U once a week, is usually sufficient. For patients with more severe osteomalacia as evidenced by bone pain, extensive skeletal involvement, or markedly elevated alkaline phosphatase, initial treatment doses of vitamin D should be about 50,000 U/day. In patients with chronic renal failure, **calcitriol** (Rocaltrol, 1,25(OH)$_2$ D) is used, initially in a dose of 0.25 µg/day. Since calcitriol can induce hypercalcemia in just a few days, close monitoring (twice weekly) of the serum calcium concentration is indicated. A daily calcium intake of 1000 mg/day should accompany the vitamin D. Success in treating osteomalacia is indicated by a lessening of bone pain and normalization of serum calcium, phosphorus, and alkaline phosphatase. The dosage of vitamin D should be reduced when the 24-hour urine calcium approaches hypercalciuric levels, i.e., over 4 mg/kg/day.

D. **Drug-Induced Osteopenia.** Phenytoin, barbiturates, and glucocorticoids can contribute to osteopenia—the anticonvulsants by interfering with the hydroxylation of vitamin D in the liver and glucocorticoids by inhibiting both intestinal absorption of calcium and new bone formation. If long-term treatment with these drugs is anticipated, steps to prevent bone loss should be considered, especially in older patients. Vitamin D, 2000–4000 U/day, in combination with calcium, 500 mg/day, may retard the bone loss otherwise caused by these medications.

Aloia JF, Cohn SH, Ostuni JA, et al: Prevention of involutional bone loss by exercise. Ann Intern Med 89:356–358, 1978.

Bikle DD: Osteomalacia and rickets. In Wyngaarden JB, Smith LH (eds): Cecil's Textbook of Medicine. Philadelphia, WB Saunders Co., 1985, pp. 1425–1430.

Nordin BE, Heyburn PJ, Peacock M, et al: Osteoporosis and osteomalacia. Clin Endocrinol Metab 9:177–205, 1980.

Riggs BL, Hadgson SF, O'Fallon WM, et al: Effect of fluoride treatment on the fracture rate in postmenopausal women with osteoporosis. N Engl J Med 322:802–809, 1990.

Riggs BL: Osteoporosis. In Wyngaarden JB, Smith LH (eds): Cecil's Textbook of Medicine. Philadelphia, WB Saunders Co., 1985, pp. 1425–1430.

Storm T, Thamsborg G, Steiniche T, et al: Effect of intermittent cyclical etidronate therapy on bone mass and fracture rate in women with postmenopausal osteoporosis. N Engl J Med 322:1265–1271, 1990.

VIII. DIABETES MELLITUS

A. **Diabetic Ketoacidosis.** The basic defect in ketoacidosis is a severe deficiency of insulin with accelerated hepatic gluconeogenesis and ketogenesis, increased release of free fatty acids from adipose tissue, and decreased utilization of glucose. Hyperglycemia leads to osmotic diuresis, which produces volume and electrolyte depletion, acidosis causes outmigration of intracellular potassium. The clinical indications of ketoacidosis include malaise, mental obtundation, nausea, and vomiting, which aggravate the volume and electrolyte depletion. Clinically, ketoacidosis is easily recognized (Table 12–6).

1. TREATMENT. This consists of (1) insulin in adequate dosage, (2) correction of fluid and electrolyte abnormalities, and (3) identification and treatment on any underlying or associated illnesses. The following measurements should be recorded on a bedside flow sheet: Bedside **blood glucose test** every 1–2 hours and urine output measurement

TABLE 12–6. DIAGNOSIS OF DIABETIC KETOACIDOSIS

SYMPTOMS	SIGNS	LABORATORY DATA
Polyuria, polydipsia	Tachycardia, postural	Hyperglycemia (blood glucose
Postural dizziness	hypotension	> 300 mg/dL)
Anorexia, nausea,	Drowsiness, stupor, or	Acidosis (pH < 7.3 and/or
vomiting, and	coma	serum bicarbonate
abdominal pain	Kussmaul's breathing,	< 15 mEq/L)
Dyspnea	odor of ketones on	Ketonemia (strongly positive
Malaise, drowsiness	breath	nitroprusside reaction in
	Hypothermia	serum diluted to half
	Facial flushing	strength with water)

every 2 hours, and serum pH or bicarbonate and potassium levels every 2–4 hours until the biochemical situation has stabilized.

2. **INSULIN ADMINISTRATION.** Various methods of insulin administration have been used successfully. The dose, frequency, and route of administration of insulin are probably less important than familiarity with a single protocol of proven effectiveness. Continuous IV infusion is widely used because of its flexibility and effectiveness. We use the protocol given below (dosages are for averaged-sized adults).

---

1. An IV bolus of 10 U of regular insulin is given.
2. An infusion of 50 U of regular insulin in 500 ml of NS (i.e., 0.1 U of insulin/milliliter of NS) is started. The initial infusion rate is 60 mL (6 U of insulin) per hour. The rate is maintained until the blood glucose level is recorded at or below 240 mg per deciliter. At that point, the insulin infusion rate is reduced to 30 ml (3 U) per hour.
3. A separate infusion of NS is started simultaneously with the insulin infusion and administered at 500 to 1000 mL/hour. When the blood glucose level falls below 240 mg/dL, the saline is replaced by D_5NS administered at a rate of approximately 150 mL per hour.
4. With the dextrose solution running, the blood glucose level is monitored at intervals of 1 or 2 hours, and the insulin infusion rate is adjusted up or down, usually 1 U per hour, in order to maintain a blood glucose level between 100 and 240 mg/dL.
5. The course is maintained until the blood glucose level becomes stable between these limits and the patient is asymptomatic and eating normally. At that stage, the patient is given a dose of intermediate-acting insulin. If it is given in the morning, the customary daily dose is used; but if it is administered later in the day, the dose is reduced in proportion to that part of the day that has elapsed. The insulin infusion is discontinued 1–2 hours after the intermediate-acting insulin is given. Booster doses of rapid-acting insulin are given at 6-hour intervals, if necessary, to keep the blood glucose level below 240 mg/dL. The size of the booster doses is usually about one fourth of the usual daily dose of intermediate-acting insulin.
6. The patient is usually kept in the hospital another day or so for stabilization of the blood glucose level and observation on a maintenance insulin program.

---

3. **FLUID AND ELECTROLYTE REPLACEMENT.** Patients with ketoacidosis show varying degrees of acidosis and depletion of saline, water, potassium, and phosphate. Fluid and electrolyte replacement must be individualized and guided by the results of monitoring. The degree of **volume depletion** is estimated clinically by assessing jugular vein pressure and by the degree of orthostatic hypotension. A drop in mean blood pressure of more than 20 mm Hg when the patient shifts from lying to standing indicates extracellular volume (ECV) depletion of at least 30%; in a patient weighing 70 kg, this would be 4.6 liters $(70 \times 0.22 \times 0.30 = 4.61)$.

Saline repletion is begun with NS. In the average adult patient, the initial infusion rate is 1000 mL for the first hour, then 500 mL per hour until postural hypotension is corrected. At this point, 0.45% saline can be substituted for NS. As saline depletion is corrected, the infusion rate is reduced. Most adult patients with diabetic ketoacidosis require 4–5 liters of fluid in the first 8 hours.

Bicarbonate therapy should be reserved for those patients with severe acidosis (a venous pH of less than 7.1). When bicarbonate is given, the initial IV solution should contain ½ NS with 2 ampules of sodium bicarbonate (each ampule contains 44.6 mEq bicarbonate) added per liter. Bicarbonate administration is discontinued when the serum pH reaches 7.1.

Serum **potassium** does not accurately reflect total body potassium in the presence of acidosis because of the transfer of potassium from the intracellular to the extracellular space. Most patients with ketoacidosis have profound deficits of total body potassium despite normal or even elevated serum potassium concentrations. On average, the potassium deficit in patients in diabetic ketoacidosis is approximately 5 mEq/kg of body weight (350 mEq in a 70-kg person). When the serum potassium level is elevated, potassium replacement is withheld until improvement in the acidosis brings about a fall in serum potassium into the normal range. Then potassium chloride is added to the IV solution to deliver 10 to 20 mEq per hour. This replacement dose is used from the beginning if the serum potassium level is normal initially. If the initial serum potassium level is low, the replacement rate should be 20 to 40 mEq per hour. Potassium replacement must be done with caution in patients with renal failure or oliguria.

Diabetic ketoacidosis is also associated with depletion of **phosphate**. Theoretically, phosphate deficiency could delay recovery, but in practice, phosphate repletion has not been shown to be of benefit in the routine treatment of diabetic ketoacidosis.

4. **IDENTIFICATION AND TREATMENT OF UNDERLYING ILLNESS.** Patients develop diabetic ketoacidosis for a reason, although that reason often escapes identification. The precipitating factor may be an acute illness, such as urinary tract infection, bronchitis, pneumonia, gastroenteritis, myocardial infarction, or appendicitis. All patients should be evaluated for intercurrent illness, which, if detected, should be treated simultaneously with the ketoacidosis. Perhaps the most common cause of diabetic ketoacidosis is the failure to increase insulin dosage during the stress of minor illness.

B. **Hyperglycemic, Hyperosmolar Coma.** Hyperosmolar coma is less common than ketoacidosis but carries a greater risk of death. Most patients are elderly and have either no history of diabetes or mild diabetes controlled by diet or oral drugs. Hyperosmolar coma is rarely seen in patients with established insulin-dependent diabetes mellitus (Table 12–7). Focal neurologic defects and seizures are also common. Complications include vascular thrombosis, acute hepatocellular necrosis, and other sequelae of hypotension and circulatory collapse. The overall mortality from hyperosmolar coma and the frequently present underlying illness may be as high as 50% in elderly patients.

Treatment is the same as that outlined for diabetic ketoacidosis, except for emphasis on correcting hyperosmolarity. Treatment is designed to correct volume depletion, hyperglycemia, potassium depletion, acidosis, and any precipitating illness. Establishing a well-designed flow chart and

**TABLE 12–7. CONDITIONS THAT MAY LEAD TO
HYPEROSMOLAR COMA**

Drugs
    Glucocorticoids
    Phenytoin
    Thiazide diuretics
Volume loss
    Vomiting
    Diarrhea
High-glucose intake in a patient with diabetes
Renal failure
Other illnesses (infection, myocardial infarction) that increase
    insulin needs

recording the amounts of insulin and IV fluids administered, as well as vital signs, fluid intake, urine output, blood glucose level, electrolytes, and creatinine concentration, are essential to proper management.

Fluid and electrolyte replacement must be tailored to the individual patient. Often the most immediate threat in hyperosmolar coma is shock from volume depletion. The degree of volume depletion is assessed by noting jugular vein distention and an orthostatic drop in blood pressure. If orthostatic hypotension is present, the ECV is decreased by at least 30% (4.6 L in a 70-kg patient). For signs of orthostatic hypotension, initial fluid therapy should be NS, 500–1000 mL/hour, although faster rates may be necessary if hypotension is severe. Most patients with hyperosmolar coma require at least 5 L of saline within the first 12 hours.

After volume depletion has been corrected with NS, the infusion should be changed to 0.45% saline and continued at 500 mL/hour to correct hyperosmolarity. The degree of hyperosmolarity (water depletion) may be estimated by the following formula:

$$\text{Plasma osmolarity} = 2(\text{Na} + \text{K}) + \frac{\text{glucose}}{18} + \frac{\text{blood urea nitrogen (BUN)}}{2.8}$$

(normal range: 280 to 300 mOsm per liter)

Because most of these patients are elderly and often have diminished cardiac reserve, great care must be taken to avoid volume overload. Monitoring of central venous or pulmonary capillary wedge pressure is frequently indicated.

C. Management of Hospitalized Patients During Medical and Surgical Illnesses. The physiologic reaction to acute illness involves release of humoral agents antagonistic to the action of insulin. Volume depletion may occur as a result of diaphoresis, anorexia, vomiting, diarrhea, and/or hyperglycemia-induced polyuria. These mechanisms lead to progressive hyperglycemia, ketosis, and volume depletion in patients with type I diabetes. The diabetes usually can be managed quite successfully with a straightforward protocol, the essentials of which are the following: (1) frequent monitoring of volume status and of glycemia and ketonuria (generally before meals and at bedtime if the patient is eating; every 6 hours in patients receiving IV nutrition), (2) supplemental rapid-acting insulin as indicated by the blood glucose readings, and (3) adequate intake of saline and carbohydrate.

1. **PATIENTS TREATED WITH INSULIN.** The patient's usual daily insulin dose is given at the customary times. The blood glucose level is measured, and additional rapid-acting insulin is given whenever the glucose reading is 240 mg/dL or higher. The dosage of supplemental rapid-acting insulin is typically one fourth of the usual total daily dosage of insulin. The goal is to maintain blood glucose concentration between 120 and 240 mg/dL. Intake of at least 150 grams of carbohydrate per 24 hours and enough saline to restore and/or maintain normal fluid volume is important. Patients with milder illnesses are usually able to take the requisite volume of fluid and allotment of carbohydrate by mouth.

2. **PATIENTS WHOSE DIABETES IS MANAGED WITH DIET ALONE OR ORAL HYPOGLYCEMIC AGENTS.** For patients with non–insulin-dependent diabetes mellitus, the management is the same as that already described, except that no intermediate-acting insulin is given, at least initially. Rapid-acting insulin is used when the blood glucose level before meals or at bedtime is 240 mg/dL or above. Initial doses of 4, 6, or 8 U are generally effective for small-, medium-, or large-framed persons, respectively. These doses can be adjusted up or down by 2 to 4 U, depending on the initial therapeutic response. The dose should be adjusted to maintain the blood glucose level between 120 and 240 mg/dL.

3. **PATIENTS TREATED ON CONTINUOUS SUBCUTANEOUS INSULIN INFUSION (INSULIN PUMP).** Patients receiving insulin by an insulin pump can often be managed during illness in or out of hospital by increasing the insulin infusion rate. For blood glucose readings of 240 mg/dL or more, the basal rate is increased by 50%. In addition, boluses equal to the usual bolus given before dinner are administered at the 4-hour checkpoints whenever the blood glucose level is 240 mg/dL or higher. The accelerated basal rate is maintained until a blood glucose reading of under 150 mg/dL is noted at a 4-hour blood glucose checkpoint.

4. **BLOOD GLUCOSE MANAGEMENT DURING HYPERALIMENTATION.** In the diabetic patient receiving parenteral hyperalimentation with concentrated glucose solutions, we recommend the addition of rapid-acting insulin to each liter of hyperalimentation fluid. A commonly chosen starting dose is 10 U/L. Substantially larger doses are often necessary, and amounts of 25 to 50 U/L sometimes are required to

control hyperglycemia. Even higher doses may be needed. IV infusions of dextrose should be continued for several hours after discontinuation of hyperalimentation to prevent hypoglycemia as a result of residual insulin action.

5. **MANAGEMENT OF DIABETES DURING SURGERY.** The goals of diabetes management in the perioperative period are to avoid extremes of glycemia and to prevent ketosis. Blood glucose concentrations between 120 and 240 mg/dL are desirable but difficult to achieve, and in many cases less stringent standards of between 100 and 300 mg/dL may have to be accepted.

On the morning of surgery, an IV infusion is started, using D_5 (usually in one-half NS), at 125 mg/hour. The object of providing 150 gm of glucose over 24 hours is to prevent excessive fat mobilization and ketone production and to protect against hypoglycemia. One half of the usual total daily dose of insulin is administered as intermediate-acting insulin (lente or NPH). Each time the blood glucose level is 240 mg/dL or more, rapid-acting insulin is given in an amount equivalent to ¼ of the patient's usual total daily dose. This protocol is continued until the patient is able to eat, when the patient's usual insulin dose is restarted while continuing the supplemental regular dose for blood glucose concentrations of 240 mg/dL or higher.

For the diabetic patient treated with oral agents or diet alone, an IV infusion is started using the same fluids and is administered at the same rate as described earlier. Blood glucose is measured every 6 hours, and rapid-acting insulin is given when the blood glucose level is 240 mg/dL or higher. For the average-sized person, a dose of 6 U of rapid-acting insulin is usually adequate, but large patients or those undergoing very extensive surgery may require substantially larger doses. The oral antidiabetic agents are omitted the day of surgery and restarted only when the patient is eating again. The contingency doses of rapid-acting insulin at the 6-hour checkpoints should be continued until the blood glucose level is consistently below 240 mg/dL.

D. **Iatrogenic Hypoglycemia.** Patients who take insulin or an oral hypoglycemic medication can develop hypoglycemia causing confusion, stupor, coma, and/or convulsions. Patients with hypoglycemia and depressed levels of consciousness should not be given oral glucose because of the risk of aspiration. Glucagon, 1 mg IM, will usually correct hypoglycemia within 30 minutes, by stimulating hepatic glycogenolysis. If qualified personnel are available, initial therapy in the obtunded or unconscious patient should be IV glucose, 50 ml or 50% dextrose (D_{50}). All patients should be observed until they are fully alert and have eaten a snack or meal. Patients with hypoglycemia caused by insulin may then be sent home if they are fully capable of taking their usual meals and a bedtime snack.

Hypoglycemic coma caused by sulfonylureas may be profound and long lasting. Patients who take sulfonylureas and who have severe, symptomatic hypoglycemia should be hospitalized and kept under close observation, including frequent blood glucose monitoring, for at least 24 hours. If hypoglycemia recurs, an infusion of D_{10} should be maintained at a rate sufficient to maintain the blood glucose concentration between 100 and 200 mg/dL.

Some patients who have been profoundly hypoglycemic remain unconscious even after the blood glucose level has been restored to normal. In such patients, cerebral edema may be responsible for the persisting coma. Mannitol, 200 ml of 20% solution given IV over 20 minutes, and dexamethasone, 10 mg IV, have been used with some apparent success in the treatment of persistent coma following hypoglycemia.

After treatment, the circumstances surrounding the episode of hypoglycemia must be reviewed with the patient and measures to prevent recurrences implemented.

IX. HYPERLIPIDEMIAS

A. Hypercholesterolemia. Reducing hypercholesterolemia lowers the risk of coronary artery atherosclerosis. Two groups of experts, operating as a National Institutes of Health (NIH) Consensus Development Conference and the National Cholesterol Education Program, provided clinically useful recommendations for dealing with hypercholesterolemia.

Before deciding on a specific treatment program for the individual patient with hypercholesterolemia, the physician should follow these steps:

---

1. Confirm the initial laboratory results. Variation in the levels of cholesterol and high-density lipoprotein cholesterol (HDLC) from both biologic and analytic causes is considerable.
2. Search for specific and potentially remediable conditions that may be causing the hypercholesterolemia. Hypothyroidism, certain medications (especially thiazide diuretics and beta blockers), obstructive biliary disease, the nephrotic syndrome, and dysproteinemia all may affect plasma cholesterol concentrations.
3. Identify and eliminate other possible coronary artery disease risk factors, such as hypertension, cigarette smoking, sedentary lifestyle, and extreme obesity.
4. Take into account the patient's age, attitude to therapy, response to previous therapy, if any, and presence of other conditions that may limit life expectancy in making treatment decisions.

The recommended treatment program is based on plasma cholesterol and low-density lipoprotein cholesterol (LDLC) concentrations. The total cholesterol level is used for initial case finding and for monitoring; LDLC is used for certain therapeutic decisions. LDLC is calculated by the equation given below.

$$LDLC = \text{total cholesterol} - (\text{triglycerides} \div 5 + HDLC)$$

Also taken into account in making treatment decisions are coronary artery disease risk factors, which, in addition to those already mentioned, include a family history of coronary artery disease, diabetes, and HDLC concentrations below 35 mg/dL (Fig. 12–1).

1. **DIET.** The foundation of treatment is a diet low in saturated fat and limited in cholesterol and, for overweight persons, restricted in calories. The American Heart Association has recommended that the total fat content of the diet should not exceed 30% and the saturated fat should not exceed 10% of caloric intake. Cholesterol should be limited to 300 mg/day. This is the so-called step 1 diet. If a more stringent diet is considered necessary, the step 2 diet limits the saturated fat to less than 7% of total calories and the cholesterol intake to less than 200 mg per day. Dietary therapy may be quite effective, especially in obese individuals and in patients with mixed hyperlipidemias (such as familial combined hyperlipidemia). Since the relationship between plasma cholesterol levels and atherosclerosis is less clear in patients in the 7th decade of age and beyond, it seems reasonable to be cautious about using medication in these older patients.

2. **MEDICATIONS FOR TREATING UNFAVORABLE PLASMA LIPID CONCENTRATIONS.** The primary objective of treating hypercholesterolemia is to reduce the patient's risk of atherosclerotic coronary artery disease. Therefore, raising HDLC may be at least as important as lowering total cholesterol and LDLC concentrations. Patients more suitable for treatment with the fibric acid derivatives, which primarily raise HDLC, are those with mild to moderately severe hypercholesterolemia (240 to 300 mg/dL) and those whose HDLC concentration is below 40 mg/dL. The concomitant presence of hypertriglyceridemia (unresponsive to diet) would strengthen the indication for use of fibric acid derivatives. Patients with more severely elevated plasma cholesterol concentrations might best be treated with agents that primarily reduce LDLC. Medications available are considered below.

    a. Fibric Acid Derivatives. In a population of younger middle-aged men, treatment with **gemfibrozil** (600 mg bid) resulted in favorable changes in the levels of total cholesterol, LDLC, and HDLC of about 10%. Fatal and nonfatal coronary events were reduced by 34%.

    New third-generation (**clofibrate** having been the first and gemfibrozil the second generation) fibric acid derivatives, including **fenofibrate** and **bezafibrate**, may become available. The newer agents are more potent, are more effective in lowering LDLC, and still retain their capacity to raise HDLC levels. Fibric acid derivatives are almost always well tolerated, side effects being infrequent and generally mild.

    b. Compactin Derivatives. These agents competitively inhibit 3-hydroxy-3-methylglutaryl coenzyme A reductase, the rate-limiting step in cholesterol synthesis. The most studied of these agents to date is **lovastatin**, which markedly reduces plasma LDL concentrations both in familial and in less clearly categorized types of

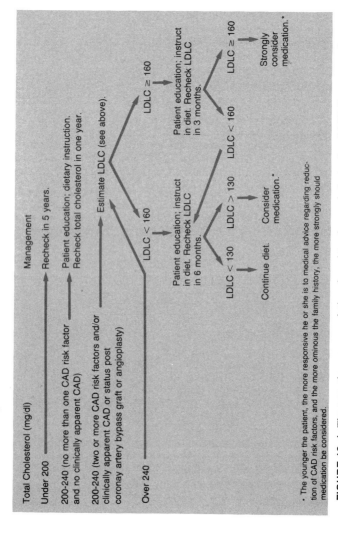

Total Cholesterol (mg/dl)   **Management**

Under 200 → Recheck in 5 years.

200-240 (no more than one CAD risk factor and no clinically apparent CAD) → Patient education; dietary instruction. Recheck total cholesterol in one year.

200-240 (two or more CAD risk factors and/or clinically apparent CAD or status post coronary artery bypass graft or angioplasty) → Estimate LDLC (see above).

Over 240 → Estimate LDLC (see above).

- LDLC < 160 → Patient education; instruct in diet. Recheck LDLC in 6 months.
  - LDLC < 130 → Continue diet.
  - LDLC > 130 → Consider medication.*
- LDLC ≥ 160 → Patient education; instruct in diet. Recheck LDLC in 3 months.
  - LDLC < 160 → Consider medication.*
  - LDLC ≥ 160 → Strongly consider medication.*

* The younger the patient, the more responsive he or she is to medical advice regarding reduction of CAD risk factors, and the more ominous the family history, the more strongly should medication be considered.

FIGURE 12–1. Therapeutic recommendations keyed to plasma cholesterol and LDLC concentrations.

hypercholesterolemia. In a small-scale study, lovastatin, in a dose of 20 mg bid, lowered the mean serum cholesterol level from 258 to 191 mg/dL and raised the mean HDLC level from 43 to 50 mg/dL. These medications seem to be well tolerated; minor elevations of liver enzyme concentration and corneal opacities are infrequent side effects. Otherwise, no serious side effects have appeared to date. In familial hypercholesterolemia, the combination of lovastatin with a bile acid-sequestrating resin appears to be considerably more effective than either agent alone.

   c. **Bile Acid–Sequestrating Resins. Cholestyramine** and **colestipol** act by binding bile salts in the intestine, thereby preventing their enterohepatic recirculation. The need for increased synthesis of bile acids depletes hepatic cholesterol, their metabolic precursor, which in turn induces up-regulation of hepatic B and E apoprotein receptors. This action has the effect of enhancing LDL clearance but also induces increased hepatic cholesterol synthesis, thereby tending to limit the efficacy of these agents. Therapy is usually started with a daily dose of 2 or 3 packets, each of which contains either 4 gm of cholestyramine or 5 gm of colestipol, stirred into water or juices. The dose is increased as indicated by serum cholesterol levels, to a maximal dosage of 24 or 30 gm daily, in divided doses before meals. These agents are expensive and unpleasant to take because of taste and insolubility. Many patients complain of bloating, constipation, or queasiness, and compliance is often suboptimal. At maximal doses, resins may reduce LDL by as much as 10 to 30 per cent. Resins can be used in combination with other agents, such as compactin derivatives or nicotinic acid.

   d. **Nicotinic Acid.** Nicotinic acid inhibits very low-density lipoprotein (VLDL) production and, as a result, also decreases LDL production. The plasma cholesterol level may be reduced up to 25% by nicotinic acid, depending on the mechanism of the hypercholesterolemia. Frequent undesirable side effects include flushing and pruritus (ameliorated by taking aspirin before each dose until tachyphylaxis eliminates the flushing) and upper GI discomfort. Aggravation of peptic ulcer disease, gout, and non–insulin-dependent diabetes mellitus may occur. The initial dosage is usually 250–500 mg daily, increased every week or two, as tolerated, to a full therapeutic dosage of 2.0–7.5 gm daily. Nicotinic acid is usually combined with a resin in the treatment of hypercholesterolemia.

B. Hypertriglyceridemia

   1. GENERAL CONSIDERATIONS. The role of hypertriglyceridemia in atherogenesis is less certain. Several studies have failed to identify a relationship. However, members of some families with a high prevalence of hypertriglyceridemia seem to be susceptible to atherosclerosis.

   Hypertriglyceridemia often reflects the interaction of a genetic cause, such as familial hypertriglyceridemia or familial combined hyperlipidemia, and an acquired cause, such as poorly controlled diabetes mellitus, certain medications (estrogens, beta-blocking agents, thiazide diuretics, or glucocorticoids), alcohol consumption, obesity, hypothyroidism, or uremia. The combination of excessive endogenous triglycerides and hyperchylomicronemia may result in triglyceride concentrations of more than 1000 mg/dL or even 20–30 times that high. Patients with such high levels of triglycerides are in danger of developing the chylomicronemic syndrome, the manifestations of which include acute pancreatitis, nonspecific abdominal or, infrequently, chest pain, impairment of recent memory, hepatomegaly, and eruptive xanthomatosis.

2. **APPROACH TO TREATMENT.** Guidelines for treating hypertriglyceridemia are given below.

---

1. Always search for and treat conditions that may cause or aggravate hypertriglyceridemia. Estrogen therapy and alcohol consumption, even in very modest amounts, may greatly elevate triglyceride concentrations in susceptible individuals. Improving diabetes control, using alternative therapy in place of thiazides and beta-adrenergic blocking agents, dietary therapy for obesity, and elimination of alcohol may make specific treatment for hypertriglyceridemia unnecessary.
2. Patients with slightly to moderately elevated triglyceride levels (250–500 mg/dL) should be treated with dietary modification only.
3. In patients with more severe hypertriglyceridemia (500–1000 mg/dL) who do not respond to diet alone and who have a family history of hypertriglyceridemia-associated atherosclerosis, the addition of medication to dietary therapy warrants consideration. In the absence of a family history of atherosclerosis, it is generally preferable not to use medication.
4. Patients with severe hypertriglyceridemia (in excess of 1000 mg/dL) who do not respond to diet alone, including complete abstention from alcohol, should be treated with medication.

---

3. **THERAPEUTIC MODALITIES**

a. **Diet.** The dietary treatment of hypertriglyceridemia is essentially the same as that for hypercholesterolemia described above. The essential feature is limitation of total fat and saturated fat and correction of obesity. Addition of fish oils rich in omega-3 fatty acids should be considered in patients not responding to standard dietary therapy.

b. **Fibric Acid Derivatives.** Gemfibrozil (600 mg bid) and clofibrate (1 gm bid) are often quite effective in lowering plasma triglyceride levels. In patients with familial combined hyperlipidemia or in those with family histories characterized by the combination of hypertriglyceridemia and atherogenesis, therapy using a resin in combination with either nicotinic acid or gemfibrozil may be preferable. Clofibrate has been shown to promote gallstone formation, cardiac arrhythmias, and venous thromboembolism. Gemfibrozil may be less lithogenic and seems to be more effective in lowering VLDL and raising HDL than is clofibrate.

c. Nicotinic Acid. See relevant section under "Hypercholesterolemia."

Brown G, Albers JJ, Fisher LD, et al: Regression of coronary artery disease as a result of intensive lipid-lowering therapy in men with high levels of apolipoprotein B. N Engl J Med 323:1289–1298, 1990.

Brown WB (ed): Fenofibrate, a third generation fibric acid derivative. Am J Med 83 (Suppl 5B):1–89, 1987.

Frick MH, Elo O, Haapa K, et al: Helsinki Heart Study: Primary-Prevention Trial with Gemfibrozil in Middle-Aged Men with Dyslipidemia. N Engl J Med 317:1237–1245, 1987.

Grundy SM: Cholesterol and coronary heart disease. JAMA 264:3053–3059, 1990.

Hegsted DM, Nicolosi RJ: Individual variation in serum cholesterol levels. Proc Natl Acad Sci USA 84:6259, 1987.

Hoeg JM, Brewer HB: 3-Hydroxy-3-methyglutaryl-co-enzyme A reductase inhibitors in the treatment of hypercholesterolemia. JAMA 258:3532–3536, 1987.

Vega GL, Grundy SM: Treatment of primary moderate hypercholesterolemia with lovastatin (mevinolin) and colestipol. JAMA 257:33–38, 1987.

13 13 13 13 13 13 13 13 13

NUTRITIONAL THERAPEUTICS

A. HILLARY STEINHART
JEFFREY P. BAKER
ALLAN S. DETSKY

13 13 13 13 13 13 13 13 13 13 13

I. NORMAL NUTRITIONAL REQUIREMENTS

Normal dietary intake should provide a balanced supply of energy, protein, fluid and electrolytes, vitamins, minerals, and trace elements. Table 13–1 lists a summary of **recommended daily nutrient intakes** for people of both sexes and all ages. Individual variation in nutrient requirement does exist, depending on the person's level of activity, rate of growth, concomitant stress, or illness. This variation must be considered when tables such as these are used. Table 13–2 lists characteristics of therapeutic diets.

A. Energy. The average energy intake required to maintain body weight in adults is in the range of 25–35 kcal/kg/day. Energy expenditure can

TABLE 13–1A. AVERAGE DAILY ENERGY REQUIREMENTS

AGE	SEX	AVERAGE WEIGHT (kg)	AVERAGE DAILY ENERGY REQUIREMENT (kcal/kg)	(kcal/d)
Months				
0–2	Both	4.5	120–100[a]	500
3–5	Both	7.0	100–95	700
6–8	Both	8.5	95–97	800
9–11	Both	9.5	97–99	950
Years				
1	Both	11	101	1100
2–3	Both	14	94	1300
4–6	Both	18	100	1800
7–9	M	25	88	2200
	F	25	76	1900
10–12	M	34	73	2500
	F	36	61	2200
13–15	M	50	57	2800
	F	48	46	2200
16–18	M	62	51	3200
	F	53	40	2100
19–24	M	71	42	3000
	F	58	36	2100
25–49	M	74	36	2700
	F	59	32	1900
50–74	M	73	31	2300
	F	63	29	1800
75 +	M	69	29	2000
	F	64	23	1500

[a]1st and 2nd figures are averages at the beginning and the end of the period.
Data from Canada Health and Welfare: Nutrition Recommendations. The Report of the Scientific Review Committee, 1990.

TABLE 13–1B. RECOMMENDED DAILY NUTRIENT INTAKE BASED ON AGE AND BODY WEIGHT

AGE	SEX	WEIGHT (kg)	PROTEIN (gm)	THIAMINE (mg)	RIBO-FLAVIN (mg)	NIACIN (NE[a])	n-3 PUFA[b] (gm)	n-6 PUFA (gm)	VIT A (RE[c])
Months									
0–4	Both	6.0	12[c]	0.3	0.3	4	0.5	3	400
5–12	Both	9.0	12	0.4	0.5	7	0.5	3	400
Years									
1	Both	11	19	0.5	0.6	8	0.6	4	400
2–3	Both	14	22	0.6	0.7	9	0.7	4	400
4–6	Both	18	26	0.7	0.9	13	1.0	6	500
7–9	M	25	30	0.9	1.1	16	1.2	7	700
	F	25	30	0.8	1.0	14	1.0	6	700
10–12	M	34	38	1.0	1.3	18	1.4	8	800
	F	36	40	0.9	1.1	16	1.1	7	800
13–15	M	50	50	1.1	1.4	20	1.4	9	900
	F	48	42	0.9	1.1	16	1.2	7	800
16–18	M	62	55	1.3	1.6	23	1.8	11	1000
	F	53	43	0.8	1.1	15	1.2	7	800
19–24	M	71	58	1.2	1.5	22	1.6	10	1000
	F	58	43	0.8	1.1	15	1.2	7	800
25–49	M	74	61	1.1	1.4	19	1.5	9	1000
	F	59	44	0.8	1.0	14	1.1	7	800
50–74	M	73	60	0.9	1.3	16	1.3	8	1000
	F	63	47	0.8[h]	1.0[h]	14[h]	1.1[h]	7[h]	800
75 +	M	69	57	0.8	1.0	14	1.0	7	1000
	F	64	47	0.8[h]	1.0[h]	14[h]	1.1[h]	7[h]	800
Pregnancy (additional)									
1st Trimester			5	0.1	0.1	0.1	0.05	0.3	100
2nd Trimester			20	0.1	0.3	0.2	0.16	0.9	100
3rd Trimester			24	0.1	0.3	0.2	0.16	0.9	100
Lactation (additional)			20	0.2	0.4	0.3	0.25	1.5	400

be measured by means of indirect calorimetry. However, in most instances this is impractical and an easier alternative is to calculate the **basal energy expenditure** (BEE) by means of the Harris and Benedict equations for men and women:

$$\text{Men: BEE (kJ/d)} = 66 + 13.8W + 5H - 6.8A$$
$$\text{Women: BEE (kJ/d)} = 655 + 9.6W + 1.8H - 4.7A$$

where W is body weight (kg), H is height (cm), and A is age (yrs). The calculated BEE should be adjusted upward approximately 10% to account for the thermogenic effect of feeding (REE = resting energy expenditure). An adjustment should also be made for the degree of stress and activity. It appears that, for patients on total parenteral nutrition, the maximum hypermetabolism secondary to stress, is approximately 30%.

Nonprotein energy requirements can be provided in the form of either carbohydrate or fat. **Carbohydrate** provides 4 kcal/gm whereas fat provides 9 kcal/gm. Current recommendations suggest reducing fat intake to 30% of total energy requirements with ⅓ of the fat in the form of saturated fats, ⅓ as monounsaturated fats and ⅓ as polyunsaturated fats. A minimum amount of the essential n-3 and n-6 **polyunsaturated fatty acids** should be present in the diet (Table 13–1B). **Cholesterol**

TABLE 13–1B. RECOMMENDED DAILY NUTRIENT INTAKE BASED ON AGE AND BODY WEIGHT *Continued*

VIT D (µg)	VIT E (mg)	VIT C (mg^d)	Folate (µg)	VIT B$_{12}$ (µg)	CAL-CIUM (mg)	PHOS-PHORUS (mg)	MAG-NESIUM (mg)	IRON (mg)	IODINE (µg)	ZINC (mg)
10	3	20	50	0.3	250^f	150	20	0.3^g	30	2^g
10	3	20	50	0.3	400	200	32	7	40	3
10	3	20	65	0.3	500	300	40	6	55	4
5	4	20	80	0.4	550	350	50	6	65	4
5	5	25	90	0.5	600	400	65	8	85	5
2.5	7	25	125	0.8	700	500	100	8	110	7
2.5	6	25	125	0.8	700	500	100	8	95	7
2.5	8	25	170	1.0	900	700	130	8	125	9
5	7	25	180	1.0	1100	800	135	8	110	9
5	9	30	150	1.5	1100	900	185	10	160	12
5	7	30	145	1.5	1000	850	180	13	160	9
5	10	40	185	1.9	900	1000	230	10	160	12
2.5	7	30	160	1.9	700	850	200	12	160	9
2.5	10	40	210	2.0	800	1000	240	9	160	12
2.5	7	30	175	2.0	700	850	200	13	160	9
2.5	9	40	220	2.0	800	1000	250	9	160	12
2.5	6	30	175	2.0	700	850	200	13	160	9
5	7	40	220	2.0	800	1000	250	9	160	12
5	6	30	190	2.0	800	850	210	8	160	9
5	6	40	205	2.0	800	1000	230	9	160	12
5	5	30	190	2.0	800	850	210	8	160	9
2.5	2	0	300	1.0	500	200	15	0	25	6
2.5	2	10	300	1.0	500	200	45	5	25	6
2.5	2	10	300	1.0	500	200	45	10	25	6
2.5	3	25	100	0.5	500	200	65	0	50	6

^{a}NE = Niacin Equivalents (1 NE = 1 mg niacin = 60 mg tryptophan).
^{b}PUFA = Polyunsaturated fatty acids.
^{c}RE = Retinol Equivalents (1 RE = 1 µg (3.33 IU) retinol, 2 µg beta-carotene or 12 µg of other carotenoid provitamins).
^{d}Smokers should increase vitamin C by 50%.
^{e}Protein is assumed to be from breast milk and must be adjusted for infant formula.
^{f}Infant formula with high phosphorus should contain 375 mg calcium.
^{g}Breast milk is assumed to be the source of the mineral.
^{h}Level below which intake should not fall.
Data from Canada Health and Welfare: Nutrition Recommendations. The Report of the Scientific Review Committee, 1990.

should probably be restricted to less than 300 mg daily. Increasing the amount of complex carbohydrates, such as starches and fibers, and decreasing the amount of simple sugars in the diet should be promoted.

B. Protein. Adequate daily protein intake for adults should be at least 0.6 gm/kg, according to the World Health Organization. In North America, this amount is generally greatly exceeded. Requirements are higher for children, adolescents, and pregnant and lactating women. Although most of the population far exceed the recommended protein intake there exists a significant proportion—primarily children, the poor and socially disadvantaged, the elderly—who do not have adequate protein intake.

Foods high in protein include meats, poultry, fish, eggs, milk and milk products, nuts, seeds and some legumes, grains and cereals. However,

TABLE 13–2. THERAPEUTIC DIETS

TYPE	INDICATION(S)	MAIN FEATURES	COMMENTS
Diabetic	Diabetes–Types I and II Gestational diabetes Impaired glucose tolerance	Increased CHO (50–55%) in form of soluble fiber Lower saturated fats Lower simple sugars	Timing of meals and snacks important (especially for patients on insulin) Weight loss for obese type II diabetics Diets based on food group substitutions
Lipid lowering	Prevention of coronary heart disease in moderate to high risk groups Blood cholesterol > 75th percentile Blood trigylceride > 90th percentile	20–30% of total calories as fat Cholesterol 100–300 mg/d Decrease or eliminate alcohol and sugars for hypertriglyceridemias Polyunsaturated/saturated fatty acid ratio > 1	Degree of restriction depends on cholesterol and triglyceride levels and previous intake
Sodium restricted	Congestive heart failure Liver disease with ascites Salt-sensitive hypertension Renal disease with sodium retention Excess mineralocorticoid states	Degree of Sodium Restriction 22 mmol (500 mg)—very strict 44 mmol (1 gm)—strict 87 mmol (2 gm)—moderate 130–217 mmol (3–5 gm)—no added salt	No salt added to foods Foods prepared and cooked without salt Low-sodium breads and butters may be required depending on restriction Dairy products and certain vegetables used in limited quantities
Controlled energy	Obesity (weight > 20% above ideal)	Reduced caloric intake of nutritionally balanced foods Avoid diets of < 4000 KJ (1000 Kcal)/day	Gradual weight loss is best (1–2 lbs per week) Physical activity important adjuvant Behavioral treatment often helpful
Renal	Renal insufficiency Chronic renal failure Acute renal failure	Energy, protein, fluid, electrolytes, vitamin and mineral intakes individualized depending on degree and type of renal impairment, use of dialysis and concomitant illnesses such as diabetes, sepsis, hypertension	Moderate protein restriction may slow progression of renal failure (0.55–0.6 gm/kg/d); increase protein for increased urinary protein losses; anorexia often a problem in chronic renal failure

Diet	Indication	Description	Comments
Liver	Hepatic failure End-stage liver disease with encephalopathy Portacaval shunt	Protein restriction for encephalopathy (0–40 gm/d) depending on stage Sodium (<2 gm/d) and water (<1500 mL/d) restriction for ascites and hyponatremia	Plant protein sources may produce less encephalopathy Hypoglycemia complicating hepatic failure generally requires IV glucose
Restricted lactose	Primary lactase deficiency Secondary lactase deficiency	Eliminate milk, milk products and some processed foods; individual tolerance determined by adding foods containing small amounts of lactose; some yogurts, fermented cheeses, and lactose-reduced milks can be tolerated	May require calcium, riboflavin and/or vitamin D supplementation
Gluten-free	Celiac disease Dermatitis herpetiformis	Eliminate barley, wheat, rye, triticale, and usually oats, wheatstarch, and beer; may have secondary lactose deficiency early in course	Individual variation exists in sensitivity to oats, malt extracts, and derivatives
Antireflux	Gastroesophageal reflux disease ? Nonulcer dyspepsia	Avoid coffee, tea, alcohol, mints, cola, cocoa, chocolate, fat, onion, garlic; small, frequent meals; avoid lying down for 2–3 hrs after meals; weight loss in obesity	Drugs, (NSAIDs, aspirin, anticholinergics) and smoking may be aggravating factors; individual tolerance to spicy foods and acidic fruit juices should be determined; elevate head of bed 4–6 inches on blocks
Post-gastrectomy	Postoperative partial or total gastrectomy, vagotomy and pyloroplasty Dumping syndrome	Small, frequent dry meals; separation of liquids and solids; low in simple carbohydrate with sufficient fat and protein	Can attempt gradual return to normal diet as tolerated; monitor weight, iron, folate and B_{12} status; watch for lactose intolerance and or steatorrhea in some patients with diarrhea

not all proteins are of equal quality. Some sources of protein, especially the vegetable sources, are lacking in one or more of the **essential amino acids**. These proteins are considered incomplete and must be taken with complementary sources of protein that provide the deficient essential amino acid(s). This is very important for people such as vegetarians, whose major protein intake is from nonanimal sources.

C. **Fluid and Electrolytes.** **Fluid intake** should be 1500–2000 mL daily. There is no fixed requirement for dietary **sodium** since normally functioning kidneys can adapt to either dietary sodium deficiency or excess. However, most sources advise avoidance of excessive sodium intake by keeping it in the range of 1.4–2.0 mmol (32–46 mg)/kg daily. Recommended daily intake for children is approximately 0.4 mmol (9 mg)/kg. **Potassium** is required for anabolic processes such as protein synthesis and cellular glucose uptake. Recommended daily potassium intake is 0.75 mmol (29 mg)/kg for adults and 1.75 mmol (68 mg)/kg for children. Recommendations for fluid and electrolyte intake in normal subjects vary according to physical activity and environmental conditions such as temperature and humidity.

D. **Vitamins and Minerals.** Recommended daily intakes of selected vitamins and minerals are listed in Table 13–1b. These micronutrients are required for maintenance of normal metabolic processes. A lack of one is often associated with a specific deficiency syndrome. The food sources of the various vitamins and minerals and the signs and symptoms of the deficiency syndromes are listed elsewhere (see References).

E. **Trace Elements.** Trace elements are present in the diet in only extremely small amounts. Deficiency syndromes are rare but do occur. The importance of the trace elements is in the fact that these syndromes can occur if trace elements are not added to parenteral nutrition solutions given to patients who are not eating.

II. NUTRITIONAL ASSESSMENT

Before nutritional support is provided for the patient at risk of developing, or who has already developed, a nutrition-associated complication, the physician must first know whether nutritional support is required for this patient at the time. To determine this, it is first necessary to assess the patient's nutritional status. Assessment may range from a simple screening procedure based on data in the patient's history and physical examination to more elaborate laboratory techniques.

A. **Diet History.** This may be performed in a number of ways such as observation of the patient's intake, determining food preferences and frequency of intake, keeping a 3–7 day record of food intake, or obtaining a 24-hour dietary recall. With these methods, one can determine if the patient's nutritional needs are being met based on standard requirements with allowances made for the underlying disease(s) and stress.

B. Physical Examination. Physical examination can provide indicators of nutritional deficiencies. Some indicators of protein-calorie malnutrition are cachexia, muscle wasting, loss of subcutaneous fat, and edema or ascites. In addition, other signs of specific nutrient or vitamin deficiency syndromes may be detected.

C. Anthropometric Measurements

1. **WEIGHT.** There are a number of methods of expressing body weight in order to determine nutritional status. The current weight or **percentage of ideal body weight** based on height and body frame size, as outlined in the Metropolitan Life Insurance Company tables, can be used, but they do not make allowances for obese patients who have lost lean body mass although their total body weight may still be greater than ideal. This problem is avoided by the use of the **percentage of usual body weight** or by **recent weight change**. Weight loss of 20–25% of the usual body weight is associated with increased morbidity and mortality. However, when using these measurements one must be aware that changes in body water, such as an increase in edema, can easily mask changes in muscle and fat content.

   The **body mass index** (BMI) is a simple way of expressing body weight in a standard manner. It is obtained by dividing the body weight (kg) by the square of the height (m). The resulting value correlates well with body fat. The normal range is 20–25 kg/m^2 with values below 18 indicating risk of nutrition-associated complications and values over 27 indicating risk of obesity-related complications. The BMI is difficult to use in the elderly, muscular athletes, and pregnant and lactating women. It should not be used in children or adolescents.

2. **SUBCUTANEOUS FAT MEASUREMENTS.** The use of calipers to measure **skinfold thickness** at various body sites—triceps, subscapular, suprailiac, anterior thigh, and umbilical—provides an indirect but reliable measurement of body fat stores. Standardized techniques performed by trained personnel using proper equipment must be ensured so that the results obtained are reliable. These measurements are not sufficiently sensitive to detect small or acute changes in body fat but can be used in monitoring chronic situations. Results can be compared with standard tables, and patients' percentiles can be determined. **Body fat depletion** is indicated by a result below the 15th percentile. However, the results are limited by the fact that they do not account for differences in fat distribution, edema fluid, and hydration status.

3. **SOMATIC PROTEIN MEASUREMENTS.** Mid-arm muscle circumference (MAMC) is an indirect measure of muscle mass calculated based on the mid-arm circumference and the triceps skinfold thickness. Errors are due to failure to account for individual variation in skin compressibility and humerus diameter and for the incorrect assumption in the model that the arm and underlying muscle are cylindrical. The MAMC is not a reliable measure of acute changes in somatic proteins but,

like subcutaneous fat measurements, can be used in monitoring chronic changes.

4. **GROWTH CHARTS.** The assessment of nutritional status in infants, children, and adolescents can be performed by means of following the growth patterns over time. Standard charts are available for plotting height, weight, or growth velocity. Deviations below the 5th percentile or a significant change in the growth pattern may indicate a nutritional deficiency, although numerous underlying disease processes can also alter growth without directly affecting nutritional status.

D. Biochemical Measurements

1. **SOMATIC PROTEINS.** These are indirect measures of the somatic protein compartment and include the **creatinine height index** and the **urinary excretion of 3-methylhistidine**. The creatinine height index involves 3 24-hour urine collections to determine the creatinine excretion as an indicator of muscle protein stores. The results are compared with standard tables for creatinine excretion and a percentage of ideal is determined. Creatinine excretion may be increased in patients with trauma or infection or in those who have undergone surgery. Excretion is decreased with increasing age, decreased GFR, and degenerative disease.

2. **VISCERAL PROTEINS.** A number of proteins that are synthesized in the liver can be measured in the serum (Table 13–3). These vary in their sensitivity and specificity for indicating malnutrition and in their circulating half-life in serum. Generally, the proteins with the shortest half-lives are the best indicators of acute or early changes in nutritional status.

E. Subjective Global Assessment (SGA).

The SGA is an easily derived measure based on data obtained from a screening history and physical examination (Table 13–4). These include patterns of weight change, dietary intake, gastrointestinal symptoms, functional capacity, the underlying disease process and its relation to nutritional needs, loss of subcutaneous fat, muscle wasting, edema, and ascites. The factors are weighted according to the examiner's subjective impression of their relative importance in that patient and the patient is then given an overall rating of either well nourished (A), moderate or suspected malnutrition (B), or severe malnutrition (C).

The SGA can be performed easily by properly trained physicians, house officers, dieticians, and nurses. It has been shown to be reliable among different observers to accurately predict the occurrence of nutrition-associated complications such as infection, and it correlates well with more objective measures of nutritional status.

F. Prognostic Nutritional Index (PNI).

The PNI is a weighted index based on 4 objective measurements: **serum albumin, triceps skinfold thickness, serum transferrin and delayed hypersensitivity reaction to 3 recall antigens**. This index can be determined in nontrauma surgical patients at the time of admission. It accurately predicts the risk of postoperative complications in this patient population.

TABLE 13-3. NUTRITIONAL ASSESSMENT: VISCERAL PROTEINS

PROTEIN	CONDITIONS CAUSING INCREASE	CONDITIONS CAUSING DECREASE	COMMENTS
Serum albumin	Dehydration	Malnutrition Maldigestion Malabsorption Protein-losing states Liver disease Congestive heart failure Cancer Acute stress Hypothyroidism Overhydration Prolonged bed rest	Serum half-life of 14–20 days Not sensitive to early deficiency or malnutrition Not specific for malnutrition
Transferrin	Iron deficiency Chronic blood loss Hypoxia Pregnancy	Malnutrition Iron overload Pernicious anemia Chronic infection Liver disease Protein-losing enteropathy	Normal range 2.0–2.6 gm/L Serum half-life of 7–10 days Not sensitive to early deficiency or malnutrition
Thyroxine-binding prealbumin	Renal disease Hodgkin's disease	Malnutrition Liver disease Inflammatory bowel disease Hyperthyroidism Burns	Normal range 1.6–3.0 gm/L Serum half-life of 2 days More sensitive to malnutrition than albumin or transferrin
Retinol-binding protein	Renal disease	Nephrotic syndrome Malnutrition Liver disease Acute metabolic stress Hyperthyroidism Cystic fibrosis	Normal range 0.3–0.8 gm/L Serum half-life of 10–12 hours Synthesized in the liver and catabolized in the kidney Very sensitive to early nutritional changes

TABLE 13–4. SUBJECTIVE GLOBAL ASSESSMENT (SGA)

(Select appropriate category with a checkmark, or enter numerical value where indicated by "#")

A. History
  1. Weight change
    Overall loss in past 6 months: amount = #_____kg; % loss = #_____
    Change in past 2 weeks: _____increase
                        _____no change
                        _____decrease

  2. Dietary intake change (relative to normal)
    _____No change
    _____Change _____duration = #_____weeks
             _____type: _____suboptimal solid diet
                          _____full liquid diet
                          _____hypocaloric liquids
                          _____starvation

  3. Gastrointestinal symptoms (that persisted for > 2 weeks)
    _____none, _____nausea, _____vomiting, _____diarrhea, _____anorexia

  4. Functional capacity
    _____No dysfunction (e.g., full capacity)
    _____Dysfunction _____duration = #_____ weeks
             _____type: _____working suboptimally
                        _____ambulatory
                        _____bedridden

  5. Disease and its relation to nutritional requirements
    Primary diagnosis (specify)_____
    Metabolic demand (stress): _____no stress _____low stress
                       _____moderate stress _____high stress

B. Physical (for each trait specify: 0 = normal, 1+ = mild, 2+ = moderate, 3+ = severe)
    #_____loss of subcutaneous fat (triceps, chest)
    #_____muscle wasting (quadriceps, deltoids)
    #_____ankle edema
    #_____sacral edema
    #_____ascites

C. SGA rating (select one)
    _____A = Well nourished
    _____B = Moderately (or suspected of being) malnourished
    _____C = Severely malnourished

PNI (% risk of complications) =
$$158 - 16.6 \text{ (ALB)} - 0.78(\text{TSF}) - 0.2(\text{TFN}) - 5.8(\text{DH})$$

where ALB = serum albumin (g/dL), TSF = triceps skinfold (mm), TFN = serum transferrin (mg/dL) and DH = maximal delayed hypersensitivity reaction to any of 3 antigens (0 = nonreactive, 1 = 5 mm reaction, 2 = greater than 5 mm reaction).

III. ENTERAL NUTRITION

When it has been determined that a patient has, or is at risk of developing, a nutrition-associated complication, a therapeutic approach must be selected. If the GI tract is functional, nutrition can often be provided orally or via tube feedings. Oral supplementation can be used if patients are able to take in enough by mouth to meet their needs. Consultation with a dietician may be needed to design an adequate diet that is acceptable to the patient. In some cases, supplementation with one of the nutritionally complete commercially available formulae (e.g., Sustacal, Meritene, Ensure, Osmolite, Isocal) or with one of the specific supplements (e.g., potassium, magnesium, calcium, zinc, vitamins) will be indicated. If the patient is still unable to meet nutritional requirments, additional support—either in the form of enteral tube feedings or parenteral nutrition—is indicated.

A. Indications for Enteral Tube Feedings

1. Patient has a functioning GI tract.
2. Patient is unable to meet nutritional requirements by means of oral feeding (anorexia, nausea, impaired swallowing, esophageal obstruction, major upper GI surgery, increased nutritional requirements, and so on.)
3. Growth retardation in children with inflammatory bowel disease (feeds given nocturnally at home) and primary therapy of inflammatory bowel disease.
4. Short bowel syndrome (more than 60 cm of functioning small intestine) or chronic partial bowel obstruction. Continuous pump infusion must be used in these situations.

B. Contraindications to Enteral Tube Feedings

1. Any cause of a nonfunctioning GI tract (e.g., obstruction, perforation, ileus, some diarrheal states such as short bowel syndrome and severe active inflammatory bowel disease).
2. High output fistula(s)
3. Inability to obtain tube access to the GI tract.
4. Refusal of patient or legal guardian.

C. Methods of Administration

1. **METHODS OF ACCESS TO THE GI TRACT**

   a. **Nasogastric (NG) tubes** are soft, narrow-bore Silastic or polyurethane tubes with weighted tips placed in the gastric antrum, ideally.

Their position in the stomach should be confirmed fluoroscopically prior to the initiation of feeding. These tubes have a tendency to clog and require frequent flushing. They are not suitable for high-viscosity formulas such as the blenderized diets but can be used for intermittent feeding.

   b. Nasoenteral (NE) Tubes. These are similar to but longer than the nasogastric tubes. They are placed in the distal duodenum or proximal jejunum under fluoroscopic control or guided by a gastroscope, and are useful in patients with delayed gastric emptying, especially when complicated by reflux and aspiration. They require continuous infusion of formula as opposed to intermittent feedings.

   c. Gastrostomy. These tubes can be inserted percutaneously under local anesthetic assisted by a gastroscope (PEG = percutaneous endoscopic gastrostomy) or under ultrasound and/or fluoroscopic guidance. They are considered to be the method of choice when long-term enteral feeding is required. They are useful when nasal irritation or necrosis occurs with NG or NE tubes and can be used for a blenderized diet. These tubes are easy to replace once the tract has matured. A smaller, mercury-tipped catheter can be passed through the gastrostomy tube down into the jejunum in order to avoid problems of impaired gastric emptying and reflux.

   d. Jejunostomy is usually performed at the time of major upper GI surgery such as a Whipple's procedure. It allows relatively early initiation of enteral feeding when the patient probably will not be able to eat for an extended period. It also avoids the problems of gastric retention and reflux or aspiration.

2. **METHODS OF FEEDING ADMINISTRATION**

   a. Intermittent Feeding. The total daily nutritional requirement is divided over 4–8 separate feedings aiming for a maximum volume of 300 mL per feeding. Each feeding is given over a minimum of 30 minutes and the feeding tube is flushed and capped after completion. This technique allows greater patient freedom between feedings *but cannot be used for tubes in the duodenum or jejunum.*

   b. Continuous Infusion. Formula is continuously infused over all or part of the day depending on individual patient requirements and tolerance. Usually there is no need to initiate infusion with diluted formulas; rather, a slower infusion rate (50 mL/hr) should be used with gradual increase to the target rate as tolerated. Some patients, such as those with short bowels or those in the ICU, may be sensitive to variation in the infusion rate and will require administration by a pump to avoid diarrhea and metabolic complications of enteral feeding.

D. **Enteral Formulas.** There are numerous enteral formulas available for use. They can be divided into several broad categories: **blenderized, polymeric,** (both milk-based and lactose-free), **elemental** (defined), **modular feedings**, and **formulas with altered amino acids**. For practical purposes, most clinicians need only be familiar with one or two formulas in each category (Table 13–5). Each nutritionally complete formula has a recommended daily volume. If this volume is not achieved, the patient is at risk of developing vitamin, mineral, or trace element deficiencies even though caloric intake may be adequate. Therefore, volumes should be continuously monitored and specific supplementation given accordingly.

E. Complications of Enteral Tube Feedings

1. MECHANICAL (TUBE) PROBLEMS

a. **Improperly Placed Tube.** All NG and NE tubes should have their position confirmed radiographically prior to initiation of feedings. Percutaneous feeding tubes are placed under direct vision, but can dislodge or migrate, especially during the first 10 days. This may result in pneumoperitoneum or leakage of gastric contents if the tract has not matured.

b. **ENT Irritation.** NG and NE tubes may result in local irritation to the nasal passageways, pharynx, and larynx. In extreme cases this may result in necrosis and infection. When these complications arise, percutaneous tube insertion should be considered.

c. **Tube Clogging.** This problem occurs primarily with small-bore tubes, but can happen with larger-bore tubes. To avoid tube clogging use low viscosity formulas, flush the tube with water or soda water after all feeds and medications, and use liquid suspensions of medications when available. Medications not available in suspension form should be crushed (except for slow-release or enteric-coated formulations).

2. GASTROINTESTINAL COMPLICATIONS

a. **Gastric Retention, Gastroesophageal Reflux, and Aspiration.** Tubes that traverse the lower esophageal sphincter may cause an increase in gastroesophageal reflux and result in esophagitis, esophageal stricture formation, and pulmonary aspiration. These complications are less common with small-bore tubes and tubes placed in the jejunum. Gastric residual volumes should be checked when gastric feedings are used; if they are greater than 100 mL, corrective action should be taken. Prokinetic agents, such as metoclopramide, domperidone or cisapride, can be used to avoid or treat gastric retention, but resistant cases may require percutaneous gastrostomy or jejunostomy. However, placement of a PEG may result in worsened gastric emptying, further aggravating reflux. This can be avoided by giving smaller feedings, keeping the head of the bed elevated, and by passing a smaller-bore tube through the gastrostomy tube into the jejunum. Small bowel feeding tubes usually get around the problem of gastric retention but are not suitable for bolus feedings.

b. **Nausea and Vomiting.** This is often associated with gastric retention and reflux but may be due to bowel obstruction, ileus, or numerous central causes of nausea and vomiting.

TABLE 13–5. ENTERAL FORMULAS

CATEGORY	DESCRIPTION	INDICATIONS AND ADVANTAGES	DISADVANTAGES
Blenderized formulas (Compleat Formulae)	Purée of beef, vegetables, fruits, nonfat dry milk, sucrose, corn oil; variations can be prepared at home for less cost but content not standardized; provides approximately 1 kcal/mL	Requires functional GI tract; contains complex carbohydrate and fiber sources; variations can be prepared at home for less cost	High lactose content; may contain gluten; high viscosity; high osmolarity; commercial preparations are expensive
Milk-based polymeric formulas (Sustacal Powder, Sustagen, Meritene)	Whole proteins (caseinates, egg albumin, soy) carbohydrates (corn syrup, maltodextrins, disaccharides), fats (vegetable oils), vitamins, and minerals; nutritionally complete; most provide approx. 1 kcal/mL but Sustagen provides 1.6 kcal/mL	Requires functional GI tract; palatable for oral use; low viscosity; consistent standardized formulation	High lactose content; high osmolarity
Lactose-free polymeric formulas (Ensure, EnsurePlus, Enrich, Isocal, Osmolite, Isosource, Precision Isotonic, Portagen, Resource Liquid, Isotein, Sustacal Liquid, Sustacal HC, Sustacal with Fiber, Jevity)	Protein isolates (12–16%), oligosaccharides (50–55%), medium and long chain triglycerides (30%), vitamins and minerals; all nutritionally complete (approximately 1 kcal/mL) but EnsurePlus, Sustacal HC, and others have higher caloric density (1.5–2.0 kcal/mL); low residue (except Enrich, Jevity, and Sustacal with Fiber)	Requires a functional GI tract; palatable for oral use; low viscosity; consistent standardized formulation; tend to be lower osmolarity (300–400 mOsm/L) than lactose-containing formulas	Not palatable for all patients May not be practical in patients with short bowel, partial bowel obstruction, fistulas (these often require elemental formulas)

478

Elemental (defined) formulas (Vivonex, Flexical, Vital, Travasorb, Peptamen Liquid, Criticare)	Nutrients in elemental or hydrolyzed form (amino acids and oligopeptides, glucose, and oligosaccharides); most calories provided by carbohydrates; very little fat as medium- or long-chain triglycerides (except Peptamen Liquid, which has 30% of calories as fat)	Indicated for short bowel (more than 60 cm functional bowel), malabsorption/maldigestion, partial bowel obstruction; requires minimal digestion; very low residue; low viscosity	Unpalatability restricts oral use; high osmolarity (from high concentration of simple sugars) results in higher incidence of GI intolerance and metabolic complications; low fat content results in potential risk of essential fatty acid deficiency
Modular feedings (Pro-Mix, Polycose, MCT oil)	Contain single nutrients (protein, carbohydrate or fat); vitamin/ mineral supplemented	Can be combined with elemental or polymeric formulas in order to individualize a patient's nutritional prescription; useful for patients with special needs (liver disease, renal, cardiac, and respiratory failure)	Preparation of specialized formula is labor intensive; combination of formulas must be carefully planned in order to avoid deficiency states and metabolic complications

    c. Diarrhea. Causes specific to enterally fed patients include an excessive rate or volume of feeding, use of hyperosmolar formulas, and bacterial contamination of the formula (especially if the hang time is more than 8 hours). Some evidence exists that patients with a low serum albumin (less than 27 gm/L) have an increased incidence of diarrhea when they are enterally fed. These patients may require parenteral nutrition until their serum albumin is sufficiently high to allow enteral feeding. The use of concomitant medications—especially antibiotics—can be associated with diarrhea in enterally fed patients. Specific malabsorptive syndromes may also result in diarrhea (e.g., lactose intolerance, pancreatic insufficiency, celiac disease, inflammatory bowel disease).

    d. Constipation. This is uncommon but can occur secondary to inadequate fluid or free water intake, the use of low residue formulations, and the concomitant use of constipating agents. Water can be added to the daily feeding regimen and a higher fiber formula (e.g., Enrich) can be used.

  3. METABOLIC COMPLICATIONS

    a. Disturbances of Water, Sodium, Potassium, Phosphate, Magnesium and Glucose Balance. Patients should be monitored periodically for occurrence of these imbalances. More frequent monitoring is indicated in very sick patients and in patients just starting enteral feeds.

    b. Drug-Nutrient Interactions. Enteral feeding may slow the absorption and/or alter the metabolism of some medications. The high vitamin K content of most formulas can make patients resistant to usual doses of coumadin.

    c. Essential Fatty Acid Deficiency. Patients on elemental formulas can theoretically develop this deficiency because of their low fat content. In practice, this rarely occurs.

IV. PARENTERAL NUTRITION

A. Indications for parenteral nutrition (PN) can be thought of as falling into one of three broad categories. Some patients may have more than one of these indications (e.g., patients with inflammatory bowel disease):

    1. Previously well-nourished patients who are unable to tolerate adequate oral intake or enteral feeding (for whatever reason) and will be unlikely to do so for at least 7–10 days.

    2. Malnourished patients who are unable to tolerate oral or enteral feeds (e.g., short bowel syndrome with less than 60 cm small intestine remaining).

    3. Gastrointestinal disorders in which "bowel rest" is a primary mode of therapy (e.g., inflammatory bowel disease, enterocutaneous, and pancreatic fistulas).

B. Contraindications

    1. Adequate oral or enteral intake to meet nutritional requirements.

    2. Lack of intravenous access (rare)

    3. Less than 5 to 7 days of PN likely required

4. Terminal illness when aggressive management is not indicated
5. Potential risks outweigh expected benefits
6. Refusal of patient or legal guardian

C. Routes of Parenteral Nutrition

1. **PERIPHERAL PARENTERAL NUTRITION.** PN solutions are infused into a peripheral vein and must therefore be of relatively low osmolarity to prevent irritation and thrombosis. The concentration of dextrose and amino acids should not exceed 5%. The major source of nonprotein energy (80–85% of total nonprotein calories) is provided as lipid, which can be given in 10 or 20% concentrations because of its isotonicity. This method requires giving larger volumes of fluid to be nutritionally complete and should not be used for more than 7 days. If parenteral nutritional support is required for more than 7 days, the central route of PN administration should be used.

2. **CENTRAL PARENTERAL NUTRITION.** Solutions of high osmolarity are infused via a catheter placed into a central vein, usually the superior vena cava (SVC). The high blood volume flowing through the SVC allows the use of high-osmolarity solutions without irritative effects. Higher concentrations of dextrose (up to 25%) can be used as an energy source. This reduces the daily fluid volume required to meet nutritional requirements. Such fluid restriction is important in congestive heart failure, renal disease, and liver failure. In most cases, approximately 50% of the nonprotein energy is provided as dextrose and 50% as lipid. This ratio can be varied depending on the individual patient characteristics. For example, in patients with respiratory failure and CO_2 retention, it would be advantageous to use an energy source with a low respiratory quotient in order to minimize CO_2 production. This is achieved by increasing the relative percentage of calories provided by lipid.

D. Central Venous Catheter Insertion.
The best route of access to the SVC is via the subclavian vein. The catheter should be inserted using strict sterile technique (gowns, masks, surgical scrubs, skin preparation) by an experienced operator. This can be performed with either the Seldinger technique or a catheter through a cannula.

The catheter, once inserted and the position in the vein confirmed by return of blood, should be sutured in position with povidone-iodine ointment prophylaxis and a small gauze placed over the exit site and an Op-Site creating a watertight seal over the dressing. A chest x-ray, to verify position of the catheter tip in the SVC just above the right atrium, must be obtained before initiation of PN. For long-term PN, such as home PN, a Hickman catheter or Port-A-Cath is indicated.

E. The Parenteral Nutritional Prescription.
Once it is decided to provide parenteral nutritional support for a patient, the daily fluid, protein, energy, electrolyte, mineral, trace element, and vitamin requirements for that patient should be determined. Since the requirements will vary according to the individual patient's previous nutritional status and underlying disease process, it is not possible to provide a set prescription appropriate for all patients.

F. Parenteral Nutrition Solutions

1. **AMINO ACIDS.** Balanced amino acid solutions are commercially available in concentrations ranging from 3.5–10% (Travasol, Aminosyn). These solutions are also provided in premixed forms containing dextrose and/or electrolytes (sodium, potassium, magnesium, acetate, chloride, and phosphorus). However, the use of premixed solutions sacrifices individual flexibility for ease of administration. The osmolarity of amino acid solutions is approximately equal to the amino acid concentration multiplied by 100 (expressed in mOsm/L).

2. **DEXTROSE.** The range of dextrose concentrations most frequently used in PN varies from 5% (peripheral) to 25% (central). The osmolarity is approximately equal to the dextrose concentration multiplied by 50. Dextrose (as monohydrate) provides 3.4 nonprotein kcal/gram. The use of dextrose as the exclusive source of nonprotein energy can result in the development of fatty liver. The dextrose is often provided by the hospital pharmacy in a single bag, mixed together with amino acids, electrolytes, vitamins, minerals, and trace elements.

3. **LIPID.** Lipid is provided in 10% and 20% emulsions. It provides a good source of nonprotein energy (1000 kcal/500 ml for the 20% emulsion and 550 kcal/500 ml for the 10% emulsion) and should be used in all patients except those with chylomicronemia. Both concentrations are isotonic and can be given via a peripheral vein without local irritation. It is also a useful source of nonprotein energy in patients with respiratory failure and CO_2 retention because of its low respiratory quotient as compared with dextrose. The lipid emulsions are usually infused via a Y-connector into the amino acid/dextrose administration tubing.

4. **ELECTROLYTES.** Sodium, potassium, calcium, magnesium, chloride, phosphate, and acetate are usually added to maintain electrolyte balance. PN solutions should be individually formulated by addition or withdrawal of specific electrolytes as appropriate. Special attention needs to be paid to potassium, magnesium, phosphorus, and zinc, especially early in the course of PN, since these ions are taken up and utilized by cells as the patient becomes anabolic, thus resulting in low serum levels and potential complications. In addition, when malnourished patients are initially refed they may have excessive sodium and water retention and the resulting risk of congestive heart failure. Thus, refeeding should be started gradually, avoiding large carbohydrate loads and carefully monitoring sodium and fluid balance.

5. **VITAMINS.** Standard multivitamin mixtures (e.g., Solu-Zyme, MVI–1000, MVI–12) should be added to PN solutions to provide water- and fat-soluble vitamins and prevent deficiency states (Table 13–6). A water-soluble multivitamin preparation (e.g., Solu-Zyme) should be added 6 days/week, and the preparation containing both fat- and water-soluble vitamins (MVI–1000) should be added once weekly in most instances. Vitamin K_1, 10 mg, can be administered IM once

TABLE 13–6. VITAMIN REQUIREMENTS ON PARENTERAL NUTRITION

VITAMIN	RECOMMENDED DAILY IV ADMINISTRATION	AMOUNT PROVIDED IN:		
		Soluzyme (5 ml)	MVI–1000 (10 ml)	MVI–12 (10 ml)
A	2500 IU (= 750 μg retinol or 750 retinol equivalents)	—	10,000 IU	600 IU
D	? (see text)	—	1000 IU	40 IU
E	10 IU	—	10 IU	2 IU
K	10 mg/wk (intramuscular)	—	—	—
B₁ (Thiamine)	5 mg	10 mg	45 mg	0.6 mg
B₂ (Riboflavin)	5 mg	10 mg	10 mg	0.72 mg
Niacinamide	50 mg	250 mg	100 mg	8 mg
B₆ (Pyridoxine)	5 mg	5 mg	12 mg	0.8 mg
B₁₂ (Cobalamin)	12 μg	25 μg	—	1 μg
Pantothenic acid	15 mg	45 mg	26 mg	3 mg
Folic acid	600 μg	5 mg	—	80 μg
C (ascorbic acid)	300–500 mg	500 mg	1000 mg	20 mg
Biotin	60 μg	—	—	12 μg

weekly. There is some evidence that IV vitamin D is associated with hypercalcemia and pancreatitis in those receiving PN and should not be given in doses of more than 2500 IU/day.

    6. TRACE ELEMENTS. See Table 13–7 for administration guidelines.

G. Monitoring

1. Catheter exit site should be monitored daily and the dressing changed at least once a week. If there is evidence of infection at the exit site, swabs of the site are sent for culture. Infusion tubing is changed every 48–72 hours.
2. Bloodwork should be done periodically following initiation of PN. Electrolytes, glucose, urea, and creatinine should be tested daily for the first 3 days and then 3 times weekly following that. Calcium, magnesium, phosphorus, AST, alkaline phosphatase, bilirubin, cholesterol, triglycerides, serum proteins, and complete blood count with differential count should be tested weekly. Monitoring of bloodwork should be more frequent in unstable patients or when specifically indicated.
3. Urine is checked for glucose and ketones every 6 hours.
4. Body weight is checked.
5. Fluid intake and output is monitored.
6. Nutritional status should be reassessed periodically in order to confirm that nutritional goals are being achieved.

H. Complications

    1. TECHNICAL
        a. Pneumothorax occurs during catheter insertion. If small and not

TABLE 13–7. TRACE ELEMENT REQUIREMENTS IN TPN

ELEMENT	RECOMMENDED DAILY IV ADMINISTRATION	COMMENT
Zinc	2.5–4 mg	Increase for GI losses (12 mg/L for small intestinal fluid or 17 mg/L for stool)
Iron (iron dextran)	1 mg	Increase to 2 mg/d in menstruating females; increase for other causes of blood loss; monitor iron stores periodically (especially in long-term PN)
Copper	0.5 mg	Increased GI losses in diarrheal illnesses; decreased excretion with impaired hepatic function (especially obstructive jaundice)
Chromium	10–20 μg	Deficiency associated with glucose intolerance
Selenium	40–120 μg	Deficiency associated with cardiomyopathy and muscle pain
Manganese	0.8 mg	Should not be given in obstructive jaundice
Iodine (potassium iodide)	120 μg	—

enlarging, it can be managed expectantly but sometimes requires insertion of a chest tube. If the catheter is properly within the SVC, it may be left in place.

b. Laceration of Subclavian Artery or Vein. Such injuries should be treated with local pressure and insertion of a chest tube if hemothorax occurs.

c. Injury to Thoracic Duct. Remove the catheter and remove any resulting chylothorax by means of repeated thoracentesis until leakage of lymph stops.

d. Injury to Brachial Plexus.

e. Catheter Embolization. This occurs when a catheter placed through a metal cannula is withdrawn with the cannula still in the vein, shearing off the catheter.

f. Air Embolism. This potentially fatal complication can occur during catheter insertion or later if the infusion tubing becomes disconnected from the catheter. The catheter should be immediately covered and the patient placed in the Trendelenburg position with the right side up.

g. Venous thrombosis around the tip of the catheter or in the SVC may be related to improper catheter position or to long-term usage. It is often associated with an underlying catheter infection and can sometimes be treated with streptokinase or urokinase to dissolve the fibrin clot and daily antibiotics but may require removal of the catheter. Urokinase is given as 7500 IU dissolved in 3 mL of normal saline which is then injected into the catheter, up to a maximum of 2.5 mL. The catheter is capped for 3 hours and then flushed with 10 mL of normal saline containing 1000 units of heparin.

2. **SEPTIC.** Catheter sepsis is an episode of sepsis that resolves after removal of the catheter. It is more commonly observed with the use of multilumen catheters and should be suspected when a patient receiving PN has a fever (even low grade), leukocytosis, or hyperglycemia. It is confirmed by a positive culture from blood or from the removed catheter tip. Not all episodes of sepsis occurring in patients on PN are catheter sepsis; efforts should be made to find other potential sources. If other sources are ruled out and catheter sepsis is suspected, infusion of the PN solutions should be discontinued and maintenance glucose/saline solution started. Cultures should be taken of the PN solution, the exit site, and blood (both peripheral and retrograde through the catheter). If blood cultures are positive, the sepsis can be treated by removal of the catheter in most cases unless the sepsis is due to *Candida* infection, in which case IV amphotericin B is indicated. If fever persists despite removal of the catheter, the patient should receive the appropriate intravenous antibiotic(s) as indicated by culture and sensitivity results. The catheter should not be replaced until the sepsis is controlled (no fever for at least 48 hours and negative blood cultures).

3. **METABOLIC**

   a. Hyperglycemia. This is due to an excessively high rate of glucose administration and/or impaired glucose utilization. Impaired utilization is often associated with sepsis, trauma, stress, diabetes, liver disease, pancreatitis, and corticosteroid administration. Hyperglycemia can result in hyperosmolar nonketotic coma and dehydration when severe. The rate of dextrose infusion should be reduced and underlying conditions corrected when possible. If hyperglycemia persists, insulin therapy should be started. A constant IV insulin infusion allows close control of the blood glucose level, especially in the unstable patient.

b. **Hypoglycemia.** This usually occurs when the infusion of dextrose is not constant throughout the day because of either mechanical infusion problems or when the dextrose infusion is suddenly stopped (usually when very high concentrations are used). Infusion pumps ensure constant rates of dextrose infusion. Avoid sudden discontinuation of dextrose infusion (e.g., for medications). When hypoglycemia occurs, constant infusion of the dextrose should be immediately resumed. Severe hypoglycemia should be treated with boluses of 50% dextrose.

c. **Electrolyte Disturbances.** Hypokalemia, hypophosphatemia, and hypomagnesemia are the most common electrolyte imbalances. They tend to occur early in the course of PN as these ions are taken up by cells during the process of protein synthesis. Additional supplementation of ions as necessary is adequate treatment.

d. **Acid-Base Disturbances.** Hyperchloremic metabolic acidosis is the most common acid-base disturbance secondary to PN. It is due to the administration of excessive chloride or to the loss of bicarbonate through GI or renal routes. To treat, reduce chloride in the PN solution and substitute acetate (which is metabolized to bicarbonate). Treat sources of bicarbonate loss if possible.

e. **Vitamin and Trace Element Deficiencies.** These should be added to PN solutions on a daily basis as recommended and appropriate adjustments made for individual patients.

f. **Hyperlipidemia.** Hypertriglyceridemia is due to excessive calorie administration (as either lipid and/or dextrose). Elevated cholesterol levels can be seen with very high rates of lipid infusion. Treatment is reduction of daily caloric and/or lipid intake.

g. **Essential Fatty Acid Deficiency.** This syndrome, characterized by dry, scaly skin and hair loss, is not seen in patients receiving lipid emulsion.

h. **Pancreatitis.** Pancreatitis occurring in patients on PN may be due hypertriglyceridemia or hypercalcemia. If it is due to hypercalcemia, vitamin D should be withdrawn from the PN solution.

i. **Liver Enzyme and Liver Function Abnormalities.** Mild abnormalities of the serum alkaline phosphatase, AST, and ALT (less than 2–3 times normal) are common. These tend to be self-limited. Fatty infiltration of the liver is related to excessive calories being provided as dextrose. Cholestatic jaundice can also occur, but its cause is not clear. It may be related to underlying sepsis in the patient receiving PN. Fatty infiltration should be treated by reducing the caloric intake and replacing about 50% of dextrose with lipid emulsion. If cholestatic jaundice occurs, a search should be made for a source of sepsis.

V. HOME PARENTERAL NUTRITION

Occasionally, a patient will have an indication for parenteral nutrition that does not resolve over the course of a hospital stay. In these cases, PN is continued at home. The most common **indications** include short bowel syndrome, radiation enteritis, extensive Crohn's disease, and diffuse intestinal hypomotility. Home PN should be provided only by an experienced multidisciplinary group consisting of physicians, nurses, pharmacists, and dieticians. Not all patients who have an indication for home PN will be suitable for the program—usually because of poor social supports and inability or unwillingness to follow the strict aseptic techniques required. Patients should be trained in the techniques while in the hospital. This takes an average of 2 weeks depending on the complexity of the prescription and the patient's aptitude.

A. Infusion of the PN Solutions—usually via a Hickman catheter or Port-A-Cath placed in the SVC—is carried out overnight, thus allowing the patient to "cap" the catheter during the day to permit usual activities. The exact composition of the infusion solutions varies. For example, some patients with short bowel syndrome are able to eat and absorb sufficient calories and protein but require infusion of fluid and electrolytes in order to prevent imbalances due to excessive losses from their stomas. Such patients may also require once-weekly lipid infusions in order to avoid essential fatty acid deficiency. Although patients are receiving PN, they are also free to eat as tolerated, according to their underlying condition. Such intake should be accounted for when determining the PN prescription.

B. Complications of home PN are similar to those experienced with in-hospital PN. Line sepsis is a frequently occurring complication often treated with urokinase, as described above, and 4 weeks of systemic antibiotics, thereby avoiding catheter removal. Stiffening and fracturing of the catheter are also more likely with prolonged PN. Certain metabolic complications such as metabolic bone disease, iron deficiency, and trace element deficiencies are more likely to develop when patients are receiving long-term home PN.

FAO/WHO/UNU: Energy and protein requirements: report of a joint FAO/WHO/UNU Expert Consultation. Technical Report No. 724. Geneva, World Health Organization, 1985.

The National Research Council: Recommended Dietary Allowances, 10th edition. Washington D.C., National Academy of Sciences, 1989.

Canada Health and Welfare: Nutrition Recommendations. The Report of the Scientific Review Committee, 1990.

Ontario Dietetic Association–Ontario Hospital Association. Nutritional Care Manual, 6th ed., Don Mills, Ontario, Ontario Hospital Association, 1989.

Shils ME, Young VR (eds.): Modern Nutrition in Health and Disease. Philadelphia, Lea & Febiger, 1988.

Detsky AS, McLaughlin JR, Baker JP et al: What is subjective global assessment of nutritional status? JPEN 11:8–13, 1987.

Baker JP, Lemoyne M: Nutritional support in the critically ill patient: if, when, how and what. Crit Care Clin 3:97–113, 1987.

ASPEN Board of Directors: Guidelines for use of enteral nutrition in the adult patient. JPEN 11:435–439, 1987.

ASPEN Board of Directors: Guidelines for use of total parenteral nutrition in the hospitalized adult patient. JPEN 10:441–445, 1986.

ASPEN Board of Directors: Guidelines for use of home total parenteral nutrition. JPEN 11:342–344, 1987.

14 14 14 14 14 14 14 14 14

RHEUMATIC DISORDERS

BRUCE C. GILLILAND
GREGORY C. GARDNER

14 14 14 14 14 14 14 14 14 14

I. RHEUMATOID ARTHRITIS

Rheumatoid arthritis (RA) is a chronic inflammatory disorder of unknown cause that affects predominantly peripheral joints in a symmetric distribution. The peak onset is in the third and fourth decades. Its U.S. incidence is 1–2%. The course of disease is highly variable, with some patients having only mild joint swelling with long remissions while others have a destructive joint disease interrupted by periods of relative inactivity. About 10% of patients have progressive joint destruction that leads eventually to significant crippling.

The clinical features of RA are presented in Tables 14–1 and 14–2. Morning stiffness is also characteristic of RA, as for all forms of inflammatory arthritis, and usually lasts longer than 30 minutes with active disease.

The diagnosis is based on the presence of arthritis for more than 6 weeks in the pattern of involvement typically seen in RA. Laboratory data and x-rays help confirm the diagnosis.

A. Treatment. The ultimate goal is to maintain the patient's ability to function. This is achieved by reducing joint pain and swelling and subsequent joint damage. **Drugs, physical and occupational therapy,** and **orthopedic surgery** are all important in management of RA. One must also deal with the psychological and social needs of a patient with this chronic disorder.

1. **ASPIRIN AND NONSTEROIDAL ANTI-INFLAMMATORY DRUGS.** Patients are initially started on an aspirin product or one of the NSAIDs. Patients may respond to one drug better than another, and the choice is empiric. They usually note improvement of symptoms within the first few days or week of treatment.

   a. **Mechanism of Action.** Aspirin and NSAIDs reduce joint inflammation by inhibiting cyclo-oxygenase, which acts on arachidonic acid to produce prostaglandins, including prostacyclin and thromboxane. They also interfere with granulocyte and monocyte func-

TABLE 14–1. CLINICAL CHARACTERISTICS OF RHEUMATOID ARTHRITIS

Joint areas potentially involved
    PIPs, MCPs, wrists, elbows, shoulders, hips, knees, ankles, MTPs,
      cervical spine
Joint pattern
    Symmetric polyarthritis (peripheral joints predominantly)
Laboratory
    Rheumatoid factor present in 80%; anemia; elevated ESR
Immunogenetics
    HLA-DR4 present in over 70%

TABLE 14–2. EXTRA-ARTICULAR FEATURES OF RHEUMATOID ARTHRITIS

Ocular
  Episcleritis, scleritis, scleromalacia
Pulmonary
  Effusions, nodules, fibrosis
Cardiovascular
  Small and medium-sized vessel vasculitis, aortitis (rare), pericarditis
Felty's syndrome
  Neutropenia and splenomegaly
Sjögren's syndrome (secondary)
  Dry eyes and mouth (sicca)

tion, and suppress bradykinin release. Table 14–3 lists the nonsteroidal anti-inflammatory drugs classified according to duration of action.

b. Dosing. Salicylates are effective in treatment of RA. The plasma half-life is 3–6 hours but increases with increasing serum concentration up to 20 hours when serum levels are elevated. The best effect is achieved with blood levels between 20 and 30 mg/dL, obtained with a dose of aspirin in the range of 4 gm/day given in divided doses. A dosage of 2 gm/day is started and gradually

TABLE 14–3. NONSTEROIDAL ANTI-INFLAMMATORY DRUGS

DRUG	DAILY DOSE (MG) RANGE	SCHEDULE (DOSES PER DAY)	UNIT SIZE (MG)
Short-acting*			
Ibuprofen	1200–3200	3–6	300, 400, 600, 800
Fenoprofen	800–3200	3–4	200, 300, 600
Ketoprofen	150–300	3–4	25, 50, 75
Indomethacin	50–200	2–4	25, 50†, 75‡
Tolmetin	600–2000	3–6	200, 400
Meclofenamate	200–400	4	50, 100
Diclofenac	100–200	2–4	25, 50, 75
Intermediate-acting*			
Naproxen	500–1500	2	250, 375, 500
Sulindac	300–400	2	150, 200
Diflunisal	500–1500	2	250, 500
Acetylsalicylic acid	1000–6000	3–4	325§
Long-acting*			
Piroxicam	20	1–2	10, 20
Phenylbutazone	300–400	1–4	100

*Drugs in the short-acting group have serum half-lives of about 1 to 4 hours, in the intermediate-acting group about 10 to 20 hours (dose dependent), and in the long-acting group about 45 hours for piroxicam and 72 hours for phenylbutazone.
†Also comes as a suppository.
‡Timed-release preparation.
§Standard size. Other unit sizes are avilable, depending on brand. Timed-release preparations are available.

increased every few days until the blood level is in the therapeutic range. It may take from 2–4 weeks for the salicylate level to reflect the daily maintenance dose.

The NSAIDs are started at a dose in the mid range and gradually increased until there is improvement. If the patient does not respond to the lower doses, the dose is increased to the maximum allowable amount and continued 2–4 weeks before another NSAID is tried. Elderly patients should be given the lowest effective dose and monitored for adverse side effects.

  c. **Adverse Reactions** are presented in Table 14–4. The major toxicities are GI and renal. Aspirin and NSAIDs can cause gastric ulceration because of inhibition of gastric prostaglandins. Gastric ulceration and bleeding and perforation may be silent, especially in the elderly. Misoprostol, a PGE_1 analogue, has been shown to be protective for the gastropathy.

  NSAIDs reduce renal blood flow in patients with underlying renal disease, congestive heart failure, cirrhosis, or hypovolemic conditions and lead to renal failure, sodium retention, and peripheral edema. Sulindac has been shown to have less effect on renal prostaglandins and probably is the drug of choice in patients with these disorders. Salicylates bind irreversibly to the platelet cyclooxygenase and interfere with platelet aggregation and blood clotting. NSAIDs also interfere with platelet function, but the effect is reversible within 5 half-lives after stopping the drug. Aspirin should be avoided in patients on anticoagulants.

2. **DISEASE-MODIFYING DRUGS.** These are drugs that can alter the rate of disease progression, slowing radiographic juxta-articular bone erosions as well as suppressing signs and symptoms of inflammation. These drugs are also referred to as slow acting, since they may require

TABLE 14–4. ADVERSE REACTIONS TO ASPIRIN AND NSAIDS

CNS
  Headaches, cognitive dysfunction, psychosis, confusion, aseptic meningitis
Pulmonary
  Exacerbation of asthma, pneumonitis
Gastrointestinal
  Dyspepsia, nausea, ulceration, perforation, diarrhea, elevated transaminases, hypersensitivity hepatitis
Renal
  Renal insufficiency, hyperkalemia, hypertension, interstitial nephritis, papillary necrosis
Hematologic
  Impaired platelet function, aplastic anemia, agranulocytosis, thrombocytopenia
Cutaneous
  Urticaria/angioedema, erythema multiforme, photosensitive eruptions, toxic epidermal necrolysis
Drug Interactions
  Increase blood levels of oral hypoglycemics, phenytoin, anticoagulants, lithium, methotrexate

4–6 months to produce clinical improvement. The accepted disease-modifying drugs are **gold salts, hydroxychloroquine, penicillamine,** and **sulfasalazine.**

a. **Gold Compounds.** When synovial proliferation involving several joints has persisted for several weeks to months, a disease-modifying agent is usually added. Gold, often the first of this group to be used, is available as **gold sodium thiomalate** and **gold sodium thioglucose.** The schedule for their administration is as follows: A test dose of 10 mg IM is given to exclude an idiosyncratic reaction. 25 mg is given the next week, and then 50 mg is given weekly until a total of 1 gm is reached. If there is no response, gold is stopped.

If the patient has had a good response before or after receiving 1 gm, then 50 mg is given every 2 weeks for 2 months, then every 3 weeks for 2 months, then finally once every 4 weeks indefinitely. If the patient shows signs of increased disease activity, the gold can be increased to weekly injections. If the patient does not respond to a course of 1 gm after reinstitution of weekly therapy, gold is then stopped. The patient's white blood cell count, platelet count, and urine are carefully monitored during therapy. With the weekly schedule, a CBC, including a platelet count, is done 1 week and urinalysis the next. When the patient is on a maintenance dose the CBC and urinalysis are obtained before the drug is given.

Auranofin is an oral gold preparation. The usual dose is 3 mg bid. The dose can be increased to 9 mg/day in divided doses if response is inadequate by 6 months. CBC and urinalysis are determined monthly. Diarrhea is the most common side effect, occurring in approximately ⅓ of patients.

Adverse Reactions to Gold. About ⅓ of the patients experience an **adverse reaction** to intramuscular gold, the most common being a rash. Since the rash can lead to generalized exfoliative dermatitis, gold should be stopped immediately. If the rash is mild and rapidly resolves, gold can be restarted with close monitoring at a lower dosage of 5–10 mg/week, which can be increased to 25 mg/week. Gold can cause **nephrotic syndrome;** in a patient with urinary protein greater than 300 mg in 24 hours, gold is usually stopped. Gold can be restarted once the urine is clear of protein, and some patients may subsequently tolerate it. The most serious gold toxicity is **aplastic anemia.** A decrease in any of the cell counts below normal requires termination of gold therapy. When the count returns to normal, rechallenge may be cautiously attempted with a lower dose of gold.

b. **Antimalarials. Hydroxychloroquine** and **chloroquine** are effective in some patients. These drugs take several weeks to months before benefit is observed. Response may take up to 6 months. The dose of hydroxychloroquine is 200–400 mg/day and that of chloroquine is 250 mg/day. The ideal patient who might respond to antimalarials is one who has not developed radiographic juxta-articular bone erosions. Antimalarials can be given indefinitely in the absence of significant side effects.

Adverse Reactions to Antimalarials. The most serious result of toxicity of antimalarials is retinal damage, which can lead to loss of vision even after the drug has been stopped. Thus, an eye examination by an ophthalmologist should be done before the start of therapy, and subsequently every 6 months. Loss of vision appears to be related more to the level of the daily dose than to the total cumulative dosage. Approximately 10% of patients experience nausea, vomiting, and/or diarrhea. Hyperpigmentation and bleaching of the hair can occur on sun exposure. Dark-skinned persons are more likely to become darker. Antimalarials also are associated with neuromyopathy, dermatitis, leukopenia, and granulocytopenia.

c. Penicillamine. This disease-modifying agent can be given after gold therapy has failed, but because of its toxicity is used only after lack of response to other agents. The drug takes several weeks to months before clinical improvement. Penicillamine is started at 250 mg/day, and if there is no improvement after 3 months, the dose is increased to 500 mg/day for another 3 months; if there is no response, it is stopped. If the response is incomplete, the dose can be increased by 125 mg every 8–12 weeks to a maximum of 750 mg daily. If there is response at these higher doses, the dose is reduced slowly to 500 mg/day.

A CBC and urinalysis are done every 2 weeks for the first 6 weeks of therapy and then monthly.

Adverse Reactions of Penicillamine. The side effects of penicillamine usually are encountered during the first 18 months of therapy. The most frequent is a rash, which when extensive requires stopping the drug. Patients also have an alteration or loss of taste perception. Aplastic anemia, leukopenia, and thrombocytopenia can develop. A white count of less than 3000 or a platelet count below 100,000/mm^3 requires immediate discontinuation. Membranous glomerulonephropathy manifested by proteinuria and nephrotic syndrome can complicate penicillamine treatment. Urinary protein greater than 2 gm/24 hours requires discontinuing penicillamine. Patients with lesser degrees of proteinuria may be able to continue penicillamine at reduced dosage. Hematuria necessitates stopping the drug. When an autoimmune syndrome (myasthenia gravis, polymyositis, systemic lupus erythematosus, Sjögren's syndrome, Goodpasture's syndrome, or pemphigoid) develops in association with penicillamine, the drug should be discontinued.

d. Sulfasalazine. Sulfasalazine has demonstrated clinical effectiveness similar to that of gold salts and penicillamine. The initial dose is 0.5 gm daily, increased weekly by 0.5-gm increments to an eventual maintenance dose of 2 gm/day. Therapeutic response is expected by 3 months. The drug is usually better tolerated than gold salts or penicillamine, its major side effects being nausea, vomiting, abdominal pain, rash, and oral ulcers. Rarely, neutropenia, anemia, and hepatotoxicity develop. This drug is considered by some to be a disease-modifying agent. As it is better tolerated, it is sometimes used before gold or penicillamine.

3. **CYTOTOXIC AGENTS.** Azathioprine, cyclophosphamide, and methotrexate are classified as cytotoxic disease-modifying agents (Table 14–5). Azathioprine and methotrexate have both been approved by the FDA for use in RA. Cyclophosphamide, however, requires informed consent for its use in RA.

   a. **Azathioprine** is a purine analogue that is metabolized to 6-mercaptopurine. The dose of azathioprine is 1–1.25 mg/kg/day. This dose can be increased to a maximum of 2.5 mg/kg/day when there has been no clinical response by 4 months. CBC and liver enzymes are determined weekly for the first 8 weeks, and then every other week, after which the interval of testing may be cautiously increased to 1 month. The drug is stopped if the white blood cell count falls below 3000/mm^3. Nausea and vomiting occur in approximately 10% of patients. Cholestatic hepatitis rarely occurs. To avoid toxicity in a patient receiving both azathioprine and allopurinol, the dose of azathioprine is reduced by at least ⅓, since the breakdown of the active form of azathioprine depends on xanthine oxidase.

   b. **Cyclophosphamide** is effective in RA, but because of its toxicity, is not recommended except under exceptional circumstances.

   c. **Methotrexate.** This has replaced gold in the therapeutic regimens of some rheumatologists as the initial disease-modifying agent. It has more rapid onset of action than the other disease-modifying agents, and a flare usually occurs within a month when the drug is discontinued for any reason other than ineffectiveness. The

TABLE 14–5. CYTOTOXIC DRUGS IN RHEUMATIC DISORDERS

DRUG	DOSE SCHEDULE	TOXIC SIDE EFFECTS
Azathioprine	Oral: 1–4 mg/kg/ day	Marrow suppression, nausea, hepatitis, pancreatitis, oncogenesis, infection
Cyclo-phosphamide	Oral: 1–4 mg/kg/ day IV: 0.5–1.0 gram/ m^2 of body surface area*	Marrow suppression, nausea and vomiting, infertility, hemorrhagic cystitis, bladder fibrosis, bladder carcinoma, infection, oncogenesis, pulmonary interstitial disease, alopecia
Chlorambucil	Oral: 0.1–0.2 mg/ kg/day	Marrow suppression, nausea and vomiting, infertility, oncogenesis, hepatotoxicity
Methotrexate	Oral: 7.5 mg–15.0 mg once a week† IV: 7.5 mg–25.0 mg once a week	Marrow suppression, nausea and vomiting, diarrhea, stomatitis, cirrhosis, interstitial pulmonary disease

*Given at 1- to 3-mo intervals; see text.
†Given once a week in three divided doses, each separated by 12 hr.

starting dosage of methotrexate is 7.5 mg divided into 3 doses given 12 hours apart once a week or given as a single dose weekly. This dosage is continued for 2–3 months. If there is no response, the dose is increased to 10 mg/week. If again there is no response after 6 weeks, the dose is increased to 12.5 mg for 6 weeks, and subsequently to 15 mg/week. Once clinical improvement is noted and sustained, the dose is gradually reduced to maintain the clinical response. The drug can be given IM as a single dose once a week. The initial dose is 7.5 mg, which is increased at the intervals outlined above. CBC, BUN, and blood creatinine are checked monthly. Methotrexate is given cautiously in reduced doses to patients with an elevated creatinine level or reduced creatinine clearance. The drug should probably not be given to patients whose creatinine level is 2 mg/dL or greater. The dose should be reduced in elderly patients.

Weak organic acids such as aspirin interfere with renal excretion of methotrexate, leading to higher and potentially toxic blood levels. NSAIDs are also weak organic acids and might have a similar effect. Drugs that displace methotrexate from albumin (e.g., phenytoin) also can produce toxic blood levels of methotrexate.

Adverse Reactions of Methotrexate. Hepatotoxicity leading to fibrosis is a concern in patients on long-term methotrexate treatment. Cirrhosis is seldom observed before a total dose of 1.5 gm. The clinical utility of performing liver biopsies regularly to look for fibrosis in patients receiving chronic methotrexate therapy is unresolved. Patients who drink alcohol excessively or who have underlying liver disease should not be given methotrexate. Bronchiolitis and interstitial pulmonary disease are uncommon complications of methotrexate and necessitate stopping the drug. Stomatitis and leukopenia also can occur.

4. **GLUCOCORTICOIDS.** Low doses of prednisone can be beneficial in patients with RA. The daily morning dose should not exceed 7.5 mg. Once there is response, prednisone is decreased by 1-mg decrements to achieve the lowest possible dose that will maintain clinical improvement. Other clinical situations in which low-dose glucocorticoids are beneficial: In a patient with active joint disease being started on a disease-modifying agent, low-dose prednisone will produce immediate clinical improvement and allow functioning during the time it takes the disease-modifying drug to become effective. Low-dose prednisone therapy also is justified in a patient whose continued functioning is necessary for maintaining a home or providing an income. Elderly patients with recent onset of RA often respond well to low-dose prednisone therapy alone.

Even with low-dose prednisone treatment, patients may be at risk for developing osteoporosis. Thus, these patients can be given supplemental calcium and vitamin D, and estrogens should be considered in postmenopausal women. Recent prospective data suggest that oral doses of glucocorticoids of 8 mg or less may not increase the risk of osteoporosis.

a. **Pulse intravenous methylprednisolone** therapy has been given to patients who are experiencing severe exacerbations. Methylprednisolone 1 gm IV is given over 30 minutes. The patient's blood pressure should be carefully monitored during this infusion, since both hypotension and hypertension have been reported. IV therapy is usually given once a month for several months.

b. **Intra-articular Glucocorticoids.** Intra-articular injection of glucocorticoids particularly helps the patient who has one or two swollen joints that have not responded to treatment. Joint injections are done under sterile conditions. The site of injection is anesthetized with 1% lidocaine; a small amount of lidocaine is also injected into the joint. The glucocorticoid preparations for intra-articular injection are in suspension and remain largely confined to the joint. The amount of steroid injected depends on joint size. The equivalent of 40 mg prednisone is recommended for injection of a knee, 10–20 mg for ankles, 5 mg for small joints of the hands or feet. In injection of the knee, 1–2 cc of 1% lidocaine can also be added. Care must be taken not to inject steroid into the soft tissue, since this will cause atrophy of the overlying tissue. Joint pain several hours after injection due to chemical synovitis can be treated with an anti-inflammatory drug or analgesic.

5. **OCCUPATIONAL AND PHYSICAL THERAPY.** Occupational and physical therapy are important in RA. Patients should be instructed in joint protection and exercises to maintain strength and joint motion. Splinting of inflamed wrists relieves pain and permits continued use of the fingers. Splints are removed at least once a day so wrists can be exercised gently through a range of motion. Wrist splints worn at night often relieve symptoms of carpal tunnel syndrome. Diet instruction and sexual counseling are also important.

6. **SURGERY.** Synovectomy at selected sites may lead to improvement and prolongation of joint function. Synovectomy might be indicated in a knee with persistent synovitis of 6 months' duration refractory to treatment. Synovectomy of the wrist and dorsal tendon sheath with resection of the ulnar styloid can reduce the risk of later extensor tendon rupture. Carpal tunnel release is indicated in patients with persistent symptoms or nerve conduction abnormalities of the median nerve. Prostheses are now available for most joints, the most successful have been the hip and knee. Metatarsal-head resection is indicated in patients with subluxation and pain not satisfactorily relieved by a metatarsal bar orthosis.

B. Treatment of Extra-articular Manifestations of RA

1. **VASCULITIS.** Patients with RA can develop symptomatic vasculitis, usually involving vessels ranging from small arteries to capillaries and venules. Manifestations include nailfold and volar pad infarcts of fingers, leg ulcers, mesenteric or coronary artery arteritis, and mono-

neuritis multiplex. Patients experiencing significant symptoms and organ damage require high doses of glucocorticoids: prednisone (60 mg/day) in divided doses initially, then gradually tapered to a single morning dose as dictated by clinical response. Cyclophosphamide 1–2 mg/kg/day may be given to patients who fail to respond to high doses of prednisone or require continued high doses of prednisone. Leg ulcers resulting from vasculitis present a difficult management problem requiring careful local care and elevation of the leg to minimize edema. Large skin ulcers may need skin grafts.

2. FELTY'S SYNDROME, characterized by RA, splenomegaly, and leukopenia, usually occurs in patients who have had RA for at least 10 years and in whom the titer of rheumatoid factor is high. Glucocorticoids may increase the neutrophil count but may not prevent infection. In most patients, splenectomy improves the neutrophil count and reduces the frequency of infection. Patients are given antipneumococcal vaccine (Pneumovax) before splenectomy.

3. SJÖGREN'S SYNDROME (SECONDARY). Patients who develop Sjögren's syndrome, manifested by dry eyes and/or mouth, are advised to use artificial tears or ointment regularly, especially at night, and to have regular dental care. Sjögren's syndrome in RA is usually not accompanied by the more severe system manifestations seen in the primary form of the disease.

II. ANKYLOSING SPONDYLITIS

Ankylosing spondylitis (AS) is characterized by bilateral sacroiliitis and varying degrees of spine involvement. The onset is usually in the 2nd or 3rd decade, beginning often insidiously with low-back pain or poorly localized discomfort. Pain may radiate down into either buttock and posterior thigh. The course of the disease and extent of back involvement are variable. The disease usually evolves over several years, moving up the spine. Some patients may have only bilateral sacroiliac involvement with minimal if any spondylitis, while others have ankylosis of the entire spine (poker spine).

A. Clinical Characteristics. These are presented in Tables 14–6 and 14–7. The HLA-B27 antigen should not be used as a routine diagnostic test

TABLE 14–6. CLINICAL CHARACTERISTICS OF ANKYLOSING SPONDYLITIS

Joint Areas Potentially Involved
  Wrists, elbows, shoulders, hips, knees, ankles, spine, sacroiliac, sternoclavicular
Joint Pattern
  Symmetric sacroiliitis; progressive spinal involvement; asymmetric peripheral joint involvement in ⅓; inflammation at insertion of Achilles tendon, plantar fascia, intercostal muscles
Laboratory
  Anemia; elevated ESR
Immunogenetics
  HLA-B27 in 90% of patients

TABLE 14–7. EXTRA-ARTICULAR MANIFESTATIONS OF ANKYLOSING SPONDYLITIS

Ocular
    Episodes of acute uniocular iritis
Pulmonary
    Fibrosis of upper lobes
Cardiovascular
    Aortic insufficiency, conduction abnormalities
Neurologic
    Cauda equina syndrome

in the evaluation of a low-back pain. X-rays of the sacroiliac joints initially show blurring, then erosions, and later fusion. Vertebral bodies become squared, and syndesmophytes eventually form bridges between the adjacent vertebrae and with diffuse involvement produce the "bamboo spine."

B. Treatment. The goal is to maintain joint function and a straight back through the use of an **anti-inflammatory agent** and **back exercises.** Treatment is started with **indomethacin** 150 mg daily in divided doses. If it is not tolerated, another NSAID can be given. Phenylbutazone has been reported to be the most effective agent in the treatment of ankylosing spondylitis; however, because of its toxicity, this drug should be used only for short periods in situations in which other agents have failed.

Sulfasalazine has been shown to be useful in peripheral arthritis and may have utility in the spinal disease as well. The dosing is similar to that in RA. Intra-articular glucocorticoids are helpful for the peripheral arthritis, but oral glucocorticoids do not have a role in AS. The hip is the most common peripheral joint affected. In severe cases, hip arthroplasty may greatly increase mobility and decrease pain. A frequent complication of hip replacement surgery in patients with spondyloarthropathy is heterotopic bone formation, which might limit mobility of the prosthesis and can be avoided by preoperative low-dose radiation.

The importance of good posture is emphasized to the patient, who should perform exercises to strengthen the extensor muscles of the back and neck. Swimming is excellent. The patient is encouraged to watch television lying on the stomach. In addition, the patient is instructed to sleep on a firm bed, lying prone as long as possible, and to use a thin or no pillow. A physical therapist should occasionally observe that the patient is doing back exercises properly.

III. REITER'S SYNDROME

Reiter's syndrome (RS) is defined as inflammatory arthritis of at least 1 month's duration associated with urethritis or cervicitis. Conjunctivitis or mucocutaneous lesions also appear in the course of this syndrome.

TABLE 14–8. CLINICAL CHARACTERISTICS OF REITER'S SYNDROME AND EXTRA-ARTICULAR MANIFESTATIONS

CLINICAL
Joint Areas Potentially Affected
  Hands, wrists, elbows, shoulders, hips, knees, ankles, toes, spine, sacroiliac
Joint Pattern
  Monoarthritis or asymmetric oligoarthritis, unilateral sacroiliitis, variable spinal
  involvement, inflammatory enthesitis at insertion of Achilles tendon, plantar
  fascia, intercostal muscles
Laboratory
  Anemia, elevated ESR
Immunogenetics
  HLA-B27 in 80% of patients

EXTRA-ARTICULAR
Ocular
  Conjunctivitis, uveitis
Urogenital
  Urethritis, prostatitis, cervicitis
Mucocutaneous
  Painless oral ulcers, circinate balanitis, keratoderma blennorrhagica on palms and
  soles, nail changes
Cardiovascular
  Aortic insufficiency, conduction abnormalities

RS may follow enteric infections with *Shigella flexneri, Salmonella,* or *Yersinia enterocolitica,* or urethritis, which, in certain cases, appears to be associated with *Chlamydia* or *Mycoplasma* infection.

A. **Clinical Characteristics** (Table 14–8). The onset of arthritis is usually acute and involves several joints in an asymmetric pattern. The knees and ankles are most often affected. Dactylitis or "sausage digit" involves the toes or fingers. Involved joints are often swollen with large effusions. The course of RS is highly variable. Some patients have a self-limited illness, while others have either persistent or recurrent arthritis.

B. **Treatment.** The arthritis is treated with indomethacin 150 mg/day in divided doses or with another NSAID. Local steroid injection may relieve plantar fasciitis or Achilles tendinitis. In persistent disease, sulfasalazine or methotrexate has been used. In more severe disease, azathioprine 1–2 mg/kg/day can be utilized.

IV. PSORIATIC ARTHRITIS

Arthritis is seen in 5% of patients with psoriasis. There is not a good association between the severity of skin disease and arthritis. Several patterns of arthritis are seen in association with psoriasis (Table 14–9).

The course of psoriatic arthritis is variable, with some patients having intermittent episodes of joint swelling, whereas others have persistent and destructive disease. Overall, the outcome of the joint disease is more favorable than in RA.

TABLE 14–9. PATTERN OF JOINT INVOLVEMENT IN PSORIATIC ARTHRITIS

Distal Interphalangeal Joints
  Occurs in 5–10% of patients, associated with psoriatic nail changes
Oligoarthritis
  Occurs in 50–60% of patients, can affect any peripheral joint
Spondylitis
  Can occur in conjunction with other joint patterns, asymmetric sacroiliac
    involvement, variable spinal involvement
Rheumatoid Arthritis-like
  Occurs in 25% of patients
Arthritis Mutilans
  Occurs in 5% of patients, severe destructive arthritis involving peripheral joints

A. Treatment. Salicylates or NSAIDs are initially given. In persistent polyarticular disease, a gold salt or methotrexate can be used in doses similar to those for RA. Methotrexate may also help the skin disease. See pages 494–495 for dosage of methotrexate.

V. ARTHRITIS OF INFLAMMATORY BOWEL DISEASE

Ulcerative colitis and regional enteritis (Crohn's disease) may be associated with arthritis. Patients can have intermittent acute arthritis of peripheral joints or sacroiliitis and spondylitis. Back involvement is indistinguishable radiographically from primary ankylosing spondylitis. Bowel disease usually precedes ankylosing spondylitis. Peripheral joint disease involves episodes of acute arthritis in one or few joints, often the knee, that last a few weeks and then usually resolve completely without residual damage. Acute peripheral arthritis responds to a nonsteroidal drug or aspirin. These drugs also alleviate the pain of spondylitis. NSAIDs must be used cautiously because they have been reported to exacerbate the bowel disease. Sulfasalazine can serve a dual function in these patients, favorably affecting the inflammatory bowel disease as well as the arthritis.

VI. VASCULITIS

The vasculitides are a group of inflammatory disorders involving blood vessels, from capillaries and venules to large arteries. The disorders are classified according to the size of vessel primarily involved and the organ system(s) affected into 4 major groups: (1) hypersensitivity vasculitis, (2) polyarteritis and related disorders, (3) Wegener's granulomatosis, and (4) giant cell arteritis (temporal arteritis and Takayasu's disease).

A. Hypersensitivity Vasculitis. Hypersensitivity vasculitis (also called small-vessel vasculitis, allergic vasculitis, or leukocytoclastic vasculitis) affects capillaries, venules, and arterioles. Immune-mediated inflamma-

TABLE 14–10. DIFFERENTIAL DIAGNOSIS OF HYPERSENSITIVITY VASCULITIS

Drugs
Bacterial endocarditis
Hypocomplementemic vasculitis
Henoch-Schönlein purpura
Mixed cryoglobulinemia
Connective tissue diseases
Malignant diseases

tion of small blood vessels can be induced by infection, collagen vascular disease, malignant disease, or drugs (Table 14–10).

Vasculitic skin lesions are palpable purpura (petechiae), vesicles, urticaria, erythema multiforme, or erythema nodosum, frequently appearing on the lower extremities below the knees. Other features include arthritis or arthralgias, myalgias, abdominal pain, GI bleeding, glomerulitis, pulmonary infiltrates, pleuritis, pericarditis, and peripheral neuropathy.

Therapy is initially directed to removing or treating any responsible stimulus for the vasculitis. Infections such as subacute bacterial endocarditis are investigated and treated appropriately. A careful drug history should be obtained; however, usually the antigen or stimulus cannot be identified. **No treatment** of the vasculitis is necessary when it is mild and transient. In patients with more severe lesions, particularly those leading to skin ulceration or internal organ involvement such as glomerulonephritis, **prednisone** 40–60 mg/day is recommended. The dose is gradually tapered based on clinical response. Prognosis is good in most cases of hypersensitivity or small-vessel vasculitis. Agents such as dapsone and colchicine have also been used.

B. Polyarteritis Nodosa and Related Disorders. Polyarteritis nodosa (PAN) involves medium-sized arteries mainly in middle-aged patients. The vasculitis is segmental and has a predilection for branching points and bifurcations of arteries. Lesions are at different stages of development. Hepatitis B and hepatitis C are associated with the vasculitis in some patients. Symptoms are often nonspecific and include fever, malaise, myalgias, weakness, and weight loss. Tender nodules representing aneurysms can sometimes be palpated along the artery. Narrowing or occlusion of small arteries can cause digital gangrene or infarction of viscera such as bowel or gallbladder. Kidney involvement can lead to hypertension and hematuria. Myocardial infarction and cerebrovascular accidents are other manifestations of PAN; the lungs are spared. Vasculitis of the lung occurs in the disorder termed allergic angiitis and granulomatosis (Churg and Strauss). These patients usually have a history of asthma and peripheral blood eosinophilia.

A variant of PAN called microscopic polyarteritis affects predominantly small arteries. Organs involved tend to be kidney, lung, and skin. This form of PAN is characterized by a positive antineutrophil cytoplasmic antibody test.

TREATMENT. This is started with **prednisone** 60 mg/day in divided doses, and **cyclophosphamide** 1–2 mg/kg/day is added. Once the patient's condition is stabilized, the dose of prednisone is gradually tapered to the lowest possible that will control symptoms. After the condition has been stable for several months the dose of cyclophosphamide is cautiously reduced, and a close watch is kept for exacerbation. In some patients the vasculitis is short-lived, whereas others may require treatment for months or longer. Although experience is limited, pulse cyclophosphamide treatment might be a reasonable alternative to daily cyclophosphamide and may reduce the risk of fibrosis and cancer of the bladder. Intervals between pulse treatment vary from 1–3 months, depending on the clinical response (see discussion of pulse cyclophosphamide treatment, "Systemic Lupus Erythematosus").

C. Wegener's Granulomatosis. This is characterized by necrotizing and granulomatous vasculitis involving the upper and lower respiratory tract and kidneys. A history of chronic sinusitis is frequent. Symptoms include cough (often productive of purulent sputum), hemoptysis, purulent nasal discharge, fever, myalgias and arthralgias, and weight loss. Hematuria, proteinuria, and a rising creatinine level indicate renal disease. Destruction of nasal cartilage produces saddle nose. Purpuric skin lesions can occur. The antineutrophil cytoplasmic antibody (ANCA) test is a new, useful diagnostic test and indicator of disease activity, but diagnosis is based on biopsy.

TREATMENT. Recognition of Wegener's granulomatosis is important, since untreated disease has a high mortality. Treatment is started with **prednisone** 60 mg/day in divided doses and **cyclophosphamide** 2 mg/kg/day. Prednisone will reduce constitutional symptoms but is not sufficient treatment. The dose of prednisone is tapered to the lowest that controls constitutional symptoms. Cyclophosphamide is continued for several months, and the dose then can be tapered slowly. A reasonable alternative to daily cyclophosphamide might be pulse therapy given at intervals of 1–3 months, depending on the clinical response. Trimethoprim-sulfamethoxazole has been used in localized upper respiratory tract disease with some success.

D. Temporal Arteritis. Temporal arteritis, also referred to as cranial or giant cell arteritis, is granulomatous vasculitis affecting medium-sized arteries, primarily of the head. Headache is a common symptom, as are temporal artery and localized scalp tenderness. Patients may also experience decreased vision, diplopia, sudden blindness, vertigo, fever, malaise, weight loss, arthralgias, and jaw claudication. Temporal arteritis can involve symptoms of **polymyalgia rheumatica** (stiffness, aching pain, and soreness of the muscles of the shoulders, neck, and hip girdles). Patients often can give the exact time the symptoms started. The sedimentation rate is usually elevated above 50 mm/hr and often higher (Westergren's method). When this diagnosis is considered, prednisone 60 mg/day in divided doses is immediately started, and a temporal artery biopsy is obtained within a few days. If it is negative, a biopsy is obtained from the other side. If this also is negative, a search should be made for other causes of these signs and symptoms.

1. **TREATMENT.** At least 40 mg prednisone per day is used for the first 4–6 weeks after diagnosis. If the patient is asymptomatic, very slow tapering of the prednisone dose is then started. Usually the patient will receive prednisone for an average of 2 years. Prednisone dosage is determined by signs and symptoms and not by the sedimentation rate. A modest elevation of sedimentation rate frequently occurs when prednisone is decreased and usually does not indicate a flare of disease. After the first several weeks of treatment, prednisone can be given as a single morning dose.

2. **POLYMYALGIA RHEUMATICA.** Patients may have polymyalgia rheumatica without clinical manifestations of temporal arteritis. For them treatment with prednisone 10–15 mg/day is started. Dramatic improvement usually occurs in 4–5 days or possibly a week. An excellent response to low doses of prednisone is typical of polymyalgia rheumatica. Low-dose prednisone is continued for several weeks and then is gradually tapered. Average treatment is 1–2 years, and attempts should be made to find the lowest possible maintenance dose.

E. **Takayasu's Arteritis.** This is a disease of young adults (especially women) but can affect all ages. The disease usually involves the aorta and its major branches, with CNS ischemia, arm claudication, renal ischemia with hypertension, and mesenteric ischemia.

TREATMENT. Prednisone 60 mg/day in divided doses is started. The dose should be kept at 40 mg or more per day for at least 6 weeks, when slow tapering is begun. It is difficult to monitor treatment of this disorder because symptoms and signs are highly variable. The patient is observed for recurrent ischemic episodes. Vascular graft surgery is necessary in some patients to restore flow and prevent tissue infarction. Preliminary data suggest methotrexate may be useful.

Chumlley LC, Harrison GG, DeRennee RA: Allergic granulomatosis and angiitis (Churg-Strauss syndrome). Mayo Clin Proc 52:477, 1977.

VII. OSTEOARTHRITIS

Osteoarthritis is the most common form of arthritis in the United States. The disease is characterized clinically by pain, restricted joint movement, and joint deformity. The disease affects predominantly middle and older-age persons and increases with age. A number of conditions that alter cartilage or joint mechanics can lead to osteoarthritis. Injury to articular cartilage, torn meniscus, or ligamental instability can cause incongruity of joint surfaces and subsequently osteoarthritis. Classification of osteoarthritis is given in Table 14–11.

A. **Clinical Characteristics.** Commonly affected joints are hips, knees, lumbar and cervical spine, the distal and proximal interphalangeal joints of the hands, and the first carpal-metacarpal and first metatarsal-

TABLE 14-11. CLASSIFICATION OF OSTEOARTHRITIS

Primary
    Localized, generalized (three or more joint areas affected), erosive (inflammatory
    form of OA of the hands)
Secondary
    Trauma, congenital anomaly (Perthes' disease, congenital hip dysplasia),
    metabolic (CPPD, ochronosis, hemochromatosis, acromegaly, gout),
    postinflammatory arthritis (rheumatoid arthritis, infection, etc.), other
    (avascular necrosis, Charcot joint)

phalangeal joint. Pain usually begins insidiously and has a deep aching quality (sometimes poorly localized), initially brought on by activity and relieved by rest. It eventually becomes more constant and can be present at night. Pain, contractures, and deformity of joints limit physical activities. On physical examination, the involved joint is swollen and tender and may be slightly warm and erythematous. The joint is enlarged because of both bony expansion and effusion. Crepitus may be felt on joint movement.

In primary osteoarthritis, routine laboratory tests including the erythrocyte sedimentation rate are normal. In secondary osteoarthritis, the laboratory reflects the underlying disease. X-rays initially are normal, but as the disease progresses joint space narrowing, subchondral bone sclerosis, periarticular bone cysts, and osteophytes are observed.

B. Treatment. The goal is to reduce pain, improve range of motion, and maintain the patient's ability to function. The involved joint should not be overused and high-impact exercises should be avoided. Flexibility should be maintained by stretching exercises. Muscle tone is achieved by activities such as walking, swimming, and bicycle riding. Overweight patients should be encouraged to lose weight. Physical therapy is directed to strengthening the muscles around the joint and improving range of motion. Use of a cane can greatly increase mobility.

Salicylates or **other NSAIDs** are effective in reducing pain and swelling (see Table 14-3). **Intra-articular glucocorticoid injections** can be given into a knee or ankle under special circumstances when the joint is already either badly damaged or pain and swelling are incapacitating. Injection of the 1st metacarpal-phalangeal joint can produce dramatic relief of pain. In addition, short-term splinting of this joint can be quite helpful.

Surgical treatment of a damaged joint is indicated when the patient's physical ability is limited by pain and loss of mobility. A change in alignment of the knee and hip joints by osteotomy can relieve pain and improve function. Total joint replacement, especially of the hip, knee, or shoulder, can dramatically decrease pain and improve function and the patient's outlook on life.

Moskowitz RW, Howell DS, et al: Osteoarthritis: Diagnosis and Management. Philadelphia, WB Saunders Co., 1984.

VIII. GOUT

Gout comprises a group of disorders that have in common clinical features caused by deposition of monosodium urate from supersaturated extravascular fluid. Gout is characterized by episodes of acute arthritis, macroaggregates of monosodium urate (tophi) primarily in articular and surrounding tissue leading sometimes to crippling arthritis (chronic tophaceous gout), and by formation of urinary urate calculi. Any of these disorders can occur alone or in combination. Gout affects middle-aged and older men and is uncommon in women until after the menopause, when its frequency approaches that in men.

A. **Causes of Hyperuricemia.** The hallmark is hyperuricemia defined as a level 2 SD above the mean. The normal serum urate concentration in men is 5.1 mg ± 1.0 mg/dL and in women is 4.0 ± 1.0 mg/dL. Approximately 5% of normal persons are hyperuricemic, and only a few will develop gout. Hyperuricemia results from overproduction or underexcretion or both. The normal amount of urate excreted by the kidney in 24 hours is 600 mg. Approximately 90% of persons with primary gout have decreased renal clearance of urate, whereas about 10% are overproducers, excreting more than 1000 mg in 24 hours. This group is at greater risk of urinary calculi.

Hyperuricemia and gout are classified as secondary when they are associated with another disorder (renal failure, polycythemia, myeloproliferative and lymphoproliferative disorders, multiple myeloma, and a hereditary disorder, G-6-PD deficiency). Certain drugs and toxins decrease renal clearance of urate, including low-dose aspirin (less than 2 gm/day), proximal loop diuretics (thiazide and furosemide), alcohol, and lead.

B. **Clinical Characteristics.** Acute gouty arthritis tends to affect distal joints in the lower extremities. The first metatarsal-phalangeal joint is most often involved, followed by tarsal joints, ankle, knee, and wrist. Urate-induced inflammation can also occur in bursae, in particular the olecranon and prepatellar. The onset of an attack is sudden. Untreated, the pain and swelling reach a peak in 24–36 hours and then subside over 3–10 days, usually without residual joint damage. Chronic tophaceous gout is characterized by aggregates of urate (tophi) in subchondral bone, cartilage, synovium, olecranon and other bursae, and in soft tissue over the extensor surface of the upper forearm and over small joints of the hand, with insidious progressive joint destruction. Tophaceous gout becomes clinically apparent 10 or more years after the initial attack of gout.

C. **Diagnosis.** This is established definitively by identifying the characteristic rod- or needle-shaped crystal either free in synovial fluid or in leukocytes under compensated polarized light.

D. **Treatment.** Goals are to (1) relieve pain and swelling of acute arthritis, (2) prevent future attacks of acute arthritis, (3) prevent and/or decrease the formation of tophi, and (4) prevent formation of urinary urate calculi.

1. **ANTI-INFLAMMATORY DRUGS.** Acute arthritis is treated with any one of several NSAIDs. Maximum daily dose schedule of NSAID is begun for 24–48 hours. Therapeutic blood levels are achieved faster with short-acting NSAIDs given in the recommended maximum daily dose. After 2 or 3 days, the dose is reduced to a midrange for the next 7–10 days. For example, indomethacin 50 mg is given every 6 hours for 24–48 hours followed by 25 mg qid for 7–10 days.

2. **GLUCOCORTICOIDS.** These are quite effective in treating acute gout and are a reasonable alternative in patients in whom large doses of NSAIDs are contraindicated. Treatment is started with 40 mg/day of prednisone, which can be given in a single dose. The dose is tapered by 5-mg decrements over the next 7 days. To prevent a poststeroid withdrawal flare of arthritis, a low dose of an NSAID (e.g., indomethacin 25 mg bid) or oral colchicine 0.6 mg bid is administered, beginning on the 3rd day of treatment and continuing for 1–2 weeks after prednisone has been stopped.

3. **INTRA-ARTICULAR GLUCOCORTICOIDS.** In a situation in which systemic steroids or other medications are contraindicated, intra-articular steroids can be effective. The joint is first thoroughly aspirated when possible, then an intra-articular steroid preparation is injected. The injection dose for the knee is the equivalent of 40 mg of prednisone; for the ankle or wrist, 10–20 mg; and for the small joints of the hands and feet, 5 mg. Lidocaine 1% can be used to anesthetize the overlying skin and soft tissue; however, this additional step may bring further discomfort and may not reduce the pain of injection. When possible, prophylactic colchicine therapy should be instituted to prevent rebound flare.

4. **COLCHICINE.** Oral colchicine has been replaced by other drugs in acute gout. However, in a patient experiencing several attacks of acute gout a year, low doses of oral colchicine (0.6 mg bid) will reduce the number and severity of episodes. An acute attack can be aborted by increasing colchicine to 0.6 mg hourly for 3–5 doses when joint pain is first experienced. In patients with renal insufficiency or liver disease, the dose of colchicine should be reduced and white counts closely monitored.

When a patient is unable to take anything by mouth, IV colchicine can be used to treat an acute attack; it does not cause the GI side effects of oral therapy. Colchicine 2 mg is diluted in 20 ml of saline and given over a 10-minute interval to reduce the possibility of severe thrombophlebitis. A secure IV line is important to prevent extravasation of colchicine, which can cause tissue necrosis. An additional 1 mg appropriately diluted can be given in 6 hours and in another 6 hours if required. Patients should not receive more than 4 mg IV for an attack of gout. IV colchicine should not be given to patients who have renal insufficiency, liver disease, or neutropenia. The dose should be reduced by ⅓ to ½ in elderly patients with decreased creatinine clearance. Colchicine toxicity includes marrow suppression, hepatocellular damage, myopathy, and neuropathy.

5. HYPOURICEMIC THERAPY. Drugs to decrease serum uric acid are indicated in patients who have tophaceous gout, frequent attacks of gout not controlled by prophylactic colchicine or NSAIDs, or recurrent urinary urate calculi. In addition, an antihyperuricemic drug is indicated in overproducers of uric acid, who are at risk of developing renal calculi. The 24-hour uric acid excretion in these patients is usually more than 1000 mg. Asymptomatic hyperuricemia or acute gout without apparent tophi does not usually require treatment with an antihyperuricemic drug, although some researchers disagree with this approach. Some recommend that uric acid be normalized in patients with nontophaccous gout. Renal disease due to parenchymal urate deposition is uncommon in patients with longstanding hyperuricemia. The antihyperuricemic drugs are probenecid, sulfinpyrazone, and allopurinol.

  a. Uricosurics. Probenecid and sulfinpyrazone are uricosuric agents. These drugs are preferably given to patients who are underexcreters of uric acid, have normal renal function, and have no renal calculi.

  (1). *Probenecid* is started at 500 mg/day in 2 divided doses and increased by 500 mg/week until serum uric acid is normalized. Most patients will respond to a dose between 1 and 3 gm/day. Fluid intake should be increased for at least the 1st month of treatment and urine alkalinized to a pH of 6.5 to prevent stone formation. Sodium bicarbonate or potassium citrate in doses up to 7.5 gm/day is given to alkalinize urine. Once serum uric acid is normal, alkalinization is not as critical. Probenecid interferes with renal excretion of a number of drugs, raising their serum levels. These include NSAIDs, sulfonamides, sulfonylureas, methotrexate, penicillin, and ampicillin. Salicylates block the action of probenecid. Adverse reactions include rash, nausea, vomiting, and anaphylaxis.

  (2). *Sulfinpyrazone* dosage is started at 100 mg/day in 2 divided doses. The dose is increased by 100 mg/week until serum uric acid is normalized. Dosage can be increased to a maximum of 800 mg if necessary. The usual maintenance dosage is around 400 mg/day in 3–4 divided doses. The same precautions regarding fluid and alkalinization apply as for probenecid. Sulfinpyrazone interferes with the excretion of sulfonamides and sulfonylureas and can potentiate the hypoglycemic effects of the latter. The drug also potentiates the action of Coumadin. Salicylates antagonize the uricosuric effect of sulfinpyrazone. Side effects include exacerbation of peptic ulcer disease and rash. Marrow suppression is rare. The drug also interferes with platelet aggregation. When probenecid or sulfinpyrazone administration is started, **colchicine** 0.6 mg/bid or low-dose NSAID is given to prevent flares of acute arthritis. Colchicine or an NSAID is continued for several months until the serum uric acid has normalized.

b. Allopurinol is an antihyperuricemic drug that blocks the formation of uric acid by inhibition of xanthine oxidase. Since the drug is excreted in the urine, the dose of allopurinol should be reduced by at least 50% in those with significantly reduced renal function. Allopurinol is the antihyperuricemic drug of choice in patients with widespread tophaceous gout and reduced renal function and in those with renal calculi. It should be used in patients with a history of stones who are overexcreters of urate, since they are at risk of developing more stones. Allopurinol should not be used to treat asymptomatic hyperuricemia. The starting dose of allopurinol is 100 mg/day and is increased by 100 mg/day until the serum uric acid concentration is less than 7 mg/dL. The dose can then be adjusted to the amount required to maintain a normal serum uric acid value. The maximum recommended daily dose is 800 mg/day. Most cases can be controlled with 300 mg/day.

An important drug interaction of allopurinol is with the chemotherapeutic drug 6-mercaptopurine and its derivative azathioprine. Because these drugs are inactivated by xanthine oxidase, allopurinol will result in increased serum levels and potential toxicity. The dose of these chemotherapeutic drugs should be reduced by at least one-third for a patient on allopurinol. Approximately 5% of patients on allopurinol will have a serious adverse reaction requiring discontinuation. The most serious side effect is a life-threatening hypersensitivity reaction with fever, rash, and hepatocellular injury. Types of rashes include pruritic maculopapular eruptions, erythema multiforme, toxic epidermal necrolysis, and generalized exfoliation. Patients with renal failure or receiving diuretics appear to be at greater risk of developing this serious drug reaction. Other side effects include nausea and diarrhea. An antihyperuricemic drug should not be started until after the acute gout attack resolves. These agents can prolong the attack by mobilizing urate from tissue sites to joint fluid. This same mechanism accounts for arthritis flares during the first several months of treatment. Patients with large tophaceous deposits may need to receive prophylactic doses of colchicine for a year or longer. In general, colchicine 0.6 mg bid or a low-dose NSAID should be given along with an antihyperuricemic drug until the uric acid level is normalized and tophi have resolved.

c. Allopurinol with Chemotherapy. Allopurinol is also used to prevent acute uric acid nephropathy in patients undergoing chemotherapy for malignant disease. The patient should first be well hydrated and given a diuretic to increase urine flow and sodium bicarbonate to alkalinize the urine. Allopurinol 8 mg/kg is given in a single daily dose for 3–4 days. To prevent a gouty arthritis attack, colchicine 0.6 mg bid is also started; it is continued until allopurinol is stopped.

Kelley WN, Fox IH, Palella TD: Gout and related disorders of purine metabolism. *In* Kelley WN, Harris ED Jr, Ruddy S, Sledge CB: Textbook of Rheumatology. 3rd ed. Philadelphia, WB Saunders Co., 1989, pp 1395–1448.

IX. CALCIUM PYROPHOSPHATE DIHYDRATE DEPOSITION DISEASE

Deposition of calcium pyrophosphate dihydrate (CPPD) crystals within articular hyaline cartilage and fibrocartilage can result in articular damage. Table 14–12 classifies CPPD crystal deposition disease.

A. **Clinical Characteristics.** Several different syndromes have been described in patients with CPPD crystal deposition disease.

1. **Pseudogout** is marked by episodes of acute arthritis, often as severe as urate gout, principally affecting the knees; wrists, elbows, and even first metatarsophalangeal joints can also be affected.

2. **Pseudorheumatoid** is associated with polyarticular involvement, morning stiffness, synovial thickening, and in some cases, elevation of the sedimentation rate.

3. **Pseudoosteoarthritis** consists of degenerative changes in multiple joints, most often, knees, wrists, metacarpophalangeal joints, hips, shoulders, ankles, and spine.

4. **Pseudoneuropathic** is a severe destructive joint disease, especially in the knees, and can be seen in the absence of a neurologic disorder.

5. **Asymptomatic CPPD.** Chondrocalcinosis, a radiographic sign of CPPD arthropathy, may be seen in the absence of symptoms.

B. **Diagnosis.** This is established by finding crystals either free in synovial fluid or in synovial fluid neutrophils. Crystals, appearing as small rods, cuboids, and rhomboids, can also be identified on synovial biopsy. They show weakly positive birefringence. X-rays show stippled or punctate deposits in articular cartilage and fibrocartilage. Calcifications can also be seen in tendons, ligaments, and joint capsules.

C. **Treatment** is similar to that for acute gout. For prophylaxis, colchicine 0.6 mg bid or daily low doses of an NSAID will decrease the number and duration of attacks. Patients with chronic forms of disease are treated with an NSAID. Treatment of the underlying metabolic disorder does not affect the clinical expression of CPPD crystal deposition disease. Intra-articular injections of glucocorticoids are also quite effective in treating this disorder. Weight-bearing joints should be injected only 2–3 times a year to prevent the possibility of accelerating joint damage.

TABLE 14–12. CLASSIFICATION OF CPPD CRYSTAL DEPOSITION DISEASE

1. Familial forms
   Most autosomal dominant and associated with early osteoarthritic joint changes
2. Associated with metabolic disease
   Hyperthyroidism, hemochromatosis, hemosiderosis, hypophosphatasia, hypomagnesemia, hypothyroidism
3. Idiopathic
   Accounts for majority of cases

X. SYSTEMIC LUPUS ERYTHEMATOSUS

SLE is an immune-mediated disorder that affects multiple organ systems. It strikes the young and old of both sexes. The female/male ratio is 9:1. The incidence is greater in black Americans than in whites.

The effects of estrogen on the immune system contribute to the high incidence of SLE in women during childbearing years. UV light, infections, and drugs are environmental factors that can trigger SLE. Abnormal immune regulation plays a critical role in SLE development. B cell hyperactivity results in hypergammaglobulinemia and autoantibodies, which are directed against antigens in the cytoplasm, nucleus, or on the surface of cell membranes. Autoantibodies directed to cell membrane antigens cause hemolytic anemia, thrombocytopenia, or neutropenia. The serologic hallmark of SLE is antinuclear antibodies, in particular antibodies to double-stranded DNA that are highly specific for SLE. Immune complexes are deposited in tissue, resulting in nephritis, arthritis, serositis, and vasculitis.

A. Clinical Characteristics. Table 14–13 lists the diagnostic criteria for SLE; clinical expression and course are highly variable. Patients may have only one or a few features, such as rash, arthritis, or pleuritis, while others have multiple organ system involvement at presentation. Likewise, manifestations vary during the course, characterized by remissions and exacerbations. Fever, anorexia, weight loss, and/or fatigue

TABLE 14–13. REVISED DIAGNOSTIC CRITERIA FOR CLASSIFICATION OF SYSTEMIC LUPUS ERYTHEMATOSUS

CRITERIA*	DEFINITION
1. Malar rash	Erythematous rash over malar eminences
2. Discoid rash	Erythematous patches with adherent keratotic scaling and follicular plugging
3. Photosensitivity	Rash as result of sun exposure
4. Oral ulcers	Oral or nasal ulceration
5. Arthritis	Nonerosive arthritis of 2 or more joints
6. Serositis	Pleuritis or pericarditis
7. Renal disorder	Persistent proteinuria >0.5 gm/day or cellular casts
8. Neurologic disorder	Seizures or psychosis not associated with medications or metabolic derangement
9. Hematologic disorder	Hemolytic anemia or leukopenia (<4000/mm^3) or lymphopenia (<1500/mm^3) or thrombocytopenia (<100,000/mm^3)
10. Immunologic disorder	Positive LE cell preparation or anti-DNA antibodies or anti-SM antibodies or false-positive VDRL
11. Antinuclear antibodies	

*For study purposes, a patient with 4 or more of these criteria simultaneously or serially is considered to have SLE.

From Tan EM, Cohen AS, Fries JF, et al: The 1982 revised criteria for the classification of systemic lupus erythematosus (SLE). Arthritis Rheum 25:1271–1277, 1982.

occur frequently. Even after years of apparent inactivity, lupus can exacerbate and progress to death. Survival of SLE patients is 86% at 5 years and 76% at 10 years.

1. **MUSCULOSKELETAL.** The most frequent symptoms are arthritis and arthralgias. Arthritis is usually symmetric and nonerosive, involving small joints of hands and feet, wrists, knees, and ankles. Arthritis can be persistent or transient. Tenosynovitis can occur alone. Muscle pain and weakness can be due to inflammatory myositis or secondary to glucocorticoids, hydroxychloroquine, or hypokalemia.

2. **SKIN.** The most typical cutaneous manifestation of SLE is a butterfly erythematous facial rash over the malar areas and bridge of nose, which is often photosensitive and usually does not lead to scarring. SLE patients can also have lesions of **discoid lupus** that can cause severe disfiguring scars. Other skin manifestations include erythema multiforme, papulosquamous lesions, petechiae, vesicles, bullae, urticaria, angioedema, and panniculitis. Reversible or scarring alopecia can also occur. Small-vessel vasculitis can appear as palpable purpura, nailfold or volar fingerpad infarcts, erythema multiforme or nodosum, or livedo reticularis.

3. **RENAL.** Clinically apparent renal disease occurs in more than half of SLE patients. Presenting signs of lupus nephritis are hematuria, proteinuria, and an active urine sediment consisting of red cell, white cell, and hyaline casts. Hypertension, nephrotic syndrome with either diffuse proliferative or membranous glomerulonephritis, and the complication of renal vein thrombosis also occur. Administration of an NSAID can worsen renal function.

Lupus nephritis is classified pathologically into pure mesangial, focal segmental, diffuse proliferative, membranous, and advanced sclerosing glomerulonephritis. There may be overlap between these major histologic types. Of the first 4 types, diffuse proliferative glomerulonephritis carries the worst prognosis. Membranous glomerulonephritis can remain static for years. Histologic indices of activity and chronicity guide treatment decisions. Glomerular hypercellularity, fibrinoid necrosis, leukocyte exudation, hyaline thrombi, and interstitial inflammation are features of disease activity and usually respond to treatment. A high chronicity index based on glomerular sclerosis, fibrous crescents, tubular atrophy, and interstitial fibrosis portends irreversible disease, especially with azotemia.

4. **PULMONARY.** The most common pulmonary manifestation is pleurisy, occurring in more than half the patients. Pleural effusions are usually slight and show mononuclear cells. Patients can also develop acute lupus pneumonitis manifested by bilateral alveolar infiltrates. Infections should always be excluded because they account for most of the pulmonary infiltrates seen in SLE. Diffuse interstitial pneumonitis occasionally is observed. Pulmonary hypertension due to vascular involvement of pulmonary arteries is a serious complication of lupus and results in death in 1–2 years. Peripheral emboli resulting from

peripheral thrombophlebitis also occur with greater frequency in lupus patients. Thrombophlebitis is associated with lupus anticoagulant or anticardiolipin antibodies.

5. **CARDIAC.** Pericarditis is the most commonly observed cardiac manifestation of SLE, occurring in about a third of patients. Fever, rub, tachycardia, and atrial fibrillation or flutter are clinical features. Tamponade is an uncommon complication. Patients can also develop myocarditis; Libman-Sacks endocarditis (nonbacterial verrucous vegetations) is usually asymptomatic and rarely diagnosed clinically. Coronary artery disease also occurs in SLE. Glucocorticoids, hypercholesterolemia, hypertension, and underlying coronary artery vasculitis are contributing factors.

6. **CENTRAL NERVOUS SYSTEM.** CNS disease covers a wide spectrum of manifestations ranging from subtle behavioral and cognitive abnormalities to strokes, seizures, and severe psychiatric disturbances. Other manifestations include aseptic meningitis, transverse myelitis, chorea, ataxia, and peripheral and cranial nerve neuropathies. Headache, often typical of migraine, is common in SLE. In patients with cerebrovascular accidents due to thrombosis there appears to be a relationship with the lupus anticoagulant or anticardiolipin antibodies.

7. **GASTROINTESTINAL.** Nausea and anorexia are common symptoms. Vasculitis of the bowel wall can cause abdominal pain, diarrhea, and melena, which can progress to bowel infarction or perforation. Acute pancreatitis can also occur as a feature of SLE or as a complication of glucocorticoid treatment.

8. **OCULAR.** Ocular manifestations are dryness (sicca syndrome), episcleritis, retinal artery vasculitis, and optic neuritis. Posterior capsule cataracts result from glucocorticoid treatment. Thrombotic glaucoma can occur in patients with anticardiolipin antibodies.

B. **Treatment.** An understanding of the disease by the patient and a good relationship among physician, patient, and family are essential. Patients should generally be seen by their physician about every 3–6 months to monitor the disease and adjust treatment. More frequent visits are needed during disease flares. Early recognition of disease flares or complications such as infections or drug reactions followed promptly by appropriate treatment can reduce morbidity and mortality. Patients should be told that estrogens used for birth control can increase the risk of lupus exacerbation. Fatigue is a common symptom in SLE. Patients should be encouraged to rest during the day and get a good night's sleep.

Since some patients experience flares of systemic disease and/or rash with exposure to ultraviolet (UV) light, they should be advised to stay out of the sun during peak hours (10 AM–3 PM) of UV light, wear appropriate clothing, and use a high-grade sunscreen, which should be applied several times a day. Patients should also be warned about artificial sources of UV light.

The risk of infection is increased in SLE patients, especially those on glucocorticoids or cytotoxic drugs. Patients should be immunized with **pneumococcal** and **influenza vaccines,** the latter yearly. Prophylactic antibiotics are indicated in patients undergoing dental procedures and should also be considered in those having invasive diagnostic studies. Intrauterine devices also carry an increased risk of infection.

1. **ARTHRITIS.** Arthritis is treated with a salicylate or NSAIDs. The dose is adjusted within the recommended range to control the symptoms. NSAID inhibition of prostaglandins within the kidney in lupus nephritis may worsen renal function. Occasionally, low-dose prednisone (5–10 mg/day) may be needed to control arthritis. For patients with persistent symptoms, hydroxychloroquine (200–400 mg/day) is useful.

2. **PERICARDITIS/PNEUMONITIS.** Pleurisy or pericarditis may respond to an NSAID but often requires glucocorticoids. The initial dose of prednisone is 20–40 mg/day. Symptoms usually respond in a few days, when dosage can be tapered by 5-mg decrements every 3–5 days, depending on the symptoms. A persistent pleural effusion should be aspirated to exclude other causes. Pericardial effusions can occasionally progress to tamponade, requiring pericentesis and instillation of glucocorticoids into the pericardium. Lupus pneumonitis also responds to the above doses of glucocorticoids after infection has been excluded.

3. **RASH.** Skin lesions may respond to topical steroids. Fluorinated steroids, however, should not be used on the face because they will lead to thinning and atrophy of the skin. Hydroxychloroquine can be used for more extensive disease, especially in patients with discoid lesions and with subacute cutaneous SLE lesions. The initial dose is 400 mg/day. Once rash is under control, this can be reduced to 200 mg/day, and eventually to 200 mg every other day. Because of the danger of retinal toxicity, the patient should have a careful baseline ophthalmologic examination, which should be repeated every 6–9 months. Prednisone beginning at 40 mg in 2–3 divided doses may be required when there is no response. The dose should be tapered as soon as possible to the lowest dose that will control the skin disease (see guidelines for steroid tapering under treatment of renal disease). Injection of glucocorticoids into the skin lesion can be quite effective but may lead to skin atrophy.

4. **RENAL DISEASE.** See Chapter 6 for treatment of lupus nephritis.

5. **CEREBRITIS.** Both the diagnosis and treatment of CNS lupus are difficult. In patients with severe cognitive abnormalities and neuropsychiatric disturbances prednisone can be tried in dosages ranging from 60–100 mg/day in 2–3 divided doses. When the patient improves, prednisone is given as a single morning dose, which is then tapered by 10-mg decrements at 5–7-day intervals until the dose is 40 mg and then by 5-mg decrements at 5–7-day intervals, depending on response.

When the patient's symptoms cannot be controlled with prednisone 10 mg/day or less, alternative treatments should be considered.

Patients already taking glucocorticoids may develop symptoms similar to those in CNS lupus. The distinction clinically between steroid psychosis and CNS lupus is difficult. When there is a question, the patient can be treated with high-dose prednisone (up to 100 mg/day) for 1 week. The prednisone dose is tapered slowly if the patient improves. If not, the symptom may be due to steroid psychosis, and prednisone should be tapered as quickly as possible. Haloperidol in doses of 1–4 mg bid or tid may help control psychiatric symptoms.

Seizures can usually be controlled with phenytoin 100 mg bid or tid. Prednisone 60 mg/day in 2 divided doses is also started; the dosage is then slowly tapered, as previously described. It is difficult to know the end point of steroid therapy in this situation when seizures are the only evidence of activity. Patients with transverse myelitis and peripheral neuropathies can also be treated with prednisone.

Strokes may be caused by vasculitis or possibly thrombosis secondary to a lupus anticoagulant or anticardiolipin. Patients should be treated with prednisone 40–60 mg/day in 2 divided doses, which is tapered slowly. In a stroke patient who has a lupus antiphospholipid antibody, anticoagulation with heparin followed by Coumadin is probably indicated, assuming there is no evidence of bleeding. An alternate treatment is low-dose aspirin 325 mg/day or every other day.

6. **CYTOPENIA.** Hemolytic anemia and thrombocytopenia usually respond to **prednisone** 40–60 mg in 2–3 divided doses. Occasionally a patient may require 80–100 mg/day in divided doses. The initial dose is continued until the platelet count or hematocrit has risen to a safe level. Prednisone dosage is then consolidated into a single morning dose, which is then tapered slowly. **Splenectomy** should be considered in thrombocytopenia or hemolytic anemia when cell counts cannot be controlled with glucocorticoids. When surgery is contraindicated, a patient with thrombocytopenia can be given **vincristine** or **vinblastine.** Danazol 300–600 mg/day in divided doses is also effective in some patients with thrombocytopenia or hemolytic anemia. IV gammaglobulin 40 mg/kg/day for 5 days has been beneficial for some patients.

7. **PULSE GLUCOCORTICOID TREATMENT.** An alternative treatment to daily high doses of glucocorticoid in severe SLE is IV boluses of glucocorticoids. **Methylprednisolone** sodium succinate 1 gm IV is given over a 30-minute period and the dose repeated on 3 consecutive days. Pulse therapy can be repeated in 3 months, depending on the patient's clinical status. After IV pulse therapy, the maintenance glucocorticoid dose is resumed; this can be further tapered on the basis of clinical parameters. Side effects include hypertension, hyperglycemia, and facial flushing. Rare complications are anaphylaxis, cardiac arrhythmias, and seizures.

TABLE 14–14. DRUGS ASSOCIATED WITH LUPUS-LIKE SYNDROME

MOST COMMONLY REPORTED	LESS COMMONLY REPORTED
Procainamide	Quinidine
Hydralazine	Practolol
Isoniazid	Penicillin
Hydantoin	Tetracyclines
	Sulfonamides
	Chlorpromazine
	D-Penicillamine
	Phenylbutazone
	Allopurinol
	Propylthiouracil

C. **SLE and Pregnancy.** Recent data question the long-held notion that pregnancy exacerbates SLE. Nevertheless, it is clear that the incidence of adverse fetal outcomes is increased at least twofold in SLE. The most common problems are miscarriage, prematurity, and stillbirth. In the presence of lupus nephritis, the risk of fetal loss is even higher. The presence of anticardiolipin antibodies also seems to be a risk factor.

Since fetal survival is improved when lupus is under control, pregnancy should be planned at a time when the disease has been inactive for several months. In patients who have had recurrent spontaneous abortions and who have been shown to have antibodies to anticardiolipin, special steps should be taken. The pregnancy should be carefully monitored and treated as high-risk. Early induction or cesarean section may be needed. Fetal survival has improved in some patients who were treated with prednisone and aspirin. Subcutaneous heparin also has been used. Glucocorticoids (prednisone, prednisolone, hydrocortisone) are metabolized by the placenta and do not affect the fetus. Dexamethasone should not be used during pregnancy. NSAIDs, antimalarials, and cytotoxic drugs should be avoided in patients contemplating pregnancy and during the pregnancy. Breast-feeding is considered safe in women who receive less than 30 mg/day of prednisone.

D. **Drug-Induced Lupus.** Several drugs can induce a lupus-like syndrome (Table 14–14). Procainamide is by far the most frequent cause of drug-induced lupus. The most common symptoms associated with drug-induced lupus are arthritis, arthralgias, pleurisy, and pericarditis. Renal and CNS disease are rare. Antinuclear antibodies (ANAs), most notably antihistone and anti–single-stranded DNA antibodies, are found in these patients. ANAs are also present in asymptomatic patients. Symptoms usually disappear a few weeks after stopping of the drug but occasionally will last for several months. The ANA test may remain positive for months to years. While symptoms usually disappear after stopping of the drug, patients may require salicylates or an NSAID. When symptoms are severe, glucocorticoids 20–40 mg/day in 2 divided doses are usually effective.

Klippel JH (ed): Systemic Lupus Erythematosus. Rheum Dis Clin North Am vol. 14, April 1988.

XI. POLYMYOSITIS AND DERMATOMYOSITIS

Polymyositis (PM) and dermatomyositis (DM) are inflammatory disorders of unknown cause involving primarily proximal muscles of the upper and lower extremities. PM/DM occurs more often in women. The mean age of onset in adults is about 50 years. ANAs are frequently present with anti-Jo-1, anti-PM/SCL, and anti-Mi appearing to have specificity for myositis. PM/DM occurs as a primary idiopathic disorder (type I and type II, respectively), in association with malignant disease (type III), in childhood (type IV), and in association with other collagen vascular diseases (type V). Inclusion, eosinophilic, and localized nodular myositis are classified as type VI.

A. Clinical Characteristics. PM or DM usually presents as symmetric proximal muscle weakness causing difficulty in climbing stairs, rising from a couch, lifting heavy objects over the head, and combing the hair. Symptoms are often present for several months before the patient sees a physician. Some patients experience muscle pain and tenderness. Weakness of the muscles of the esophagus or pharynx produces dysphagia or dysphonia. Cardiac manifestations include cardiac arrhythmias, heart failure, and pericarditis. Interstitial fibrosis develops in about a third of patients. Patients are also at risk of aspiration pneumonitis. Raynaud's phenomenon, arthralgias, or arthritis may be experienced, as well as constitutional symptoms of malaise, weight loss, and fever.

In DM, rash can precede, coincide with, or follow the onset of muscle weakness. Typically the patient develops an erythematous facial rash, often with a butterfly distribution, periorbital edema, and a dusky purple discoloration of the upper eyelids referred to as heliotrope. Scaly, purplish-red papules develop over the dorsal surfaces of the interphalangeal joints, elbows, knees, and medial malleoli. Diagnostic tests for PM/DM are elevated muscle enzymes (CPK, aldolase, SGOT), myopathic changes on EMG (short-amplitude polyphasic potentials, fibrillations, irritability), and positive muscle biopsy (fiber necrosis, inflammatory infiltrate).

The course is highly variable. The cumulative survival rate is greater than 70% at 8 years, but therapy can be stopped in 75% of patients.

B. Treatment. Initial treatment is with **prednisone** 60–80 mg/day in 3 divided doses. After the first week the dosage can be consolidated into a single morning dose. This dose is maintained until muscle enzymes are normal. Improvement should occur within the first few weeks or month of treatment, at which time the dosage is tapered by 10 mg-decrements every 5–7 days until it is 30 mg, and then by 5-mg decrements at the same intervals. The patient's clinical state, muscle strength, and serum enzyme values are closely monitored and used as guidelines for reducing prednisone. Most cases respond to prednisone, and a low daily dose or alternate-day schedule can be used for maintenance. A cytotoxic agent should be added when myositis cannot be controlled with prednisone 20 mg/day or less after 2–3 months of starting prednisone. The most experience with cytotoxic drugs in PM/DM has been with azathioprine and methotrexate. The dose of **azathioprine** is 1.5–3 mg/kg/day. The initial dose of **methotrexate** is 7.5 mg/week given in 3 divided doses 12 hours apart once a week. This dose can be gradually increased to 15 mg weekly. When a patient is unable to tolerate oral methotrexate because of GI upset, the drug can be given IM beginning with 10 mg once a week, which can be increased up to 25 mg once a week depending on clinical response. Methotrexate should not be given to those with a creatinine value greater than 2.0 mg/dL or with liver disease. Concomitant aspirin or an NSAID, which are weak organic acids, can raise the blood level of methotrexate by interfering with its excretion and increase the risk of toxicity. (See Rheumatoid Arthritis). When the rash in DM does not respond to prednisone, **hydroxychloroquine** can be used, beginning with a dose of 400 mg/day (See Rheumatoid Arthritis).

Steroid **myopathy** can complicate the clinical course of PM/DM and is likely when muscle weakness progresses in the face of normal muscle enzymes. The dose of prednisone is reduced to a level that will keep muscle enzymes normal. Steroid myopathy can also contribute to muscle weakness in a patient with active myositis, in which case, the dose of steroid is maintained and a cytotoxic drug (methotrexate) is added with the expectation that prednisone can later be reduced.

During active disease, patients should regularly receive passive range-of-motion exercises to prevent contractures. Once the disease is under control, physical activity and muscle strengthening can gradually be increased.

Bradley WG, Tandan, R: Inflammatory diseases of muscle. *In* Kelley WN, Harris ED, Jr, Ruddy S, Sledge CB: Textbook of Rheumatology. 3rd ed. Philadelphia, WB Saunders Co, 1989, vol 2, pp 1283–1287.

XII. SYSTEMIC SCLEROSIS

Systemic sclerosis (scleroderma) is a chronic inflammatory disorder of unknown cause characterized by fibrosis of the skin and visceral organs, including the GI tract, lungs, heart, and kidney. Its onset is usually in the 3rd to 5th decades; women are affected 4 times more often than men. ANAs are often present, most notably antitopoisomerase (SCL-70), anticentromere, and antinucleolar antibodies. Anticentromere is highly specific for limited cutaneous scleroderma or CREST syndrome.

The degree and extent of skin and visceral involvement vary greatly. Systemic sclerosis can be divided into a diffuse cutaneous form and a limited cutaneous form with some overlap. Those with the diffuse cutaneous form have involvement of both distal and proximal aspects of the extremities, face, and trunk and are more likely to develop serious visceral disease. In the limited cutaneous form, skin involvement is usually restricted to the distal extremities and progresses slowly over years. Significant renal involvement is rare. This limited form of disease is also referred to as CREST syndrome (*c*alcinosis, *R*aynaud's phenomenon, *e*sophageal dysmotility, *s*clerodactyly, and *t*elangiectasia). The prognosis is worse in patients with diffuse cutaneous involvement. Although limited cutaneous disease is usually a more benign form, a few patients develop progressive pulmonary arterial hypertension, which is often fatal.

A. Clinical Characteristics

1. **SKIN.** The first symptom of systemic sclerosis is usually Raynaud's phenomenon. The skin over the hands eventually becomes thickened, leathery, and tightly bound to underlying tissue. Digital ulcers, gangrene, and resorption of the distal phalanx may occur. Skin later becomes shiny, taut, and pigmented, with areas of hypopigmentation. Punctate telangiectasias appear over the fingers, hands, face, mouth, lips, and tongue. Calcium deposits may appear in the volar pads of fingers and over extensor surfaces of the forearms, elbows, and knees. After many years, skin eventually softens in most patients but remains atrophic. Arthritis/arthralgias, joint contractures, fibrosis of tendon sheaths, and muscle atrophy may be present.

2. **GASTROINTESTINAL.** Systemic sclerosis affects the lower ⅔ of the esophagus and lower esophageal sphincter. Patients complain of dysphagia, especially with solids. Reflux leads to esophagitis and strictures. Hypomotility of the small intestine produces bloating and abdominal pain, suggesting obstruction (pseudo-obstruction). **Bacterial overgrowth** in the atonic small bowel is responsible for causing malabsorption syndrome, manifested by steatorrhea, hypoalbuminemia, hypocalcemia, anemia, and weight loss. In the large bowel, wide-mouthed diverticula occur along the antimesenteric border of the transverse and descending colon. Hypomotility of the large bowel leads to obstipation.

3. **PULMONARY.** Pulmonary manifestations include interstitial pulmonary fibrosis, reduced diffusion capacity, and less commonly pleurisy. Pulmonary arterial hypertension also occurs and is seen mostly in patients with limited cutaneous involvement or CREST syndrome.

4. **CARDIAC.** Features of cardiac involvement are left ventricular dysfunction, heart failure due to myocardial fibrosis, pericarditis, and varying degrees of heart block and arrhythmia.

5. **RENAL.** Kidney disease is the most common cause of death in patients with systemic sclerosis. Scleroderma renal crisis most often occurs in patients with rapidly progressing diffuse cutaneous scleroderma and is usually manifested by malignant hypertension, proteinuria, and microscopic hematuria. If not treated, renal function rapidly deteriorates.

6. **MISCELLANEOUS.** Patients can also develop **hypothyroidism,** due to fibrosis of the thyroid gland or associated with Hashimoto's thyroiditis. **Biliary cirrhosis** is present in some patients with CREST syndrome. **Sjögren's syndrome,** with dry eyes and dry mouth, can also occur.

B. Treatment.
While no cure exists for systemic sclerosis, treatment of the involved organ system can be beneficial. The patient should be seen at least every 3 months or more often, depending on the severity of the illness and medications. Throughout their illness, patients will need

repeated explanations and reassurances. Early recognition of scleroderma renal crisis can prevent potential renal damage.

1. **PENICILLAMINE.** Penicillamine is the most widely used drug for this disorder. Retrospective studies show that patients on penicillamine have less skin thickening and reduced rate of new visceral organ involvement. To reduce adverse reactions, the dose is started low and increased slowly. The starting dose is 250 mg once a day, which is increased at 1–3 month intervals up to 1.5 gm/day as tolerated. Since few patients can tolerate 1.5 gm/day, a maintenance dose between 0.5 and 1 gm/day is used for most. Doses of 500 mg or less can be given once a day. Higher amounts are given in 2 or 3 divided doses. The drug should be taken on an empty stomach. CBC and urinalysis are done monthly.

2. **RAYNAUD'S PHENOMENON.** Patients are instructed to avoid frequent exposure to cold, to dress warmly, and to keep their body and face as well as their extremities warm. Beneficial **vasodilator** drugs include reserpine, alpha-methyldopa, phenoxybenzamine, prazosin, and **calcium channel blockers (nifedipine, diltiazem).** Nitroglycerin paste applied to hands and feet is useful in some. The dose of nifedipine is usually 10 mg tid and of diltiazem 60 mg tid or qid. Surgical sympathectomy can lead to transient improvement. Some patients benefit from learning **biofeedback** techniques for increasing skin temperature. Digital ulcers should be kept clean and protected from trauma by wearing of a finger guard.

3. **ESOPHAGEAL DYSMOTILITY/REFLUX.** Patients with esophageal reflux are advised to eat smaller meals, not to lie down for a few hours after a meal, to have the head of the bed elevated, and to avoid coffee, tea, and chocolate, which relax the lower esophageal sphincter. Antacids and **H₂ blockers** are also given. **Metoclopramide,** a smooth muscle stimulator, can improve esophageal motility. Esophageal dilation may be necessary in patients with strictures. Patients with malabsorption syndrome, often caused by bacterial overgrowth, improve with intermittent use of broad-spectrum antibiotics (tetracycline, metronidazole, or trimethoprim-sulfamethoxazole). In patients with constipation, stool softeners and mild laxatives are usually adequate.

4. **ARTHRITIS.** Polyarthritis is treated with an NSAID. The patient should do daily flexibility exercises to maintain range of motion.

5. **RENAL CRISIS.** This is treated immediately with a potent antihypertensive agent. The angiotensin-converting enzyme inhibitors (e.g., captopril) are effective in controlling blood pressure and improving renal function and are the treatment of choice. Overdiuresis should be avoided, since it might decrease the effective plasma volume and renal blood flow. Patients with progressive renal failure should be prepared for the possibility of dialysis and renal transplantation.

6. **PULMONARY HYPERTENSION/FIBROSIS.** There is no long-term effective treatment for pulmonary arterial hypertension. Calcium channel blockers may provide transient improvement. Patients with lung involvement should receive Pneumovax and yearly influenza vaccinations. Home oxygen therapy may be necessary for patients with significant diffusion abnormality.

C. **Overlap Syndromes.** Diagnostic criteria for more than one collagen vascular disease may be present. Overlap syndromes include systemic sclerosis and PM, SLE and RA, SLE and systemic sclerosis, and systemic sclerosis and RA. Myositis is also seen in conjunction with RA and SLE. Sjögren's syndrome may accompany almost any of the collagen vascular diseases.

1. **MIXED CONNECTIVE TISSUE DISEASE.** The term "mixed connective tissue disease" (MCTD) was originally used to define a disorder with features of SLE, systemic sclerosis, polymyositis, and rheumatoid arthritis. In addition, patients also had in common high titers of antibodies to ribonucleoprotein (RNP). Clinical manifestations include Raynaud's phenomenon, puffy hands, tight skin, esophageal dysmotility, rash, arthritis/arthralgias, pleurisy, pericarditis, aseptic meningitis, and myositis. These features appear sequentially over months and years. Eventually, about half of the cases of MCTD evolve into a clinical picture most consistent with systemic sclerosis, while others resemble SLE, RA, or Sjögren's syndrome or remain undifferentiated. The term "undifferentiated connective tissue disorder" has been suggested for cases that do not have diagnostic criteria for any one collagen vascular disease.

The inflammatory features of MCTD respond to **glucocorticoids,** but treatment does not prevent this disorder from evolving into systemic sclerosis or other disorders. Inflammatory features of MCTD such as pleurisy, pericarditis, or myositis respond to **prednisone** 40–60 mg/day. Mild disease can be managed with low doses of prednisone or an NSAID. Treatment of overlap syndrome is directed to the individual collagen vascular disease components.

2. **EOSINOPHILIC FASCIITIS.** This is characterized by rapid onset of pain, tenderness, and swelling of upper and lower extremities that develops after strenuous physical exercise in many patients. It affects both sexes equally. Onset is mostly between ages 30 and 65. Eosinophilic fasciitis is associated in a few patients with hematologic disorders, most often aplastic anemia and thrombocytopenia. The swelling progresses to brawny induration, followed subsequently by retraction of subcutaneous tissue leading to a cobblestone or puckered appearance. Biopsy consisting of skin, fascia, superficial muscles shows inflammation consisting of histiocytes, eosinophils, lymphocytes, and plasma cells involving the dermis and deep fascia. Patients also may experience polyarthralgias, arthritis, fever, fatigue, and weight loss. In some patients there is spontaneous improvement or improvement with glucocorticoids. Others go on to develop chronic fibrotic and

atrophic skin changes and joint contractures, involving most often elbows, knees, ankles, wrists, and hands.

Treatment consists of **prednisone** 40–60 mg/day in divided doses and reduced gradually as previously described (see "Systemic Lupus Erythematosus, Rash"). Glucocorticoids should be given only for treatment of the acute inflammatory phase of disease and are of no benefit for chronic fibrotic cutaneous lesions. The response to prednisone is variable. Hydroxychloroquine 400 mg/day has also been effective in some cases.

Bennett RM: Mixed connective tissue disease and other overlap syndromes. *In* Kelley WN, Harris ED, Jr, Ruddy S, Sledge CB, Textbook of Rheumatology. 3rd ed. 1989, vol 2, pp 1147 1165.
Seibold JR: Scleroderma. *In* Textbook of Rheumatology. 2nd ed. 1985, vol 2, pp 1215–1244.

XIII. EOSINOPHILIA-MYALGIA SYNDROME

The eosinophilia-myalgia syndrome (EMS) occurs in people using the amino acid L-tryptophan. For diagnostic purposes, it consists of eosinophilia, often dramatic, and debilitating myalgias, usually affecting the proximal muscles, in the context of tryptophan ingestion. Other features include cough; pulmonary infiltrates; diffuse swelling of the extremities, progressing to eosinophilic fasciitis-like skin changes; alopecia; and axonal polyneuropathy. Biopsy of affected muscles often discloses cellular infiltrates of lymphocytes, histocytes, and less often, eosinophils in muscle and fascia. The majority of the 1400 reported cases have been in women (90%). Some patients developed EMS after they stopped taking L-tryptophan. The drug has been withdrawn from the market. At present, the cause is thought to be chemical or bacterial contamination that occurred during the manufacture of L-tryptophan. Treatment in severely affected patients has consisted of high-doses of prednisone, some patients requiring more aggressive treatment with cytotoxic drugs, plasmapheresis, and even high doses of immunoglobulin. So far, 16 deaths have been reported, most often from severe lung or nerve involvement. Since the disease was recognized only in October 1989, long-term outcome data are still pending, but it appears that many patients may have sequelae.

15 15 15 15 15 15 15 15 15

DERMATOLOGIC DISEASES

MARK BERNHARDT
KENNETH A. ARNDT

15 15 15 15 15 15 15 15 15 15 15

I. GENERAL PRINCIPLES OF SKIN CARE

The two principal variables in dispensing topical medication—the medication itself and the vehicle—must both be appropriate for the condition under treatment. In general, **acute inflammation is best treated with aqueous, drying preparations and chronic inflammation is treated with hydrophobic, more occlusive, lubricating compounds. Open wet dressings** cool and dry through evaporation. The resulting vasoconstriction decreases the augmented local blood flow present in inflammation. In addition, wet dressings cleanse the skin of exudates, crusts, and debris; help maintain drainage of infected areas; and decrease pain and/or pruritus. They are indicated in the therapy for acute inflammatory conditions, erosions, and ulcers. **Powders** promote drying by increasing the effective skin surface area. They are primarily used in intertriginous areas to reduce moisture, maceration, and friction. **Lotions** consist of suspensions of a powder in water. **Solutions** are lotions in which the active ingredients are dissolved, and consequently they are clear. **Tinctures** are alcoholic or hydroalcoholic solutions. As lotions and tinctures evaporate, they cool and dry; lotions leave a uniform film of medication on the skin. Sprays and aerosols act similarly. A **gel** is a transparent, semisolid emulsion that liquefies on contact with the skin, drying as a thin, greaseless, nonocclusive film. Lotions and gels are particularly useful for hairy areas. **Creams** are semisolid emulsions of oil in water. Although creams are often more cosmetically acceptable to patients, they may not be as effective for dry chronic dermatoses as **ointments,** which consist of an emulsion of water droplets suspended in oil or as an inert base such as petrolatum.

An important consideration in topical therapy is dispensing the proper amount of medication. When inadequate amounts are prescribed, the patient may apply the medication too sparingly or less frequently than necessary. Table 15–1 gives conservative amounts needed for single or multiple applications of a cream, ointment, or lotion.

Bickers DR, Hazen PG, Lynch WS: Clinical Pharmacology of Skin Disease. New York, Churchill Livingstone, 1984.

Fitzpatrick TB, Eisen AZ, Wolff K (eds): Dermatology in General Medicine. 3rd ed. New York, McGraw-Hill, 1987.

Moschella SL, Hurley HJ (eds): Dermatology. 2nd ed. Philadelphia, WB Saunders Co., 1985.

Rook A, Wilkinson DS, Ebling FJG (eds): Textbook of Dermatology. 4th ed. Oxford, England, Blackwell, 1986.

II. TREATMENT OF DERMATITIS

Dermatitis is the most common inflammatory reaction pattern of the skin. The morphologic and histopathologic changes in all forms of dermatitis and eczema, terms that are used interchangeably, are similar. The earliest and mildest changes are erythema and edema. These may

TABLE 15–1. AMOUNT OF TOPICAL MEDICATION NEEDED FOR SINGLE OR MULTIPLE APPLICATIONS

AREA TREATED	ONE APPLICATION (GM)	TWICE DAILY FOR 1 WK (GM)	THREE TIMES DAILY FOR 2 WK (GM)
Hands, head, face, anogenital area	2	28	90
One arm, anterior or posterior trunk	3	42	120
One leg	4	56	180
Entire body	30–60	420–480	1.26–2.52 kg (42–84 oz)

progress to vesiculation and oozing and then to crusting and scaling. Finally, if the process becomes chronic, the skin will be lichenified (thickened with accentuated skin markings), excoriated, and either hypopigmented or hyperpigmented. The factors that may initiate dermatitis are numerous, and its patterns dictate both the clinical classification and the therapy.

Atopic dermatitis is an intensely pruritic, chronic eruption. Although it may disappear with time, it is estimated that 30–80% of patients with atopic dermatitis will continue to have. intermittent exacerbations throughout life, often when under physical or emotional stress. Approximately 70% of patients with atopic dermatitis have a family history of atopy, and about 50% of children with atopic dermatitis develop either rhinitis or asthma. **Lichen simplex chronicus** is a localized, chronic pruritic disorder resulting from repeated scratching and rubbing. Well-circumscribed lichenified plaques usually are located on ankles, anterior area of the tibia, and neck. Dry, keratotic papules and giant "scratch papules," or prurigo nodularis, are also a response to the repeated trauma of scratching. **Contact dermatitis** may be produced by primary irritants or allergic sensitizers. It is not the specific morphology that distinguishes contact dermatitis from other types of eczema but rather its distribution and configuration. This type of dermatitis is located in exposed or contact areas and typically has bizarre or artificial patterns characterized by sharp, straight margins, acute angles, and straight lines. **Hand dermatitis** is a common, chronic disorder that has as its most characteristic lesion myriads of small vesicles scattered on the sides of the fingers, and less often, throughout the palms. More severe changes include bulla formation and extreme inelasticity of the skin, with deep, painful fissures. **Nummular dermatitis** is characterized by round (coin shaped), eczematous plaques most commonly located on the dorsa of the hands and forearms, lower aspect of the legs, and buttocks.

A. **General Principles.** **Topical corticosteroids** are the primary agents in treatment. Effectiveness is related to the potency of the drug and its percutaneous penetration. Potency is most often assessed in vivo by their ability to produce vasoconstriction on human skin, and results of this bioassay correlate well with clinical trials (Table 15–2). **Ointment** vehicles generally impart better biologic activity to the incorporated steroids than do creams or other vehicles. Occluding the treated area with nonporous plastic wraps dramatically raises the effectiveness of topical corticosteroids by increasing the hydration of the horny layer and the surface area of the skin, thereby both enhancing percutaneous absorption and inducing a reservoir of the medication in the stratum corneum. Folliculitis, miliaria, and maceration may occur from excessive occlusion.

Multiple **adverse effects** can be associated with use of topical corticosteroids. Burning, itching, and dryness are usually related to the vehicle: ointments are better tolerated when applied to inflamed skin than are creams or gels. Atrophy, telangiectasia, striae, and purpura may occur if potent preparations are applied over a week to a few months. The more potent the corticosteroid preparation, the more rapid and severe the adverse effects will be, especially if it is applied to those areas (face and intertriginous and anogenital areas) where there is greater absorption. Less common side effects include acneiform lesions, hypertrichosis, hypopigmentation, and ocular hypertension from application around the eyes. The greater absorption that occurs with occlusive techniques increases the risk of local steroid side effects as well as hypothalamic-pituitary-adrenal (HPA) axis suppression. It should be assumed that all patients undergoing substantial occlusive therapy have temporary suppression of the HPA axis. If used injudiciously, even without occlusion, the most potent formulations may induce mild hypercortisolism, HPA axis suppression, or rarely Cushing's syndrome. Although the optimal frequency of corticosteroid application is unknown, there is probably no advantage to more than twice-daily usage. Repeated appli-

TABLE 15–2. POTENCY OF SELECTED TOPICAL CORTICOSTEROIDS

1 (most potent)	Betamethasone dipropionate ointment (optimized vehicle) (Diprolene)
	Clobetasole propionate ointment (Temovate)
2	Fluocinonide cream, ointment, gel (Lidex)*
	Halcinonide cream (Halog)
3	Betamethasone valerate ointment (Valisone)*
	Triamcinolone acetate cream (Aristocort-HP)*
4	Fluocinolone acetonide ointment (Synalar)*
	Hydrocortisone valerate ointment (Westcort)
5	Hydrocortisone butyrate cream (Locoid)
	Betamethasone dipropionate lotion (Diprosone)*
6	Desonide cream (Tridesilon)
	Fluocinolone acetonide solution (Synalar)*
7 (least potent)	Hydrocortisone (Hytone)*

Modified from Cornell RC, Stoughton RB: Correlation of the vasoconstriction assay and clinical activity in psoriasis. Arch Dermatol 121:63–67, 1985.

*Available as generic products. Studies to date have found that most generic topical corticosteroids are *not* biologically equivalent to the brand name products.

cation of a topical corticosteroid may result in a diminished effect (tachyphylaxis). It is therefore best to treat effectively for days to 2 weeks and then have steroid-free intervals of 4–7 days or more.

All forms of dermatitis are intensely pruritic, and scratching may exacerbate atopic dermatitis and lichen simplex chronicus. Therapy with topical corticosteroids has some antipruritic effects, but specific measures aimed at reducing pruritus are also worthwhile. **Topical antipruritics** work either through decreasing sensitivity of the cutaneous nerve endings (e.g., phenol) or through a counterirritant effect of substituting one sensation such as cooling for another, that is, itching (menthol). Dermatitic skin frequently will not tolerate application of such compounds owing to a concomitant stinging or burning sensation or to the greater chance of sensitization when a topical agent is applied to already inflamed skin. **Oral antihistamines** often alleviate pruritus, allay anxiety, and allow sleep, even when itching is not directly related to histamine effects. The several chemical classes of antihistamines show only minor variations in their properties, and a side effect such as somnolence, which might preclude their use in one situation, may be advantageous in another. To be used most effectively, antihistamines should be gradually increased until either clinical remission occurs or side effects become bothersome (or intolerable).

B. Specific Treatments

1. ATOPIC DERMATITIS

a. Preventive Measures. The environment should be kept at a constant temperature—comfortable, but not hot. Humidifiers will help alleviate skin dryness, especially during the winter; excess humidity should be avoided. Clothing worn next to the skin should be absorbent and nonirritating, laundered with bland soaps, and thoroughly rinsed. Overly frequent bathing, which promotes xerosis, must be eliminated. Emollients or medications should be applied immediately after bathing to "trap" water in the skin and enhance absorption. Frequent application of bland lubricants soothes and physically protects the skin and is the most important single measure in atopic dermatitis therapy.

b. Treatment of Active Dermatitis. Compresses with aluminum acetate (Burow's) solution should be placed on exudative areas for 20 minutes 4–6 times a day. Alternatively the patient should be placed in a tub 2 or 3 times a day, to which an antipruritic colloid such as oatmeal (Aveeno, 1 cup to ½ tub of tepid water), has been added. Twice-daily application of a potent corticosteroid preparation will quickly quell inflammation and pruritus. If maintenance therapy is needed, it is advisable to use the least potent preparation (e.g., 1% hydrocortisone) that is effective. Tar compounds (Estar gel, T/Gel) are useful as adjunctive therapy in patients with chronic dermatitis (see "Treatment of Psoriasis" below). They may be used alternately with corticosteroids or applied at the same time to the skin. Bath oil (Balnetar, 4 capfuls) is also helpful. Oral antihistamines should be used in an attempt to suppress pruritus. Hydroxyzine (Atarax, 10–25 mg po (q4h–q6h) is usually the best initial choice. A newer, less sedating antihistamine, terfenadine (Seldane 60 mg po bid), is an alternative when sedation is an intolerable side effect. Conversely, diphenhydramine (Benadryl, 25 mg po q4h–q6h) may be appropriate when some degree of sedation is desirable.

Acute flares of atopic dermatitis may be suppressed by a short course of prednisone (40–60 mg po daily, tapered over a 10–14-day period) or a single IM injection (e.g., triamcinolone acetonide [Kenalog] 40 mg). Long-term administration of systemic corticosteroids plays no part in treatment of atopic dermatitis. Photochemotherapy (psoralen-UVA [PUVA]) can induce remission in selected patients with recalcitrant chronic atopic dermatitis. Impetiginization should be managed with appropriate oral antibiotics. Treatment of *Staphylococcus aureus* infection (e.g., erythromycin, 250 mg po q6h) may be helpful in selected patients.

2. **LICHEN SIMPLEX CHRONICUS.** Potent topical corticosteroids, usually applied under airtight occlusive dressings, are extremely effective. Intralesional injection of corticosteroids (e.g., triamcinolone acetonide [Kenalog] 2.5–10.0 mg/mL) is often the therapy of choice. Intralesional therapy has the potential risks of long-term potent topical corticosteroid use. Antihistamines may occasionally be of value, especially when administered immediately before bedtime.

3. **CONTACT DERMATITIS**

   a. **Preventive Measures for Primary Irritant or Hand Dermatitis.** Exposure to household and work irritants such as soaps, detergents, solvents, bleaches, ammonia, and moist vegetables and fruits should be decreased. Without such avoidance, all other treatment is bound to be suboptimal. Patients need to receive frequent reinforcement in this rather tedious and difficult aspect of their care. Rings that occlude the underlying skin must be removed before any hand work is done. Waterless hand cleansers will remove stubborn soils and greases and are preferable to the use of other solvents. The skin should be lubricated frequently with a bland cream or lotion. If possible, heavy-duty vinyl or plastic gloves should be worn during work. Thin, white cotton liners may be worn underneath the gloves to absorb sweat. Some allergens (e.g., nickel) and high concentrations of irritants (e.g., 10% potassium hydroxide) may penetrate rubber-based gloves. Furthermore, patients may occasionally become allergic to the rubber in lined rubber gloves. There are various barrier protective creams designed for use against aqueous compounds (Kerodex no. 71, SBS-44, and West no. 311), solvents (Kerodex no. 51, SBS-46, and West no. 411), or dusts (West no. 211). Barrier creams applied before work and during work breaks are moderately effective.

   b. **Preventive Measures for Allergic Contact Dermatitis.** The patient should wash thoroughly as soon as possible after exposure to the allergen. Clothing or implements that may have become exposed should also be cleansed before being used again. Hyposensitization to allergic contact antigens such as poison ivy and oak (and others) is of negligible, if any, benefit.

c. **Treatment of Acute Dermatitis.** Topical compresses or tub baths, such as those described for atopic dermatitis, are helpful for exudative, vesicular, or bullous lesions. After vesiculation subsides, topical corticosteroids will generally suffice for mild to moderate inflammation. For more severe cases, early aggressive treatment with systemic corticosteroids is indicated; prednisone, 60 mg po daily, tapered over a 15–20-day course, should be used. Some improvement in the rash and discomfort is usually observed within 48 hours after therapy is initiated. If inadequate amounts of systemic steroids are given for too short a time, a rebound reaction with generalized exacerbation may occur. Acute reactions to a strong irritant should be treated with forceful and prolonged irrigation by water. Acid burns should not be rinsed with alkali, and vice versa; doing so causes an exothermic reaction and further tissue damage. Industrial toxicity texts should be consulted concerning specific therapy for offending chemicals. Oral antihistamines should be administered as needed.

d. **Treatment of Chronic Contact or Hand Dermatitis.** The affected area should be soaked for 5 minutes in water, and then a hydrophobic emollient (e.g., petrolatum) or a potent topical corticosteroid ointment should be immediately applied. Tar preparations may be useful. The affected area should be soaked in a solution of 2 capfuls of Balnetar or other tar compound in tepid water for 15 minutes and then rinsed; a topical steroid ointment should be applied immediately. Phototherapy is frequently helpful in chronic hand dermatitis.

4. **NUMMULAR DERMATITIS.** Nummular dermatitis is treated as outlined above. In addition, iodochlorhydroxyquin (Vioform), which has mild antibacterial and antifungal effects, may help, especially when used in combination with a tar and/or a corticosteroid preparation. As is true with any dermatitis, bacterial superinfection may occur and should be treated with appropriate topical and systemic antibiotics.

Cowan MA: Nummular eczema: A review, follow-up and analysis of 325 cases. Acta Derm Venerol 41:453–460, 1961.
Epstein E: Hand dermatitis: Practical management and current concepts. J Am Acad Dermatol 10:395–424, 1984.
Hanifin JM: Atopic dermatitis. J Am Acad Dermatol 6:1–13, 1982.
Jorizzo JL, Gatti S, Smith EB: Prurigo: A clinical review. J Am Acad Dermatol 4:723–728, 1981.
Tan PL, Barnett GL, Flowers FP, et al: Current topical corticosteroid preparations. J Am Acad Dermatol 14:79–93, 1986.

III. TREATMENT OF PSORIASIS

Psoriasis is a chronic, proliferative epidermal disease that affects 2–8 million people in the United States. Age of onset is most often in the 3rd decade, though psoriasis may appear at any time from infancy to old age. A family history is found in 30% of patients, and a polygenic mode of inheritance appears most likely. The pathogenesis of psoriasis remains unclear, despite the elucidation of numerous biochemical abnormalities affecting cyclic nucleotides, polyamines, and arachidonic acid metabolites, as well as immunologic, especially leukocyte, aberrations. The psoriatic lesion is an erythematous, sharply circumscribed plaque covered by loosely adherent, silvery (micaceous) scales. Any area of the body may be involved, but lesions tend to occur most often on the elbows, knees, scalp, genitalia, and intergluteal cleft. In most patients, the disease remains localized as discrete plaques, though generalized involvement may develop.

A. General Principles

1. **PHOTOTHERAPY.** This is the treatment of choice for most cases of moderate to severe psoriasis. It should be administered only by a qualified dermatologist. The ultraviolet (UV) spectrum is subdivided into three bands: UVC (200–290 nm), UVB (290–320 nm), and UVA (320–400 nm). UVC radiation has virtually no medical applications except as used in germicidal lamps. UVB radiation is responsible for most of the therapeutic effects of sunlight. Although exposure to sunlight is certainly less expensive and more pleasant than acquiring UV light in medical surroundings, inherent difficulties in its control and monitoring dictate that UVB phototherapy be administered via an artificial source in phototherapy booths. Numerous protocols involving repeated exposure to UVB light alone or with prior application of tar compounds (the Goeckerman regimen) have demonstrated effectiveness. The disadvantages of UVB phototherapy derive from the known deleterious effects of UV radiation on the skin. Long-term exposure has been clearly related to actinic keratoses, basal cell carcinoma, and squamous cell carcinoma and has been demonstrated to promote the epidermal and dermal changes popularly ascribed to "aging." Since UVB light is that portion of the solar spectrum that is most responsible for sunburning (erythemogenic), patients for whom phototherapy is being considered should be properly advised and periodically observed for atypical keratinocytic or melanocytic lesions. UVA light is most frequently administered in combination with a photoactive drug, psoralen, to reduce the increased epidermal turnover characteristic of psoriasis. Psoralen-UVA (PUVA) photochemotherapy, as well as more conventional UVB light treatment, has numerous cutaneous and even systemic immunologic effects. In photochemotherapy, the psoralen is administered orally 2 hours before exposure to UVA light, but patients remain photosensitive for up to 24 hours. Phototoxicity, both acute and cumulative, is an even greater concern for PUVA than for UVB therapy.

2. **TAR COMPOUNDS.** If phototherapy is one of the more recent advances in the treatment of psoriasis, tar compounds must be considered one of the oldest. The ability of coal tars to inhibit epidermal DNA synthesis might account for their effectiveness in treating psoriasis. Coal tars are carcinogenic for the skin of experimental animals and are photosensitizing. The risk of developing skin cancer from the therapeutic use of coal tars with or without phototherapy, however, appears to be low. Coal tars are available in a wide range of vehicles,

including creams, ointments, gels, shampoos, and bath preparations. Patient acceptance is often limited by their distinctive odor and propensity for staining.

B. **Specific Treatments.** Potent topical corticosteroids applied twice daily are very effective. Ointments are preferable, except for use on the scalp, where a gel or liquid vehicle is easier to use and more acceptable cosmetically. Overnight occlusion with plastic wrap, body suit, or shower cap may facilitate the initial response but should be discontinued once the lesions subside. Injection of corticosteroids (e.g., triamcinolone acetonide [Kenalog] 2.5–5.0 mg/mL) beneath individual plaques will cause involution within 7–10 days and is particularly helpful in patients with just a few lesions. Coal tar therapy may be used alone or in conjunction with topical corticosteroids. **Anthralin** (Drithocreme, Lasan), a synthetic derivative of a substance originally extracted from the *Andira araroba* tree of Brazil, reduces epidermal mitotic activity, perhaps through interference with mitochondrial DNA. Anthralin preparations may be irritating and will stain both skin and clothing. Initially, the lowest strength (0.1%) should be applied for 4–6 hours/day, and both the concentration of the anthralin and the duration for which it is applied should gradually be increased until a therapeutic effect is seen. Alternatively, the higher concentrations (0.5–1.0%) may be used for shorter periods (10 minutes–1 hour/day). **Salicylic acid** acts like a keratolytic and thus helps remove adherent scales from psoriatic lesions. This removal in turn promotes the penetration and efficacy of other modalities, including corticosteroids, tars, and phototherapy. Keralyt gel (6% salicylic acid, 60% propylene glycol, and 20% ethyl alcohol) is particularly useful when applied under occlusion to hydrated skin overnight.

Phototherapy is the treatment of choice for widespread or recalcitrant psoriasis. Antimetabolites (hydroxyurea, methotrexate) and immunomodulating drugs (cyclosporine) should be reserved for patients with serious disease unresponsive to other treatments in whom economic or social consequences justify the side effects. The same considerations apply to the use of etretinate (Tegison), a synthetic retinoid particularly useful in the most severe erythrodermic and pustular variants of psoriasis. All of these forms of therapy are generally administered by dermatologists familiar with their use.

Ashton RE, Andre P, Lowe NJ, et al: Anthralin: Historical and current perspectives. J Am Acad Dermatol 9:173–192, 1983.
Farber EM, Abel EA, Charuworn A: Recent advances in the treatment of psoriasis. J Am Acad Dermatol 8:311–321, 1983.
Rook AJ, Maibach HI: Psoriasis. Semin Dermatol 4:271–326, 1985.

IV. TREATMENT OF ACNE

The clinical spectrum of acne lesions ranges from mild and purely comedonal (whiteheads and blackheads) to more moderate inflammatory (papules and pustules) to severe cystic (cysts and nodules). Therapy for acne not only must be appropriate for the predominant clinical type and severity of disease but must also take into consideration any aggravating (e.g., androgen excess) or complicating (e.g., gram-negative folliculitis) factors. The diverse agents that have been successfully used for acne reflect its multifactorial nature.

A. **Mild Involvement (Few to Many Comedones, Few or No Inflammatory Lesions).** Tretinoin (Retin-A) is the most effective comedolytic agent. Its irritant effect sometimes limits its usefulness, though this can be minimized by proper application and a gradual increase in the potency of the formulation until the therapeutic effect is achieved. Therapy should be started with either the 0.01% gel or the 0.025% cream. If no improvement is seen after 12 weeks, a higher concentration (0.025% gel, 0.05% cream) is used. A small amount should be applied once daily to all affected areas, avoiding the periorbital and perioral areas. The skin should be thoroughly dry before application; if the patient has washed, at least 15 minutes should pass before tretinoin is administered. Some patients will sunburn more easily, and excessive sun exposure must be avoided when using this product.

Bacteriostatics are thought to improve acne by decreasing the formulation of harmful by-products as well as the actual number of *Propionibacterium acnes* bacteria. There are numerous gel-based benzoyl peroxide products (Desquam-X, Benzagel, and Persa-Gel). The lower concentration (2.5%) is usually better tolerated and is often as effective as the higher (5–10%) ones. Benzoyl peroxide washes are also useful adjuvants in any acne treatment regimen. These agents should be applied twice daily; if excessive erythema and dryness develop, the concentration and frequency of application should be decreased, or an alternative therapy should be adopted. Topical antibiotics are most effective for papular and pustular lesions. Clindamycin and erythromycin appear to be the most effective and easiest to use. All topical antibiotics are applied twice daily. Clindamycin phosphate (Cleocin T) is available in solution, lotion, or gel form. Erythromycin base is available as a solution (Staticin, A/T/S), pledgets (Erycette), gel (Emgel), or combined with benzoyl peroxide (Benzamycin). Combined tretinoin-benzoyl peroxide therapy is very effective for comedonal and papular acne. These agents must be applied at different times, not simultaneously, because mixing the highly unsaturated tretinoin with the reactive oxidant benzoyl peroxide inactivates both. The irritant response to this regimen limits its use.

B. **Moderate Involvement (Numerous Inflammatory Lesions or Cysts).** Topical therapy should be initiated, as suggested above. Oral antibiotics work through reduction of the normal cutaneous flora (particularly *P. acnes*) and direct anti-inflammatory effects. The results of antibiotic therapy cannot be adequately assessed for at least 6–8 weeks. If antibiotic is given for long periods, every attempt must be made to decrease to the lowest effective dose. Numerous oral antibiotics are useful; the choice of a particular drug is empiric and should take into consideration cost, convenience, and effect of previous treatments. **Tetracycline** (250 mg po qid) is usually the drug of choice. It is inexpensive and, except for GI irritation and candidal vaginitis, relatively free of side effects. Erythromycin (250 mg po qid) is usually the next drug of choice. Minocycline is quite effective, though its higher cost precludes use as a first-line therapy. Transient dizziness and nausea are usually avoidable if treatment is initiated with a dosage of 50 mg po bid, increasing to a maximum of 100 mg po bid, as needed. Ampicillin (250 mg po qid) is useful in certain patients, particularly pregnant women, in whom the use of tetracycline or minocycline must be avoided. An occasional complication of long-term broad-spectrum antibiotic therapy is gram-negative folliculitis. Patients will notice the sudden appearance of numerous pustules or inflammatory cysts infected with *Proteus, Pseudomonas,* or *Klebsiella* species. Any sudden change in clinical severity or morphology warrants Gram stain and bacterial culture.

C. **Severe Involvement Unresponsive to Other Therapy.** Estrogens (administered as anovulatory agents) may help young women with severe acne. Most or all of the estrogen effect is the result of inhibition of adrenal androgen production. Thus, combination oral contraceptives should contain a nonandrogenic progestin, such as ethynodiol diacetate (Demulen). Estrogen therapy is rarely indicated before age 16, after which time there will be no problem with growth retardation. **Prednisone** (5.0–7.5 mg po every evening) is helpful in female patients with severe acne unresponsive to conventional therapy who suffer from overproduction of androgens by the adrenal glands. **Spironolactone** (100–200 mg po daily), an aldosterone antagonist with antiandrogenic side effects, is an alternative for women with androgen excess who cannot use oral contraceptives or corticosteroids.

Patients with severe cystic acne unresponsive to high–dose antibiotic therapy should be considered for treatment with **isotretinoin** (Accutane), a drug that inhibits sebaceous gland function and alters the inflammatory response. Isotretinoin is administered on a basis of 0.5–1.0 mg/kg/day for 5 months. Aside from its known teratogenic effects, most of the other side effects of isotretinoin are transient and mild, including cheilitis, xerosis, alopecia, and hypertriglyceridemia. Although patients may experience a temporary flare in cystic lesions when therapy is initiated, this does not affect ultimate response. Asymptomatic vertebral hyperostoses are a recognized side effect of isotretinoin therapy that may not become apparent for 6–12 months after treatment. The therapy of choice for cystic lesions and acne abscesses is intralesional injection of small amounts of corticosteroid preparations (e.g., triamcinolone acetonide [Kenalog] 2.5 mg/mL). Most lesions will flatten and disappear within 48 hours after injection.

Dicken CH: Retinoids: A review. J Am Acad Dermatol 11:541–552, 1984.
Levine RM, Rasmussen JE: Intralesional corticosteroids in the treatment of nodulocystic acne. Arch Dermatol 119:480–481, 1983.
Melski JW, Arndt KA: Topical therapy for acne. N Engl J Med 302:503–506, 1980.
Stern RS, Pass TM, Komaroff AL: Topical versus systemic agent treatment for papulopustular acne. Arch Dermatol 120:1571–1578, 1984.

V. TREATMENT OF SKIN INFECTIONS

A. Superficial Fungal Infections

1. CANDIDIASIS. *Candida albicans* is a frequent cause of paronychial, intertriginous, oral, and vulvovaginal infections. Diagnosis can be easily confirmed by microscopic examination using potassium hydroxide or by culture. There are 4 classes of agents most commonly used

for topical treatment of candidal infections: haloprogin (Halotex); the synthetic imidazole compounds, miconazole (Monistat-Derm), clotrimazole (Lotrimin, Mycelex), ketoconazole (Nizoral), and econazole (Spectazole); ciclopirox olamine (Loprox); and the polyene antibiotic nystatin. The imidazoles are at least as effective as nystatin for treating cutaneous candidiasis and in cream form may be superior to nystatin in the treatment of candidal vulvovaginitis. Ciclopirox is probably as efficacious as the imidazoles. Creams may be used for most cutaneous and vulvovaginal infections, though patients with the latter might prefer vaginal suppositories. Oral candidiasis is best treated with oral clotrimazole troches or nystatin suspension. Paronychial and oral infections require more frequent applications, as often as 5 times a day, because the medication does not remain in contact with the skin or mucous membranes. Vulvovaginitis and other cutaneous candidal infections will respond to once- or twice-daily dosage, depending on the drug and dosage form.

Orally administered nystatin (500,000 U tid or qid) is useful when recurrent or resistant infections in the perianal, vulvar, or diaper areas are due to reinfection from gut organisms. Ketoconazole administered orally is effective for chronic mucocutaneous candidiasis, severe candidal nail infection, and recurrent vulvovaginitis but has no role in treating the more common forms of candidiasis. Candidal paronychia can be managed with amphotericin B lotion, alcoholic solutions of 1% gentian violet, or 2–4% thymol in absolute alcohol. Though esthetically unappealing, gentian violet solution is particularly useful in severe, recalcitrant oral infections. Predisposing factors, particularly excessive moisture and maceration, must be eliminated.

DeVillez RL, Lewis CW: Candidiasis seminar. Cutis 19:69–83, 1977.

2. **DERMATOPHYTE INFECTIONS.** The anatomic site, not the specific species of dermatophyte fungi, determines the appropriate treatment. Infections of the body and groin and superficial involvement of the beard area, palms, and soles can be managed by topical measures. Oral therapy is indicated when such measures fail, as well as when scalp and nails are affected. The synthetic imidazoles, haloprogin, tolnaftate, and the allylamine derivative Naftifine (Naftin) will clear most superficial dermatophyte infections within 1–4 weeks. Econazole, ketoconazole, and the newer imidazoles, sulconazole (Exelderm) and oxiconazole (Oxistat), are used once daily except for tinea pedis in which a twice-a-day dosage is more effective. The other antimycotics are applied twice a day. Therapy should be continued for 4 weeks to decrease the relapse rate. A keratolytic agent such as Keralyt gel (see "Treatment of Psoriasis" above) should be used for thick, hyperkeratotic involvement, as on the palms or soles. Open wet dressings (see "Treatment of Dermatitis" above) should be applied to acute vesicular lesions.

Griseofulvin is the drug of choice when systemic treatment of dermatophyte infections is warranted. Absorption is enhanced if an ultramicrosized form is taken with a fatty meal. The dose and duration of therapy depend on the area infected. Infections of nonhairy areas (e.g., tinea pedis, tinea corporis) respond to ultramicrosized griseo-fulvin, 500 mg po once daily, though tinea corporis may be expected to clear within 3–4 weeks, as opposed to the 3 months it may take for tinea pedis. Nail infections require 500–1500 mg daily of ultra-microsized griseofulvin for an even longer period (6–9 months for fingernails, 9–18 months for toenails). Scalp infection (tinea capitis) requires 6–8 weeks of ultramicrosized griseofulvin; approximately 5 mg/pound of body weight is the effective dose for children.

Ketoconazole is useful in treating chronic, recalcitrant, and gris-eofulvin-resistant dermatophytosis. The usual dosage is 200 mg taken daily in the morning. Although this dosage is usually well tolerated, hepatic injury, including fatal hepatic necrosis, as well as other possible adverse reactions, do occur; thus, treatment decisions must take into consideration the potential risks of this therapy.

Elewski BE, Hazen PG: The superficial mycoses and the dermatophytes. J Am Acad Dermatol 21:655–673, 1989.
Lambert DR, Siegle RJ, Camisa C: Griseofulvin and ketoconazole in the treatment of dermato-phyte infections. Int J Dermatol 28:300–304, 1989.
Lesher JL, Smith JG Jr: Antifungal agents in dermatology. J Am Acad Dermatol 17:383–394, 1987.

3. **TINEA VERSICOLOR.** This asymptomatic eruption is caused by the lipophilic yeastlike organism *Pityrosporum orbiculare,* the pathogenic form of the normal skin resident *Pityrosporum ovale.* A peculiar aspect of tinea versicolor is its propensity to cause either hypopig-mented or hyperpigmented lesions, which are highly confluent, round, finely scaled, thin plaques most often located on the upper torso. Most treatments will remove any evidence of active infection (i.e., scaling) within several days, while the pigmentary changes may take several months to resolve. In general, treatments should be used for 2 weeks, at which time a repeat application of a potassium hydroxide preparation will yield negative results if therapy has been successful. The synthetic imidazoles, ciclopirox, haloprogin, and tolnaftate, ap-plied once or twice a day, are all effective. Selenium sulfide suspension (Exsel, Selsun) is applied once daily to the affected areas, allowed to dry, and then washed off after 5 minutes. Zinc pyrithione–containing shampoos (Head & Shoulders, Zincon) are applied in a similar fashion. Tinver lotion (25% sodium hyposulfite, 1% salicylic acid, and 10% alcohol) is applied twice a day. Tretinoin (Retin-A) cream (0.05% bid; see "Treatment of Acne" above) not only will cure tinea versicolor but also will promote more rapid fading of hyperpigmented lesions. Ketoconazole (a single 400-mg dose) is effective both mycol-ogically (negative results on potassium hydroxide test) and clinically (prompt fading of the lesions). Griseofulvin is ineffective against tinea versicolor.

Savin RC: Systemic ketoconazole in tinea versicolor: A double-blind evaluation and 1-year follow-up. J Am Acad Dermatol 10:824–830, 1984.

B. Herpesvirus Infections

1. **HERPES SIMPLEX.** Cutaneous herpes simplex infections take two distinct forms: (1) the painful and disabling primary infection of previously uninfected individuals and (2) the common, bothersome

recurrent form, colloquially known as cold sores or fever blisters. Herpes simplex infections may be particularly severe and widespread in patients with certain skin disorders (e.g., atopic dermatitis) or immunodeficiencies. Infection by herpes simplex or varicella-zoster virus can be readily confirmed by cytologic examination of a scraping obtained from the base of a vesicular lesion and by culture. A Tzanck preparation will reveal characteristic multinucleated giant keratinocytes.

Acyclovir (Zovirax), a purine nucleoside analogue, has revolutionized the treatment of herpes simplex infections. Its safety and specificity depend on two factors: (1) a viral enzyme, thymidine kinase, is necessary for conversion of the drug to its active form and (2) once activated, acyclovir inhibits a virus-specific DNA polymerase required for viral replication. Treatment promptly aborts new lesion formation, reduces viral titers, promotes healing, and ameliorates pain. IV acyclovir (5 mg/kg q8h) also prevents reactivation of herpes simplex in seropositive, immunocompromised patients undergoing chemotherapy or transplantation. Oral acyclovir (200 mg 5 times daily for 5 days) promotes resolution of primary herpes simplex infections, if begun within 3 days of onset. Although treatment of the primary episode will not per se affect the frequency or severity of future recurrences, if acyclovir is given continuously (200 mg po tid) to patients with frequent recurrences (more than 6 per year), it will significantly reduce or even prevent outbreaks. Topical acyclovir (5% ointment applied q3h) has a modest effect on primary genital herpes simplex infections, if begun within 72 hours of onset. Clinical studies have failed to show any benefit from its use in nongenital or recurrent episodes. Aside from transient renal dysfunction when IV acyclovir is administered too rapidly, acyclovir appears remarkably free of side effects. The greatest concern is that its overuse will promote the emergence of resistant viral strains. Thymidine kinase–deficient mutants have been recognized but seem to be less pathogenic to humans. Open wet compresses (10 minutes tid or qid) or sitz baths are indicated for acute vesicular outbreaks. Mouthwashes (benzalkonium chloride [Zephiran] 1:1000 or tetracycline suspension 250 mg/60 ml of water) are cleansing and soothing in primary herpetic gingivostomatitis. Topical antibacterials (see "Impetigo" below) should be applied to cutaneous herpes infections to prevent bacterial superinfection. Herpes simplex infection is one of the few instances in which use of topical anesthetics is effective and justifiable. Dyclonine hydrochloride (Dyclone), elixir of diphenhydramine hydrochloride (Benadryl elixir), or viscous lidocaine (Xylocaine) may be used for oral lesions, and benzocaine aerosol (Americaine) or pramoxine hydrochloride (Tronothane) ointment may be used for the anogenital area. They can be applied as frequently as necessary.

2. **VARICELLA.** Most patients with varicella require only symptomatic therapy. A drying antipruritic lotion (calamine alone or with 0.25% menthol and/or 1% phenol) should be applied. Phenol should not be used in pregnant women. Administration of oral antihistamines may decrease pruritus (see "Treatment of Dermatitis" above). Oral acy-

clovir (10–20 mg/kg/day in a qid divided dose for 5–7 days) reduces the duration and severity of varicella in otherwise healthy children. It does not, however, affect the rate of complications (e.g., secondary bacterial infection, pneumonitis, meningoencephalitis). Immunocompetent adults with uncomplicated varicella are treated with acyclovir 1000 mg po 4 times/day for 5–10 days. Results are best if therapy is started within the first 24 hours of development of vesicles. Severe varicella, especially in the immunocompromised patient, is best treated with IV acyclovir, as is disseminated herpes zoster. High-risk susceptible patients (e.g., those with lymphoma or leukemia or immunodeficiency; the newborn child of a mother with varicella) under 15 years of age who have had close exposure to varicella or zoster should be passively immunized with varicella zoster immunoglobulin (VZIG). This immunization will moderate or even abort clinical infection if administered within 72 hours of exposure but is of no value in established infections.

3. **HERPES ZOSTER.** The more general measures described for herpes simplex and varicella are also applicable to herpes zoster. IV acyclovir (500 mg/m^2 q8h for 7 days) alleviates the discomfort and shortens the course of localized zoster. IV acyclovir can also prevent or abort dissemination in the immunocompromised patient. Herpes zoster in an immunocompetent patient responds to oral acyclovir (800 mg po 5 times/day for 7–10 days) if therapy is initiated within 48 hours of onset. Acyclovir not only shortens the duration of herpes zoster and reduces the acute pain but also it may decrease the risk of subsequent postherpetic neuralgia.

Balfour HH Jr, Kelly JM, Suarez CS, et al: Acyclovir treatment of varicella in otherwise healthy children. J Pediatr 116:633–639, 1990.
Feder HM: Treatment of adult chicken pox with oral acyclovir. Arch Intern Med 150:2061–2065, 1990.
McKendrick MW, McGill JI, White JE, et al: Oral acyclovir in acute herpes zoster. Br Med J 293:1529–1532, 1986.
Wheeler CE Jr: Antiviral drugs and vaccines for herpes simplex and herpes zoster. J Am Acad Dermatol 18:161–238, 1988.

C. Impetigo. Nonbullous streptococcal impetigo occurs most often on the face or other exposed areas. It is highly contagious among infants and children but less so in older persons. Untreated streptococcal impetigo usually resolves in about 10 days. The overall incidence of postpyodermal acute glomerulonephritis is 2% or less. Bullous staphylococcal impetigo is also seen primarily in children and is caused by group II type 71 staphylococci. These organisms produce a toxin that induces a superficial intraepidermal blister. Staphylococci may also colonize primary streptococcal impetigo. The streptococcal impetigo lesion begins as a small erythematous macule that rapidly develops into a fragile vesicle. The vesicle then breaks, leaving a red, oozing erosion surmounted by a "stuck-on," thick golden crust. Staphylococcal impetigo lesions appear as flaccid blisters, initially clear and then cloudy, that have a thin varnish-like crust when they rupture.

Mupirocin (Bactroban, applied tid) is the first topical antibiotic as effective as oral medication in the treatment of impetigo due to either

Staphylococcus or *Streptococcus*. Widespread involvement warrants systemic therapy.

Bullous staphylococcal impetigo should be treated with a semisynthetic penicillin (e.g., dicloxacillin, 250 mg po qid) or erythromycin if the organisms are sensitive to this drug. Streptococcal impetigo should be treated with one intramuscular injection of benzathine penicillin (1.2 million U). An alternative therapy is 10 days of erythromycin (250 mg po qid) or phenoxymethyl penicillin (250 mg po qid).

Lesions should be soaked 3 or 4 times a day in warm tap water, saline, or a soap solution to remove the crusts. In addition, it is advisable to have both the patient and the family bathe once or twice daily with a bactericidal (e.g., povidone-iodine [Betadine]) or bacteriostatic solution (e.g., phisoDerm, chlorhexidine gluconate [Hibiclens]). A topical antibiotic ointment (e.g., povidone-iodine [Betadine], polymyxin B–bacitracin [Polysporin]) should be applied to the base of lesions after the crust has been removed.

Dillon HC: Topical and systemic therapy for pyodermas. Int J Dermatol 19:443–451, 1980.

Mertz PM, Marshall DA, Eaglstein WH, et al: Topical mupirocin treatment of impetigo is equal to oral erythromycin therapy. Arch Dermatol 125:1069–1073, 1989.

D. Scabies is caused by infestation with the mite *Sarcoptes scabiei*. Principally acquired through close personal contact, it may be transmitted by clothing, linens, or towels. The widespread, intensely pruritic eruption of scabies represents the host's immune response to the parasite. The mite itself can be found in inconspicuous linear papules (burrows) most often located on the interdigital spaces, wrists, elbows, nipples, umbilicus, lower abdomen, genitalia, and intergluteal cleft. Microscopic examination of a thin epidermal-shave biopsy specimen of such a lesion will demonstrate the mite, its eggs, and/or mite feces (scybala). Permethrin 5% cream (Elimite) is the treatment of choice for scabies. It is applied at bedtime to the entire body from the neck down. Medication should be left on for 8–12 hours before being washed off. At that time, clothing, towels, and linens should be laundered. A second application of permethrin 1 week later is necessary only if there is evidence of residual active mites. Lindane (Kwell, Gamene) when used in the same manner as permethrin is also effective. Crotamiton (Eurax) cream, applied twice and left on during a 48-hour period, is an alternative that is more antipruritic but less scabicidal than lindane.

Persistent itching in treated patients may be due to continued infestation, residual hypersensitivity reaction to the mite, or irritation from overzealous use of lindane. If hypersensitivity is the reason, treatment with topical corticosteroids or a short, tapering course of oral corticosteroids will bring relief. Occasionally, persistent, intensely pruritic nodules remain after successful scabietic therapy. These nodules respond to intralesional corticosteroids.

Felman YM, Nikitas JA: Scabies. Cutis 33:266–284, 1984.

Haustein U-F, Hlawa B: Treatment of scabies with permethrin versus lindane and benzoyl benzoate. Acta Dermvenerol 69:348–351, 1989.

E. Warts are intraepidermal tumors of the skin caused by infection with the human papillomavirus (HPV). Numerous types of HPV have been defined. In general, there is no absolute correlation between infection by a given HPV type and any particular lesional morphology, although certain HPV types characteristically affect special target areas. Warts may be found in persons of any age but are most common in those between the ages of 12 and 16. They may spread by contact or autoinoculation; anogenital warts (condylomata acuminata) are particularly contagious. HPV types 16 and 18 in condylomata acuminata likely increase the risk of cervical and anorectal carcinoma. Electrodesiccation, curettage, cryosurgery, and laser surgery are effective treatments that require additional training and equipment.

Keratolytics, such as 5–20% salicylic acid and 5–20% lactic acid in flexible collodion (Duofilm, Occlusal), may produce good results for most types of warts except the mosaic plantar variety. Keratolytic agents act by mechanically removing infected cells and by provoking an inflammatory reaction that elicits a virus-specific immune response. Keratolytic agents are used as follows:

1. The area should be washed thoroughly with soap and water;
2. The surface of the wart should be rubbed gently with a mild abrasive such as an emery board, pumice stone, or callous file;
3. The keratolytic should be applied to the wart with a toothpick or orangewood stick;
4. The keratolytic should be allowed to dry.

This regimen is repeated nightly until a response is seen, undue irritation develops, or it is obvious that the warts are resistant. (This may take as long as 12 weeks to ascertain.)

Cantharidin (Cantharone) is a mitochondrial poison that results in an intraepidermal blister. The lesion is painted with the solution, allowed to dry, and then covered with a nonporous occlusive tape (e.g., Blenderm). The tape is removed in 24 hours, following which a blister, often hemorrhagic, develops. Any residual wart evident at a 1–2-week follow-up can be re-treated. **Podophyllum** resin (podophyllin), a cytotoxic agent that arrests mitosis in metaphase, is used primarily for treatment of condylomata acuminata. Care must be taken to avoid applying the medication to normal skin. When therapy is initiated, the podophyllin is washed off 1–4 hours after application to avoid undue inflammation and discomfort. If no response is seen at 1-week follow-up, the length of time the medication is left on is progressively increased, up to 24 hours. Podophyllin may cause systemic neurotoxic effects if absorbed. It is therefore inadvisable to apply it in large amounts on mucous membranes or to use it during pregnancy, because of its possible cytotoxic effect on the fetus.

Intralesional injection of interferon-α (Intron-A) may be considered for patients with recalcitrant condylomata acuminata, but the discomfort, side effects, and cost of this therapy severely limit its utility.

Androphy EJ: Human papillomavirus. Arch Dermatol 125:683–685, 1989.
Boot JM, Blog FB, Stolz E: Intralesional interferon alpha-2b treatment of condylomata acuminata previously resistant to podophyllin resin application. Genitourin Med 65:50–53, 1989.
Silva PD, Micha JP, Silva DG: Management of condyloma acuminata. J Am Acad Dermatol 13:457–463, 1985.

VI. TREATMENT OF PRURITUS

Itching is the cardinal symptom of most dermatologic diseases. It may be localized or generalized, paroxysmal or unremitting. Itching and pain are transmitted along similar, if not identical, peripheral neural pathways, and itching does not occur in an area insensitive to pain. Histamine is the classic but not the only mediator of pruritus, since most itchy conditions are not accompanied by other signs of histamine release (i.e., wheal and flare), nor are antihistamines always effective in reducing itch. Various proteases, peptides, and prostaglandins potentiate histamine's effect without being directly pruritogenic. Kallikrein, substance P, and serotonin may also be primary mediators. The patient with itching and no rash poses a particularly challenging diagnostic and therapeutic dilemma. Excessively dry skin (asteatosis, xerosis) can be quite pruritic. Pruritus accompanied by no skin changes other than those produced by scratching itself may also be secondary to numerous systemic diseases (Table 15–3). Especially when no definitive cure of the underlying illness may be offered, specific therapy aimed at reducing such pruritus is most welcome.

A. Xerosis. Dry skin is a common condition, especially among the elderly. When severe enough to provoke inflammation, it is also known as asteatotic eczema. Environmental factors are important: repeated exposure to solvents, soaps, and disinfectants will remove lipid from the skin, increasing transepidermal water loss up to 75 times the normal amount. Decreased relative humidity and cold, dry winds will literally pull water from the skin. Factors that decrease the relative humidity include increased ambient temperature and ventilating with cold, dry air.

1. **PREVENTIVE MEASURES.** Room temperatures must be kept as low as comfortable. Use of humidifiers (built-in or portable) should be encouraged. Bathing should be restricted to once every 1–2 days, and warm, not hot, bath water should be used. Bath oils may be used, but these can make the tub dangerously slick and are of limited therapeutic benefit. Excessive exposure to soaps, solvents, or other drying agents must be avoided. A mild soap, such as Dove, should be used. Finally, emollients should be applied frequently. These agents are most effectively applied when the skin is already moist (i.e., immediately after bathing). When choosing an emollient, one

TABLE 15–3. SYSTEMIC DISEASES ASSOCIATED WITH PRURITUS

Uremia
Obstructive biliary disease (e.g., primary biliary cirrhosis)
Myeloproliferative disorders (e.g., polycythemia vera, Hodgkin's disease)
Iron deficiency
Endocrine disorders (e.g., thyrotoxicosis)
Visceral malignancies
Neurologic disorders (e.g., brain abscess)

Modified from Denman ST: A review of pruritus. J Am Acad Dermatol 14:375–392, 1986.

should sacrifice esthetics for efficacy, because thicker, less appealing preparations (e.g., Eucerin, petrolatum) are more effective than lighter lotions (e.g., Alpha-Keri, Lubriderm).

2. **TREATMENT OF EXISTING DRYNESS.** The primary means of correcting dryness is to add water to the skin first and then apply a hydrophobic substance to keep it there. Emollients are only moderately effective at actually "moisturizing" the skin, despite advertising claims to the contrary. When used alone, hydrophobic emollients hydrate the skin simply by preventing the normal transepidermal water loss. Maximal hydration is achieved by the use of 40–60% propylene glycol in water applied under plastic occlusion overnight. Keralyt gel is a salicylic acid and propylene glycol formulation that is extremely effective at hydrating and simultaneously removing scaling. Creams containing urea and/or lactic acid (e.g., Carmol, Lac-Hydrin, and U-Lactin) are particularly helpful. Topical corticosteroid ointments used with occlusive dressings are the most effective and rapid therapy for symptomatic xerosis and associated eczematous changes.

B. **Uremic Pruritus.** Renal failure is the most prevalent of all systemic diseases associated with pruritus. Pruritus has become a much more common problem for uremic patients, though it remains unclear whether this is due to dialysis itself or is simply a product of patients' greater longevity. 80–90% of patients on hemodialysis at some time experience significant pruritus; 42% find that their itching is most severe during or immediately after dialysis treatments. The cause is unknown. Efforts aimed at correcting calcium and phosphorus abnormalities common in chronic renal failure will often, although not invariably, alleviate pruritus. Increased levels of magnesium and vitamin A within the skin have also been postulated to contribute to itching. The dry skin to which uremic patients are prone may further aggravate their itching.

SPECIFIC TREATMENTS. UVB phototherapy is almost always effective, with a decrease in itching usually seen after 8 suberythemogenic daily doses. Parathyroidectomy may result in dramatic relief of itching within 24–48 hours in patients with secondary hyperparathyroidism. The response is not invariable, and if patients become hypercalcemic postoperatively, the pruritus can recur. Activated charcoal (6 gm/day po for 8 weeks) may be effective; it will nonspecifically bind other orally administered drugs. Finally, cholestyramine (5 gm po bid) may alleviate not only hepatic but also uremic pruritus (see below).

C. **Cholestatic Pruritus.** Pruritus occurs in 25% of patients with cholestatic liver disease but is rarely seen in hepatitis without biliary obstruction. Although purified bile salts applied to the skin are pruritogenic, and lowering the serum bile concentration usually ameliorates cholestatic pruritus, no convincing evidence has been found that total or individual levels of bile salts, either circulating or within the skin, correlate with the presence or absence of itching.

SPECIFIC TREATMENTS. Cholestyramine (Questran 4 gm po 1–3 times daily), an ion exchange resin, is frequently effective, though its antipruritic effect seems separate from its ability to normalize bile salt levels. Cholestyramine is a powder that is mixed with water or another fluid before ingesting. Colestipol (Colestid) is another ion-exchange resin that may be substituted in patients who find choles-tyramine too constipating. Like charcoal, ion-exchange resins may bind other orally administered drugs. Oral vitamin K supplements (10 mg a week) should be given concurrently. Phenobarbital (3 to 4 mg per kilogram per day po) can reduce cholestatic pruritus, though the mechanism by which it does so remains unknown. Phenobarbital is sedating and may interfere with the metabolism of many drugs. UVB phototherapy is often helpful in treating cholestatic pruritus. Rifampin (150 mg po bid–tid) is also effective in some patients with cholestatic pruritus. The presumed mode of action is rifampin's inhibition of intrahepatic bile acid uptake or stimulation of microso-mal enzymes that detoxify nonbile salt pruritogens or both.

D. **Hematologic Pruritus.** Fourteen to 52% of patients with polycythemia vera have pruritus. Though elevated plasma and urine histamine levels, correlating with an increased number of basophils, have been found in $\frac{2}{3}$ of patients with polycythemia vera, antihistamines are usually inef-fective at controlling their pruritus. Iron deficiency, with or without anemia, may also be associated with pruritus. Pruritus is frequently seen in Hodgkin's disease, often before the correct diagnosis is evident; severe, generalized pruritus may indicate a more serious prognosis.

SPECIFIC TREATMENTS. Cimetidine, a histamine$_2$ (H$_2$) blocker (300 mg po qid), or cyproheptadine, an antihistamine and antiserotonin agent (4 mg po every four hours), may reduce the pruritus of polycythemia vera, though double-blind studies have not confirmed their effectiveness. Aspirin (500 mg po tid) may also reduce itching, but its use in these patients carries an unacceptably high risk of severe gastrointestinal bleeding and, therefore, cannot be recommended. Iron replacement will abolish pruritus due to iron deficiency, often before any measurable change in the hematologic status.

General Treatment Measures. Antihistamines are usually ineffective for pruritus due to systemic illness. Coexisting conditions that may aggravate the pruritus—particularly xerosis, as is frequently observed in chronic renal failure—should be appropriately managed. Dietary manip-ulation may occasionally be helpful; low-protein diets have been suc-cessful for uremic pruritus, whereas diets rich in polyunsaturated fatty acids may help cholestatic pruritus.

Denman ST: A review of pruritus. J Am Acad Dermatol 14:375–392, 1986.
Ghent CN, Carruthers SG: Treatment of pruritus in primary biliary cirrhosis with rifampin. Gastroenterology 94:488–493, 1988.
Martin J: Pruritus. Int J Dermatol 24:634–639, 1985.

16 16 16 16 16 16 16 16 16 16

NEUROLOGIC DISEASES

PHILLIP D. SWANSON

16 16 16 16 16 16 16 16 16 16 16

The number of neurologic conditions managed with medical therapy may surprise those who view diseases of the nervous system as poorly amenable to treatment. Although many therapeutic measures are not curative, a rather extensive therapeutic armamentarium is available to manage neurologic disorders.

I. SEIZURE DISORDERS

Epileptic seizures are commonly encountered in medical practice. The physician must be able to treat seizures immediately and manage patients on a long-term basis. Seizure management requires understanding of both seizure classification and anticonvulsant drugs.

A. Seizure Classification. Seizures are grouped into two principal categories: (1) primary generalized and (2) partial (Table 16–1). Three problems may lead to confusion with this classification. First, the category of primary generalized seizures includes both absences (petit mal seizures) and grand mal or other seizures associated with convulsive movements. Second, partial seizures may become secondarily generalized. Third, absence seizures and complex partial (psychomotor, temporal lobe) seizures may not be readily distinguishable on descriptive clinical grounds, in which case an incorrect anticonvulsant choice is likely to be made.

B. Seizure Treatment

1. **When to Treat a Seizure.** Certain clinical situations associated with seizures can be managed **without** anticonvulsant drugs, including uncomplicated febrile seizures and seizures due to withdrawal from alcohol or sedative/hypnotic drugs. Even in children with multiple febrile seizures, or febrile seizures that are prolonged or are partial at the onset, prophylactic medication (usually phenobarbital) is no longer recommended. Drug and alcohol withdrawal seizures are not treated prophylactically because of difficulties in following these patients and because seizures should not recur if substance abuse is terminated. A common management problem is whether to treat a person who has had a single seizure of unknown cause. Estimated risk of recurrence is 31–71% within the first 3 years. Some physicians may prefer to wait until a second seizure occurs before instituting long-term anticonvulsant therapy. Prophylactic therapy (usually with phenytoin) has been used for patients with open head injuries or documented contusions. A recent randomized study showed that phenytoin reduced seizure frequency only during the first week after a severe head injury. Thus the drug may be safely discontinued after the first week if no seizures have occurred. If a seizure has taken place, medication is continued for 6 months to a year. For concussion without evidence of contusion, anticonvulsants are not recommended.

TABLE 16–1. INTERNATIONAL CLASSIFICATION OF EPILEPTIC SEIZURES

I. Partial Seizures (seizures beginning locally)
  A. Simple partial seizures (consciousness not impaired)
    1. With motor symptoms
    2. With somatosensory or special sensory symptoms
    3. With autonomic symptoms
    4. With psychic symptoms
  B. Complex partial seizures (with impairment of consciousness)
    1. Beginning as simple partial seizures and progressing to impairment of consciousness
      a. With no other features
      b. With features as in A.1–4
      c. With automatisms
    2. With impairment of consciousness at onset
      a. With no other features
      b. With features as in A.1–4
      c. With automatisms
  C. Partial seizures secondarily generalized
II. Generalized Seizures (bilaterally symmetric and without local onset)
  A. 1. Absence seizures
     2. Atypical absence seizures
  B. Myoclonic seizures
  C. Clonic seizures
  D. Tonic seizures
  E. Tonic-clonic seizures
  F. Atonic seizures
III. Unclassified Epileptic Seizures (inadequate or incomplete data)

Abstracted from Commission on Classification and Terminology of the International League Against Epilepsy: Proposal for revised clinical and electroencephalographic classification of epileptic seizures. Epilepsia 22:489–501, 1981. This classification was approved by the International League Against Epilepsy in September 1981.

2. **Initial Anticonvulsant.** The guiding principle is to select the least toxic agent most likely to control the type of seizure being treated. To minimize toxicity, many agents are started at a dose lower than the expected final one. In general, at a fixed dose, 5 drug half-lives are needed to achieve a steady state. In the pediatric age group, the dosage is based on the patient's weight. Tables 16–2 and 16–3 list characteristics of many of the available anticonvulsant drugs.

  a. **Absence Attacks.** Ethosuximide (Zarontin) is the first drug used. Valproic acid (Depakote or Depakene) is also effective in this type of seizure. With the latter drug, hepatic function should be assessed periodically. Hepatotoxicity has almost always occurred within 6 months of beginning of therapy.

  b. **Primary Generalized Convulsions.** Phenytoin (Dilantin), valproic acid, phenobarbital, or carbamazepine (Tegretol) may be selected. Potential side effects must be considered when choosing a drug, especially in women of childbearing age. Although anticonvulsant effects on the fetus remain controversial, certain results must be

TABLE 16–2. COMPARISON OF SELECTED ANTICONVULSANTS COMMONLY USED FOR INITIAL TREATMENT OF SEIZURES

DRUG	USUAL TOTAL DAILY DOSE FOR ADULTS (mg)	TARGET PLASMA LEVEL (μg/ml)	PLASMA HALF-LIFE IN ADULTS (hr)	COMMON SIDE EFFECTS	APPROX $ COST OF 100 TABLETS OR CAPSULES	COMMENTS
Phenytoin (Dilantin)	300–400	10–20	24–72	Gingival hyperplasia, ataxia, fetal malformations	7–10 (100 mg)	
Phenobarbital (Luminal)	90–300	10–40	90–120	Drowsiness	4 (30 mg)	
Carbamazepine (Tegretol)	600–1200	6–12	10–20	Dizziness, leukopenia	20–30 (250 mg)	Blood counts necessary
Ethosuximide (Zarontin)	750–2000	40–100	30–50	Nausea	25–35 (250 mg)	Agent of choice for absence (petit mal) seizures
Primidone (Mysoline)	500–1500	5–15 (phenobarbital, major metabolite)	7–14	Sedation	8–25 (250 mg)	Do not use with phenobarbital
Valproic acid (Depakote)	1000–3000	50–100	10–12	GI disturbances, sedation	25–50 (250 mg)	Can raise serum level of phenobarbital

Data from Swanson PD: Anticonvulsant therapy. Postgrad Med 65:147–154, 1979; and Bleck TP: Convulsive disorders: The use of anticonvulsant drugs. Clin Neurophysiol 13:198–209, 1990.

TABLE 16–3. SELECTED ANTICONVULSANTS WITH LIMITED APPLICATION

DRUG	COMMENTS
Mephenytoin (Mesantoin)	Useful for generalized and partial seizures; bone marrow suppression possible
Mephobarbital (Mebaral)	No advantage over phenobarbital
Methsuximide (Celontin)	Ancillary drug for generalized or partial seizures
Clonazepam (Clonopin)	Used for myoclonic seizures; high incidence of drowsiness and ataxia
Phenacemide (Phenurone)	Uncommonly used because of side effects of aplastic anemia, liver damage, and psychiatric disturbances
Clorazepate (Tranxene)	Longer acting than diazepam
ACTH	Used for infantile spasms
Lorazepam (Ativan)	Because of short half-life, usefulness limited to status epilepticus
Diazepam (Valium)	
Paraldehyde	Used IV or rectally for status epilepticus

Adapted from Swanson PD: Anticonvulsant therapy. Postgrad Med 65:147–154, 1979.

discussed with the patient: (1) severe midline defects such as meningomyelocele have been reported in children born of mothers taking valproic acid; (2) phenytoin and other agents such as phenobarbital may produce a syndrome called the fetal hydantoin syndrome; and (3) probably any anticonvulsant increases the risk for birth defects severalfold. Phenytoin also is known to produce gingival hyperplasia, hirsutism, and probably some coarsening of the skin, side effects that are of particular concern for women and children. Thus, in a young woman, carbamazepine might be chosen as a first drug, even though it is more expensive than phenytoin and may be no more effective for seizure control. Pregnant patients taking valproic acid should have amniotic alpha-fetoprotein levels measured and ultrasonic monitoring at about 16 weeks' gestation.

  c. **Partial Seizures.** Carbamazepine is becoming the first-line drug. The danger of serious hematologic abnormalities is low. The total white blood cell count may drop to around 4000/cu mm in patients on long-term carbamazepine. Blood counts should be done at intervals, at first monthly, then less frequently. Carbamazepine should be started at a low dosage. For an adult, an appropriate beginning dose is ½ tablet (100 mg) bid. After a week the dosage is increased by ½ tablet, and increases continue every 3 or 4 days as tolerated, until a dose of 1 tablet (200 mg) tid is reached. At this time, the blood level of the drug should be determined. If the level is in the range of 6 μg/mL, the dosage is maintained at 3/day. If it is significantly below this range, the daily maintenance dose is increased to 4 tablets. Phenytoin is often the first drug used for **generalized tonic–clonic convulsions** or **partial seizures.**

It is relatively inexpensive. The total daily dose can be given once a day because of a long half-life. At higher doses the plasma levels of phenytoin rise more rapidly (saturation kinetics), and smaller increments and longer intervals should be used for increases. Other drugs such as phenobarbital and primidone (Mysoline) are used less frequently because of sedative side effects. Phenobarbital is one of the major metabolites of primidone; the two drugs should not be used together.

3. **WHEN SHOULD A SECOND DRUG BE USED?** Usually, a second drug should be considered when the patient has had another seizure in spite of treatment that has produced therapeutic levels. The serum level of the first drug should be measured, and if it is below the accepted therapeutic range or if the patient has no signs of toxicity, one should first increase the dosage of the initial drug. If seizures continue, a second drug is then added. In contrast to past practice, it now is recommended that the first drug be tapered if addition of the second drug achieves seizure control. However, many patients prefer to continue with 2 drugs if they are seizure free, because of concern that stopping the first drug will increase the chances of another seizure.

4. **HOW LONG SHOULD AN ANTICONVULSANT BE CONTINUED?** Duration of treatment with anticonvulsants has not been established. In approximately 40% of patients who have been seizure free for 2 or more years, seizures recur within 1½ years of discontinuing medication, a risk that should be explained to a patient before discontinuance. Discontinuation should be gradual over a few weeks to minimize the likelihood of withdrawal seizures. **If epileptiform discharges are present on an EEG, stopping the drug is risky.**

C. **Status Epilepticus.** A state of repetitive focal or generalized seizures with incomplete neurologic recovery between seizures is called status epilepticus. Rarely the only manifestation is altered consciousness (absence or complex partial status). Possible causes include meningitis; cessation of anticonvulsant therapy; withdrawal from ethanol or sedative drugs; electrolyte disturbances; hypoglycemia; subarachnoid hemorrhage; uremia; toxicity from drugs such as high-dose penicillin, meperidine, or theophylline; and recreational drug (cocaine) ingestion. Aggressive anticonvulsant therapy is indicated; there is no single accepted regimen.

Initial management consists of establishing an airway; positioning the patient to avoid aspiration of stomach contents; inserting an IV line; obtaining blood for estimation of glucose, electrolyte, and creatinine levels; and administering 50 mL of 50% glucose. Rapidly acting anticonvulsants are given IV. Commonly, a rapidly acting benzodiazepine (diazepam or lorazepam) is used, followed by a loading dose of a longer-acting agent such as phenytoin. IV diazepam, in 2-mg increments to a total dose of 10 mg, is often used. Lorazepam, which may have a longer anticonvulsant effect and be less likely to produce respiratory depression, is given in 1- to 4-mg increments, to a total dosage of 9 mg. With either drug, injections are spaced 5 minutes apart.

The most popular long-acting anticonvulsant is **phenytoin,** which can be administered IV in a slow push at a rate **no greater than 50 mg/ minute.** Up to 1 gm may be administered over an hour to a patient who has not already been taking this agent. The IV line should contain **normal saline only.** Phenytoin must never be administered intramuscularly, because it will precipitate in the muscle and not be reliably absorbed. IV phenytoin can produce cardiac arrhythmias, conduction defects, and hypotension. Blood pressure and pulse are checked frequently and ECG monitoring is continuous. An alternative long-acting drug, phenobarbital, can also be administered IV in 250-mg doses. Two doses are usually well tolerated. However, respiratory arrest may occur more frequently when phenobarbital is given with a benzodiazepine than when phenobarbital is given alone. Other agents that can be used when seizures continue include paraldehyde (IV, by nasogastric tube, or rectally), lidocaine, and general anesthetics. IV paraldehyde is rarely necessary. 50 mL is diluted with 250 mL of saline solution and given IV using inert tubing. If given by nasogastric tube or rectally, 5- to 10-mL boluses can be used. Intravenous pentobarbital has been successfully used to stop refractory status epilepticus. The drug is given initially as a bolus of 5 mg/kg. This is followed by 25- to 50-mg boluses every 2–5 minutes until a burst-suppression pattern is seen on EEG. An IV infusion is continued at a rate of 5 mg/kg/h, with gradual decreases after 12–24 hours.

Brown TR, Mikati M: Status epilepticus. *In* Ropper AH, Kennedy SF: Neurological and Neurosurgical Intensive Care. 2nd ed. Rockville Md, Aspen Publishers, 1988, pp 269–288.

Delgado-Escueta AV, Wasterlain CG, Treiman JDM, et al (eds): Status Epilepticus. Adv Neurol, vol 34, 1983.

Farwell JR, Lee YJ, Hirtz DG, et al: Phenobarbital for febrile seizures—effects on intelligence and on seizure recurrence. N Engl J Med 322:364–369, 1990.

Gress D: Stopping seizures. Emergency Medicine 22:22–29, 1980.

Hauser WA, Rich SS, Annegers JF, et al: Seizure recurrence after a first unprovoked seizure: An extended follow-up. Neurology 40:1163–1170, 1990.

Johnson LC, DeBolt WL, Long MT, et al: Diagnostic factors in adult males following initial seizures: a 3-year follow-up. Arch Neurol 27:193–197, 1972.

Juul-Jensen P: Frequency of recurrence after discontinuance of anticonvulsant therapy in patients with epileptic seizures. Epilepsia 5:352–363, 1964.

Levy RJ, Krall RL: Treatment of status epilepticus with lorazepam. Arch Neurol 41:605–611, 1984.

Pierelli F, Chatrian GE, Erdly WW, et al: Long-term EEG video-audio monitoring: detection of partial epileptic seizures and psychogenic episodes by 24-hour EEG record review. Epilepsia 30:513–523, 1989.

Temkin NR, Dikmen SS, Wilensky AJ, et al: A randomized, double-blind study of phenytoin for the prevention of post-traumatic seizures. N Engl J Med 323:497–502, 1990.

II. SLEEP DISORDERS

Daytime sleepiness is a complaint that may require special EEG monitoring before a definitive diagnosis is made. It is important **not** to treat patients with stimulant drugs if a precise diagnosis has not been established. The disorders that do require specific management are narcolepsy and sleep apnea. A specialized sleep laboratory is often required to establish the correct diagnosis.

A. Narcolepsy. The narcolepsy syndrome has four components: episodes of irresistible daytime sleepiness (narcolepsy), episodes of sudden loss of postural tone (cataplexy), brief episodes of inability to move upon awakening (sleep paralysis), and vivid hallucinations upon going to sleep or awakening (hypnagogic hallucinations). Many patients have only 1 or 2 of these symptoms. Patients with the narcoleptic syndrome often enter rapid eye movement (REM) sleep almost immediately. **Methylphenidate** (Ritalin) in dosages of 5–10 mg tid is considered to be the most effective drug. An alternative agent is pemoline (Cylert) 18.75 mg each morning, which can be increased as needed up to 6 tablets/day in divided doses. Drugs should not be prescribed unless the diagnosis is well established. The physician should monitor the number of prescribed pills and use the lowest effective dose. If cataplectic symptoms are bothersome, imipramine (Tofranil) or an analogue is often very effective at a dosage of 25 mg bid or tid.

B. Sleep Apnea. This most commonly is due to obstruction to air flow in overweight persons who are snorers. A prolonged sleep EEG, with monitoring of air flow and intraesophageal pressure, is used to confirm the diagnosis. Although surgical procedures such as tracheostomy and uvulopalatopharyngoplasty are sometimes necessary, less invasive therapy is often satisfactory. Approaches include weight loss, use of tongue-restraining devices, continuous positive airway pressure, and treatment with agents such as protriptyline and medroxyprogesterone.

Bliwise DL: Sleep-related respiratory disturbance in elderly persons. Compr Ther 10:8–14, 1984.
Kryger M, Roth T, Dement W: Principles and Practice of Sleep Medicine. Philadelphia, WB Saunders Co., 1989.

III. COMA AND ALTERED MENTAL STATUS

Stupor, coma, and delirium are presenting symptoms of cerebral dysfunction due to multiple potential causes. Proper management involves simultaneously establishing a correct diagnosis and instituting measures to prevent complications and to treat rapidly correctable conditions such as hypoglycemia. Altered mental status implies bilateral cerebral dysfunction or disturbance at the level of the high brain stem, the location of the reticular activating system. Metabolic, toxic, vascular, space-occupying, traumatic, and seizure disorders lead the list of conditions that may manifest in this way. Usually, historical clues are more helpful than physical examination in coming to a rational diagnostic conclusion. Since patients brought to medical attention usually cannot provide accurate information, efforts should be made to seek out relatives, neighbors, or friends who can.

A. Coma. The first measures to be taken when a comatose patient arrives in the emergency room include vital sign assessment, IV line placement, blood withdrawal for determining glucose and electrolyte levels, and IV administration of glucose with thiamine. Taking appropriate measures to maintain blood pressure and respiration then allows time to assess the patient's neurologic and clinical status further. Examination of the head and ear canals for signs of trauma and flexion of the neck to evaluate nuchal rigidity are two quick diagnostic observations to be made. The level of consciousness is assessed by use of verbal commands and, if necessary, noxious stimuli. Assessment of the pupils, visualization of the fundi for papilledema and subhyaloid hemorrhages (the latter common with subarachnoid hemorrhage secondary to rupture of a berry aneurysm), examination of eye movements, and detection of lateralizing motor signs are the most important parts of the neurologic assessment. The most valuable radiologic test is CT scan, but if the patient is febrile and meningitis is strongly suspected, a delay of CSF examination to carry out CT may be unwarranted.

1. **COMA DUE TO ISCHEMIA, HYPOXIA, OR CARBON MONOXIDE POISONING.** Ways to improve survival of cerebral tissues after cardiorespiratory arrest or after exposure to high levels of carbon monoxide are being actively investigated. Hyperbaric oxygen treatment is indicated for patients in deep coma who have been exposed to high doses of carbon monoxide. For less severely affected persons or for those who have had cerebral ischemia from cardiorespiratory arrest, oxygen is given by endotracheal tube. No drug has been shown to improve outcome in such patients. Use of barbiturates, calcium entry blockers, or blockers of excitatory amino acid (glutamate, aspartate) receptors has been advocated in an attempt to reduce brain damage. Results of animal studies support the use of each of these agents. Thus far, however, only barbiturates have been tested extensively in humans, and results are not encouraging. Studies of calcium entry blockers are in progress, while the search for useful excitatory amino acid blockers is an active area for investigation.

2. **COMA DUE TO FAT EMBOLISM.** Diffuse encephalopathy from fat embolism occurs in some patients after fracture of a long bone. After a delay of several hours to a few days, the patient becomes stuporous or comatose, often having developed petechiae of skin, conjunctivae, or retina, as well as respiratory distress. Prophylactic use of high-dose methylprednisolone in patients with long-bone fractures has been reported to reduce the incidence of fat embolism (Ann Intern Med 146:969–973, 1986). Once the syndrome has developed, intensive respiratory care is the most important therapy. The use of heparin, steroids, or other agents does not appear to improve the clinical outcome.

B. Delirium. Sudden onset of confusion, often associated with visual hallucinations and impaired consciousness, indicates the presence of delirium. Obtaining a history of previous psychiatric problems, use of medications, substance abuse, the presence of other medical problems such as diabetes mellitus or thyroid disease is especially important. The presence of fever may suggest the onset of encephalitis or meningitis. In an alcoholic, Wernicke's encephalopathy due to thiamine deficiency is suggested by the presence of nystagmus and ophthalmoplegia. The physician will obtain a blood sample for glucose, electrolytes, CBC, cultures, and drug screen. CT will usually be done to rule out a structural lesion or subarachnoid hemorrhage. Measures similar to those taken with a comatose patient (see above) are carried out. Tremulousness, confusion, hallucinosis, seizures, and delirium tremens usually occur in individuals who have been drinking ethanol heavily for several weeks and who have recently reduced the amount of ethanol consumption. Similar symptoms occur in persons who are addicted to barbiturates or other sedative drugs. Withdrawal from narcotics also may be accompanied by similar symptoms, though seizures are unusual. Distinguishing delirium from acute psychosis can be difficult.

Management of the delirious patient requires hospital admission and close observation. The patient should be in a quiet private room with orienting objects such as a clock and a calendar. The presence of a family member or close friend may be reassuring and should be encouraged. Frequent observation for changes in consciousness and vital signs and monitoring of intake and output are routine. When the patient is in bed, side rails should be raised. Waist and limb restraints may be needed if the patient is combative, is likely to wander, or is being fed parenterally. Medications are used in the lowest doses necessary to keep the patient calm.

Antipsychotic drugs such as haloperidol (2–5 mg), chlorpromazine (50–100 mg), or thiothixene (20 mg) are used for rapid tranquilization. Lower doses should be used in the elderly. These drugs should be avoided in delirium associated with ethanol or sedative withdrawal because of the danger of precipitating seizures. In this situation, a benzodiazepine is used. Lorazepam 1–2 mg IM can be administered. Chlordiazepoxide hydrochloride 25–100 mg IM can be used. Either drug can be given orally, and repeat doses may be administered every 4–6 hours. Diazepam and paraldehyde are also used by some physicians. Propranolol has been used in doses up to 540 mg/day for treating agitated delirium in brain-injured patients. Bradycardia and hypotension are limiting factors. It is important to prevent cumulative effects of whichever drug is chosen. The requirement for sedation will likely diminish within a short time, since the normal course of delirium is improvement within hours to a few days.

Goldberg RJ, Dubin WR, Fogel BS: Behavioral emergencies. Assessment and psychopharmacologic management. Clin Neuropharmacol 12:233–248, 1989.
Jacobson DM, Terrence CF, Reinmuth OM: The neurologic manifestations of fat embolism. Neurology 36:847–851, 1986.
Plum F, Posner JB: The Diagnosis of Stupor and Coma. 3rd ed. Philadelphia, FA Davis, 1980.

IV. DEMENTIAS

A. **Alzheimer's Disease.** No medication alters the course of Alzheimer's disease. Mild, transitory symptomatic improvement may occur with some drugs that increase activity in cholinergic systems. However, these agents cannot be recommended with enthusiasm. The list includes lecithin (a source of choline), physostigmine, and tetrahydroaminoacridine, which is being subjected to experimental testing. A frequently prescribed ergotamine compound (mixture of equal parts of dihydroergocornine, dihydroergocristine, and dihydrocryptine [Hydergine]) can no longer be recommended. The use of agents that have vasodilating or other rheologic effects is not supported by clinical data.

B. "Treatable" Dementias. Many papers have stressed the importance of diagnosing treatable causes of dementia before assuming a patient has a progressive untreatable disorder. Unfortunately the proportion of patients with treatable conditions is small among those in whom dementia is the primary complaint. Clinical clues may exist to alert the physician to alternative diagnoses, such as hypothyroidism, "normal-pressure" hydrocephalus (NPH), or AIDS-related dementia (Table 16–4). Shunting in patients with NPH is most likely to result in improvement in cognitive function when the cause is known and when the duration of symptoms is short (less than 6 months) (Ann Neurol 20:304–310, 1986).

Assuming no specific treatment is available for the dementia, in what areas can the physician assist the patient? In general, it is best to use as few medications as possible. Bothersome hallucinations or nocturnal agitation may respond to a neuroleptic such as haloperidol. Drugs with anticholinergic actions, such as those used to treat depression and even diphenhydramine for "sundowning" (nocturnal confusion), can aggravate the dementia or delirium. Urinary retention can also result. Long-term management usually involves assessment of medical, psychologic, and social needs in conjunction with the family and caregivers. Caregiver education is valuable. Optimal outcomes in progressive dementias depend on measures designed to preserve caregiver strength and stamina (respite care, recognition of depression) and minimize excess disability due to coexistent illness.

Barry PP, Moskowitz MA: The diagnosis of reversible dementia in the elderly: a critical review. Arch Intern Med 148:1914–1921, 1988.
Thompson TL II, Filley CM, Mitchell WD et al: Lack of efficacy of Hydergine in patients with Alzheimer's disease. N Engl J Med 323:445–448, 1990.

V. HEADACHE AND OTHER NEUROLOGIC CAUSES OF PAIN

A. Headache. A patient with **acute** headache should be managed differently from a patient with **chronic** headache.

    1. ACUTE HEADACHE. Sudden onset of headache can be an incapacitating and worrisome problem. Perhaps the most important piece of information is whether the headache is of new onset or whether it is one episode of a longstanding pattern. Headache of recent onset should alert the physician to several conditions: acute sinusitis, acute glaucoma, subarachnoid hemorrhage from a leaking berry aneurysm, or bacterial or viral meningitis. The presence of other symptoms or signs, such as tenderness over the frontal or maxillary sinuses, nasal congestion, visual symptoms, fever, and neck stiffness, may make the diagnosis apparent. However, the characteristics of the headache itself may not be specific. Index of suspicion must be high enough so that the appropriate laboratory test (CT, lumbar puncture, and sinus films) is obtained. Patients with subarachnoid hemorrhage sometimes

TABLE 16–4. DIFFERENTIAL DIAGNOSIS OF DEMENTIA

CAUSE	CLINICAL CLUES	CONFIRMATORY TESTS*
Alzheimer's disease	No other neurologic signs	
Pick's disease	Symptoms less global than in Alzheimer's disease	
Multi-infarct dementia	Pseudobulbar palsy, episodic worsening	CT may show lacunar infarcts
Depression	Depressed mood	Response to antidepressants
Drugs (tranquilizers, antiparkinsonian agents)	History of drug use, slurred speech, ataxia, lethargy, withdrawal symptoms, or improvement in hospital	Toxicology screen
Chronic subdural hematoma	History of drinking, anticoagulant therapy, lethargy, headache	CT, brain scan
Vitamin B_{12} deficiency	Ataxia, posterior column signs	CBC, B_{12} level, Schilling's test
Hydrocephalus	Incontinence, gait disturbance	CT, isotope cisternography
Hypothyroidism	Husky voice, stiff muscles, "hung-up" reflexes	Thyroid studies
Syphilis	Tongue tremor, miotic pupils	VDRL, FTA
Chronic meningitis, (fungus, tumor, tuberculosis)	Other signs of systemic disease	LP for cells, glucose cytology, culture
Huntington's disease	Parent or siblings in mental hospital; fidgety on physical examination	CT for caudate atrophy
Creutzfeldt-Jakob disease	Progressive over months; myoclonus	EEG: triphasic sharp waves
AIDS-related dementia	History of homosexuality, promiscuity, or IV drug abuse	HIV antibody
Dialysis dementia	Appropriate clinical setting; speech problems, myoclonus, seizures	EEG: slow waves, bursts, spikes

Adapted from Swanson PD: Signs and Symptoms in Neurology. Philadelphia, JB Lippincott, 1984.

*CT = computed tomography; CBC = complete blood count; VDRL = Venereal Disease Research Laboratory; FTA = fluorescent treponemal antibody; LP = lumbar puncture; EEG = electroencephalogram; HIV = human immunodeficiency virus.

give a history of having been seen in an emergency room several days before for an occipital headache, for which analgesics were prescribed before the patient was sent home. Assuming that the patient's history and the headache's character support the diagnosis of muscle contraction or migraine headache, acute pharmacologic treatment may be indicated. Acute muscle contraction headaches should be accompanied by tenderness in the painful areas and resistance to stretch of the painful muscles. Moist heat with a towel soaked in hot water or hot packs may bring relief. Ice packs or gentle massage may also help. Injections of narcotic analgesics such as meperidine should be avoided.

IV or IM dihydroergotamine has been advocated for emergency room treatment of migraine headaches. Up to 3 doses of 1 mL (1 mg of dihydroergotamine mesylate) can be given at 30-minute or 1-hour intervals. Total weekly dosage should not exceed 6 mL. The drug is contraindicated in pregnancy and in angina, hypertension, or peripheral arterial disease. Other agents used in acute migraine include a phenothiazine such as chlorpromazine 5–10 mg IV, prochlorperazine (Compazine) 2–10 mg IV, or metoclopramide 5–10 mg IV; verapamil 5–10 mg IV; or dexamethasone 20 mg. Propranolol (20 mg po), used with acetaminophen, can be effective for mild migraine headaches. An acute migraine episode may also respond to analgesics such as aspirin or acetaminophen or to a nonsteroidal anti-inflammatory agent such as ibuprofen.

2. **CHRONIC HEADACHE.** Differentiating characteristics of the most common headache types are listed in Table 16–5. A new exhaustive headache classification scheme substitutes the term tension type for muscle contraction and lists the diagnostic criteria for each headache type and subtype (Cephalalgia [suppl 7]:1–96,1988). Tension-type or muscle contraction headaches are frequent, often occurring daily, and may be located in occipital, frontal, or temporal areas. Although usually steady, they may have a throbbing quality or associated nausea. Migraine headaches may be preceded by a visual aura or, rarely, by other symptoms suggesting cerebral ischemia (aphasia or hemisensory or hemiparetic symptoms). The headaches occur episodically, are usually throbbing, and frequently are associated with nausea and other systemic symptoms such as malaise. Subvarieties of migraine are cluster headaches (daily severe pain, retro-orbital location, lacrimation, and nasal stuffiness) and chronic cluster headaches. Temporal arteritis is suspected in older persons with symptoms of malaise, weight loss, and muscle aching. The erythrocyte sedimentation rate is almost always elevated.

   a. **Treatment of Muscle Contraction Headaches.** Understanding that the pain may relate to continued muscle contraction may be helpful to the patient. Demonstrating tenderness and increased muscle tone in painful areas assists in this understanding. Long-term use of narcotic medications should be avoided. Approaches to be encouraged are (1) simple self-administered stretching and relaxation; (2) professional instruction in relaxation, using bio-

TABLE 16–5. CLASSIFICATION OF HEADACHE

1. Vascular headache of the migraine type
   a. Classic migraine
   b. Common migraine
   c. Cluster migraine
   d. Hemiplegic migraine or ophthalmoplegic migraine
   e. Lower-half headache
2. Muscle contraction headache
3. Combined headache: vascular and muscle contraction
4. Headache of nasal vasomotor reaction
5. Headache of delusional, conversion, or hypochondriacal states
6. Nonmigrainous vascular headaches
7. Traction headaches
8. Headache due to overt cranial inflammation
9. Headache due to disease of ocular structures
10. Headache due to disease of aural structures
11. Headache due to disease of nasal and sinus structures
12. Headache due to disease of other cranial and neck structures
13. Cranial neuritides
14. Cranial neuralgias

feedback and relaxation-training techniques; and (3) for very severe pain, physical therapy with heat and massage. Low-dose tricyclic antidepressants (amitriptyline 25–50 mg hs) may help patients with a debilitating chronic pain syndrome. Nonsteroidal anti-inflammatory drugs such as naproxen (375–500 mg tid) may be tried for both muscle contraction and migraine prophylaxis.

b. **Migraine Prophylaxis.** Daily medication should be reserved for patients whose headaches occur frequently. The initial drug choice will vary with the physician's experience and will depend upon what the patient has tried in the past.

Effective antimigraine drugs have generally been shown to benefit perhaps ⅔ of patients when compared with placebos. An agent least likely to produce toxicity should be tried first. If one agent is ineffective, another may be substituted. Aspirin, naproxen, cyproheptadine (Periactin), propranolol, amitriptyline, or a calcium entry blocker may each be tried, with little danger of serious side effects. Cyproheptadine has in some instances produced increased appetite and weight gain. Beta-adrenergic blockers are sometimes poorly tolerated because of the occurrence of lassitude, alteration in sleep patterns, or depression. Tricyclic antidepressants often cause sleepiness and dry mouth. Calcium entry blockers are usually well tolerated, but their effectiveness in migraine prophylaxis may be less striking than suggested by early enthusiastic reports. Methysergide (Sansert) is used much less frequently than the others, because of the serious side effect of retroperitoneal fibrosis. It is an effective agent for true migraine, and if its use is interrupted every 4 months, there should be little danger of ureteral obstruction. Initially the dosage should be low

(2 mg bid), but if necessary, it can be increased to double this amount. Patients should be warned of side effects, which include angina and intermittent claudication.

B. Face Pain. Pain in the distribution of the face, jaw, or throat must first be diagnosed before a treatment plan can be made. Primary diagnostic considerations are (1) trigeminal and glossopharyngeal neuralgias; (2) disease of teeth, sinuses, or other structures in the head area; (3) pain due to contraction of muscles of mastication; and (4) atypical facial pain.

1. TRIGEMINAL AND GLOSSOPHARYNGEAL NEURALGIAS. These neuralgias share pain characteristics that usually make the clinical diagnosis rather straightforward. The pain occurs suddenly in brief bursts and is usually severe and lancinating. The pain of trigeminal neuralgia (tic douloureux) is almost always in the distribution of the second or third division of the trigeminal nerve; that of glossopharyngeal neuralgia is in the posterior pharynx. The pain is often triggered by stimulation of skin or mucous membrane by such activities as chewing and swallowing. Without such a trigger point the diagnosis should be questioned. The cause is not usually apparent but may be irritation of the affected nerve root by a redundant arterial branch within the posterior intracranial fossa. Although relief may be obtained by surgical intervention, in which a sponge is placed between the nerve root and adjacent artery, or by electrolytic damage to a nerve branch, many patients can be treated with antiseizure medication with good effect. Carbamazepine is begun at a dosage of 100 mg once or twice a day, and the amount gradually increased until a therapeutic level is reached. Blood levels of 6–12 μg/mL are usually tolerated without serious side effects. If the pain persists, phenytoin may be used in doses similar to those effective for seizure disorders.

2. ATYPICAL FACE PAIN. Surgical procedures must be avoided in patients whose face pain is not typical of the above neuralgias. The pain is usually more constant, is poorly localized, and is not relieved by anticonvulsant therapy. In some cases the pain is due to chronic contraction of muscles of mastication, and relief is obtained by measures used by dentists to reduce muscle tension.

C. Drug Withdrawal from Patients with Chronic Pain. Specialty clinics to deal with patients suffering from chronic pain have been established in a number of medical centers. Use of behavioral approaches for managing such patients is emphasized. Many patients with chronic pain have become dependent on narcotic and sedative drugs. A popular method for withdrawal of medications is the use of a "pain cocktail" (Pain 26:153–165, 1986). For patients taking narcotics, methadone is used in doses equivalent to those of the narcotic the patient is taking. Phenobarbital is used to replace sedative drugs. A pain cocktail is prepared in which 1 or both of these 2 drugs are added to a taste-masked liquid. The patient is given 10 mL of the pain cocktail every 6 hours. Doses of methadone and phenobarbital are then reduced each day by

15–20% and 10%, respectively. Rapid tapering may require inpatient observation.

Buckley FP, Sizemore WA, Charlton JE: Medication management in patients with chronic nonmalignant pain: a review of the use of a drug withdrawal protocol. Pain 26:153–165, 1986.

Foley KM, Payne R (eds): Current Therapy for Pain. Toronto, BC Decker, 1987.

Graham JR: Migraine headache: diagnosis and management. Headache 19:133–141, 1979.

Meyer JS, Hardenberg J: Clinical effectiveness of calcium entry blockers in prophylactic treatment of migraine and cluster headache. Headache 23:266–277, 1983.

Raskin NH, Schwartz RK: Interval therapy of migraine: long-term results. Headache 20:336–340, 1980.

Swanson PD: Signs and Symptoms in Neurology. Philadelphia, JB Lippincott, 1984.

Ziegler DK: Migraine and cluster headache. In Johnson RT: Current Therapy in Neurologic Disease-3. Philadelphia, BC Decker, 1990.

VI. BRAIN TUMORS, INCREASED INTRACRANIAL PRESSURE, AND SPINAL CORD COMPRESSION

Surgical management of space-occupying lesions of the brain or spinal cord is beyond the scope of this chapter. There are, however, certain medical aspects of therapy. The management of increased intracranial pressure is also important for other conditions such as stroke, generalized cerebral ischemia, and benign intracranial hypertension (pseudotumor cerebri).

A. Brain Tumors

1. **PITUITARY TUMORS.** Adenomas and microadenomas of the pituitary can arise from different cell types. The type most amenable to medical treatment is the **prolactinoma,** which secretes prolactin and produces galactorrhea and hypogonadism as early symptoms. This diagnosis can be confirmed by the serum prolactin levels. Tumor size is determined by radiologic studies. Bromocriptine, a dopamine agonist, causes reduction in the size of prolactin-secreting tumors. Dosages below 10 mg daily are effective and are given for several weeks before trans-sphenoidal tumor removal. Microadenomas do not require surgery. Alternative dopamine agonists such as pergolide have longer half-lives and are taken less frequently than bromocriptine.

2. **GLIOMAS.** Tumor debulking and radiation are mainstays of treatment for primary gliomas of the CNS. The tumor is classified according to probable cellular origin (e.g., oligodendroglioma, astrocytoma) and graded (grade I to IV) according to degree of malignancy. Following surgery, most patients receive radiation therapy, which may include a combination of whole-brain irradiation and a boost or radionuclide implant to the tumor site. Adjunctive therapy with chemotherapeutic agents can prolong survival in some cases. Modest success has been achieved with nitrosourea-based protocols.

3. **CEREBRAL METASTASES.** Metastases to the brain or to the leptomeningeal spaces are more common than primary brain tumors. Therapy with whole-brain irradiation may produce temporary regression. Meningeal carcinomatosis may respond to intrathecal or intraventric-

ular administration of an appropriate chemotherapeutic agent such as methotrexate. Patients with a large single metastasis may do better if this is surgically removed before irradiation. Cerebral metastases frequently are associated with cerebral edema. Long-term administration of corticosteroids is then recommended.

B. Increased Intracranial Pressure. Increases in intracranial pressure of 200 mm CSF or more can occur in any situation in which the volume of intracranial contents is increased. The success of therapy aimed at reducing intracranial pressure depends on the cause of the pressure increase. Thus, measures to reduce cerebral edema may be effective with brain tumors but much less so in edema associated with cerebral infarction.

1. CORTICOSTEROIDS. **Dexamethasone** is the steroid most often used for reducing cerebral swelling associated with primary or metastatic brain tumors. An initial dose of 10 mg, followed by 4 mg q6h is the usual dosage. However, much higher doses (1 mg/kg) have been recommended by some neurosurgeons. Marked reduction in peritumor edema may occur. H_2 receptor agonists and sucralfate should be used to prevent GI ulceration (see Chapter 6). Electrolyte and blood glucose levels need to be determined periodically.

2. HYPEROSMOLAR AGENTS. **Mannitol,** given IV as a 20–25% solution, is the most widely used agent for reducing brain swelling by increasing serum osmolality. Doses of 0.25–0.75 gm/kg body weight are used, and dramatic reduction in intracranial pressure can occur. However, the reduction is temporary, and the effects of repeated infusions of mannitol become less. Acute renal failure has developed in patients receiving total doses of more than 600 gm. An initial dose of 0.75–1.0 gm/kg can be used, followed by lower doses of 0.25–0.5 gm/kg every 3–5 hours, depending on the level of intracranial pressure and the serum osmolality, which may be raised to about 320 mosm/L. Foley catheterization and strict monitoring of intake and output are mandatory.

3. HYPERVENTILATION. Reducing the $Paco_2$ to 25–30 mm Hg can reduce cerebral blood volume and hence the intracranial pressure by 20–30%. The effect may not be long lasting. This requires an endotracheal tube and frequent monitoring of blood gases.

4. SURGICAL MEASURES. In some clinical situations (e.g., hydrocephalus associated with subarachnoid hemorrhage), removal of CSF by means of a ventriculostomy is useful. Internal decompression of an intracerebral mass (tumor or hemorrhage) may be needed to prevent transtentorial herniation. Rarely, craniectomy (with preservation of the cranial bone and later replacement at the original site) has been lifesaving in those with large hemispheral infarcts.

5. BENIGN INTRACRANIAL HYPERTENSION. This condition, also called pseudotumor cerebri, is usually of unknown cause. The patient is often young and obese and develops headaches. The only physical sign is papilledema. After known causes of increased intracranial

pressure are excluded (tumor, hydrocephalus), the diagnosis is considered. In some instances, thrombosis of a draining venous sinus is implicated (e.g., patients with mastoiditis). Other possible causes (hypervitaminosis A, tetracycline, endocrine abnormalities) are usually not present. The goal of treatment is to prevent headaches and blindness. Treatment with periodic spinal punctures for removal of CSF, best performed with an 18-gauge needle, may suffice to prevent headaches. Enough fluid is removed to reduce the pressure to 150–180 mm H_2O. Furosemide or acetazolamide in standard doses is used with success in many persons. A rare patient requires decompression of the optic nerves to prevent progressive visual loss. Lumboperitoneal shunt is an alternative in refractory cases.

C. Acute Spinal Cord Compression. Rapid onset of leg weakness is often due to spinal cord compression. Spinal cord compression due to trauma or to epidural tumor should be immediately treated with steroids. Based on a recent randomized study, a patient with traumatic spinal cord compression is immediately treated with an IV bolus of methylprednisolone 30 mg/kg body weight over 15 minutes. After 45 minutes this is followed by a 23-hour infusion of 5.4 mg/kg/hour. Patients treated within 8 hours of injury are most likely to benefit. Spinal cord compression due to epidural metastases should also be treated with corticosteroids, though in this situation, the recommended regimen is a 10-mg IV bolus of dexamethasone followed by 4 mg po q4h. Higher doses provide no additional benefit. Radiologic assessment (MRI or myelography) should be carried out rapidly. Radiation therapy is then instituted. If the patient's condition deteriorates further, neurosurgical decompression may be necessary.

Barrow DL, Tindall GT, Kovacs K, et al: Clinical and pathological effects of bromocriptine on prolactin-secreting and other pituitary tumors. J Neurosurg 60:1–7, 1984.

Bracken MB, Shepard MJ, Collins WF et al: A randomized, controlled trial of methylprednisolone or naloxone in the treatment of acute spinal-cord injury. N Engl J Med 322:1405–1411, 1990.

Burger PC: Malignant astrocytic neoplasms: classification, pathologic anatomy, and response to treatment. Semin Oncol 13:16–26, 1986.

Dorman HR, Sondheimer JH, Cadnapaphornchai P: Mannitol-induced acute renal failure. Medicine 69:153–159, 1990.

Kleinberg DL, Boyd LAE, Wardlaw S, et al: Pergolide for the treatment of pituitary tumors secreting prolactin or growth hormone. N Engl J Med 309:704–709, 1983.

Kornblith PL, Walker M: Chemotherapy for malignant gliomas. J Neurosurg 68:1–17, 1988.

Leibel SA, Sheline GE: Radiation therapy for neoplasms of the brain. J Neurosurg 66:1–22, 1987.

Patchell RA, Cirrincione C, Thaler HT et al: Single brain metastases: surgery plus radiation or radiation alone. Neurology 36:447–453, 1986.

Ropper AH, Kennedy SF: Neurological and Neurosurgical Intensive Care. 2nd ed. Rockville, Md, Aspen Publishers, 1988.

Vecht CJ, Haaxma-Reiche H, van Putten WLJ: Initial bolus of conventional versus high-dose dexamethasone in metastatic spinal cord compression. Neurology 39:1255–1257, 1989.

West CR, Avellanosa AM, Barua NR, et al: Intraarterial 1,3-bis(2-chloroethyl)-1-nitrosourea (BCNU) and systemic chemotherapy for malignant gliomas: a follow-up-study. Neurosurgery 13:420–426, 1983.

VII. CEREBROVASCULAR DISEASE

Prevention of hemorrhagic and ischemic stroke is far more effective in reducing morbidity than is treatment after the stroke has occurred.

One of the most important accomplishments in disease prevention has been reduction in stroke incidence by better control of hypertension. In contrast, morbidity and mortality figures for completed strokes have improved little if at all. In assessing a patient suspected of having a stroke, the first question is whether the event is **ischemic** or **hemorrhagic.** Treatment decisions are determined by the clinical course and by the presumed cause. Especially important is whether an ischemic event is from an embolic source. With hemorrhagic stroke, distinction between primary intracerebral hemorrhage and hemorrhage from a ruptured berry aneurysm is important in directing management of the case.

A. Ischemic Stroke

1. **TRANSIENT ISCHEMIC ATTACKS.** By convention, transient ischemic attacks (TIAs) are episodes of transient dysfunction of an area of the CNS in the distribution of a supplying artery that **last less than 24 hours.** The usual duration of an episode is 10–15 minutes. TIAs can be mimicked by partial seizures and by migraine "accompaniments" (symptoms, thought to be due to cerebral ischemia that may precede an episode of migraine headache and that occur without headache in some individuals). Presyncopal episodes producing global cerebral ischemia due to decrease in cardiac output or blood pressure should not be labeled TIAs.

Treatment strategies are designed to accomplish the following: (1) medically reduce the incidence of emboli by interfering with platelet aggregation or by reducing thrombus formation with anticoagulants and (2) surgically reduce sources of emboli, increase flow, and prevent occlusion of a major supplying vessel, usually a severely stenotic internal carotid artery.

a. **Antiplatelet Agents.** These are used for stroke prevention in both men and women with TIAs whether or not endarterectomy is performed. **Aspirin** inhibits the enzyme cyclooxygenase in platelets, thus interfering with the formation of thromboxane A_2. Platelet aggregation and adhesion to vessel walls are thereby lessened. The doses of aspirin used in many clinical studies also inhibit prostacyclin formation in the vessel endothelial cells in vitro and could thereby augment platelet adhesion. Recent studies suggest that low (300 mg/day) aspirin dosage may be as effective as high dosage (900–1200 mg/day) in preventing stroke in patients with TIAs or small strokes. Other agents such as dipyridamole (Persantine) or sulfinpyrazone (Anturane) have not potentiated the effects of aspirin when tested in large controlled studies. **Ticlopidine** is an antiplatelet agent that also works for stroke prevention in controlled studies. Side effects include diarrhea, rash, and neutropenia. The effective dose is 250 mg bid.

b. **Anticoagulants.** The use of anticoagulants for stroke prevention in patients with TIAs is controversial. A patient seen for the first time in the period soon after the onset of a TIA may be a candidate for acute anticoagulation with heparin, the rationale being that onset of TIAs may be a harbinger of an impending stroke. CT without contrast enhancement always should be done before initiation of anticoagulation. Lumbar puncture is usually not recommended because hemorrhagic complications (spinal epidural hemorrhage) are more likely to occur unless anticoagulation is delayed. Heparin is given as a constant infusion, at a dose of 1000 units/hour. The goal is to bring the partial thromboplastin time to 1.5 times the control value. Bolus heparinization may increase the risk of hemorrhage. If no further TIA occurs, there are no clear guidelines to duration of anticoagulation treatment. Some recommend switching to coumarin and maintaining anticoagulation (prothombin levels at 1.5 times control) for 3 months. Others may choose to discontinue heparin during the hospital stay after 1 or 2 weeks.

2. EVOLVING STROKE. It is rare for the physician to encounter a stroke patient in whom signs fluctuate clearly enough to justify the designation **stroke in evolution.** This term should be used for the patient in whom signs are clearly worsening upon repeated observation or improve only to worsen again. Generally accepted treatment in such patients is acute anticoagulation with heparin as outlined in the discussion of TIAs. Since most series involve relatively few patients, solid support for this approach is lacking.

3. COMPLETED STROKE. Most patients coming to the hospital for treatment belong in this category. If there is no evidence that the stroke resulted from an embolus, anticoagulation is not instituted. Fluid overload should be avoided. Attention must be paid to avoiding aspiration, to initiating range of motion to paralyzed limbs, to preventing bed sores by turning and by using protective boots and an appropriate mattress. If the infarct is large and associated with cerebral swelling, **hyperosmotic therapy** with mannitol (0.25 gm/kg IV) may be temporarily beneficial. Most studies suggest that **steroids** are not helpful and may even worsen the prognosis. **Hemicraniectomy** has been shown to be lifesaving in some patients with massive right hemisphere infarcts. Survivors often show marked functional impairment.

4. EMBOLIC STROKE. Many ischemic strokes are due to emboli that usually originate in the heart. Embolic cerebral infarctions often become hemorrhagic, but hemorrhage may not be evident in the hours immediately after onset of symptoms. If the source of emboli is evident, as in a patient with a cardiac mural thrombus or with rheumatic heart disease, mitral stenosis, and an enlarged left atrium, anticoagulation is usually recommended. Anticoagulation is not being used to influence the ischemic area but rather to lessen the likelihood of emboli recurrence. In rheumatic heart disease the estimated risk of recurrent emboli is 1%/day in the first 2 weeks. Because of the risk that anticoagulants will increase the likelihood of hemorrhage into the cerebral infarct, caution must be used in deciding when to begin anticoagulant therapy. Factors that increase the risk of deterioration, such as stupor or coma, and demonstration of a large infarct

562 / NEUROLOGIC DISEASES

with swelling or shift of hemispheral structures should alert the clinician to monitor the patient's status with repeat CT 24–48 hours before anticoagulation is begun. Heparin is usually begun IV, 1000 units/hour, and the dosage is subsequently adjusted to achieve a PTT of 1.5 times the control value.

B. Hemorrhagic Stroke

1. **PRIMARY SUBARACHNOID HEMORRHAGE.** Bleeding from a ruptured berry aneurysm usually is confined to the subarachnoid space, though in some instances the stream of blood is directed into the cerebral substance and may enter a ventricle. The diagnosis is usually confirmed by demonstrating subarachnoid blood by CT. Early neurosurgical intervention should be considered in patients who have not been devastated by the hemorrhage. The patient should be in an ICU, in a darkened room. A stool softener and an analgesic such as codeine should be given as needed. Medical management is directed at controlling hypertension, reducing intracranial pressure, and preventing spasm of intracranial arteries. There is no certain way of preventing vasospasm. However, controlled studies with **nimodipine,** a calcium entry blocker, suggest that the drug is of benefit in reducing the severity of neurologic deficits resulting from vasospasm. Nimodipine is given in a dosage of 60 mg (2 capsules) q4h for 21 consecutive days. If a nasogastric tube is required, the contents of the capsule are extracted into a syringe and washed down the tube with 30 mL of normal saline. After the aneurysm has been clipped, maintaining a mean arterial pressure of 100–120 mm Hg may help prevent vasospasm. This is achieved by intravascular volume expansion with normal saline and a plasma substitute to raise the pulmonary wedge pressure above 15 mm Hg. The use of antifibrinolytic agents such as aminocaproic acid (Amicar) is controversial.

2. **INTRACEREBRAL HEMORRHAGE.** Rupture of small penetrating arterial branches occurs most commonly in patients with chronic hypertension. Common sites of primary intracerebral hemorrhage are deep within a cerebral hemisphere (striatum or thalamus), cerebellum, and pons. There is no specific medical therapy to reduce cerebral damage. Some patients may benefit from clot evacuation. More superficial hemorrhages occur in patients who have developed **congophilic (amyloid) angiopathy** of small cerebral vessels. Surgical evacuation is not recommended because of a high risk of rebleeding.

Cerebral Embolism Study Group: Cardioembolic stroke, early anticoagulation, and brain hemorrhage. Arch Intern Med 147:636–640, 1987.

Delashaw JB, Broaddus WC, Kassell NF, et al: Treatment of right hemispheric cerebral infarction by hemicraniectomy. Stroke 21:874–881, 1990.

Estol C, Caplan LR: Therapy of acute stroke. Clin Neuropharmacol 2:91–120, 1990.

Hass WK, Easton JD, Adams HP, et al: A randomized trial comparing ticlopidine hydrochloride with aspirin for the prevention of stroke in high-risk patients. N Engl J Med 321:501–507, 1989.

Hirsh J: Therapeutic range for the control of oral anticoagulant therapy. Arch Neurol 43:1162–1164, 1986.

Millikan CH, McDowell F, Easton JD: Stroke. Philadelphia, Lea & Febiger, 1987.

VIII. MOVEMENT DISORDERS

Though one could include seizures in this group of conditions, **movement disorders** are usually restricted to movements not accompanied by alteration in consciousness. Many of these conditions arise from disease in the basal ganglia. However, **tremors** may emanate from structures in cerebellum or midbrain, and **myoclonus** may occur with disease in spinal cord, brain stem, or cerebral cortex. In this section, therapy for spasticity will also be discussed (Table 16–6).

A. Myoclonus. Myoclonic movements can be simply termed jerks. They may be focal or segmental, or they may be generalized, involving many muscles synchronously or asynchronously. They can arise by excitation or by disinhibition of neurons at spinal cord, brain stem, or thalamic level. Myoclonic jerks can be benign, as with nocturnal myoclonus, or they can occur as a sign of more serious pathology, such as CNS hypoxia or encephalitis or during the course of certain degenerative disorders. Medical treatment of myoclonic jerks depends on the mechanism of production of myoclonus and the site of pathophysiology. Generalized myoclonus associated with or preceding generalized seizures may respond to anticonvulsants such as sodium valproate. Postanoxic myoclonus may respond to drugs that affect serotoninergic systems. The drug clonazepam may be effective in this situation in dosages of 4–10 mg/day.

B. Spasticity. Spasticity is the term used to describe increased resistance of muscles to passive stretch that is accompanied by hyperactive tendon reflexes. Patients can be severely disabled by increased muscle tone.

TABLE 16–6. THERAPY OF NONPARKINSONISM MOVEMENT DISORDERS

CONDITION	TREATMENT	RESULT
Myoclonus (postanoxic)	Clonazepam, valproic acid	Variable
Spasticity	Baclofen, dantrolene	Variable
Chorea (especially Huntington's disease)	Haloperidol, reserpine	Moderate success
Torticollis, tics	Haloperidol	Variable
Dystonias	Botulinum toxin injections	Good, but temporary for focal dystonias
Neuroleptic-induced movement disorders		
Acute dystonia	Diphenhydramine	Very successful
Parkinsonism	Anticholinergics	Moderate to marked
Tardive dyskinesias	Reserpine	Fair to poor
	Choline percursors	Variable
Benign essential tremor	Beta blockers (propranolol, nadolol), sedatives (primidone)	Moderate success
Gilles de la Tourette syndrome	Haloperidol, pimozide, clonidine, sulpiride	Moderate success

Spasticity can also be accompanied by involuntary spasms of extension or flexion of muscles. Spasticity can result from damage to descending suprasegmental motor pathways at spinal cord or higher brain stem or hemispheral levels, presumably by removal of descending inhibitory influences on spinal cord activity. Though unilateral spasticity may result from hemispheral damage due, for example, to cerebral infarction, medical treatment is usually used in patients with spinal cord damage from trauma or diseases such as multiple sclerosis.

Pharmacologic treatment of spasticity is limited by side effects of potentially effective drugs. At this time, **baclofen** is considered the most effective agent. Drug administration is begun at a dosage of 5 mg tid and increased every few days. The maximum recommended dose is 80 mg daily, though some patients have required higher doses to obtain relief. Drowsiness, dizziness, and fatigue are common side effects that limit the dose that can be given. Other drugs used for treating spasticity include **benzodiazepines** such as diazepam and **dantrolene.** These agents are of limited use because of side effects. Dantrolene is thought to act peripherally on the excitation-contraction mechanism of muscle. Frequently, patients receiving enough dantrolene to reduce spasticity will develop accompanying weakness. The drug would be used in a patient with severe spasticity who did not respond to baclofen or a benzodiazepine. Treatment is begun with a dose of 25 mg daily, which is increased in 25-mg increments, as tolerated. Doses as high as 400 mg daily have been tolerated by some persons.

C. Chorea. This is an involuntary movement that occurs characteristically in Huntington's disease, inherited as an autosomal dominant trait and due to a defective gene on chromosome 4, and Sydenham's chorea, associated with rheumatic fever. Choreiform movements may also be seen in parkinsonian patients receiving excessive levodopa and in patients with tardive dyskinesias. Medical treatment of choreiform movements is not satisfactory. The movements may be lessened by the neurotransmitter-depleting agent reserpine or by neuroleptic drugs such as haloperidol. It is best not to use these agents, however, unless the choreiform movements are large and are incapacitating. Reserpine may be started at doses of 0.5 mg that are gradually increased until symptoms are improved or until side effects become a problem. The drug can be used in doses that are higher than those used to treat hypertension.

D. Dystonias. Dystonias currently are classified as **focal** or **generalized.** Focal dystonias include spasmodic torticollis and writer's cramp. Medical treatment is usually unsatisfactory. Occasionally, behavioral modification approaches are successful. An approach that appears to bring about good though temporary (3–6 months) improvement is the injection under electromyographic control of small amounts of type A botulinum toxin (Oculinum). This therapy can be used for **blepharospasm, spasmodic torticollis, spasmodic dysphonia,** other focal dystonias, and hemifacial spasm.

Generalized dystonias may occur in a variety of pathologic conditions. The principally encountered ones are (1) **tardive dyskinesias,** resulting from prolonged use of neuroleptic or antinausea medications, (2) dystonias occurring in parkinsonian patients being treated with levodopa, and (3) dystonia occurring during the course of the genetic condition termed **dystonia musculorum deformans** or **torsion dystonia.** Levodopa-related dystonias are improved by reducing the amount of antiparkinsonian medication given with each dose. Dystonias caused by neuroleptic or antinausea medication may or may not improve with removal of the offending drug. Medical treatment of these refractory movement disorders is generally unsatisfactory. Of the many medications that have been tried, anticholinergic therapy may be the most satisfactory. Trihexyphenidyl HCl is usually used. Beginning with 1- or 2-mg tablets, the dose may be increased as tolerated. Young patients are able to tolerate much higher doses than are older individuals, who can become confused or delirious with toxic amounts of anticholinergic drugs. Dry mouth is often a problem because of decreased saliva. Doses as high as 75 mg have been tolerated by some. Less success is reported with baclofen or clonazepam. Dopamine agonists, antagonists, and depleters have been relatively unsuccessful. A rare form of generalized dystonia responds to small amounts of levodopa, given in the form of Sinemet.

E. Parkinson's Disease. The cardinal symptoms and signs of Parkinson's disease are bradykinesia (slow movement), resting tremor, rigidity of muscles, and problems with balance and walking. These problems may occur individually or together. The response to therapy may be better for one symptom than for another. Some disagreement remains among specialists about which medication to use initially (Table 16–7).

1. **LEVODOPA.** Levodopa in the form of Sinemet is the most effective antiparkinsonian drug and may be chosen as the initial drug. Sinemet may be started with 1 yellow tablet (carbidopa 25 mg, levodopa 100 mg) after a meal, and 1 tablet may be added at another time every 3–4 days to a dosage of 2 tablets tid. The patient should be assessed after 2 or 3 weeks. If the drug is well tolerated, and if it is necessary to increase the dose, 1 tablet of Sinemet 25-250 tid should be substituted. Half-tablet increments can be continued until significant improvement is noted or until side effects prevent further increase. The lowest dose that produces satisfactory improvement is then continued.

Problems may occur in patients who take Sinemet: (1) Nausea is common and is best managed by reducing the amount taken at one time. (2) Some patients benefit less when the drug is taken after a meal. Absorption of levodopa in the proximal small bowel and transport from blood to brain take place through facilitated transport mechanisms for neutral amino acids. For patients who respond poorly to Sinemet, a trial of low-protein meals is warranted. (3) Although many patients will remain stable with the same Sinemet dose for a number of years, others will notice gradual worsening of bradykinesia, tremor, or balance. If there have been no medication side effects, an increased dose may be effective at that time. (4) Some patients will note that symptoms worsen after 3 hours or so and that improvement is delayed for 30 minutes after a dose of Sinemet. In such patients,

TABLE 16–7. SOME DRUGS USED TO TREAT PARKINSONISM

AGENT	MODE OF ACTION	USUAL DAILY DOSAGE	APPROX $ COST OF 100 TABLETS OR CAPSULES	SIDE EFFECTS
Levodopa	Converted to dopamine	3–6 gm	10 (500 mg)	**Peripheral:** nausea, vomiting, hypotension, glaucoma, cardiac arrhythmia; **Central:** memory loss, confusion, hallucinosis, dyskinesia
Levodopa & carbidopa combinations (Sinemet)	Carbidopa blocks peripheral metabolism of levodopa	0.4–1.5 gm levodopa	50 (10/100) 55 (25/100) 65 (25/250)	Central side effects of levodopa; on-off reaction more common
Bromocriptine (Parlodel)	Dopamine agonist	25–100 mg	113 (2.5 mg)	Confusion, hallucinosis, dyskinesia, nausea
Pergolide (Permax)	Dopamine agonist	3 mg	15 (0.05 mg) 45 (0.25 mg) 155 (1.0 mg)	Confusion, hallucinosis, dyskinesia, nausea
Anticholinergics				
Benztropine (Cogentin)	Muscarinic blockers	5–6 mg	12 (2 mg)	Confusion, memory loss, hallucinations, dry mouth, urinary retention, constipation
Trihexyphenidyl (Artane)	Muscarinic blockers	6–10 mg	7 (2 mg)	
Procyclidine (Kemadrin)	Muscarinic blockers	6–20 mg	5–8 (5 mg)	
Ethopropazine (Parsidol)	Muscarinic blockers	300 mg	7 (10 mg) 12 (50 mg)	
Selegiline (deprenyl, Eldepryl)	Monoamine oxidase B inhibitor	10 mg	200 (5 mg)	Insomnia
Antihistamines Diphenhydramine	Muscarinic blocker	50–200 mg	4–13 (50 mg)	Somnolence
Amantadine (Symmetrel)	Unknown; mild anticholinergic	200 mg	30 (100 mg)	Confusion, hallucinosis, dry mouth, peripheral edema, livedo reticularis

it may be useful to give the same total daily dosage but in smaller doses at shorter intervals, i.e., 2.5 or 3 hours. (5) The total dose may need to be reduced if choreiform movements or facial grimacing is bothersome. (6) "On-off" effects occur in a small percentage of patients. These are abrupt fluctuations in the parkinsonian symptoms and in dyskinesia that are not easily correlated with the timing of medication. Reduction in dose and shortening the interval between doses may be helpful.

Sinemet-SR, a controlled-release preparation, produces a slower rise and fall in plasma levodopa levels than does the standard form of the drug. 1 tablet contains 50 mg of carbidopa and 200 mg of levodopa (the same 1:4 ratio as in the standard Sinemet 25-100 tablet) with a 90% "release time" of 2–2.5 hours. This preparation may help with managing the patient with severe fluctuations in clinical response.

2. OTHER DRUGS FOR PARKINSON'S DISEASE. Additional medications that are sometimes beneficial include (1) the dopamine agonists bromocriptine (Parlodel) and pergolide (Permax); (2) selegiline (deprenyl, Eldepryl); (3) the anticholinergics such as trihexyphenidyl (Artane); and (4) amantadine (Symmetrel). Each of these agents can be used in combination with Sinemet. Bromocriptine is available in 2.5-mg and 5.0-mg tablets. Its plasma half-life is 3–4 times longer than that of levodopa. In controlled studies, bromocriptine improves parkinsonian symptoms, either alone or as a supplement to levodopa. Unfortunately the drug is expensive, and side effects are frequent. These include mental changes (confusion, psychosis), erythromelalgia, nausea, and dyskinesias. It is difficult to judge the appropriate dose of this agent. Doses as high as 50–100 mg/day have been given, but current recommendations by the manufacturer are to begin with very low doses of 1.25 mg/day and to increase in increments of 1.25–2.5 mg every 2–4 weeks, to the lowest dosage that produces a therapeutic response. **Pergolide** is a more recently introduced dopamine agonist that may be used as an alternative to bromocriptine. Pergolide is usually started at a dosage of 0.05 mg/day, with gradual increases in 0.1- to 015-mg increments every 3rd day up to 0.75 mg/day. If further increments are necessary, doses are then increased in 0.25-mg increments to a dosage of about 3 mg/day.

Selegiline (deprenyl, Eldepryl) is an irreversible inhibitor of the monoamine oxidase isoenzyme, MAO-B, which is the principal form in brain and blood platelets. The drug may prolong the action of levodopa and thereby benefit the patient with rapid "wearing off" of levodopa effects before the subsequent dose. Two 5-mg tablets suffice to almost completely inhibit MAO-B activity. The drug is given at breakfast and lunch to avoid nighttime insomnia. Selegiline taken early in the course of Parkinson's disease may lengthen the time before levodopa is required.

Trihexyphenidyl is one of several anticholinergic agents used for adjunctive therapy for parkinsonism (Table 16–7). These agents should be given at low initial doses and gradually increased as tolerated. Dry mouth, visual blurring, mental changes, and urinary retention are common side effects that limit the dosages. The effectiveness of these anticholinergic drugs is similar, though some neurologists prefer **ethopropazine** (Parsidol) for treating tremor. Another agent, **diphenhydramine** hydrochloride (Benadryl), has both anticholinergic and antihistaminic actions and may be useful when taken at bedtime in a dose of 25–50 mg.

Amantadine (Symmetrel) may have effect on dopamine release and reuptake from nerve endings as well as anticholinergic effects. It may be used as a supplemental drug in a dosage of 100–300 mg/day.

F. Nonparkinsonian Tremor

1. **ESSENTIAL TREMOR** is ordinarily confined to the upper extremities and head and usually increased in amplitude by dorsiflexing the wrists or performing a task such as writing or drinking from a glass. Essential tremor only rarely disappears with medical treatment. Two types of drugs are used: (1) beta-adrenergic blockers such as propranolol and (2) sedative-anticonvulsant drugs such as primidone (Mysoline). Many physicians now choose to use low dosages of primidone (50 mg hs) and gradually increase (to 250 mg/day). Others prefer to use propranolol in dosages beginning at 20–40 mg/day and increasing to 160 mg/day (40 mg qid). Dosages of 160 mg bid of long-acting propranolol have been used, as have alternative beta-adrenergic blockers such as metoprolol. Other agents, such as the anxiolytic benzodiazepines, have also been used. Drug side effects may be more bothersome to the patient than the tremor. Many may prefer not to take medications or to take a pill only at certain times, such as before a meal or when anticipating a stressful situation.

2. **ACTION OR INTENTION TREMOR** due to damage to cerebellar pathways is refractory to most medical therapy. An occasional patient will report minimal improvement with a benzodiazepine such as diazepam or lorazepam.

G. Wilson's Disease.

Hepatolenticular degeneration is inherited as an autosomal recessive disorder with tremor and dystonia seen in childhood or early adulthood. Elevated copper levels in striatum and liver presumably produce clinical symptoms. Copper chelation with D-penicillamine is the treatment of choice. The drug is given orally, beginning at 1 gm/day (250 mg qid ac and hs). The dose may be increased to 2 gm/day if negative copper balance is not achieved with the lower dose. A diet low in copper is also recommended, as is administration of 25 mg/day of pyridoxine. If symptoms worsen during the initial phase of treatment, the dosage of D-penicillamine should be reduced and later increased gradually over several weeks to months.

Cedarbaum JM: The promise and limitations of controlled-release oral levodopa administration. Clin Neuropharmacol 12:147–166, 1989.

Jankovic J, Schwartz K, Donovan DT: Botulinum toxin treatment of cranial-cervical dystonia, spasmodic dysphonia, other focal dystonias and hemifacial spasm. J Neurol Neurosurg Psychiatry 53:633–639, 1990.

Markham CH, Diamond SG: Long-term follow-up of early dopa treatment in Parkinson's disease. Ann Neurol 19:365–372, 1986.

The Parkinson Study Group: Effect of deprenyl on the progression of disability in early Parkinson's disease. N Engl J Med 321:1364–1371, 1989.

IX. MULTIPLE SCLEROSIS

This disorder of unknown cause is a source of frustration for patient and physician because of the uncertainties of prognosis and the difficulties in assessing treatment results. Its course is unpredictable. Some patients have a classic picture of multiple exacerbations and remissions. In others there is slow progression; in still others there is little progression. Since the disease is likely to have a viral or immunologic cause, most suggested treatments alter the immune system in some way. At this time, there is no convincing evidence that any treatment alters the ultimate outcome. Nonetheless, certain treatments are used by respected workers in the field. Others are considered to be of no benefit. In this section we will mainly discuss those treatments that are accepted as possibly useful and will mention some of the others that are controversial or unaccepted by most neurologists.

A. Immunosuppressant Therapy. Corticosteroid therapy is the most widely used. Its acceptance followed the report of a cooperative study that used ACTH. Most physicians now treat patients with short courses of **prednisone** in dosages of 60–120 mg/day at the onset. High doses of **IV methylprednisolone** (1000 mg) for 3–5 days have been suggested to speed recovery after an acute exacerbation of the disease. The use of **cyclophosphamide** is advocated by some. A widely cited study that was randomized, though not "blinded," reported stabilization of disease progression when patients were treated with an intense course of IV cyclophosphamide: 400 mg/day for patients under 115 pounds and 500 mg/day for heavier individuals. The final dose is that required to produce leukopenia within 10–14 days (5.0–7.5 gm). Cyclophosphamide in 250 ml of 0.5 NS is administered IV in 4 divided doses over 1–2 hours. Patients who undergo this therapy lose their hair temporarily and need to be observed for development of infection and hemorrhagic cystitis. Nausea and vomiting also complicate repeated infusions. Because of the toxicity of this approach, it is usually reserved for patients with relentlessly progressive multiple sclerosis whose disability is severe. Long-term therapy with 100–150 mg/day of **azathioprine** is used in a number of countries, though a large controlled study showed only modest benefit.

Other agents under investigation for treatment of multiple sclerosis include interferons, cyclosporin A, and copolymer I. Encouraging reports have shown lower exacerbation rates after intrathecal administration of natural beta-interferon, though chronic progression was not arrested. In contrast, gamma-interferon has been reported to increase the number of exacerbations of the disease. Another investigational therapy is total lymphoid irradiation (Neurology 38 (suppl 2):32–41, 1988). It is possible that we are nearing the time when rational treatments for multiple sclerosis will be available. At present, certain immunologic treatments are used, but none has been shown to arrest the disease irrevocably.

Hauser SL, Dawson DM, Lehrich JR, et al: Intensive immunosuppression in progressive multiple sclerosis. N Engl J Med 308:173–180, 1983.

Noseworthy JH, Seland TP, Ebers GC: Therapeutic trials in multiple sclerosis. Can J Neurol Sci 22:355–362, 1984.

Rose AS: Cooperative study in the evaluation of therapy in multiple sclerosis: ACTH vs placebo. Final report. Neurology 20:1–59, 1970.
Sibley WA: Therapeutic Claims in Multiple Sclerosis. 2nd ed. New York, Demos, 1988.
Van den Noort S: Immunosuppressant treatment in multiple sclerosis. Clin Neuropharmacol 8:58–63, 1985.
Weiner HL, Hafler DA: Immunotherapy of multiple sclerosis. Ann Neurol 23:211–222, 1988.

X. NEUROMUSCULAR DISORDERS

A. Neuropathies and Radiculopathies. Disorders that involve the peripheral nerves can be broadly classified into (1) polyneuropathies, in which peripheral nerves are affected in general; and (2) mononeuropathies, radiculopathies, and plexopathies, in which individual nerves, roots, or nerve plexuses are affected by a pathologic process. "Multiple mononeuropathies" (mononeuritis multiplex) also occur, usually in the setting of a disorder such as polyarteritis nodosa in which infarcts of multiple nerves can occur.

1. **POLYNEUROPATHIES.** Causes of polyneuropathies are multiple and include toxic (e.g., arsenic, vincristine, disulfiram, and hexane), metabolic (e.g., diabetes mellitus, uremia), genetic (e.g., Charcot-Marie-Tooth disease), neoplastic ("remote" effect of malignancies), infectious (leprosy), and immunologic (e.g., Guillain-Barré syndrome and chronic inflammatory demyelinating neuropathy) factors. When a cause is discernible, its removal may result in improvement of the polyneuropathy. Acute and chronic neuropathies of unknown cause are often assumed to be secondary to an immunologic disorder.

The term Guillain-Barré syndrome often is applied to polyneuropathies with a rapid onset over a few days. **Treatment of Guillain-Barré syndrome** is, in great part, concerned with preventing complications associated with severe weakness or respiratory paralysis. Treatment measures depend on the extent of the disability and may require admission to an ICU, institution of respiratory assistance, and physical therapy measures to prevent contractures and pressure sores. The use of more specific measures to prevent worsening of Guillain-Barré is increasing. **Plasmapheresis** has gained acceptance on the strength of a multicenter-controlled study suggesting that this treatment speeds recovery. Current recommendations are as follows: patients are considered for plasmapheresis who have developed the rapid onset of ascending paralysis thought to represent polyneuropathy of the Guillain-Barré type. Treatment within 7 days of neurologic symptom onset is encouraged. In the randomized multicenter trial reported in 1985, 3–5 exchanges were carried out over 1–2 weeks. A total of 200 mL of plasma was exchanged per kg of body weight, the replacement solution usually consisting of Plasmanate or 5% salt-poor albumin. **High-dose intravenous immunoglobulin** is a newly introduced treatment for neuropathies that are immune-mediated, and has also been used for myasthenia gravis. Rapid symptomatic improvement has been reported with both acute and chronic neuropathies, the latter sometimes associated with a monoclonal gammopathy. Improvement has not always been sustained, however. Patients receive a total of 2 gm/kg immunoglobulin (Sandoglobulin). The medication is divided into 5 doses infused in 1–2 L NS over several hours each day. Rapidly progressive weakness, usually with onset in muscles innervated by cranial nerves may be due to **botulism**. The toxin is produced by strains of the organism *Clostridium botulinum* and is usually ingested by eating tainted home-canned vegetables. For inactivation, the toxin requires heating for 30 min at 80°F or boiling for 3 min. The toxin binds irreversibly to presynaptic membranes, is taken up into cholinergic nerve endings, and prevents release of acteylcholine at neuromuscular junctions, including those of the heart and intestine. Administration of antibody is of uncertain benefit, since toxin binding has already occurred by the time the diagnosis is made. In very early cases, antibody should probably be given to minimize further toxin binding. Severely affected patients will require ventilatory support, which may be needed for weeks or months until the toxic effects eventually diminish. Anticholinesterases and guanidine hydrochloride (a drug that facilitates release of acetylcholine at synapses) are of little benefit.

2. **RADICULOPATHIES, PLEXOPATHIES, AND MONONEUROPATHIES**
   a. **Cervical or Lumbar Radiculopathy.** Acute radicular compression by herniated nucleus pulposus material is associated with pain and paresthesias in the distribution of the compressed nerve root. Avoidance of spine movement, bed rest, use of analgesics and nonsteroidal anti-inflammatory agents usually provide symptomatic relief. If pain persists and if evidence of nerve root damage occurs, x-ray and electrical diagnostic procedures are instituted and surgical decompression carried out in selected cases.
   b. **Entrapment Neuropathies.** Certain peripheral nerves are subject to entrapment as they pass through narrow passages or to compression against hard surfaces. Terms such as **carpal tunnel syndrome** (compression of the median nerve at the wrist) and **meralgia paresthetica** (compression of the lateral femoral cutaneous nerve as it passes through the inguinal ligament) are used to denote entrapment of specific nerves. In many cases, nerve compression can be reduced by identifying and eliminating aggravating factors. For example, with median nerve compression in the carpal tunnel, wearing a wrist splint and avoiding repetitive wrist movement will improve symptoms. The use of a nonsteroidal anti-inflammatory agent such as naproxen (Naprosyn), 375 mg bid, may help. Some physicians inject steroids (20 to 40 mg of methylprednisolone) into the area to reduce inflammatory swelling. This injection should be done only by those familiar with the technique, and it is probably best to refer patients who do not respond to splinting to a hand surgeon for possible surgical decompression.
   c. **Brachial Neuritis.** The cause is unknown but is presumed to be immunologic, since a similar syndrome has occurred after immunization. The affected individual rapidly develops pain and weakness in muscles of an extremity. Usually the proximal muscles of an arm are involved unilaterally. The syndrome may resemble

poliomyelitis, though CSF pleocytosis is not present. A short course of oral prednisone (e.g., 80 mg daily for 3 days, tapering over the next 9 days) is often used, though efficacy is not proven. Severe pain may require analgesics. Physical therapy may be necessary to prevent frozen shoulder.

d. Bell's Palsy. The cause of acute facial muscle weakness from dysfunction of the 7th cranial nerve usually is unclear, though herpes zoster can invade this nerve. Most Bell's palsy patients recover satisfactory function, though if axons are damaged, nerve regrowth may be accompanied by synkinetic movements of facial muscles. Controlled clinical studies have suggested that excellent recovery can occur if steroids are given within a few days of onset. One week of prednisone, 60 mg/day po, followed by a rapid taper over the next week, is recommended in such instances. Using an eye patch and artificial tears at night helps protect the globe. Surgical decompression of the facial nerve in its bony canal is not indicated.

B. Diseases of Muscle and the Myoneural Junction. The generic term for a disorder involving muscle primarily is **myopathy.** Myopathies include the genetic muscular dystrophies and acquired conditions such as polymyositis and endocrine myopathies. The periodic paralyses not associated with definite histologic changes may be included as well. Disorders of the myoneural junction such as myasthenia gravis and the Lambert-Eaton syndrome are not usually called myopathies.

1. THE MUSCULAR DYSTROPHIES. No cure is available for the genetic disorders known as the muscular dystrophies. Some studies suggest, however, that chronic prednisone therapy retards progression of weakness in patients with **Duchenne muscular dystrophy** (DMD) (Arch Neurol 44:818–822, 1987). Beginning doses were 2 mg/kg daily, shifting to an alternate-day schedule of about ⅔ of the original 2-day dose. Studies of this type have not been rigidly controlled, and results must be considered promising but not established. Weakness generally is managed in coordination with rehabilitation specialists. Prevention of contractures, use of appropriate assistive devices for ambulation, and proper nutrition require attention. Treatment of heart failure or arrhythmias may require appropriate cardiologic consultation. In DMD a muscle membrane protein, designated **dystrophin,** is deficient. Treatment trials transferring normal myoblasts into skeletal muscles of DMD patients with the hope of synthesizing the missing dystrophin are being carried out.

2. DISORDERS ASSOCIATED WITH MYOTONIA. Myotonia is the phenomenon of delay in relaxation after muscle contraction. Clinically, two disorders, both genetic, are associated with clinical myotonia: **myotonic muscular dystrophy** and **myotonia congenita.** The phenomenon of myotonia is usually less incapacitating than is weakness in the former, whereas in the latter, myotonia dominates the clinical picture. Myotonia can be lessened by drugs that act on excitable membranes: the anticonvulsant phenytoin in conventional doses and quinine (300–

600 mg tid or qid). Procainamide (3–4 gm/day in divided doses) is also effective but should be used with caution as it may potentiate heart block. These agents do not improve the weakness in myotonic dystrophy.

3. **MYASTHENIA GRAVIS.** Etiology and treatment of myasthenia gravis (MG), a condition characterized by fatiguing of skeletal muscle, have been extensively studied. Autoimmune damage to the acetylcholine receptors of the neuromuscular junction results in a decreased response to acetylcholine released by the motor neurons. Several therapeutic approaches are used and are based on the following principles: (1) increasing the concentration of acetylcholine at the neuromuscular junction with anticholinesterase drugs, and (2) altering the immunologically mediated interference with the acetylcholine receptor.

Anticholinesterase treatment is used to relieve symptoms. Pyridostigmine (Mestinon) is given orally at intervals of 3–4 hours. The long-acting drug comes in 60 mg tablets and in a sustained-release capsule containing 180 mg. To avoid overmedication, the sustained-release preparation should be used only at night in patients who have difficulty swallowing the morning tablet. The drug is begun at ½ or 1 tablet every 4 hours. Semiobjective testing of muscle fatiguing should be carried out *before* and ½–1 hour *after* the dose of pyridostigmine. Muscles shown to fatigue are tested. Ptosis is probably the most easily tested (the examiner should ask the patient to look up until ptosis occurs and then compare the width of the palpebral fissure). The most important muscles affected by the disease, those of the pharynx and of respiration, are harder to test. Detecting speech slurring or nasality after reading aloud or counting for an extended time is one assessment method. Fatigue of arm muscles can be measured by timing how long the patient can hold the arms outstretched. Pulmonary function testing can be used, as can hand dynamometers, if available. The pyridostigmine dose can then be titrated upward by increments of ½ tablet until the response is optimal. A patient's anticholinesterase requirement may change. Myasthenic patients may appear in the emergency room with increased weakness. It is then critical to determine whether the increased weakness represents a worsening of MG or whether it is due to excessive anticholinesterase medication. Weakness due to excessive anticholinesterase is often accompanied by salivation, hyperactive bowel sounds, and diarrhea, and sometimes fasciculations. Further anticholinesterase medication should be withheld to observe whether the weakness improves or worsens. Short-acting anticholinesterase given parenterally (edrophonium [Tensilon]) can be dangerous, produce marked worsening of the patient's weakness, and even lead to respiratory arrest. Patients on anticholinesterases may develop bothersome muscarinic side effects, such as intestinal hypermotility with cramps and diarrhea. Atropine sulfate, at doses of 0.4 mg q 6–8 hs, often helps. A scopolamine transdermal patch has also been used with success.

Therapies to alter the immune system in myasthenia gravis: Thymectomy may bring about a remission in MG, but it has never been subjected to a rigorous randomized trial. Some neurologists restrict thymectomy to younger patients unless there is evidence of thymoma. Some advocate early thymectomy, even when myasthenic symptoms are relatively mild. The patient must play an important role in deciding when and if the procedure will be done. Postoperatively, the need for anticholinesterase may be less than preoperatively, and the dose should be adjusted.

Prednisone has become standard when an anticholinesterase fails. One approach to initiating therapy is to begin at a low dose with gradual increases until benefit is seen, and the other is to begin at a high dose and, after benefit occurs, reduce the total dose and shift to an alternate-day regimen to lessen the severity of steroid side effects. This approach is used most frequently. Initial hospitalization is recommended because of the risk (48% in one series) of symptom exacerbation during initiation of steroid therapy. The patient is started on prednisone 60–100 mg each day. Improvement may occur in a few days or weeks, and an alternate-day regimen is used. Reduction in dose in 10-mg increments can then be instituted, as tolerated. Some neurologists recommend reduction by 10 mg every 2 months, but more rapid tapers are often tolerated well with no worsening in symptoms. If weakness recurs, the dose can be increased again, often with repeated improvement. Other immunosuppressive drugs are used if prednisone is ineffective. Azathioprine, at a dose of 2.0 to 2.5 mg/kg/day, and cyclophosphamide have been used successfully. High-dose IV immunoglobulin, and plasmapheresis are also used for providing dramatic, though usually temporary, relief (see section on Guillain-Barré syndrome, p. 570).

4. **PERIODIC PARALYSES.** These genetically determined conditions, usually inherited as autosomal dominant traits, are classified according to whether the serum potassium level falls or rises during an acute attack. The most common variety is the hypokalemic form, in which attacks of weakness are often precipitated by a high-carbohydrate meal. **Nonfamilial hypokalemic** periodic paralysis is occasionally the result of thyrotoxicosis. It is most common in Oriental males. Attacks usually cease when the patient is euthyroid. **Hyperkalemic** and **normokalemic** forms of periodic paralysis may be associated with myotonia and cardiac arrhythmias.

a. **Acute Attacks.** These are usually self-limited. Since respiratory muscles are ordinarily not affected, bed rest and fluid replacement usually suffice. Potassium is given only for clearly identified cases of the hypokalemic type. When the diagnosis has been made previously, an acute attack may be shortened by 15 mL of a sugar-free oral solution of 10% potassium chloride (20 mEq). This dose may be repeated several times at hourly intervals. For the hyperkalemic or normokalemic varieties, ingestion of high-carbonate beverages may help abort an attack. If weakness is severe, glucose plus insulin or other measures to treat hyperkalemia are used.

b. Prophylactic Therapy. For most patients with hypokalemic periodic paralysis, acetazolamide (Diamox) treatment effectively prevents attacks at doses of 125 to 1500 mg/day. Other drugs that have been used for prevention are the carbonic anhydrase inhibitor dichlorophenamide (50 mg bid or tid), and the potassium-sparing diuretics amiloride (5 mg up to 20 mg per day), triamterene (50 mg tid or qid), and spironolactone (25 mg bid or tid). Propranolol at a dose of 40–80 mg bid or tid has also been used with some success in patients with refractory disease. Hyperkalemic periodic paralysis attacks may also be prevented with acetazolamide or hydrochlorothiazide.

Bunch TW: Prednisone and azathioprine for polymyositis: long-term follow-up. Arthritis Rheum 24:45–48, 1981.

Havard CWH, Fonseca V: New treatment approaches to myasthenia gravis. Drugs 39:66–73, 1990.

Kleyweg RP, van der Meche FGA, Meulster J: Treatment of Guillain-Barré syndrome with high-dose gammaglobulin. Neurology 38:1639–1641, 1988.

Mulder DJG, Herrmann C Jr, Keesey J, et al: Thymectomy for myasthenia gravis. Am J Surg 146:61–66, 1983.

Munsat TL, Scheifer RT: Myotonia. Clinical Neuropharmacology 4:83–107, 1979.

Pascuzzi RM, Coslett HB, Johns TR: Long-term corticosteroid treatment of myasthenia gravis: report of 116 patients. Ann Neurol 15:291–298, 1984.

Riggs JE: Periodic paralysis. Clinical Neuropharmacology 12:249–257, 1989.

Rowland LP: Controversies about the treatment of myasthenia gravis. J Neurol Neurosurg Psychiatry 43:644–659, 1980.

The Guillain-Barré Syndrome Study Group: Plasmapheresis and acute Guillain-Barré syndrome. Neurology 35:2096–2104, 1985.

Van Doorn PA, Brand A, Strengers PFW, et al: High-dose intravenous immunoglobulin treatment in chronic inflammatory demyelinating polyneuropathy. Neurology 40:209–212, 1990.

APPENDIX
APPENDIX
APPENDIX

From Wyngaarden JB, Smith LH Jr, and Bennett JC (eds): Cecil Textbook of Medicine, 19th ed. Philadelphia, W. B. Saunders Co., 1992, pp 2377–2380.

DRUGS—THERAPEUTIC AND TOXIC LEVELS

Drug	Specimen		Reference Interval (Conventional Units)	Reference Interval (International Units)
Acetaminophen	Serum or plasma (hep or EDTA)	Therap:	10–30 μg/mL	66–199 μmol/L
		Toxic:	>200 μg/mL	>1324 μmol/L
Amikacin	Serum or plasma (EDTA)	Therap:		
		Peak	25–35 μg/mL	43–60 μmol/L
		Trough (severe infection):	4–8 μg/mL	6.8–13.7 μmol/L
		Toxic:		
		Peak	>35 μg/mL	>60 μmol/L
		Trough	>10 μg/mL	>17 μmol/L
ε-Aminocaproic acid	Serum or plasma (hep or EDTA); trough	Therap:	100–400 μg/mL	0.76–3.05 mmol/L
Amitriptyline	Serum or plasma (hep or EDTA); trough (>12 h after dose)	Therap:	120–250 ng/mL	433–903 nmol/L
		Toxic:	>500 ng/mL	>1805 nmol/L
Amobarbital	Serum	Therap:	1–5 μg/mL	4–22 μmol/L
		Toxic:	>10 μg/mL	>44 μmol/L
Amphetamine	Serum or plasma (hep or EDTA)	Therap:	20–30 ng/mL	148–222 nmol/L
		Toxic:	>200 ng/mL	>1480 nmol/L
Bromide	Serum	Therap:	750–1500 μg/mL	9.4–18.7 mmol/L
		Toxic:	>1250 μg/mL	>15.6 mmol/L
Caffeine	Serum or plasma (hep or EDTA)	Therap:	3–15 μg/mL	15–77 μmol/L
		Toxic:	>50 μg/mL	>258 μmol/L
Carbamazepine	Serum or plasma (hep or EDTA); trough	Therap:	4–12 μg/mL	17–51 μmol/L
		Toxic:	>15 μg/mL	>63 μmol/L
Carbenicillin	Serum or plasma	Therap:		Dependent on minimum inhibition concentration of specific organism
Chloramphenicol	Serum or plasma (hep or EDTA); trough	Toxic:	>250 μg/mL	>660 μmol/L
		Therap:	10–25 μg/L	31–77 μmol/L
Chlordiazepoxide	Serum or plasma (hep or EDTA); trough	Toxic:	>25 μg/mL	>77 μmol/L
		Therap:	700–1000 ng/mL	2.34–3.34 μmol/L
Chlorpromazine	Serum or plasma (hep or EDTA); trough	Toxic:	>5000 ng/mL	>16.7 μmol/L
		Therap:	50–300 ng/mL	157–942 nmol/L
		Toxic:	>750 ng/mL	>2355 nmol/L

Drug	Specimen	Category		
Cimetidine	Serum or plasma (hep or EDTA); trough	Therap:	0.5–1.2 µg/mL	2–5 µmol/L
Clonazepam	Serum or plasma (hep or EDTA; trough	Therap:	15–60 ng/mL	48–190 nmol/L
		Toxic:	>80 ng/mL	>254 nmol/L
Clonidine	Serum or plasma (hep or EDTA)	Therap:	1.0–2.0 ng/mL	4.4–8.7 nmol/L
Clorazepate	Serum or plasma (hep or EDTA)	As desmethyldiazepam: Therap:	0.12–1.0 µg/mL	0.36–3.01 µmol/L
Cocaine	Serum or plasma (hep or EDTA); on ice	Therap:	100–500 ng/mL	330–1650 nmol/L
		Toxic:	>1000 ng/mL	>3300 nmol/L
Cyclosporine	Serum (12 h after dose)	Therap:	100–400 ng/mL	83–333 nmol/L
		Toxic:	>400 ng/mL	>333 nmol/L
Desipramine	Serum or plasma (hep or EDTA); trough (≥12 h after dose)	Therap:	75–300 ng/mL	281–1125 nmol/L
		Toxic:	>400 ng/mL	>1500 nmol/L
Diazepam	Serum or plasma (hep or EDTA); trough	Therap:	100–1000 ng/mL	0.35–3.51 µmol/L
		Toxic:	>5000 ng/mL	>17.55 µmol/L
Digitoxin	Serum or plasma (hep or EDTA) ≥6 h after dose	Therap:	20–35 ng/mL	24–46 nmol/L
		Toxic	>45 ng/mL	>59 nmol/L
Digoxin	Serum or plasma (hep or EDTA); trough (≥12 h after dose)	Therap:	0.8–1.5 ng/mL	1.1–1.9 nmol/L
		CHF: Arrhythmias:	1.5–2.0 ng/mL	1.9–2.6 nmol/L
		Toxic:	>2.5 ng/mL	>3.2 nmol/L
Diphenylhydantoin (see Phenytoin)				
Disopyramide	Serum or plasma (hep or EDTA); trough	Therap: Arrhythmias: Atrial	2.8–3.2 µg/mL	8.3–9.4 µmol/L
		Ventricular	3.3–7.5 µg/mL	9.7–22 µmol/L
		Toxic:	>7 µg/mL	>20.7 µmol/L
Doxepin	Serum or plasma (hep or EDTA); trough (≥ 12 h after dose)	Therap:	30–150 ng/mL	107–537 nmol/L
		Toxic:	>500 ng/mL	>1790 nmol/L
Ethchlorvynol	Serum or plasma (hep or EDTA)	Therap:	2–8 µg/mL	14–55 µmol/L
		Toxic:	>20 µg/mL	>138 µmol/L
Ethosuximide	Serum or plasma (hep or EDTA); trough	Therap:	40–100 µg/mL	283–708 µmol/L
		Toxic:	>150 µg/mL	>1062 µmol/L
Fenoprofen	Plasma (EDTA)	Therap:	20–65 µg/mL	82–268 µmol/L
Flecainide	Serum or plasma (hep or EDTA); trough	Therap:	0.2–1.0 µg/mL	0.5–2.4 µmol/L
		Toxic:	>1.0 µg/mL	>2.4 µmol/L

Table continued on following page

DRUGS—THERAPEUTIC AND TOXIC LEVELS Continued

Drug	Specimen		Reference Interval (Conventional Units)	Reference Interval (International Units)
Furosemide	Serum (30 min after dose)		1–2 µg/mL	3–6 µmol/L
Gentamicin	Serum or plasma (EDTA)	Therap:		
		Peak (severe infection)	8–10 µg/mL	16.7–20.9 µmol/L
		Trough (severe infection)	2–4 µg/mL	4.2–8.4 µmol/L
		Toxic:		
		Peak	>10 µg/mL	>21 µmol/L
		Trough	>4 µg/mL	>8.4 µmol/L
Glutethimide	Serum	Therap:	2–6 µg/mL	9–28 µmol/L
		Toxic:	>5 µg/mL	>23 µmol/L
Imipramine	Serum or plasma (hep or EDTA); trough (≥12 h after dose)	Therap:	125–250 ng/mL	446–893 nmol/L
		Toxic:	>500 ng/mL	>1784 nmol/L
Isoniazid	Serum or plasma (hep or EDTA)	Therap:	1–7 µg/mL	7–51 µmol/L
		Toxic:	20–710 µg/mL	146–5176 µmol/L
Kanamycin	Serum or plasma (EDTA)	Therap:		
		Peak	25–35 µg/mL	52–72 µmol/L
		Trough (severe infection)	4–8 µg/mL	8–16 µmol/L
		Toxic:		
		Peak	>35 µg/mL	>72 µmol/L
		Trough	>10 µg/mL	>21 µmol/L
Lidocaine	Serum or plasma (hep or EDTA); ≥45 min following bolus dose	Therap:	1.5–6.0 µg/mL	6.4–26 µmol/L
		Toxic:		
		CNS or cardiovascular depression	6–8 µg/mL	26–34.2 µmol/L
		Seizures, obtundation, decreased cardiac output	>8 µg/mL	>34.2 µmol/L
Lithium	Serum or plasma (hep or EDTA); (>12 h after last dose)	Therap:	0.6–1.2 mEq/L	0.6–1.2 nmol/L
		Toxic:	>2 mEq/L	>2 mmol/L
Lorazepam	Serum or plasma (hep or EDTA)	Therap:	50–240 ng/mL	156–746 nmol/L
Meperidine	Serum or plasma (hep or EDTA)	Therap:	400–700 ng/mL	1620–2830 nmol/L
		Toxic:	>1 µg/mL	>4043 nmol/L
Meprobamate	Serum	Therap:	6–12 µg/mL	28–55 µmol/L
		Toxic:	>60 µg/mL	>275 µmol/L
Methadone	Serum or plasma (hep or EDTA)	Therap:	100–400 ng/mL	0.32–1.29 µmol/L
		Toxic:	>2000 ng/mL	>6.46 µmol/L

Drug	Specimen	Level	Concentration	SI units
Methaqualone	Serum or plasma (hep or EDTA)	Therap:	2–3 µg/mL	8–12 µmol/L
		Toxic:	>10 µg/mL	>40 µmol/L
Methotrexate	Serum or plasma (hep or EDTA)	Therap:	variable	variable
		Toxic:		
		Low-dose therapy (1–2 wk)	>9.1 ng/mL	>20 nmol/L
		High-dose therapy (48 h)	>454 ng/mL	>1000 nmol/L
Methsuximide (N-desmethyl methsuximide)	Serum	Therap:	10–40 µg/mL	53–212 µmol/L
		Toxic:	>40 µg/mL	>212 µmol/L
Methyldopa	Plasma (EDTA)	Therap:	1–5 µg/mL	4.7–23.7 µmol/L
		Toxic:	>7 µg/mL	>33 µmol/L
Methyprylon	Serum	Therap:	8–10 µg/mL	43–55 µmol/L
		Toxic:	>50 µg/mL	>273 µmol/L
Mexiletine	Serum or plasma (hep or EDTA)	Therap:	0.7–2.0 µg/mL	3.9–11.2 µmol/L
		Toxic:	>2.0 µg/mL	>11.2 µmol/L
Morphine	Serum or plasma (hep or EDTA)	Therap:	10–80 ng/mL	35–280 nmol/L
		Toxic:	>200 ng/mL	>700 nmol/L
N-Acetylprocainamide	Serum or plasma (hep or EDTA); trough	Therap:	5–30 µg/mL	18–108 µmol/L
		Toxic:	>40 µg/mL	>144 µmol/L
Nitroprusside	Serum or plasma (EDTA)	As thiocyanate:		
		Therap:	6–29 µg/mL	103–499 µmol/L
		Toxic:	10–40 µg/mL	53–212 µmol/L
Normethsuximide	Serum	Toxic:	>40 µg/mL	>212 µmol/L
Nortriptyline	Serum or plasma (hep or EDTA); trough (≥12 h after dose)	Therap:	50–150 ng/mL	190–570 nmol/L
		Toxic:	>500 ng/mL	>1900 nmol/L
Oxazepam	Serum or plasma (hep or EDTA)	Therap:	0.2–1.4 µg/mL	0.70–4.9 µmol/L
Paraquat	Whole blood (EDTA)		0.1–1.6 µg/mL	0.39–6.2 µmol/L
	Urine	Occup exp:	0.3 µg/mL	1.17 µmol/L
		Toxic:	0.9–64 µg/mL	3.50–249 µmol/L
Pentobarbital	Serum or plasma (hep or EDTA); trough	Therap:		
		Hypnotic	1–5 µg/mL	4–22 µmol/L
		Therap coma	20–50 µg/mL	88–221 µmol/L
		Toxic:	>10 µg/mL	>44 µmol/L
Phenacetin	Plasma (EDTA)	Therap:	1–30 µg/mL	6–167 µmol/L
		Toxic:	50–250 µg/mL	279–1395 µmol/L
Phencyclidine	Serum or plasma (hep or EDTA)	Toxic:	90–800 ng/mL	370–3288 nmol/L

Table continued on following page

DRUGS—THERAPEUTIC AND TOXIC LEVELS Continued

Drug	Specimen	Reference Interval (Conventional Units)	Reference Interval (International Units)
Phenobarbital	Serum or plasma (hep or EDTA); trough	Therap: 15–40 µg/mL	65–170 µmol/L
		Toxic:	
		Slowness, ataxia, nystagmus 35–80 µg/mL	151–345 µmol/L
		Coma with reflexes 65–117 µg/mL	280–504 µmol/L
		Coma without reflexes >100 µg/mL	>430 µmol/L
Phensuximide (both parent and N-desmethyl metabolites)	Serum or plasma (hep or EDTA)	Therap: 40–60µg/mL	228–324 µmol/L
Phenylbutazone	Plasma (EDTA)	Therap: 50–100 µg/mL	162–324 µmol/L
		(not well defined) Toxic: >100 µg/mL	>324 µmol/L
Phenytoin	Serum or plasma (hep or EDTA); trough	Therap: 10–20 µg/mL	40–79 µmol/L
		Toxic: >20 µg/mL	>79 µmol/L
Primidone	Serum or plasma (hep or EDTA); trough	Therap: 5–12 µg/mL	23–55 µmol/L
		Toxic: >15 µg/mL	>69 µmol/L
Procainamide	Serum or plasma (hep or EDTA); trough	Therap: 4–10 µg/mL	17–42 µmol/L
		Toxic: >10 µg/mL	>42 µmol/L
		Also consider effect of metabolite, N-acetylprocainamide,	
Propoxyphene	Plasma (EDTA)	Therap: 0.1–0.4 µg/mL	0.3–1.2 µmol/L
		Toxic: >0.5 µg/mL	>1.5 µmol/L
Propranolol	Serum or plasma (hep or EDTA); trough	Therap: 50–100 ng/mL	193–386 nmol/L
Protriptyline	Serum or plasma (hep or EDTA); trough (≥12 h after dose)	Therap: 70–250 ng/mL	266–950 nmol/L
		Toxic: >500 ng/mL	>1900 nmol/L
Quinidine	Serum or plasma (hep or EDTA); trough	Therap: 2–5 µg/mL	6–15 µmol/L
		Toxic: >6 µg/mL	>18 µmol/L
Salicylates	Serum or plasma (hep or EDTA); trough	Therap: 150–300 µg/mL	1086–2172 µmol/L
		Toxic: >300 µg/mL	>2172 µmol/L
Secobarbital	Serum	Therap: 1–2 µg/mL	4.2–8.4 µmol/L
		Toxic: >5 µg/mL	>21.0 µmol/L

Drug	Specimen	Condition		
Theophylline	Serum or plasma (hep or EDTA)	Therap:	8–20 µg/mL	44–111 µmol/L
		Toxic:	>20 µg/mL	>110 µmol/L
Thiocyanate	Serum or plasma (EDTA)	Nonsmoker:	1–4 µg/mL	17–69 µmol/L
		Smoker:	3–12 µg/mL	52–206 µmol/L
		Therap, after nitroprusside infusion:	6–29 µg/mL	103–499 µmol/L
	Urine	Nonsmoker:	1–4 mg/d	17–69 µmol/d
		Smoker:	7–17 mg/d	120–292 µmol/d
Thiopental	Serum or plasma (hep or EDTA); trough	Hypnotic:	1.0–5.0 µg/mL	4.1–20.7 µmol/L
		Coma:	30–100 µg/mL	124–413 µmol/L
		Anesthesia:	7–130 µg/mL	29–536 µmol/L
		Toxic conc:	>10 µg/mL	>41 µmol/L
Thioridazine	Serum or plasma (hep or EDTA)	Therap:	1.0–1.5 µg/mL	2.7–4.1 µmol/L
		Toxic:	>10 µg/mL	>27 µmol/L
Tobramycin	Serum or plasma (hep or EDTA)	Therap:		
		Peak (severe infection)	8–10 µg/mL	17–21 µmol/L
		Trough (severe infection)	<4 µg/mL	<9 µmol/L
		Toxic:		
		Peak	>10 µg/mL	>21 µmol/L
		Trough	>4 µg/mL	>9 µmol/L
Tocainide	Serum or plasma (hep or EDTA)	Therap:	4–10 µg/mL	21–52 µmol/L
Valproic acid	Serum or plasma (hep or EDTA); trough	Therap:	50–100 µg/mL	347–693 µmol/L
		Toxic:	>100 µg/mL	>693 µmol/L
Vancomycin	Serum or plasma (hep or EDTA); trough	Therap:	5–10 µg/mL	3–7 µmol/L
		Toxic:	>80–100 µg/mL	>55–69 µmol/L
		(not well established)		
Verapamil	Serum or plasma (hep or EDTA)	Therap:	100–500 ng/mL	220–1100 nmol/L
Warfarin	Serum or plasma (hep or EDTA)	Therap:	1–10 µg/mL	3–32 µmol/L

INDEX

INDEX

INDEX

Note: Page numbers followed by (t) refer to tables.

Allopurinol *(Continued)*
hepatic oxygenase system effect of, 6(t)
hepatotoxicity of, 332
6–mercaptopurine interaction with, 508
Alpha-antitrypsin deficiency, 338
Alpha-methyldopa (Aldomet), for
hypertension, 184, 187(t)
immune hemolytic anemia and, 355, 355(t)
lipid effects of, 180(t)
Alprazolam (Xanax), dosage for, 24(t)
in pregnancy, 38(t)
Aluminum acetate solution, for atopic
dermatitis, 526
Aluminum hydroxide (Amphojel, Basaljel),
in acute renal failure, 194
in hyperphosphatemia, 56
Aluminum silicate, hydrated (Kaolin), 16
Aluminum toxicity, in hemodialysis, 351
Alupent. See *Metaproterenol.*
Alveolar air equation, 284, 285(t)
Alzheimer's disease, 551–552, 553(t)
Amantadine (Symmetrel), adverse effects of,
66(t)
drug interactions with, 66(t)
for Parkinson's disease, 566(t), 568
Amebiasis, 126(t)
Amikacin, dosage for, 68(t)
for meningitis, 116
in renal failure, 218(t)
organism susceptibility to, 73(t)
Amiloride (Midamor, Moduretic), for
congestive heart failure, 158(t)
for hypertension, 181, 182(t)
for hypokalemic paralysis, 575
in renal insufficiency, 217(t)
Amino acids, for parenteral nutrition, 482
ε-Aminocaproic acid, reference values for,
578(t)
Aminoglutethimide, for cortisol suppression,
443
Aminoglycosides, adverse effects of, 66(t)
dosage for, 68(t)
drug interactions with, 66(t)
for meningitis, 116
for peritonitis, 214
for *Pseudomonas aeruginosa* pneumonia, 86
in hemodialysis, 222(t)
in peritoneal dialysis, 221(t)
in renal failure, 218(t)
nephrotoxicity of, 203
Aminophylline. See also *Theophylline.*
dosage for, 259, 259(t)
for severe asthma, 266(t)
intravenous, 258, 259(t)
metabolism of, 259(t)
oral, 258, 259(t)
Aminosalicylic acid, for Crohn's disease, 307
for ulcerative colitis, 313
immune hemolytic anemia and, 355, 355(t)
in renal insufficiency, 217(t)
Amiodarone, dosage for, 174(t)
drug interactions with, 176(t)

Amiodarone *(Continued)*
electrophysiologic effects of, 175(t)
for ventricular arrhythmias, 174(t)
hepatic oxygenase system effect of, 6(t)
Amitriptyline (Elavil, Endep), dosage for,
28(t)
for irritable bowel syndrome, 297(t)
in pregnancy, 36(t)
in renal insufficiency, 220(t)
reference values for, 578(t)
Ammonium chloride, for drug overdose, 34
Amobarbital (Amytal), dosage for, 24(t)
reference values for, 578(t)
Amoxapine (Asendin), dosage for, 29(t)
in pregnancy, 36(t)
Amoxicillin, dosage for, 69(t)
for bronchitis, 83
for infectious arthritis, 107
for Lyme disease, 108
for otitis media, 80
for renal failure, 218(t)
for surgical prophylaxis, 79
for urinary tract infection, 103
in hemodialysis, 222(t)
Amoxicillin-clavulanate (Augmentin), dosage
for, 69(t)
for bacterial vaginosis, 101
for chronic bronchitis, 83
for otitis media, 80
for sinusitis, 80
for urinary tract infection, 103
Amphetamine, reference values for, 578(t)
Amphojel (aluminum hydroxide), in acute
renal failure, 194
in hyperphosphatemia, 56
Amphotericin B, adverse effects of, 66(t)
dosage for, 68(t), 120(t)
drug interactions with, 66(t)
for amebic meningitis, 117
for cryptococcal meningitis, 90(t)
for cutaneous candidiasis, 533
for fungal arthritis, 108
for fungal endocarditis, 113
for fungal meningitis, 117
for fungal sinusitis, 81
for peritonitis, 214
in pregnancy, 36(t)
in renal failure, 218(t)
Ampicillin, dosage for, 69(t)
for acne, 532
for gonorrhea, 94, 95
for *Hemophilus influenzae* pneumonia, 86
for infectious diarrhea, 106(t)
for meningitis, 116
for otitis media, 80
for peritonitis, 114, 214
for pyelonephritis, 104
for surgical prophylaxis, 79
in hemodialysis, 222(t)
in pregnancy, 36(t)
in renal failure, 218(t)
organism susceptibility to, 71(t)

Milk of Magnesia (magnesium hydroxide),
    dosage for, 15(t)
    in pregnancy, 38(t)
Milrinone, for congestive heart failure, 160(t)
Miltown. See *Meprobamate.*
Minerals, daily intake of, 466(t)–467(t), 470
Minimal bactericidal concentration, in
    antimicrobial susceptibility testing, 65
Minimal-change disease, 226
Minimal inhibitory concentration, in
    antimicrobial susceptibility testing, 65
Minipress. See *Prazosin.*
Minocycline, for acne, 531
    in renal failure, 218(t)
Minoxidil (Loniten), for hypertension, 186,
    188(t)
    in renal insufficiency, 220(t)
Misoprostol, for peptic ulcer disease, 296(t),
    303
Mithramycin (plicamycin), for chronic
    myelogenous leukemia, 397
    for hypercalcemia, 55, 446, 447(t)
    for malignant hypercalcemia, 388–389
Mitomycin C (Mutamycin), 378(t), 381
    toxicity of, 378(t)
Mitral regurgitation, 163–164
Mitral stenosis, 163
Mitral valve prolapse, 164
Mixed connective tissue disease, 519
Mobilization, in malignant hypercalcemia, 388
Mobitz block, type I, 171, 172
    acute myocardial infarction and, 149(t)
    type II, 171
    acute myocardial infarction and, 149(t)
Moduretic. See *Amiloride.*
Monoamine oxidase inhibitors, dosage for,
    29(t)
    for depression, 27
MOPP (mechlorethamine [Mustargen],
    vincristine [Oncovin], procarbazine,
    prednisone), for Hodgkin's disease, 402,
    402(t)
Moraxella catarrhalis, antimicrobial agents
    for, 71(t)–74(t)
Moricizine (Ethmozine), for ventricular
    tachycardia, 169
Morphine (Roxanol), dosage for, 10(t), 11
    for myocardial infarction, 142
    in pregnancy, 36(t)
    in renal insufficiency, 220(t)
    reference values for, 581(t)
Motility, disorders of, 305–306
Motion sickness, management of, 18
Motrin. See *Ibuprofen.*
Movement disorders, 563–568
6-MP. See *6-Mercaptopurine.*
MTX. See *Methotrexate.*
Mucomyst (N-acetylcysteine), for
    acetaminophen hepatotoxicity, 332–333
Mucorales, in immunocompromised host,
    122(t)
Mucormycosis, in sinusitis, 81

Multiple myeloma, 231–233, 399–401
Multiple sclerosis, 569
    immunosuppressant therapy for, 569
Mumps, immunization for, 96(t)
    in pregnancy, 38(t)
Mupirocin (Bactroban), for impetigo, 536–
    537
Muscle, sarcoidosis of, 274(t)
    spasm of, narcotics and, 11
Muscular dystrophy, 572
    myotonic, 572–573
Mutamycin (mitomycin C), 378(t), 381
    toxicity of, 378(t)
Myasthenia gravis, 573–574
    prednisone for, 574
    thymectomy for, 574
Mycobacterium avium-intracellulare, in AIDS,
    91(t)
Mycobacterium tuberculosis, 92–93
    in osteomyelitis, 110
Myelofibrosis, agnogenic myeloid metaplasia
    with, 368
Myelogenous leukemia, chronic, 396–398
Myeloid blast crisis, 397–398
Myeloid leukemia, acute, 392–394
Myeloma, multiple, 231–233, 399–401
Myeloproliferative disorders, 368–369
    classification of, 368
Myleran. See *Busulfan.*
Myocardial infarction, 141–154
    acute, 143–146
    anisoylated plasminogen-streptokinase acti-
      vator complex for, 144, 145(t)
    arrhythmia prevention for, 142
    arrhythmias and, 147, 148(t)–149(t)
    beta-adrenergic blockers for, 142
    calcium channel blockers for, 142–143
    cardiogenic shock after, 151
    cigarette smoking and, 153
    complications of, 147–151, 148(t)–149(t)
      late, 151–152
    conduction disturbances after, 147
    congestive heart failure and, 152
    Dresssler's syndrome and, 152
    electrical disturbances after, 147, 148(t)–
      149(t)
    extension of, 150
    hypercholesterolemia and, 153
    hypertension and, 153
    intraventricular blocks after, 147
    ischemia after, 150
    laboratory findings in, 143
    left ventricular failure after, 150
    mural thrombi and, 152
    nontransmural, 146–147
    oxygen therapy for, 142
    pain relief for, 142
    pathophysiology of, 143
    percutaneous transluminal coronary angio-
      plasty for, 144, 146
    pericarditis and, 152
    perioperative, 41

Nutrition *(Continued)*
    indications for, 475
    intermittent, 476
    jejunostomy for, 476
    nasoenteral tubes for, 476
    nasogastric tubes for, 475–476
    in adult respiratory distress syndrome, 283
    normal requirements for, 465(t), 465–470
    parenteral, 480–487
      amino acids for, 482
      central, 481
      central venous catheter insertion in, 481
      complications of, 484–486
        metabolic, 485–486
        septic, 485
        technical, 484–485
      contraindications to, 480–481
      dextrose for, 482
      electrolytes for, 482
      home, 487
      indications for, 480
      lipids for, 482
      monitoring of, 484
      peripheral, 481
      prescription for, 481
      routes of, 481
      solutions for, 482–484, 483(t), 484(t)
      trace elements in, 484(t)
      vitamins for, 482, 483(t), 484
Nystatin, for candidiasis, 91(t)
  for cutaneous candidiasis, 533
  for esophageal candidiasis, 300
  for oropharyngeal fungal infection, 120(t)

O

Obesity, diet for, 468(t)
Octreotide, in Zollinger-Ellison syndrome, 305
Oculinum (botulinum toxin), for dystonia, 564
Ointment, 523, 524(t)
OKT3, in renal transplantation, 237
Omeprazole, drug interactions with, 297
  for peptic ulcer disease, 296(t), 303
  for reflux esophagitis, 296(t), 297
Oncovin. See *Vincristine.*
Ondine's curse, 272
Oophorectomy, in breast cancer, 409
Opiates, antidote for, 35(t)
Opium, in pain management, 12
  tincture of (Paregoric), dosage for, 17(t)
Oragrafin (sodium ipodate), for hypertension, 435
  for thyroid storm, 436(t)
Oral contraceptives. See *Contraceptives, oral.*
Oretic. See *Hydrochlorothiazide.*
Organophosphates, antidote for, 35(t)
Orudis (ketoprofen), dosage for, 8(t)
  for rheumatoid arthritis, 490(t)

Osalazine (Dipentum), for Crohn's disease, 307
  for ulcerative colitis, 297(t), 313
Os-Cal (oyster shell calcium), for hypocalcemia, 449, 449(t)
  for osteoporosis, 450(t)
  in acute renal failure, 194
Osmolite, 478(t)
Osteoarthritis, 503–504
Osteodystrophy, renal, in chronic renal failure, 209
Osteomalacia, treatment of, 451
Osteomyelitis, acute, 108–109
  chronic, 109–110
  contiguous foci of, 109
  fungal, 110
  hematogenous, 100, 109
  peripheral vascular disease and, 109
  tuberculous, 110
  vertebral, 110
Osteopenia, drug-induced, 451–452
Osteoporosis, 450–451
Otitis externa, 79–80
Otitis media, acute, 80
  chronic, 80
Ovary, cancer of, 412–413
  chemotherapy for, 412
    salvage, 413
  intraperitoneal chemotherapy for, 413
  palliation for, 413
  radiation therapy for, 413
  surgery for, 412
    second-look, 412–413
Overflow incontinence, 32
Overlap syndromes, 519–520
Oxacillin, in pregnancy, 36(t)
  in renal insufficiency, 220(t)
Oxazepam (Serax), 23
  dosage for, 24(t)
  in pregnancy, 38(t)
  reference values for, 581(t)
Oximetry, 239
Oxprenolol (Trasicor), dosage for, 130(t)
  properties of, 130(t)
Oxtriphylline, in pregnancy, 36(t)
Oxybutinin (Ditropan), for detrusor muscle instability, 31
Oxycodone (Percocet, Percodan, Tylox), dosage for, 10(t)
  in pregnancy, 36(t)
Oxygen, content equation for, 285(t)
  therapy with, 244–245, 246(t)–247(t)
    delivery systems for, 246(t)–247(t)
    in chronic obstructive pulmonary disease, 269
    in myocardial infarction, 142
    in pulmonary hypertension, 292
    indications for, 245
    mask for, 246(t)–247(t)
    nasal cannula for, 246(t)
    respiratory acidosis with, 244–245
    T tube for, 247(t)

Pressure, intracranial, increased, 558–559
Pressure sores, 30
Primaquine, in malaria, 124
Primidone (Mysoline), for seizures, 545(t)
  in hemodialysis, 222(t)
  reference values for, 582(t)
Prinivil (lisinopril), for hypertension, 185(t)
  in renal insufficiency, 220(t)
Prinzmetal's angina, 139–140
Pro-Banthine (propantheline bromide), for
  detrusor muscle instability, 31
Probenecid, for gonorrhea, 95
  for gout, 507
Procainamide, dosage for, 173(t)
  drug interactions with, 5(t), 176(t)
  electrophysiologic effects of, 175(t)
  for ventricular arrhythmias, 173(t)
  for ventricular tachycardia, 168
  immune hemolytic anemia and, 355, 355(t)
  in hemodialysis, 222(t)
  in peritoneal dialysis, 221(t)
  in pregnancy, 37(t)
  in renal failure, 218(t)
  lupus-like syndrome with, 515
  reference values for, 582(t)
Procardia. See *Nifedipine.*
Prochlorperazine (Compazine), dosage for,
  19(t)
  for migraine headache, 554
  for nausea, 296(t), 306
  in pregnancy, 37(t)
Proctitis, gonococcal, 319–320
  infectious, 297(t), 319–320
Proctosigmoiditis, ulcerative, 313
Procyclidine (Kemadrin), for Parkinson's
  disease, 566(t)
Progesterone (Provera), for menopause, 445
Prognostic nutritional index, for nutrition
  assessment, 472, 475
Progressive systemic sclerosis, 233
Prolactinoma, 431–432, 557
Prolixin (fluphenazine), dosage for, 21(t)
Promethazine (Phenergan), dosage for, 19(t)
  in pregnancy, 37(t)
Pro-Mix, 479(t)
Propafenone, dosage for, 174(t)
  drug interactions with, 176(t)
  for ventricular arrhythmias, 174(t)
Propantheline bromide (Pro-Banthine), for
  detrusor muscle instability, 31
Propoxyphene (Darvon), dosage for, 10(t)
  in renal insufficiency, 220(t)
  reference values for, 582(t)
Propranolol (Inderal), dosage for, 130(t),
  183(t)
  for delirium, 551
  for hypertension, 181, 183(t)
  for hyperthyroidism, 434
  for hypertrophic cardiomyopathy, 162
  for hypokalemic paralysis, 575
  for migraine headache, 554
  for myocardial infarction, 142

Propranolol (Inderal) *(Continued)*
  for paroxysmal supraventricular tachyarrhythmia, 166
  for thyroid storm, 436(t)
  hepatic oxygenase system effect of, 6(t)
  in pregnancy, 37(t)
  in renal insufficiency, 220(t)
  perioperative, 42
  properties of, 130(t)
  reference values for, 582(t)
Propylthiouracil (PTU), for hyperthyroidism,
  434
  for thyroid storm, 436(t)
  in pregnancy, 38(t), 436
  in renal failure, 218(t)
Prostaglandins, for peptic ulcer, 303
Prostate cancer, 425–426
Prostatectomy, heparin in, 43
Prostatitis, bacterial, acute, 104
  chronic, 104
Prosthesis, joint, infection of, 108
  valve, endocarditis and, 113
Protein, daily intake of, 467, 470
  daily requirement for, 466(t)
  in acute renal failure, 194
  retinol-binding, changes in, 473(t)
  somatic, measurement of, 471–472
  visceral, measurement of, 472, 473(t)
Proteus mirabilis, antimicrobial agents for,
  71(t)–74(t)
Prothrombin time, 360
Protriptyline (Vivactil), dosage for, 28(t)
  reference values for, 582(t)
Proventil (albuterol), for airway disease,
  257(t)
  for asthma, 266(t)
Provera (progesterone), for menopause, 445
Prozac (fluoxetine), dosage for, 29(t)
  in renal insufficiency, 220(t)
Pruritus, 539(t), 539–541
  cholestatic, 540–541
  hematologic, 541
  in chronic renal failure, 209
  systemic disease and, 539(t)
  treatment of, 526
  uremic, 540
Pruritus ani, 320
Pseudoephedrine, in pregnancy, 37(t)
Pseudogout, 509
Pseudohyperkalemia, 52
Pseudohyponatremia, 50
Pseudomembranous colitis, 315–316
  chronic, 297(t)
Pseudomonas aeruginosa, antimicrobial agents
  for, 71(t)–74(t)
Pseudomonas pseudomallei, 87
Pseudoneuropathic disease, 509
Pseudoosteoarthritis, 509
Pseudorheumatoid disease, 509
Psittacosis, 86
Psoriasis, 528–530
Psoriatic arthritis, 499–500, 500(t)